Community and Public Health
Nutrition

Sari Edelstein, PhD, RDN
Professor, Retired
Nutrition and Dietetics Department
Simmons University

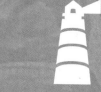
JONES & BARTLETT
LEARNING

World Headquarters
Jones & Bartlett Learning
25 Mall Road
Burlington, MA 01803
978-443-5000
info@jblearning.com
www.jblearning.com

Jones & Bartlett Learning books and products are available through most bookstores and online booksellers. To contact Jones & Bartlett Learning directly, call 800-832-0034, fax 978-443-8000, or visit our website, www.jblearning.com.

32332-0

Production Credits

Vice President, Product Management: Marisa R. Urbano
Vice President, Content Strategy and Implementation: Christine Emerton
Director of Product Management: Matthew Kane
Product Manager: Whitney Fekete
Director, Content Management: Donna Gridley
Manager, Content Strategy: Carolyn Pershouse
Content Strategist: Rachael Souza
Director, Project Management and Content Services: Karen Scott
Manager, Project Management: Jessica deMartin
Project Manager: Erin Bosco
Digital Project Manager: Angela Dooley

Director of Marketing: Andrea DeFronzo
Vice President, Manufacturing and Inventory Control: Therese Connell
Composition: Exela Technologies
Project Management: Exela Technologies
Cover Design: Briana Yates
Media Development Editor: Faith Brosnan
Rights & Permissions Manager: John Rusk
Rights Specialist: Liz Kincaid
Cover Image (Title Page, Part Opener, Chapter Opener): © olies/Shutterstock.
Printing and Binding: LSC Communications

Library of Congress Cataloging-in-Publication Data

Names: Edelstein, Sari, author.
Title: Community and public health nutrition / Sari Edelstein, PhD, RDN, Professor, Retired, Nutrition and Dietetics Department, Simmons College.
Other titles: Nutrition in public health.
Description: Fifth edition. | Burlington, MA : Jones & Bartlett Learning, [2023] | Revision of: Nutrition in public health / edited by Sari Edelstein, PhD, RDN, Professor, Retired, Department of Nutrition, School of Health Sciences, Simmons College, Boston, Massachusetts. 2018. Fourth edition. | Includes bibliographical references and index.
Identifiers: LCCN 2021039001 | ISBN 9781284234237 (paperback)
Subjects: LCSH: Nutrition–United States–Handbooks, manuals, etc. | Public health–United States–Handbooks, manuals, etc. | Nutrition policy–United States–Handbooks, manuals, etc.
Classification: LCC RA601.N84 2023 | DDC 362.17/6–dc23
LC record available at https://lccn.loc.gov/2021039001

6048

Printed in the United States of America
26 25 24 23 22   10 9 8 7 6 5 4 3 2 1

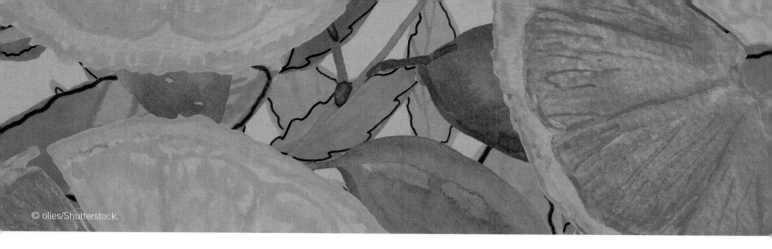

To many of my past students, who stepped up and wrote these chapters now that they are professionals in their own right.

Brief Contents

Preface xvii

Features of This Text xix

Acknowledgments xxiii

Contributors xxv

Reviewers xxvii

Part I Applying Nutrition in Community and Public Health 1

Chapter 1 Applying Nutrition Science to the Community and Public's Health 3

Chapter 2 Nutritional Epidemiology: An Introduction 47

Part II Shaping the Policies that Affect the Public's Health 69

Chapter 3 Creating and Influencing Public and Nutrition Policy 71

Chapter 4 The Role of the Federal Agencies in Community and Public Health Nutrition 99

Part III Assessing and Intervening in the Community's Nutrition Needs 125

Chapter 5 Community Needs-Assessment 127

Chapter 6 Planning and Evaluating Nutrition Services for the Community 157

Chapter 7 Serving Those at Highest Nutrition Risk 183

Chapter 8 Intervening to Change the Public's Eating Behavior 209

Part IV Promoting the Public's Nutritional Health 249

Chapter 9 Growing a Healthier Nation: Maternal, Infant, Child, and Adolescent Nutrition with an Emphasis on Childhood Overweight and Health Equity 251

Chapter 10 The Importance of Community and Public Health Nutrition Programs in Preventing Disease and Promoting Adult Health 305

Chapter 11 Promoting Older Adult Nutrition 343

Chapter 12 Providing Nutrition Services in Community and Public Health Primary Care 367

Part V   Protecting the Public's Nutritional Health   403

Chapter 13   Food Security and Adequate Food Access for the Public   405

Chapter 14   Safeguarding the Food Supply and Securing the Food Supply   423

Part VI   Managing Programs   493

Chapter 15   Grant Writing in Community and Public Health Nutrition   495

Chapter 16   Staffing, Managing, and Leading Community and Public Health Nutrition
                Personnel   527

Chapter 17   Team Nutrition Members in Community and Public Health Nutrition   545

Part VII   Surviving in a Competitive World   567

Chapter 18   Networking for Nutrition and Earning Administrative Support   569

Chapter 19   Marketing Nutrition Programs and Services   587

Chapter 20   Striving for Excellence and Envisioning the Future   609

Glossary   621
Index   627

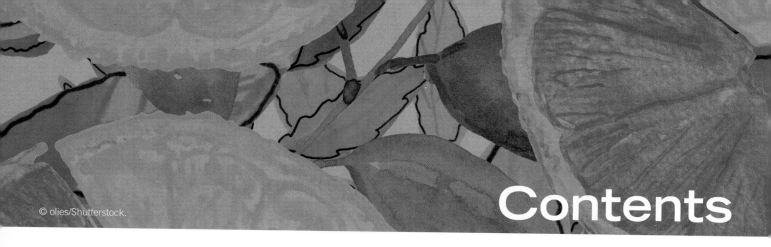

Contents

Preface   xvii

Features of This Text   xix

Acknowledgments   xxiii

Contributors   xxv

Reviewers   xxvii

**Part I
Applying Nutrition in Community
and Public Health   1**

**Chapter 1
Applying Nutrition Science to the
Community and Public's Health   3**

Nina Current, MS, RDN, LDN

List of Abbreviations   4

Introduction   5

**Community and Public Health Nutrition and Public
Health Dietitians/Nutritionists   7**

Peer-Reviewed Literature and Evidence-Based Practice   8

Finding Peer-Reviewed Literature   8
Assessing Article Quality   10

Nutrition Monitoring   12

Nutrition Screening and Assessment   13
Population Surveillance   15

Study Designs and Uses   21

Epidemiologic Studies   21
Metabolic Diet Studies   23
Clinical Trials   24
Animal Studies   24

Community and Public Health Services   25

Healthy People 2030   25
Nutrient Requirements   28
The Center for Nutrition Policy and Promotion   29

Summary   39

Learning Portfolio   40

Key Terms   40

Issues for Discussion   40
References   40

**Chapter 2
Nutritional Epidemiology:
An Introduction   47**

Lisa S. Brown, PhD, RDN, LDN

Elizabeth Newton, MS

Introduction   48

Overview of Epidemiology   48

Overview of Nutritional Epidemiology   49

**Types of Study Designs Used in Nutritional
Epidemiology   51**

Guidelines for Causality   52
Incidence and Prevalence   56
Measuring Dietary Exposure: Dietary Assessment
   Methods   57
Validity of Dietary Data   59

**General Considerations in Nutritional Epidemiologic
Studies   60**

The Role of Nutritional Epidemiology in Public Health   61

Summary   62

Learning Portfolio   63

Key Terms   63
Issues for Discussion   63
Practical Activities   63
Resources   64
References   64

**Part II
Shaping the Policies that Affect the
Public's Health   69**

**Chapter 3
Creating and Influencing Public and
Nutrition Policy   71**

Jody L. Vogelzang, PhD, RDN, FAND, CHES

Introduction   72

Characteristics of Public Policy 72

U.S. Public Health Policy 74

Nutrition Policy: A Brief History 74
Nutrition Policy: Goals and Methods 76

Policy Formulation 77

Agenda Setting 78
Policy Formulation 79
Policy Implementation 80
Policy Evaluation 81

Policy Creation at the Federal Level 81

Policy Development at All Levels of Government: Federal, State, and Local 83

The Role of the Federal Government in Policy
  Development 84
The Role of Public Agencies in Policy Development 85
The Role of State Government in Policy
  Development 86
The Role of Local Government in Policy
  Development 87

Leadership Roles for Nutritionists 88

Advocating and Influencing Health and Nutrition Policies 88

Influencing Legislation 89

Importance of Building an Infrastructure of Support 93

Advocacy Activities and Skills for Individuals 93

The Future of Public Health 94

Summary 95

Learning Portfolio 96

Key Terms 96
Issues for Discussion 96
Resources 97
References 97

**Chapter 4
The Role of the Federal Agencies in Community and Public Health Nutrition 99**

Juliana Ross Gilenberg, RDN, CSO, CNSC, LDN

Introduction 100

Overview of Food, Nutrition, and Consumer Services 100

Food and Nutrition Service 100
Center for Nutrition Policy and Promotion 103

Overview of the Food Safety and Inspection Service 105

Overview of Research, Education, and Economics 105

Agricultural Research Service 105
National Agricultural Library 106
National Programs in Human Nutrition 106
National Institute of Food and Agriculture (NIFA) 109

History of Nutrition Education at the USDA 112

Nutrition, Agriculture, and Health of Americans 113
History of the USDA's Research Role in Public
  Health Nutrition 113

U.S. Food and Drug Administration 114

Centers for Disease Control and Prevention 116

Environmental Protection Agency 118

Summary 120

Learning Portfolio 121

Key Terms 121
Issues for Discussion 121
Practical Activities 121
Resources 122
References 122

**Part III
Assessing and Intervening in the Community's Nutrition Needs 125**

**Chapter 5
Community Needs-Assessment 127**

Melinda Boyd, DCN, MPH, MHR, RDN, FAND

Introduction 128

Community Needs-Assessment: Definition and Overview 128

Steps to Conduct a Community Needs-Assessment 130

Phase 1: Needs-Assessment Planning 130
Phase 2: Methodology Development 134
Plan to Obtain Community Data 135
Plan to Obtain Data on the Target Population 137
Methods for Obtaining Data on the Target
  Populations (Primary Data Collection) 141
Phase 3: Data Collection and Analysis 147
Phase 4: Using the Needs-Assessment Results 148
Needs-Assessment in Practice: Baltimore City 149
Health Indicators Evaluated 149
Socioeconomic Indicators 149

Summary 151

Learning Portfolio 152

Key Terms 152
Issues for Discussion 152
Practical Activities 152

Resources   154
Sample Community Needs Assessments   154
References   155

**Chapter 6
Planning and Evaluating Nutrition
Services for the Community   157**

Julie M. Moreschi, MS, RDN, LDN

Introduction   158
Types of Planning   158
The Need for and Benefits of Planning   159
Choosing a Program Planning Model   160
Project Models   161
Ecological Models   161
PATCH and APEX-PH   162
Consumer-based Model   166
The Health Communication
  Process   167
Mobilizing for Action Through Planning &
  Partnerships   168
MAP-IT   169
**Guide for Effective Nutrition Interventions and
Education (GENIE)   170**
Intervention Mapping   170
Community Health Assessment and Group
  Evaluation (CHANGE)   170
Protocol for Assessing Community
  Excellence in Environmental Health
  (PACE-EH)   171
Program Implementation   172
Determining Team Membership   174
Health Program Evaluation   175
Benefits of Evaluation   175
Types of Evaluations   175
PRECEDE-PROCEED Evaluation Model   175
**Sustaining Your Program Planning
Efforts   178**
Program Planning During COVID-19   178
Summary   178
Learning Portfolio   179
Key Terms   179
Issues for Discussion   179
Practical Applications   179
Resources   179
Online Resources   179
References   180

**Chapter 7
Serving Those at Highest Nutrition
Risk   183**

Julie M. Moreschi, MS, RDN, LDN

Introduction   184
Defining High-Risk Factors   184
Poverty   184
Unemployment and Underemployment   187
Inadequate Education and Literacy   188
Cultural Barriers   189
Substandard Housing and Homelessness   190
Hunger and Food Insecurity   192
Geographic and Social Isolation   197
Limited or Inadequate Health Care   198
Transportation Environment   198
Neighborhood and Built Environment   199
Improving Services to At-Risk Families   199
Ethics of Health   199
Summary   202
Learning Portfolio   204
Key Terms   204
Issues for Discussion   204
Practical Activities   204
Resources   205
References   205

**Chapter 8
Intervening to Change the Public's
Eating Behavior   209**

Jessica L. Garay, PhD, RDN, CSCS, FAND

April Pelkey, BS

Introduction   210
Models & Theories of Health Behavior   211
Diffusion of Innovation Theory   211
Health Belief Model   212
Knowledge-Attitude-Behavior Model (KAB)   212
PRECEDE-PROCEED   213
Social Cognitive Theory/Social Learning Theory   213
Socioecological Model   214
Theory of Reasoned Action/Planned Behavior   215
(Transtheoretical) Stages of Change Model   215
Current Eating Trends   215
Food Away from Home Is Impacting the Food
  Environment   217
Food Fads and Emerging Dietary Practices   217

Changing Eating Behavior   218

Healthy People 2030   219
Dietary Guidelines for Americans   220
The Influence of Media on Eating Behavior   221
The Food Industry   222
Schools   223
Organizational and Worksite Interventions   226
Family and Friends   227
Community Interventions   230
Places of Worship   231
Reaching Older Adults   231
Individual and Group Counseling   232
Role of Government   233
Price Adjustments, Taxation, and Subsidies   236
Social Marketing   237
Health Communication Technology   239

Summary   240

Learning Portfolio   241

Key Terms   241
Issues for Discussion   241
Practical Activities   241
Resources   242
References   243

**Part IV
Promoting the Public's Nutritional
Health   249**

**Chapter 9
Growing a Healthier Nation: Maternal,
Infant, Child, and Adolescent Nutrition
with an Emphasis on Childhood
Overweight and Health Equity   251**

Meg Bruening, PhD, MPH, RDN

Gabriela Martinez, BS

Molly Jepson, BS

Introduction   252

Healthy People 2030 Objectives   252

Maternal Health   254

Preconceptional Period   255
Nutritional Assessment and Intervention During the
  Preconceptional Period   255
Prenatal Care   256
Nutritional Assessment and Intervention in
  Pregnancy   258
Special Conditions   259

Infancy   260

Breastfeeding   260
Formula Feeding   262

Infant Growth and Development   263
Complementary Foods   263
Important Nutrients in Infancy   264
Nutritional Assessment and Intervention
  in Infancy   265

Childhood and Adolescence   266

Nutrient Requirements for Children and
  Adolescents   266
Assessment of Growth and Weight Status   268
School-based Weight Screening   269
Early Childhood Specifics   270
Nutritional Assessment and Intervention in Early
  Childhood   270
School-Aged Child Specifics   272
Changes in the Food Environment   272
Nutritional Assessment and Intervention
  in School-Aged Children   274
Nutrition Education in Schools   277
Screen Time   277
Adolescence Specifics   278
Physiologic Changes   279
Nutritional Assessment and Intervention in
  Adolescence   281
Physical Activity   282
Physical Inactivity Affecting Overweight Status in
  Children   283
School Physical Education   284
Family Mealtime   284
Impact of Families on Childhood Weight Status   285
Household Food Insecurity   286
Supplemental Nutrition Assistance Program Education
  (SNAP-Ed)   286

**Overweight in Children from a Public Health
Perspective   287**

Overweight Rates in the United States   287
Health Effects of Overweight   288
Health Disparities   288
Economic Effects of Overweight   288

**Environmental Influences on Children Who Are
with Overweight   289**

Societal Factors   289
Overweight and Energy Balance   289
Programs and Resources That Support Evidence-Based
  Practices in Preventing Overweight in Children   290

Public Health Initiatives   291

Special Supplemental Nutrition Program for Women,
  Infants and Children   291
Bright Futures   293

**Opportunities for Community and Public Health
Dietitians/Nutritionists to Intervene and Prevent
Overweight in Children   293**

WIC   294
Head Start/Preschool/Daycare   294
School Systems   294
After-School Care   295
Other Possible Venues   295

Opportunities for Community and Public Health Dietitians/Nutritionists to Promote Health Equity   295

Envisioning the Future of Public Health Nutrition for Maternal, Infant, Child, and Adolescent Health   295

Summary   296

Learning Portfolio   298

Key Terms   298
Issues for Discussion   298
Resources   299
References   300

**Chapter 10
The Importance of Community and Public Health Nutrition Programs in Preventing Disease and Promoting Adult Health   305**

Marianella Herrera-Cuenca DSc, MD

Introduction   306

Chronic Diseases: The Leading Causes of Death and Disability   306

Determinants of Health, Risk Factors, and Chronic Disease   307

Prevention Strategies   308

Primary Prevention: Health Promotion   308
Secondary Prevention: Risk Appraisal and Risk Reduction   309
Tertiary Prevention: Treatment and Rehabilitation   310
Early prevention: Developmental Origins of Health and Disease and Life Course Approach   310
Implications of Prevention Levels   311

Dietary Guidelines for Disease Prevention   312

Diet and Health: Nutrition Strategies, Health Determinants, and Risk Factors   315

Obesity   316
Cardiovascular Disease   319
Cancer   325
Diabetes   327
Osteoporosis   330
Chronic Kidney Disease   332

Summary   334

Learning Portfolio   335

Key Terms   335
Issues for Discussion   335
Practical Activities   335
Resources   336
References   336

**Chapter 11
Promoting Older Adult Nutrition   343**

Shirley Y. Chao, PhD, RDN, LDN, FAND

Amy Sheeley, PhD, RDN

Introduction   344

The Older Population and Improvements in Health and Nutrition   344

Characteristics and Demographics of the Older Adult Population   345
Baby Boomers   345

Unique Features of Baby Boomers   346

Educational Demands of Older Adults   347

State of Health of Older Adult Population   347

Health Insurance and Screening   349

Aging-In-Place   349

Wellness Screening and Interventions   349

Screening   349
Nutrition   350
Physical Activity   351

Nutrition Support Services for Older Adults   352

Feeding America's Elderly   352

Factors that Promote Program Success   355

Program Evaluation   357

Other Community and Public Health Nutrition Interventions   359

Supplemental Nutrition Assistance Program   359
The Commodity Supplemental Food Program   359
The Child and Adult Care Food Program   360
Seniors Farmer's Market Nutrition Program   360
Medicaid & Nutrition Services   360

The Future   360

Evidence-Based/Self-Management   361
Internet/Social Media Learning   361

Summary   362

Learning Portfolio   363

Key Terms   363
Issues for Discussion   363

Practical Activities   363
Online Resources   364
References   364

Chapter 12
Providing Nutrition Services in Community and Public Health Primary Care   367

Lauren Melnick, MS, RDN, LDN

Introduction   368

Room for Nutrition in Primary Care   369

Telemedicine/Telenutrition in Primary Care   370

Agency for Healthcare Research and Quality   371

Barriers to Providing Nutrition Services in Primary Care and Strategies for Increasing Services   372

Physician Confidence and Skills   374
Physician's Time Constraints   375
Compensation and Reimbursement   377

Systemwide Change Strategies for Reducing the Cost of Medical Care   377

Chronic Disease Management and Self-Management   378

Summary of Health Insurance Plans   380

Indemnity (fee-for-service)   380
Managed Care   381
Government Programs   382

Representative Programs That Deliver Nutrition Services in Primary Care Settings   384

The Indian Health Service   384
Type 2 Diabetes—an Epidemic among American Indian/Alaskan Native Populations   385

Health Resources and Services Administration, Bureau of Primary Health Care   387

Bureau of Primary Health Care   388
Migrant Health Centers   390
Public Housing Primary Care Program   390
Health Care for the Homeless   391

Summary   393

Learning Portfolio   395

Key Terms   395
Issues for Discussion   395
Student Activities   395
References   399

Part V
Protecting the Public's Nutritional Health   403

Chapter 13
Food Security and Adequate Food Access for the Public   405

David H. Holben, PhD, RDN, LD, FAND

Introduction   406

Measuring the Food Security Status of the Public   407

Food Security in the United States   411

Coping Strategies Used by the Public to Avoid Food Insecurity   414

Impact of Food Insecurity on the Public   417

Strategies to Assist the Public in Securing Adequate Food   417

Summary   418

Learning Portfolio   419

Key Terms   419
Issues for Discussion   419
Practical Activities   419
Resource List   420
Key Term References   420
References   420

Chapter 14
Safeguarding the Food Supply and Securing the Food Supply   423

Chloe Giraldi, MS, RDN, LDN

Introduction   424

Food Safety Defined   424

Protecting the Food Supply   425

Federal Agencies   425
State and Local Collaboration   428

Food Safety Laws   428

Federal Meat Inspection Act of 1906   428
Federal Food, Drug, and Cosmetic Act of 1938   430
Food Additives Amendment, 1958   430
Color Additives Amendment, 1960   431
The Nutrition Labeling and Education Act of 1990   431
Dietary Supplement Health and Education Act of 1994   431
Food Quality Protection Act of 1996   431
Public Health Security and Bioterrorism Preparedness and Response Act of 2002   432

Food Allergen Labeling and Consumer Protection Act, 2004   432

Food, Conservation, and Energy Act of 2008   432

Food Safety Modernization Act of 2011   433

Hazard Analysis and Critical Control Points   433

Good Manufacturing Practices   434

Hazards to Food Safety   434

Biologic Hazards   434

Bacteria   439

Supply-Chain, Food and COVID   443

COVID-19 Impact on Food Industry-Related Businesses   443

Food Purchasing Habits During the COVID-19 Pandemic   444

USDA Actions During the COVID-19 Pandemic   445

Testing and Emergency Vaccine Use Authorization   446

Physical Hazards   453

Food Safety in the 21st Century   454

Blockchain and the Food System   454

Industrial Internet of Things (IIoT) and Food Safety   455

Agroterrorism and Bioterrorism   456

Food as a Target   456

Physical   456

Psychological   457

Economic   458

Political   459

Public Health Preparedness for Food Biosecurity   459

Potential Agents   459

Foods at Risk   460

Food Biosecurity Triad: Food Systems Security, Public Health Vanguard, and Consumer Engagement   464

Food System Security   464

Public Health Vanguard   467

Consumer Engagement   469

From Awareness to Security   473

Terms Relevant to Public Health Preparedness   473

Summary   476

Learning Portfolio   477

Key Terms   477

Issues for Discussion   477

Practical Activities   477

Online Resources   479

References   479

**Part VI
Managing Programs   493**

**Chapter 15
Grant Writing in Community and Public Health Nutrition   495**

Kathleen Cullinen, PhD, RDN

Introduction: Financing Community and Public Health Nutrition Programs and Services   496

General Revenue   498

Grants   498

Third-Party Reimbursement   500

Public Health Department Accreditation   501

Developing Skills in Grant Writing   501

Preparing Your Grant Application   502

Concept Paper   502

Data in Grant Writing for Program Planning and Evaluation   507

Accessing Existing Data Sources   509

Problem   510

Place   510

Person   510

Time Period   511

Data-Driven Program Planning   512

Prioritizing Health Needs   513

Data in Program Management and Evaluation   514

Nutrition Monitoring and Surveillance   515

Protection of Human Subjects   516

Data Compilation   516

Data Requirements, Collection, and Management   516

Prior to Submitting Your Grant Proposal   518

Summary   519

Learning Portfolio   521

Key Terms   521

Issues for Discussion   521

Practical Activities   521

Resources   525

References   526

**Chapter 16
Staffing, Managing, and
Leading Community and
Public Health Nutrition
Personnel   527**

Erin Gilfillan, MS, RDN, CDN

Hannah Husby, MS, RDN, CDN

Stephanie Cook, RDN, CSO, LDN

Introduction   528

**The Role of a Public Health Nutrition
Director/Manager   528**

**The Role of a Public Health Nutrition
Director/Manager During Public Health
Emergencies   539**

Summary   540

Learning Portfolio   541

Key Terms   541
Issues for Discussion   541
Practical Activity   541
Resources   542
References   542

**Chapter 17
Team Nutrition Members
in Community and Public Health
Nutrition   545**

Megan Lehnerd, PhD

Joycelyn Faraj, PhD, RDN

Introduction   546

**Members of the Community and Public Health
Nutrition Team   546**

Nutritionists/Dietitians and Dietetic Technicians   547
Health and Nutrition Educators   549
Foodservice Professionals   550
Public Health Nutrition Program
   Director/Manager   551
Community Health Worker   552
Consultant   552
Medical Professionals   553
Social Workers   555
Psychologists   555
Researcher/Academic   556
Policymakers   556
The Public   556

Education Programs   557
Bachelor's or Master's in Public Health   557
Nutrition Education for Public Health Nutrition
   Team Members   557
Professional Societies and Continuing
   Education   558

Teamwork   559
Developing an Effective Public Health Team   559
Strategies and Characteristics of a Properly
   Functioning and Effective Team   560
Cultural Considerations for the Public Health
   Nutrition Team   561

Chapter Summary   562

Learning Portfolio   563
Key Terms   563
Issues for Discussion   563
Practical Activities   563
References   564

**Part VII
Surviving in a Competitive World   567**

**Chapter 18
Networking for Nutrition and
Earning Administrative Support   569**

Farrell Frankel, MS, RDN

Introduction   570

**Networks, Alliances, Coalitions,
and Consortiums   570**
Networks   570
Alliances   571
Consortia and Coalitions   571

Collaborating with Others for Nutrition Networks   572
Resources   573
Access   573
Constraints   573
Knowledge   574

Developing a Community-Based Nutrition Network   574

Professional Networking   574
Networking Tips   576

Earning Administrative Support   577

The Administration's Perspective   578

**Understanding the Agency Vision and Strategic
Plan   578**

Synergizing with the Strategic Plan 579

Partnering to Achieve Shared Goals 580

Relations with the Policy Board 580

Communications with the Media 581

Preparing and Distributing Press Kits 581
Promoting Nutrition Messages Through Media 581
Obtaining Financial Support for Nutrition
 Programs and Initiatives 582

Summary 582

Learning Portfolio 584

Key Terms 584
Issues for Discussion 584
Practical Activities 584
References 584

**Chapter 19
Marketing Nutrition Programs
and Services 587**

Federika Garcia Muchacho, MS, RDN, LDN

Gisela Alvarez, RDN, LDN

Introduction 588

Business Marketing Versus Social Marketing 588

Marketing Research 589

Data Collection 590

Secondary Data 590

Primary Data 591

Qualitative and Quantitative Data 592

Market Segmentation 592

The Social Marketing Mix 593

Product 593
Place 594
Price 594
Promotion 595

Evaluation 596

Formative Evaluation 597
Process Evaluation 597
Outcome Evaluation 597

Social Media and Technology; Opportunities
for Business and Social Marketing for Nutrition
Professionals 598

Social Media Analytics 600

Marketing Ethics 601

Summary 602

Learning Portfolio 604

Key Terms 604
Issues for Discussion 604
Resources 605
References 606

**Chapter 20
Striving for Excellence and Envisioning
the Future 609**

Christina Ypsilantis, RDN, LDN

Introduction 610

Multidisciplinary Roles of the Community and Public
 Health Dietitian/Nutritionist 610
Nutrition Educator 610
Nutrition Researcher 611
Nutrition Advocate 612
Education in Public Health and Nutrition 612
Maintaining Currency in the Profession 613
Utilizing Technology 615
Collaborations 615

Future Challenges in Public Health Nutrition 616

Summary 617

Learning Portfolio 618

Key Terms 618
Issues for Discussion 618
Practical Activities 618
Online Resources 619
References 619

Glossary 621
Index 627

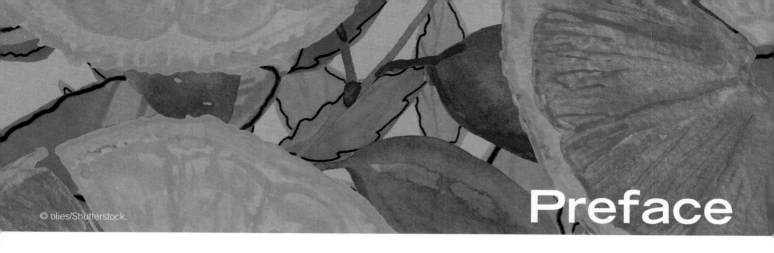

Preface

What Is Community and Public Health Nutrition?

Community and public health nutrition is a complex, multi-faceted set of programs dedicated to improving the health of the population through improved nutrition. In more detail, community and public health nutrition primarily exists to:

- Improve the health of the whole population and teach high-risk subgroups within the population improved nutrition
- Emphasize health promotion and disease prevention through improved nutrition
- Provide integrated community efforts for improved nutrition with leadership demonstrated by local, state, and federal government offices

To accomplish these three primary elements of community and public health nutrition, the U.S. Public Health Service has delineated 10 Essential Public Health Service Functions.[1] Each of these 10 elements will assist the reader in understanding the steps that must be taken by public health professionals to bring about definitive qualitative and quantitative results.

1. Monitor health status to identify and solve community health problems
2. Identify and investigate the causes of health problems and health hazards in the community
3. Mobilize community partnerships and action to identify and solve health problems
4. Develop policies and plans that support individual and community health
5. Enforce laws and regulations that protect health and ensure safety
6. Link people to needed personal health services and assure the provision of health care when otherwise unavailable
7. Inform, educate, and empower people about health issues
8. Evaluate effectiveness, accessibility, and quality of personal and population-based health services
9. Assure a competent public health and personal healthcare workforce
10. Research for new insights and innovative solutions to health problems

When these 10 elements are expanded to full explanations, we create a compendium of information that mirrors the table of contents in this book. The organization of *Community and Public Health Nutrition, Fifth Edition* embraces the essential public health service functions.

Organization of This Text

The structure of *Community and Public Health Nutrition* has been completely reorganized not only to encompass public health nutrition but also to include community nutrition.

Part I, "Applying Nutrition in Community and Public Health," creates the necessary foundation for readers to understand community and public health nutrition. These chapters include:

- An explanation that community and public health goals are built on a foundation of sound research, wherein peer-reviewed studies provide the groundwork
- A journey through studying populations utilizing epidemiology and how problems and solutions are questioned and acted upon

Chapters 3 through 8 comprise Part II, "Shaping the Policies That Affect the Community and Public's Health," and Part III, "Assessing and Intervening in the Community's Nutrition Needs." These chapters illustrate the landscape of community and public health, including:

- The role of the local, state, and federal government in supporting community and public health nutrition
- How researchers and others determine the need for community and public health nutrition in areas of the United States
- How researchers determine the needs of each community and focus on its nutritional problems
- An explanation of how nutritional services are planned and evaluated for a community
- Changing the public's eating behavior

[1] www.cdc.gov/publichealthgateway/publichealthservices/essential healthservices.html

In Part IV, "Promoting the Public's Nutritional Health," Chapters 9 through 12, we strive to educate the reader about local, state, and federal programs that provide community and public health nutrition for those at risk. These include:

- Promoting maternal, infant, child, and adolescent nutrition
- Assessing and providing for adult nutrition
- Caring for older adults and their nutritional problems
- Explaining nutritional programs in public health

Part V, "Protecting the Public's Nutritional Health," delineates 21st century issues in providing safe and secure food supplies for the public. These include:

- Providing food security and adequate food access for the public
- Safeguarding and securing the food supply

Part VI, "Managing Programs," and Part VII, "Surviving in a Competitive World," address the administrative and managerial portion of community and public health nutrition and programs. These include:

- Grant writing for funding of community and public health nutrition programs
- Staffing, managing, and leading community and public health nutrition personnel
- Leveraging nutrition education through a community and public health team
- Networking for nutrition by earning administrative support
- Marketing nutrition programs and services
- Striving for excellence and envisioning the future

Features of This Text

An effort has been made to ensure that pedagogical features are consistent from chapter to chapter. At the beginning of each chapter, the reader will find the following:

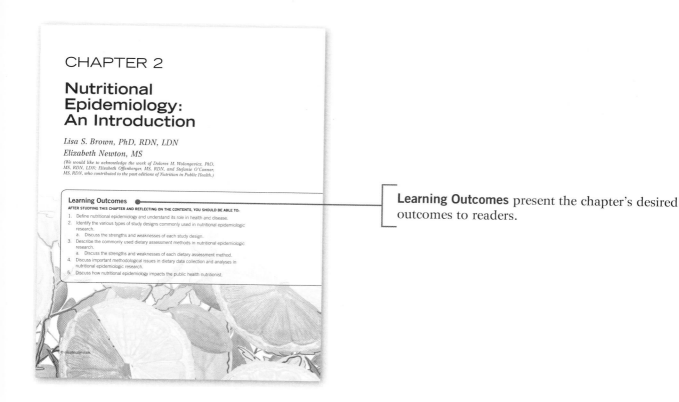

CHAPTER 2

Nutritional Epidemiology: An Introduction

Lisa S. Brown, PhD, RDN, LDN

Elizabeth Newton, MS

(We would like to acknowledge the work of Dolores M. Wolongevicz, PhD, MS, RDN, LDN; Elisabeth Offenberger, MS, RDN, and Stefanie O'Connor, MS, RDN, who contributed to the past editions of Nutrition in Public Health.)

Learning Outcomes

AFTER STUDYING THIS CHAPTER AND REFLECTING ON THE CONTENTS, YOU SHOULD BE ABLE TO:

1. Define nutritional epidemiology and understand its role in health and disease.
2. Identify the various types of study designs commonly used in nutritional epidemiologic research.
   a. Discuss the strengths and weaknesses of each study design.
3. Describe the commonly used dietary assessment methods in nutritional epidemiologic research.
   a. Discuss the strengths and weaknesses of each dietary assessment method.
4. Discuss important methodological issues in dietary data collection and analyses in nutritional epidemiologic research.
5. Discuss how nutritional epidemiology impacts the public health nutritionist.

Learning Outcomes present the chapter's desired outcomes to readers.

Key Terms help the reader quickly identify critical new terms, with definitions included in the end-of-text Glossary.

Epidemiology assesses the occurrence of a disease within a set population. This field also looks at the factors that prevent and hasten the disease's development.

Nutritional epidemiology utilizes the processes of epidemiology to look at the influence of dietary factors on a disease or health condition in the population.

In the middle of each chapter, the reader will find the following:

Discussion Prompts provide practical application questions for readers to ponder and find solutions for as future community and public health personnel.

Discussion Prompt

Describe the factors that prevented the recognition of a nutrition link and good health. How did epidemiology change this thinking?

Strategy Tips encourage readers to take the chapter material further and call to action what health professionals should do in a situation.

Strategy Tips

Contacting elected officials

Vote in elections to influence who will represent your views in government.
- Join a professional association or advocacy group(s) that advocates for public health. Many voices are generally louder than one. Be active in the group and encourage policy involvement.
- Conflicts arise. Don't take them personally. Learn from your opponent's position; it may strengthen your own position. Accept that some people may reject you for your position on an issue.
- Write letters to the editor of the newspaper when you have a strong position on a health or nutrition issue.
- Identify and know your audience. Adjust your message to better target their concerns and needs.
- Be persistent. Learn from your own mistakes and move on with that knowledge to do a better job next time.
- Take the time to comment on policy proposals and changes. The government often requests written comments on new policies and policy changes. These requests for comments are printed in the Federal Register for comment periods of 30 to 90 days. This is one of those unusual times when someone is required to read your letter and comments. Federal employees are required to read and compile all comments received during a comment period. These compiled comments are then used to support approval, change, or rejection of proposed policies.

Pandemic Learning Opportunity

If epidemiologists were able to act faster than what occurred in 2021, how would the outcome change? Going further, how important is it to have a fully functioning epidemiology unit working in the United States?

Pandemic Learning Opportunity asks the readers to recognize problem-solving situations that occurred during the pandemic for future use.

At the end of each chapter, the reader will find the following:

Case Studies provide a real-world dimension to chapter content, illustrating how public health nutrition issues and programs can affect real people. Each chapter now has two case studies.

Case Study: Type 2 Diabetes Epidemiology Study

This case study will provide a scenario in which a nutritional epidemiologic study is warranted. Following the case, there will be questions based upon the scenario presented.

You are a nutritionist working at a community health center providing basic nutrition education through general nutrition group education courses. Prior to the beginning of each course, you ask your clients to fill out a questionnaire that asks about various chronic diseases they have to better tailor your education throughout the course. You notice that over the last year, there has been an increased number of individuals who have reported new onset type 2 diabetes mellitus. You wonder if the increase in this disease is just in the clients whom you are seeing or if this is occurring within the greater community of your health center and that community food and exercise habits may be impacting the trend you have noticed. Your supervisor decides that it would be beneficial for you to look into the trend that you are seeing and conduct a small study using health center resources.

1. What is the purpose of your study?

2. Which type of study design should you choose for your study? What are the strengths and weaknesses of the study design chosen?

3. Which type of dietary assessment method would best fit with your design and purpose? What are the advantages and disadvantages to using this type of method?

4. Would your study result in significant causality? Is that necessary for your purpose?

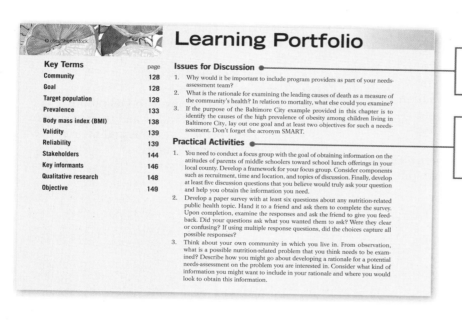

© olios/Shutterstock.

Learning Portfolio

Key Terms	page
Community	128
Goal	128
Target population	128
Prevalence	133
Body mass index (BMI)	138
Validity	139
Reliability	139
Stakeholders	144
Key informants	146
Qualitative research	148
Objective	149

Issues for Discussion

1. Why would it be important to include program providers as part of your needs-assessment team?

2. What is the rationale for examining the leading causes of death as a measure of the community's health? In relation to mortality, what else could you examine?

3. If the purpose of the Baltimore City example provided in this chapter is to identify the causes of the high prevalence of obesity among children living in Baltimore City, lay out one goal and at least two objectives for such a needs-sessment. Don't forget the acronym SMART.

Practical Activities

1. You need to conduct a focus group with the goal of obtaining information on the attitudes of parents of middle schoolers toward school lunch offerings in your local county. Develop a framework for your focus group. Consider components such as recruitment, time and location, and topics of discussion. Finally, develop at least five discussion questions that you believe would truly ask your question and help you obtain the information you need.

2. Develop a paper survey with at least six questions about any nutrition-related public health topic. Hand it to a friend and ask them to complete the survey. Upon completion, examine the responses and ask the friend to give you feedback. Did your questions ask what you wanted them to ask? Were they clear or confusing? If using multiple response questions, did the choices capture all possible responses?

3. Think about your own community in which you live in. From observation, what is a possible nutrition-related problem that you think needs to be examined? Describe how you might go about developing a rationale for a potential needs-assessment on the problem you are interested in. Consider what kind of information you might want to include in your rationale and where you would look to obtain this information.

Issues for Discussion encourage readers to discuss topics relevant to the chapter with their peers.

Practical Activities suggest activities that allow readers to apply what has been learned in the chapter, either individually or as part of a group.

Online Resources direct readers to websites relevant to the chapter content.

Online Resources

1. Administration on aging: http://www.aoa.gov
2. American Association of Retired Persons: http://aarp.org
3. American Geriatrics Society: http://americangeriatrics.org
4. Centers for Medicare and Medicaid Services: http://cms.hhs.gov/
5. Meals on Wheels Association of America: https://www.mealsonwheelsamerica.org/
6. Mini Nutritional Assessment: https://www.mnaelderly.com/forms/mini/mna_mini_english.pdf
7. National Association of Nutrition and Aging Services Programs: http://www.nanasp.org
8. National Institute on Aging: https://www.nia.nih.gov/
9. National Institutes of Health Seniors Health: https://www.nia.nih.gov/health
10. Older Americans Act Nutrition Program: https://acl.gov/sites/default/files/news%202017-03/OAA-Nutrition_Programs_Fact_Sheet.pdf
11. U.S. Food and Drug Administration – Food Safety for Older Adults: https://www.fda.gov/media/83744/download

These pedagogical features assist in bringing the chapter material to life as students will need to use critical thinking to solve public health nutrition problems through application.

New to this Edition

Community and Public Health Nutrition, Fifth Edition has maintained the cutting-edge relevance of previous editions, while adding several enhancements:

- New Box Features were created for this edition including **Discussion Prompts, Lessons Learned from the Pandemic**, and **Strategy Tips** which were developed to help the reader with critical thinking and practical application.

- **Additions to the Table of Contents.** The Table of Contents has added material to reflect the addition of community nutrition to each chapter. The text can now be fully utilized for both community nutrition and public health nutrition courses.

- **Thoroughly revised and in-depth content.** Each chapter has been updated and enhanced to give the reader a vast supply of background information and a full understanding of community and public health nutrition. In addition, new and expanded topics have been added to the *Fifth Edition* to reflect current community and public health issues. These include:
  - Updated *Dietary Guidelines for Americans, Healthy People 2030*, and other nutrition indexes

  - Updated community and federal nutrition policies and services
  - Updated approaches to disease prevention and new disease statistics, including current U.S. statistics and census information
  - Newly added grant-writing procedures
  - New, comprehensive, end-of-text Glossary

- **Added Case Studies.** Two case studies are now found at the end of each chapter, reinforcing key concepts by presenting real-life examples. An Answer Key for all case study questions is available for qualified instructors.
- A **Study Guide** is now provided Online featuring numerous activities for students to complete in writable PDFs.

Instructor and Student Resources

Qualified instructors can receive access to the full suite of instructor resources, including the following:

- Slides in PowerPoint format, featuring more than 300 slides
- Test Bank, containing 600 questions
- Study Guide containing the following for each chapter:
  - Learning Outcomes
  - Practical Activities
  - Matching Key Terms with Definitions
  - Additional Case Studies and their answers
  - Fill-in-the-blank Questions and their answers
  - Critical Thinking Questions
  - Issues for Discussion

Acknowledgments

The editor of *Community and Public Health Nutrition, Fifth Edition* would like to recognize the chapter contributors and the Jones & Bartlett Learning staff for their diligence and hard work to make this edition possible.

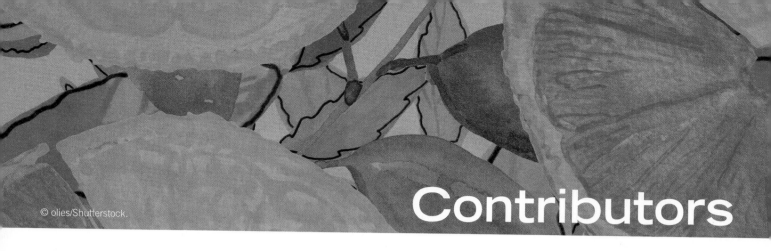

Contributors

Nina Current, MS, RDN, LDN

Lisa S. Brown, PhD, RDN, LDN

Elizabeth Newton, MS

Jody L. Vogelzang, PhD, RDN, FAND, CHES

Juliana Ross Gilenberg, RDN, CSO, CNSC, LDN

Melinda Boyd, DCN, MPH, MHR, RD, FAND

Julie M. Moreschi, MS, RDN, LDN

Jessica L. Garay, PhD, RDN, CSCS, FAND

April Pelkey, BS

Meg Bruening, PhD, MPH, RD

Gabriela Martinez, BS

Molly Jepson, BS

Marianella Herrera-Cuenca DSc, MD

Shirley Y. Chao, PhD, RDN, LDN, FAND

Amy Sheeley, PhD, RDN

Lauren Melnick, MS, RDN, LDN

David H. Holben, PhD, RDN, LD, FAND

Chloe Giraldi, MS, RD, LDN

Kathleen Cullinen, PhD, RDN

Erin Gilfillan, MS, RDN, CDN

Hannah Husby, MS, RDN, CDN

Stephanie Cook, RDN, CSO, LDN

Megan Lehnerd, PhD

Joycelyn Faraj, PhD, RDN

Farrell Frankel, MS, RDN

Federika Garcia Muchacho, MS, RDN, LDN

Gisela Alvarez, RDN, LDN

Christina Ypsilantis, RD, LDN

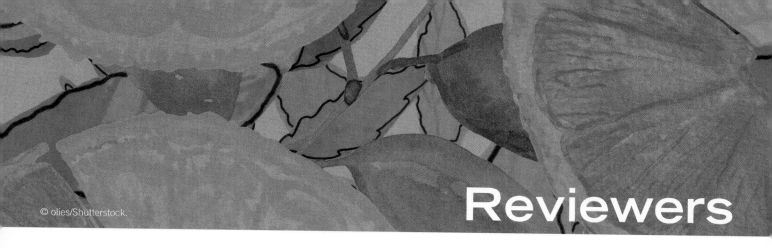

Reviewers

Amir Alakaam, PhD
Associate Professor
The University of Tennessee at Chattanooga

Kelly Burgess, MBA, RD, LDN
Licensed and Registered Dietitian
Adjunct Professor
Better Health LLC

Natalie Caine-Bish, PhD, RD
Associate Professor, Didactic Program Director
Kent State University

Mary Beth Gilboy, PhD, MPH, RDN
Associate Professor of Nutrition
West Chester University of Pennsylvania

Krystal Lynch, PhD, MPH
Assistant Professor, Nutrition and Dietetics
Eastern Illinois University

Colleen Tewksbury, PhD, MPH, RD, CSOWM, LDN
Senior Research Investigator
University of Pennsylvania

PART I

Applying Nutrition in Community and Public Health

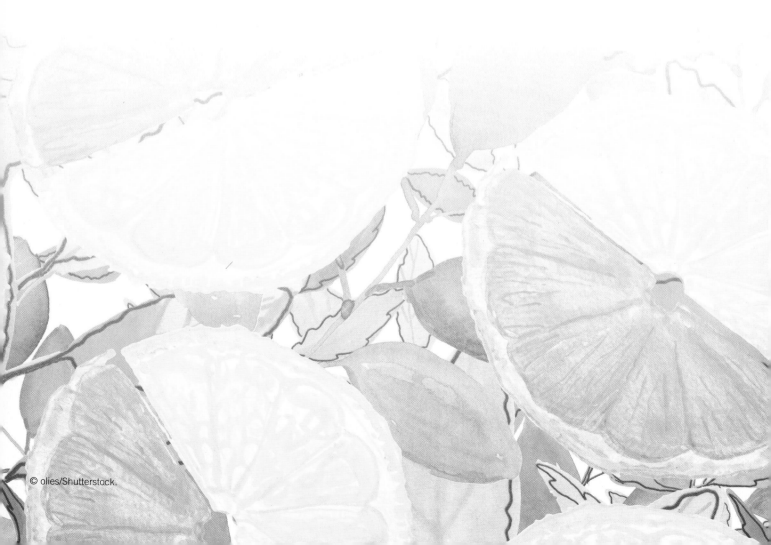

CHAPTER 1

Applying Nutrition Science to the Community and Public's Health

Nina Current, MS, RDN, LDN

(We would like to acknowledge the work of Carol E. O'Neil, PhD, MPH, RDN, LDN, and Theresa A. Nicklas, DrPH for their work on past editions of Nutrition in Public Health.)

Learning Outcomes

AFTER STUDYING THIS CHAPTER AND REFLECTING ON THE CONTENTS, YOU SHOULD BE ABLE TO:

1. Explain how and why nutrition policies, programs, and practice must be evidence-based.
2. Evaluate the peer-reviewed literature and assess bodies of evidence used to form nutrition policies and recommendations.
3. Compare and contrast different types of research studies and explain how they are used to form policies, programs, and consumer information.
4. Explain how and why nutrition policies, recommendations, and programs are changed at regular intervals.
5. Use the same resources as community and public health dietitians/nutritionists to keep up with current research or available programs that are grounded in research.

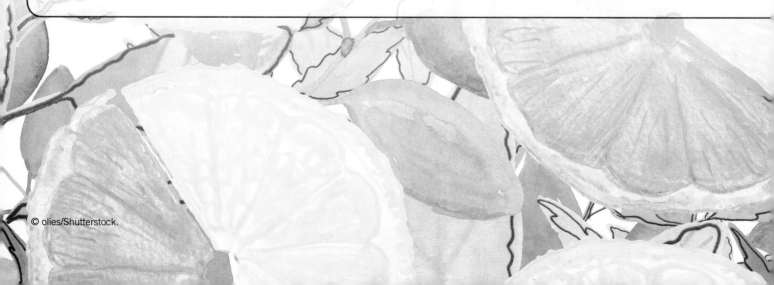

List of Abbreviations

Academy: The Academy of Nutrition and Dietetics

AI: Adequate Intake

ARS: Agricultural Research Service

ATBC: Alpha-Tocopherol, Beta-Carotene Cancer Prevention Study

BHS: Bogalusa Heart Study

BMI: Body Mass Index

BRFSS: Behavioral Risk Factor Surveillance System

CARDIA: Coronary Artery Risk Development in Young Adults

CARET: Carotene and Retinol Efficacy Trial

CNPP: Center for Nutrition Policy and Promotion

CDC: Centers for Disease Control and Prevention

CHD: Coronary Heart Disease

CSFII: Continuing Survey of Food Intake by Individuals

CVD: Cardiovascular Disease

DASH: Dietary Approaches to Stop Hypertension

DGA: Dietary Guidelines for Americans

DHKS: Diet and Health Knowledge Survey

DRI: Dietary Reference Intakes

DV: (Percent) Daily Value

EAL: Evidence Analysis Library

EAR: Estimated Average Requirement

ERS: Economic Research Service

FAO: Food and Agriculture Organization of the United Nations

FFQ: Food Frequency Questionnaire

FHS: Framingham Heart Study

FNB: Food and Nutrition Board (Health and Medicine Division, National Academies of Sciences, Engineering, and Medicine)

FNS: Food and Nutrition Service (USDA)

HHANES: Hispanic Health and Nutrition Examination Survey

HHS: (Department of) Health and Human Services

HMD: Health and Medicine Division (National Academies of Science, Engineering, and Medicine

HNIS: Human Nutrition Information Service (USDA)

HP: Healthy People

IOM: Institute of Medicine (National Academies of Sciences, Engineering, and Medicine)

LDL-C: Low-density Lipoprotein Cholesterol

NCCDPHP: National Center for Chronic Disease Prevention and Health Promotion (CDC)

NCI: National Cancer Institute

NCHS: National Center for Health Statistics

NFCS: Nationwide Food Consumption Survey

NESR: Nutrition Evidence Systematic Review

NHANES: National Health and Nutrition Examination Survey

NHLBI: National Heart, Lung, and Blood Institute

NIA:	National Institute on Aging
NIH:	National Institutes of Health
NHIS:	National Health Interview Survey
NHS:	Nurses' Health Study
NLEA:	Nutrition Labeling and Education Act of 1990
NNMRRP:	National Nutrition Monitoring and Related Research Program
OCPHP	Office of Disease Prevention and Health Promotion
PedNSS:	Pediatric Nutrition Surveillance System
PL:	Public Law
PNSS:	Pregnancy Nutrition Surveillance System
QHC:	Qualified Health Claims
RACC:	Reference Amount Customarily Consumed
RDA:	Recommended Dietary Allowances
RCT:	Randomized Controlled Trial (or Randomized Control Trial)
SNDA:	School Nutrition Dietary Assessment Study
SNAP:	Supplemental Nutrition Assistance Program
TDS:	Total Diet Study
UL:	Tolerable Upper Intake Level
USDA:	United States Department of Agriculture
WHO:	World Health Organization
WIC:	Special Supplemental Program for Women, Infants, and Children
YRBSS:	Youth Risk Behavioral Surveillance System

Introduction

Prior to the 1970s, community and public health nutrition was primarily focused on feeding programs and preventing nutrient deficiency diseases. Early in the 20th century, there was a general lack of understanding of the relationship between diet and disease, and diseases such as pellagra (niacin deficiency) and rickets (vitamin D deficiency) were common. As food availability improved and the prevalence of deficiency diseases decreased, there was a growing awareness that dietary excess and imbalance increased the risk of developing chronic disease, such as coronary heart disease (CHD), hypertension, type 2 diabetes mellitus, and cancer.[1]

In 1977, the US Senate Select Committee on Nutrition and Human Needs, under Senator George McGovern, issued *Dietary Goals for the* United States.[2] The goals engendered controversy among health professionals and the food industry because of how they were conceived and presented. At that time, there was also a lack of consensus on the impact of food/nutrients on chronic disease risk. In retrospect, the authors of these dietary goals were remarkably perspicuous. The statement by Dr. C. Edith Weir, Assistant Director of the Human Nutrition Research Division, U.S. Department of Agriculture (USDA), that "Most all of the health problems underlying the leading causes of death in the U.S. could be modified by improvements in diet"[2] remains the cornerstone of public health nutrition and nutrition policy in the United States.

Today, the preponderance of epidemiologic, clinical, and laboratory data have clearly linked both diet and physical inactivity with chronic disease.

Pandemic Learning Opportunity

Since the COVID-19 pandemic, the leading causes of death may have changed, with the corona virus landing in the top five. This has been a community and public health disaster.

National Health and Nutrition Examination Survey Is a program of studies designed to assess the health and nutritional status of adults and children in the United States. The survey combines interviews and physical examinations and is free to the public.

The World Health Organization's report on the Commission on Ending Childhood Obesity can be found online at https://apps.who.int/iris/bitstream/handle/10665/204176/9789241510066_eng.pdf

Information on obesity and obesity trends in the United States can be found on the website of the CDC: http://www.cdc.gov/obesity/data/prevalence-maps.html

Five of the 10 leading causes of death—heart disease, cancer, stroke, diabetes mellitus, and kidney disease—are related directly to poor diet, physical inactivity, and other lifestyle factors.[3] The cost of these diseases, both in terms of direct patient care and lost productivity, to the United States is staggering; for example, in 2014, heart disease and stroke cost approximately $329.7 billion dollars with $199.2 billion dollars being spend on direct patient care.[4] In 2010, cancer care cost $157 billion dollars.[5] In 2017, diagnosed diabetes mellitus cost $327 billion dollars with $237 billion dollars going to direct medical costs.[6] All stages of chronic kidney disease (including end-stage) cost Medicare $120 billion. The chronic disease cost calculator provides additional information about the cost of chronic diseases at the state level.[7]

Not included among the five major causes of death, but a major contributor to these and other health problems, is obesity. Obesity has reached epidemic proportions. **National Health and Nutrition Examination Survey (NHANES)** data from 2015 to 2016 showed that among adults, 38.0% of males and 41.5% of females were obese or had a body mass index (BMI $\geq$30).[8] The prevalence of obesity among U.S. children 2–19 years of age was 18.5% from 2015–2016. The prevalence of obesity among children 2–5 years of age (13.9%) was lower than among children 6–11 years (18.4%) and adolescents 12–19 years (20.6%). The same pattern was seen in males and females, with the exception of boys aged 6–11 years (20.4%) roughly equal to boys 12–19 years (20.2%)—girls in those age groups were more similar to the total trend.[9] Obesity in children is calculated differently than in adults since the relationship between BMI and body fat in children varies with age and pubertal maturation; thus, a single cutoff cannot be used for all ages. For children, a percentile range on the Centers for Disease Control and Prevention (CDC) growth charts is used: less than the 5th percentile is underweight, the 5th to <85th percentile is normal weight, 85th–<95th percentile is considered obese, and $\geq$95th percentile is considered obese.[10]

A significant increase in obesity in adults and children was seen from 1999–2000 through 2015–2016; however, no change was seen in children between 2003–2004 and 2013–2014. No significant change in obesity prevalence among adults or children was seen between 2013–2014 and 2015–2016.[9] In the United States, current estimated total medical costs of obesity in 2013 was $342.2 billion.[11] It is crucial to work toward reducing disease risk and promoting healthy behaviors in all individuals. Read more about childhood obesity in Chapter 9.

These health problems are not unique to the United States. Globally in 2016, noncommunicable (chronic) diseases accounted for 71% of all deaths (41 million people), 85% of whom lived in low- or middle-income countries.[12] Over the next decade, it is estimated that 55 million annual deaths worldwide will occur as a result from these diseases. The World Health Organization (WHO) has acknowledged the priority for addressing noncommunicable diseases globally. Achieving better health outcomes for these diseases "is a precondition for, an outcome of and an indicator of" economic development, environmental sustainability, and social inclusion.[13] The WHO finalized a global strategy to improve diet and increase physical activity to reduce the risk of chronic noncommunicable diseases while continuing to carry forward the long-term WHO goals in other nutrition-related areas, including undernutrition.

Relatively few modifiable risk factors—such as lack of fruit and vegetable intake, abnormal weight gain, smoking, inappropriate use of alcohol, and physical inactivity—cause the majority of the chronic disease burden. Changes in diet and physical activity patterns can significantly reduce disease risk, often in a surprisingly short time period. In 2018, a large proportion of cardiovascular disease in the United States was attributable to just seven risk factors: dietary risks, high systolic blood pressure, high BMI, high total cholesterol levels, high fasting plasma glucose levels, tobacco smoking, and low levels of physical activity. The largest contribution to cardiovascular disease risk comes from dietary factors.[14] However, healthy diet is the least likely heart healthy behavior to be achieved by American adults. In 2012, nearly 10% of cardiometabolic deaths (66,508 of 702,208 total cardiometabolic deaths) were attributed to high sodium intake; this represents a 6% increase over a 10-year period. A total of 318,656, or 45%, of cardiometabolic deaths are attributable to poor dietary habits in general. The role of **public health dietitians/nutritionists** is crucial in working to reduce risk for this and other chronic diseases in this country.

Community and Public Health Nutrition and Public Health Dietitians/Nutritionists

The National Academy of Medicine Initiative, as part of the *Vital Directions for Health and Health Care* series, released a 2016 discussion paper (*Advancing the Health of Communities and Populations*) defining public health as "[a]ddressing social, behavioral, and environmental factors that discourage healthy eating patterns or promote unhealthy exposures like smoking" in a manner that "ensures conditions in which people can be healthy."[15] In 2011–2012, the Institute of Medicine's (now known as the Health and Medicine Division of the National Academies of Sciences, Engineering, and Medicine) Board on Population Health and Public Health Practice redefined public health and clinical medicine as simply "the health system" public health dietitians/nutritionists are a vital part of that system.[16] Priorities for health care in America in 2021 include addressing health costs and financing, optimizing health and well-being for women and children, transforming mental health and addiction services, actualizing better health and health care for older adults, and improving the country's resilience against future infectious disease threats.[17]

Community and public health dietitians/nutritionists need to be able to understand what drives food and physical activity choices by consumers. Eating motivations involve many elements besides hunger including physiological factors, psychological factors (e.g., emotional state, disordered eating), social reasons (e.g., cultural, religious), socioeconomic factors (e.g., accessibility, availability, and affordability), and food sensation (e.g., smell, appearance, taste).[18-22] The decision not to engage in regular physical activity may be driven by lack of knowledge and attitudes about physical activity recommendations, lack of a safe place to exercise or of social support, lack of access to programs, and time.[23,24] However, there also may be strong psychological factors related to initiation and maintenance of exercise.[25]

Without the knowledge of why different populations choose healthy foods or choose not to exercise, it is difficult to understand why people eat what they do, why they do or do not engage in physical activity, or why they are or are not able to plan interventions and design policies and recommendations that change behavior that will lead to a healthier lifestyle.

Community and public health dietitians/nutritionists need to have a broad grasp of the sciences, including the pathophysiology of disease, genetics, biotechnology and its impact on sustainable agriculture, nutritional biochemistry and molecular biology, nutrigenomics, informatics, biostatistics, epidemiology, psychology, sociology, and nutritional sciences. Finally, community and public health dietitians/nutritionists need to know what information and resources

Public health nutritionist An expert in food and nutrition who applies this expertise to nutrition research, practice, and policy to improve the health of populations.

are available to them to help plan and assess programs at the national, state, local, or individual levels.

Today, for consumers and health professionals alike, there is a bewildering array of diet and physical promotion information available on the Internet, social media, and through other media channels and it can be difficult to determine fact from false claims.[26,27] On discussion forums for online nutrition courses, over 50% of the sources that learners used for food- and nutrition-related information came from online websites and only 5% of food- and nutrition-related information shared on the forums was written by a nutritional professional.[28] It is vital that health professionals, including registered dietitians, provide timely, accurate online information,[29] and help consumers understand that not all available information is accurate and help them understand how to distinguish sound science from less credible information. To do this, we, as health professionals, need to understand how to evaluate information.

In this chapter, we will look at examples of how to interpret and evaluate the professional literature to 1) make **evidence-based practice** decisions in community and public health; 2) learn the science behind nutrition recommendations, policy, and legislation; and 3) find ways for nutritional science to be translated into messages for consumers.

Evidence-based practice Is the conscientious effort to use the best available evidence when making clinical decisions.

Nutrigenomics Is the study of the effects of food or food components on gene expression and how individual genetic differences can affect the way we respond to foods or nutrients.

Discussion Prompt: **Research**

nutrigenomics. Nutrigenomics is the study of the effects of food or food components on gene expression and how individual genetic differences can affect the way we respond to foods or nutrients. Need to know more? The CDC provides information through the Public Health Genomics and Precision Health Knowledge Base (v7.0) https://phgkb.cdc .gov/PHGKB/phgHome.action?action=home

Strategy Tip

The second edition of detailed recommendations for physical activity were published in 2018 by the Department of Health and Human Services (available at health.gov/our-work/physical-activity /current-guidelines)

Strategy Tip

Anybody can post anything on the Internet—and very little information is removed. To determine if the site you've chosen for information is accurate, reliable, and timely, get in the habit of evaluating websites and teaching your clients to evaluate them. Need help? Learn how to do it from a reliable source: https://guides.library.cornell.edu/evaluating _Web_pages>

Peer-Reviewed Literature and Evidence-Based Practice
Finding Peer-Reviewed Literature

Peer-reviewed literature Literature, including nutrition literature, that has been subjected to scholarly review by experts in the field and revision by the author to address any comments or concerns of these scholars prior to publication in a scientific journal or textbook.

Peer-reviewed literature is the *gold standard* for scientific information provided to the public as well as the information used for setting recommendations and policies, designing and evaluating nutrition programs, and conducting ethical evidence-based nutrition and dietetics practice. Unfortunately, the literature can be difficult to understand and results from different studies can be contradictory. Use of different study designs, populations, or methods—including statistical analyses—contribute to the confusion.

Assessing the science behind the policies, programs, practice, and consumer information begins with asking a question and finding, reading, and evaluating the articles needed to answer it. **PubMed** is the premiere database for articles on nutrition topics. This database is composed of more than 19 million citations for biomedical articles from MEDLINE and life science journals. Many citations in PubMed include links to full-text articles from PubMed Central or publisher websites. Important databases for nutrition-related research are shown in **Table 1–1**.

> **PubMed** The premiere database for peer-reviewed articles on nutrition and medicine. Many citations in PubMed include links to full-text articles from PubMed Central or publisher websites.

TABLE 1–1
Databases Important for Nutritional Sciences Literature Searches

Database	Purpose
AGRICOLA AGRICultural OnLine Access	Provides citations in agriculture and related fields; produced by the National Agricultural Library (NAL).
AGRIS International System for Agricultural Science and Technology	International information system for the agricultural sciences and technology; created by the Food and Agriculture Organization of the United Nations (FAO).
BRFSS Behavioral Risk Factor Surveillance System: Survey Data	Includes eight databases on specific illnesses or aspects of chronic disease prevention and health promotion; designed to help public health professionals and educators locate program information. Managed by the Centers for Disease Control and Prevention (CDC)
CARIS Current Agricultural Research Information System	Created by FAO to identify and facilitate the exchange of information about current agricultural research projects being carried out by or on behalf of developing countries.
The Cochrane Library	Contains reliable evidence from Cochrane and other systematic reviews, clinical trials, and more. Cochrane reviews bring you the combined results of the world's best medical research studies and are recognized as the gold standard in evidence-based health care.
Directory of Open Access Journals	This database increases the visibility and ease of use of open access journals and promotes their increased usage and impact.
Embase	The trusted resource for the most comprehensive biomedical information.
ERIC Educational Resources Information Center	Includes educational research and resources; early childhood education, junior colleges and higher education; reading and communications skills; languages and linguistics; education management; counseling and personnel services; library and information science; information resources. Sponsored by the Institute of Education Sciences.
Food Safety Research Database	The Food Safety Research Information Office is located at the NAL. This office provides information on publicly funded, and to the extent possible, privately funded food safety research initiatives to prevent unintended duplication of food safety research and to assist the executive and legislative branches of the government and private research entities to assess food safety research needs and priorities.
FSTA Food Science and Technology Abstracts	The largest collection of food science, food technology, and food-related human nutrition abstracts. It contains over 1.5 million records with approximately 1,700 new entries added every week. FSTA covers journal articles as well as patents, theses, standards, legislation, books, reviews, and conference proceedings.
Health Source: Nursing/Academic Edition	Provides 260 scholarly full text journals, including nearly 120 peer-reviewed journals focusing on many medical disciplines. Also features abstracts and indexing for 930 journals.
Index to Scientific and Technical Proceedings	Indexes the published literature of the most significant conferences, symposia, seminars, colloquia, workshops, and conventions in a wide range of disciplines in science and technology over the last 5 years.
LILACS Latin American and Caribbean on Health Sciences Literature	Comprehensive database of Latin America and Caribbean with more than 880,000 records of peer-reviewed journals, thesis and dissertations, government documents, annals of congresses and books; sponsored and managed by BIREME through the Pan American Health Organization (PAHO)

(continues)

TABLE 1–1
Databases Important for Nutritional Sciences Literature Searches *(continued)*

Database	Purpose
MEDLINE	Sponsored by the National Library of Medicine, contains citations and abstracts to international biomedical literature from over 5,200 journals on subjects in biomedicine and health used in research and clinical care, public health, health policy development, or related educational activities.
Merck Index Online	Highly authoritative, full test database of information on chemicals, drugs, and biologicals; contains over 11,500 monographs. Sponsored online by the Royal Society of Chemistry.
Nursing and Allied Health Premium	Contains over 700 scholarly journals and 360 full-length clinical skills videos to support the teaching, learning, and research needs of nursing and allied health students and educators. Developed by Proquest, formerly the Nursing and Allied Health Database.
Science Direct	Database of more than 2,500 journals and 39,000 books in scientific, technical, and medical research, including 370 full open-access publications. Offered through Elsevier.
Scopus®	The largest abstract and citation base of peer-reviewed literature.
Web of Science (Science Citation Index Expanded)	Indexes over 9,200 major journals across 178 scientific disciplines.

If your library does not have access to these databases, just ask the librarian at your college or university to help you.

Strategy Tip

Not familiar with PubMed? Work through the online tutorials to help with your literature searches (https://learn.nlm.nih.gov/documentation/training-packets/T0042010P/) or ask your college or university librarian to help you.

Assessing Article Quality

After asking a question and determining the appropriate database to use, the next stage is selecting the descriptors and conducting the search. The descriptors and the search limits depend on the question(s) you are asking. For example, if your question is, "What is the effect of 100% fruit juice consumption on weight in children?" your descriptors could be "fruit juice" OR "fruit" AND "weight" OR "BMI" AND "children" OR "adolescents." The search might be easier if your search limit is "All Children," in which case the last two descriptors could be eliminated. Scanning the titles and abstracts will allow you to determine which articles are appropriate to answer your question. Obtaining the full-text articles, either by downloading them or visiting the library, and assessing them are the next steps (**Table 1–2**). This is not casual reading to prepare a summary

TABLE 1–2
How to Assess an Article from the Peer-Reviewed Literature

Title
1. Did the title reflect what was actually done in the study? The purpose, the populations used, the findings, and conclusions can be reflected in the title. A positive statement about the contents rather than a title that is a question is preferred.

Abstract
1. Did the abstract clearly outline all aspects of the manuscript?
   a. The purpose of the study
   b. The methods
   c. The results
   d. The conclusions
2. Was enough information provided to understand what was done and what was found?

Introduction
1. Did the authors provide enough background information to understand why the study was done?
2. Did the authors provide enough background information to let you know what others have done on this topic and where there might be gaps in the literature?*
3. Were important studies omitted from the introduction? This might suggest bias.
4. Did the authors clearly state the purpose of the study? A hypothesis or research question should have been stated. Not all study designs are appropriate for testing hypotheses; for example, cross-sectional studies are hypothesis generating.

Materials and Methods (could be referred to as Subjects and Methods)

1. Was the type of study clearly defined?
2. Did the experimental design allow the research question or hypotheses to be tested?
3. If appropriate, was a control group included? Was it comparable to the test group?
4. Was the population appropriate for the study?
5. Was the population suitable to generalize results?
6. Was the population well defined?
   a. Number/adequate sample size for appropriate statistical power
   b. Gender, age, race/ethnicity, income, etc.
   c. Inclusion/exclusion criteria for the study
   d. If the study population was a subset of a larger population, was it clear how the study population differed from the larger population? This could indicate bias.
   e. Was a convenience sample used or were the participants randomized?
7. Were there ethical concerns if human subjects or vertebrate animals were used? Was there a clear statement that the research has been approved by the appropriate committee?
8. Were the methods presented in enough detail so that the research could be repeated (or built upon) by another research team?
9. Were the methods used reliable and valid?
10. Statistical methods:
    a. Were they appropriate?
    b. Were outcome variables clearly defined?
    c. Did the authors control for potential confounding variables?
    d. Was a statistical probability level clearly stated?
11. Was it clearly stated how the data will be presented in the results (e.g., data are presented as mean ± standard error [SE])?
12. Were all terms defined?

Results

This section should present study results only. No methodology should be presented and unless it is a combined Results and Discussion section; there should be no interpretation of the information.

1. Were results organized in a logical sequence?
   a. Did the results follow the same order as the methods?
2. Were demographics presented?
3. Were the graphics appropriate?
   a. Were they needed? Should more or less be included?
   b. Was the information clearly presented in labeled tables and figures? Can the tables and figures stand alone?
   c. From a biological standpoint, were the data reasonable?

Discussion

1. Were the study objectives met?
2. Did the authors adequately interpret their results?
3. Did the authors discuss their results and compare them with the current literature?
4. Was the discussion related directly to the results or was it overly speculative?
5. If nonstandard methods were used, were they adequately discussed?
6. Were limitations of the study clearly stated?
7. Were conclusions drawn? Were they supported by the results?

References

1. Were appropriate citations listed? Were they accurate? Were they timely?
2. Were enough references presented so that a cogent whole presentation was in the manuscript?

Acknowledgments

1. Were the funding sources clearly identified?
2. Were there real or apparent conflicts of interest that could suggest bias?

---

*This is difficult for those unfamiliar with the literature but becomes easier with practice and familiarity with the topic.

of the article but a critical evaluation of the published study—try it out with a subject you're interested in. However, a single peer-reviewed article is not sufficient to make ethical evidence-based practice decisions; setting public health goals (e.g., Healthy People [HP] 2030); developing dietary recommendations, (e.g., Dietary Reference Intakes [DRI]); mandating nutrition policy (e.g., Dietary Guidelines for Americans [DGA]); or designing nutrition programs for health professionals and the public (e.g., the Produce for Better Health Foundation's Have A Plant®). To do this, the strength of a body of scientific studies must be assessed.

The Agency for Healthcare Research and Quality, through its Evidence-Based Practice Centers, sponsors the development of evidence reports and

Hierarchy of evidence Reflects the relative weight of different types of studies when making decisions about evidence based practice or clinical interventions. There is no single accepted version of the hierarchy of evidence, but there is general agreement that systematic reviews and meta-analyses rank the highest, followed by randomized controlled trials, cohort studies, and expert opinions and anecdotal experience ranks at the bottom.

Cross-sectional studies A type of observational study that involves collection and analysis of data from a population at one point in time. The National Health and Nutrition Examination Survey is an example of a cross-sectional study. These studies are used to generate hypotheses, not to test them.

Cohort studies A study design where populations (called cohorts) are followed prospectively or retrospectively with status evaluations for a disease or other outcome to determine which risk factors are associated with that outcome.

Randomized controlled trials A type of scientific study design in which the individuals being studied are randomly assigned to different treatments under study. The most rigorous of these trials is a double-blind, placebo-controlled trial, in which neither the investigator nor the study participant knows the treatment type. Results from these studies provide strong evidence in the hierarchy of evidence. This study design allows for testing of hypotheses.

Evidence Analysis Library A web-based site that provides the best available nutrition evidence on a variety of topics. Sponsored by the Academy of Nutrition and Dietetics, full access is free to Academy members.

Nutrition monitoring Collecting nutrition and health-related information from a population is critical for designing and evaluating policies and programs that improve health status and decrease risk factors.

technology assessments to assist public- and private-sector organizations in their efforts to improve the quality of health care in the United States.[30-32] There are three important domains that should be addressed to grade the strength of the evidence: 1) the quality of the studies—including the extent to which bias was minimized, 2) the quantity of the studies—including the magnitude of effect, the number of studies conducted, and the sample size or power of the study, and 3) the consistency of results—whether similar studies produce similar results.

Another critical consideration when assessing the body of evidence is the study design: what type of study was used to produce the test results, and what was the relevance to the disease/condition/program under study? Some study designs are more powerful than others in providing evidence on a topic; this has given rise to the concept of a "**hierarchy of evidence**"[33] about the effectiveness of interventions, treatments, practice protocols, or policies. From bottom (least convincing) to top (best evidence), the hierarchy is generally presented as: expert opinion, case reports, case series, case-control studies; **cross-sectional** surveys; **cohort studies** (prospective or retrospective); **randomized controlled trials (RCT)**; and systematic reviews of RCT with or without meta-analysis. It should be kept in mind; however, that this hierarchy assumes that all studies were well designed and executed. A poor RCT may not provide the same level of evidence as a very well-designed, cross-sectional survey.

To assess a body of evidence, many organizations, including the National Heart, Lung, and Blood Institute (NHLBI), the Academy of Nutrition and Dietetics (the Academy), and the American Diabetes Association, have grading scales. The NHLBI uses a four-point scale to grade the scientific evidence from different study types (**Table 1–3**). The **Evidence Analysis Library (EAL)** of the Academy uses a five-step process; the fourth of which is to summarize evidence and the last is to develop a conclusion statement and assign a grade.

For the Academy's EAL, the scoring system is somewhat different. The Academy uses Grades I, II, III, IV, and V for good/strong, fair, limited/weak, expert opinion only, and not assignable, respectively.[31] Examples of evidence statements for a wide variety of nutrition-related topics are found on the EAL's website, including: Adult Weight Management, Bariatric Surgery, Fruit Juice, Heart Failure, Hypertension, Physical Activity, and Sodium. Keep in mind with all types of evidence reviews that they are time-consuming and new studies are continually being published. Be sure the information you use in your evidence review and your practice is the most recently available.

In addition to the EAL, the U.S. Department of Agriculture's (USDA) Nutrition Evidence Systematic Review (NESR) conducts systematic reviews to inform nutrition policy and programs, including the Dietary Guidelines for Americans. The process by which the NESR evaluates a body of literature on a given topic is similar to that of the EAL. The process used by the NESR is: Recruit expert workgroup, formulate evidence analysis questions, and conduct literature review for each question, Extract evidence and critically appraise each study, synthesize the evidence, and develop and grade a conclusion statement (https://nesr.usda.gov/).

Nutrition Monitoring

Collecting nutrition and health-related information from a population is critical for designing and evaluating policies and programs that improve health status and decrease risk factors. Scientists analyze data from **nutrition monitoring** programs and use these analyses to contribute to the literature.

TABLE 1–3
National Heart, Lung, and Blood Institute's Evidence Categories

Category	Sources of Evidence	Definition
Category A	Randomized controlled trials (rich body of data)	Well-designed, randomized clinical trials that provide a consistent pattern of findings in the population for which the recommendation is made. Category A requires substantial numbers of studies involving substantial numbers of participants.
Category B	Randomized controlled trials (limited body of data)	Limited randomized trials or interventions, post-hoc subgroup analyses, or meta-analyses of randomized clinical trials. These are used when there are a limited number of existing trials, study populations are small or provide inconsistent results, or when the trials were undertaken in a population that differs from the target population of recommendation.
Category C	Observational or nonrandomized studies	Evidence is from outcomes of uncontrolled or nonrandomized trials or from observational studies.
Category D	Panel Consensus Judgment	Expert judgment is based on the panel's synthesis of evidence from experimental research described in the literature or derived from the consensus of panel members based on clinical experience or knowledge that does not meet the above criteria. This category is used only where the provision of some guidance was deemed valuable but an adequately compelling clinical literature addressing the subject of the recommendation was deemed insufficient to place in one of the other categories.

National Institutes of Health. National Heart, Lung, and Blood Institute. Clinical Guidelines on the Identification, Evaluation, and Treatment of Overweight and Obesity in Adults: The Evidence Report (Appendices). Accessed January 31, 2021. Available at https://learn.nlm.nih.gov/documentation/training-packets /T0042010P

To be useful, information must be collected in a timely manner and presented to scientists, policymakers, and the public in a readily understandable form. Without current monitoring, decisions may be made using insufficient information or incorrect assumptions. Nutrition and health-related information can be obtained using several methods, notably through nutrition screening, assessment, and surveillance; these are often collectively referred to as nutrition monitoring.

Nutrition Screening and Assessment

Nutrition screening is a systematic approach to quickly identify nutrition problems or individuals at nutritional risk that are in need of further assessment or an intervention. Screening can be done in free-living and hospitalized individuals; however, it is important to use validated instruments to maximize the chance of correctly identifying at-risk individuals.[34,35] The mini-nutritional assessment, used in screening elderly populations[36] is a widely used, valid screening instrument. Many other screening tools are available for nutrition professionals, including those designed to determine malnutrition,[37] diabetes risk,[38] and food security.[39]

Nutrition assessment collects, verifies, and interprets data used to identify nutrition-related problems and includes nutrition-related history, anthropometric measures, biochemical data, nutrition-focused physical findings, and social and medical history. This can be gathered on a population or individual level and various methods are used to collect these data.[40] To assess nutrition-related history, especially nutrition intake, community and public health, dietitians/nutritionists use such methods as 24-hour diet recalls, food frequency questionnaires (FFQs), food records (or diaries), food and nutrient screeners (also called short dietary assessments),[41] or newer technology-based dietary assessment tools such as web-based programs, mobile applications, or image-based tools.[42,43]

The 24-hour diet recall is used to capture short-term diet information about a group of people. Principal strengths of 24-hour diet recalls are

Strategy Tip

The Academy of Nutrition and Dietetics (the Academy) members have full online access to the Evidence Analysis Library at https://www.andeal.org. Members can also download the Evidence Analysis Manual.

Strategy Tip

Stay on top of nutritional monitoring and other events in public health by subscribing online to the *Morbidity and Mortality Weekly Report* at http://www.cdc .gov/mmwr/mmwrsubscribe.html

Center for Nutrition Policy and Promotion The center within the U.S. Department of Agriculture (USDA) where scientific research is linked to the nutritional needs of the American public. Projects include, but are not limited to: the Dietary Guidelines of Americans, MyPlate, the Healthy Eating Index, the USDA Food Patterns, and the USDA Food Plans: Cost of Food.

that they provide detailed information about the types and amounts of food consumed on a given day, have a low response burden, and are cost-effective.[41] The principal limitations are that they rely on specific memory, respondents may under- or over-report consumption, and need multiple nonconsecutive recalls in order to estimate usual dietary intake. Additionally, 24-hour diet recalls are not valid for individuals; collection of group data from 24-hour diet recalls with mean reporting, for example, as used by What We Eat in America, the dietary component of the NHANES, is an appropriate use of 24-hour diet recalls;[44] however, it has long been recognized that 24-hour diet recalls may not reflect usual intake.[41] In 2003, staff members of NHANES began collecting two recalls, the first in person in the Mobile Examination Center and the second 3 to 10 days later by telephone. The National Cancer Institute (NCI), coupled with the **Center for Nutrition Policy and Promotion (CNPP)**, developed a statistical method to calculate usual intake using both recalls.[45] The multiple-pass method for the 24-hour dietary recalls[46] should be used to avoid underreporting of intake (**Table 1–4**). The standard for assessing intake is multiple

TABLE 1–4
Information Collected During National Health and Nutrition Examination Survey Diet Interviews

5-Step Multiple-Pass Approach			
Step	**Purpose**		
Quick List	Collect a list of foods and beverages consumed the previous day.	For each food and beverage consumed during previous 24-hour period	Detailed description
			Additions to the food
			Amount consumed
			What foods were eaten in combination
			Time eating occasion began
			Name of eating occasion
Forgotten Foods	Probe for foods forgotten during the Quick List.		Food source (where obtained)
			Whether food was eaten at home
			Amounts of food energy and 60+ nutrients/food components provided by the amount of food (calculated)
Time & Occasion	Collect time and eating occasion for each food.	For each respondent on each day	Day of the week
			Amount and type of water consumed, including total plain water, tap water, and plain carbonated water
Detail Cycle	For each food, collect detailed description, amount, and additions. Review 24-hour day.		Source of tap water
			Daily intake usual, much more or much less than usual
			Use and type of salt at table and in preparation
			Whether on a special diet and type of diet
Final Probe	Final probe for anything else consumed.		Frequency of fish and shellfish consumption (past 30 days)
			Daily total intakes of food energy and 60+ nutrients/food components (calculated)

U.S. Department of Agriculture. Accessed January 31, 2021. Retrieved from https://www.ars.usda.gov/northeast-area/beltsville-md-bhnrc/beltsville-human-nutrition-research-center/food-surveys-research-group/docs/ampm-usda-automated-multiple-pass-method

24-hour dietary recalls using the multiple-pass method. Intake can change from weekday to weekend, from season to season, and between holiday and nonholiday days; it is important to get a proper sample of the study group using 24-hour diet recalls at different times of the week and year to better capture these differences. The NCI's Dietary Assessment Primer contains recommendations for data capture for 24-hour diet recalls, in addition to other dietary assessment tools.[41]

It should also be noted that NHANES collects information on supplement and prescription medication intake, food security, some consumer behaviors, as well as anthropometrics. These data can be used with the data collected from the recalls not only to further the nutrition assessment but also to look for associations among variables.

Food Frequency Questionnaires (FFQs), in contrast to 24-hour diet recalls or food records, are designed to measure dietary intake over longer periods. FFQs vary in the number of food items, food groups, and food portion assessments—all of which affect nutrient intake.[41] Similar to 24-hour diet recalls, FFQs often underestimate intake of total energy, and energy adjustment can be used to reduce the effects of measurement error, that is, regression dilution. It is also important that appropriate racial and ethnic foods consumed by the targeted population be included when designing FFQ. Although a wide variety of FFQs are in use, some have not been validated against 24-hour recalls or direct observation. Using meta-analyses, FFQs with longer food lists (200 items) were shown to have 0.01 to 0.17 higher correlation coefficients than FFQs with shorter food lists (<100 items) for most nutrients.[47] An advantage of FFQs is that they can be self-administered and thus are suitable for large epidemiologic studies.

Newer methods of dietary intake measurement include digital photography entered by either a researcher or self-recording from a mobile application.[42] An example is the Remote Food Photography Method, which uses a smartphone to capture images of food selection and plate waste, which are sent to a server for intake estimation.[48] These digital photography methods are appealing because they use technology, but accuracy is dependent on training staff, study participants, or clients to take consistent photographs. Other methods used to determine intake include direct observation, plate waste, and food records with or without weighing foods.

Determining intake accurately is critical. Intake of food groups can be determined from using instruments as conventional as the *Start Simple with MyPlate* app[49], which is appropriate for the public, and the Food Patterns Equivalents Database,[50] which may be more appropriate for health professionals. Nutrient intake can be assessed using the USDA FoodData Central,[51] the Food and Nutrient Database for Dietary Studies,[52] and commercially available diet analysis programs. Different databases may not yield the same nutrient analyses and it is best to be consistent when using them to analyze data. Whenever possible, dietary intake should be confirmed using appropriate biomarkers; for example, folate intake should be confirmed with serum folate levels.[41] Intake of nutrients or food groups can be compared with recommended values for specific populations and, in turn, with the prevalence or incidence of chronic disease.

Population Surveillance

Surveillance comes from the French verb *surveiller*, "to watch over." In 1968, the World Health Assembly described surveillance as "the systematic collection and use of epidemiologic information for planning, implementation, and assessment of disease control."[53] Surveillance, in contrast to surveys, is

National Nutrition Monitoring and Related Research Program
Established in 1990 (PL 101-445), this is a comprehensive, coordinated program for nutrition monitoring and related research to improve health and nutrition assessment in U.S. populations.

Goals of NHANES

- Estimate the number and percentage of persons in the U.S. population, and designated subgroups, with selected diseases and risk factors
- Monitor trends in the prevalence, awareness, treatment, and control of selected diseases
- Monitor trends in risk behaviors and environmental exposures
- Analyze risk factors for selected diseases
- Study the relationship between diet, nutrition, and health
- Explore emerging public health issues and new technologies
- Establish a national probability sample of genetic material for future genetic research
- Establish and maintain a national probability sample of baseline information on health and nutritional status

continual, and data that are collected can be used to provide the framework for public health policies and rationale for intervention. Surveillance also provides a way to monitor the effectiveness of specific interventions. This completes the loop—surveillance studies that can be used to determine nutritional problems or nutritional needs, and after the intervention, they can be used to determine whether the problems remain or if the intervention was effective.

Most governments track the health and nutrition status of their population. For example, the U.S. government has tracked information on food and the food supply for more than 100 years, starting with the USDA's Food Supply Series in 1909.[54] In 1936–1937, the USDA conducted the first national survey, known as the Consumer Purchases Study, to measure distribution of food at the household and individual level and conducted follow-up surveys at roughly 10-year intervals. The 1955 Household Food Consumption Survey (later called the Nationwide Food Consumption Survey (in 1977)) was the first nationally representative survey to cover all four seasons of food intake.[55,56] Health status was initially tracked separately from nutrition; in 1960, the National Health Examination Survey was initiated[57] however, it did not include information on nutrition and its link with diet. Federal officials thus could not provide information on diet and disease or undernutrition to Congress. The nation's largest nutrition survey to date was the Ten-State Nutrition Survey conducted between 1968 and 1970 in 10 states: California, Kentucky, Louisiana, Massachusetts, Michigan, New York, South Carolina, Texas, Washington, and West Virginia; however, the data collected and analyzed were not a nationally representative sample.[58] The NHANES I and II and the Pediatric Nutrition Surveillance Systems were initiated in the 1970s.[57,59]

In 1990, the **National Nutrition Monitoring and Related Research Program (NNMRRP)** (Public Law [PL] 101-445) established a comprehensive, coordinated program for nutrition monitoring and related research to improve health and nutrition assessment in U.S. populations.[60] The NNMRRP required a program to coordinate federal nutrition monitoring efforts and assisted state and local governments in participating in a nutrition monitoring network; an interagency board to develop and implement the program; and a nine-member advisory council to provide scientific and technical advice and to evaluate program effectiveness. The NNMRRP also required that dietary guidelines (DGA) be issued every 5 years, and that any dietary guidance issued by the federal government for the general public be reviewed by the Secretaries of Agriculture and Health and Human Services (HHS).

The NNMRRP encompasses more than 50 surveillance activities that monitor and assess health and nutritional status in the United States. Monitoring efforts are divided into five overarching areas: nutrition and related health measurements; food and nutrient consumption; knowledge, attitude, and behavior assessments; food composition and nutrient databases; and food supply determinants. Important monitoring programs are summarized in **Table 1–5**. Most of the data sets generated through this program are available to the public. Some are restricted, due to confidential or disclosure rules/regulations, and can be accessed by researchers through application to the Research Data Center in the National Center for Health Statistics (NCHS) headquarters in Hyattsville, Maryland.

In 2002, the Department of HHS and the USDA integrated NHANES and the Continuing Survey of Food Intakes by Individuals (CSFII), the two major diet and health surveys, into a continuous data collection system. Diet and nutrition information thus can be linked directly to health status information. The integrated dietary component of the NHANES is titled, "*What We Eat in America.*"[61]

TABLE 1–5
National Nutrition-Related Health Assessments[a]

Survey Name	Date	Target	Data Collected	Dept/Agency
Nutritional and Related Health Measurements				
NHANES[b]	1999–present	Civilian, noninstitutionalized persons 2 months or older; oversampling of adolescents, African-Americans, Mexican-Americans, and adults >60 years of age	Survey elements are similar to NHANES III & NHIS.[c] This is a continuous monitoring system.	NCHS, CDC (HHS)
NHANES III	1988–1994	Civilian, noninstitutionalized persons 2 months or older; oversampling of adolescents, non-Hispanic blacks, Mexican-Americans, children, 6 years and adults >60 years of age	Demographics, dietary intake (24-hour recall and food frequency), biochemical analysis of blood and urine, physical examination, anthropometry, blood pressure, bone densitometry, diet and health behaviors, health conditions	NCHS, CDC (HHS)
NHANES III Supplemental Nutrition Survey of Older Persons	1988–1994	Representative U.S. elderly population	See above	NCHS, NIH/NIA
HHANES	1982–1984	Civilian, noninstitutionalized Mexican Americans in five southwestern states, Cuban Americans in Dade Co., FL, and Puerto Ricans in New York, New Jersey, and Connecticut, 6 months to 74 years of age	Demographics, dietary intake (24-hour recall & food frequency), biochemical analysis of blood and urine, physical exam, anthropometry, blood pressure, diet and health behaviors, health conditions	NCHS (HHS)
NHANES II	1976–1980	Civilian, noninstitutionalized persons 6 months to 74 years of age	Demographics, dietary intake, biochemical analysis of blood and urine, physical exam, anthropometry	NCHS (HHS)
NHANES I	1971–1974	Civilian, noninstitutionalized population of the conterminous states 1 to 74 years of age	Demographics, dietary information, biochemical analysis of blood and urine, physical exam, anthropometry	NCHS (HHS)
Food and Nutrient Consumption				
CSFII[d]	1994–1996 1989–1991 1985–1986	Individuals of all ages with oversampling in low-income households	One- and 3-day food intakes, times of eating events, sources of food eaten away from home	ARS, HNIS
TDS	1961, annual	Specific age and gender groups	Determines levels of nutrients and contaminants in the food supply—analyses are performed on foods that are "table-ready"	FDA (HHS)
Consumer Expenditure Survey	1980, continuous	Noninstitutionalized population and a portion of the institutionalized population in the United States	Demographics, food stamp use, average annual food expenditures	U.S. Bureau of Labor Statistics
NFCS	1987 1977–1978	Households in the conterminous states—all income and low income	Households: quantity (pounds), money value (dollars), and nutritive value of food eaten. Individuals: food intake, times of eating events, and sources of foods eaten away from home	HNIS (USDA) ARS (USDA)

(continues)

TABLE 1–5
National Nutrition-Related Health Assessments[a]   *(continued)*

Survey Name	Date	Target	Data Collected	Dept/Agency
Food and Nutrient Consumption				
SNDA II	1998	Public schools in the 48 contiguous states and the District of Columbia that participate in the National School Lunch Program	School and food service characteristics, nutrients by food group and relationship to the RDA and DGA by meals, source of meals, and nutrient content of USDA meals	FNS/USDA
WIC Infant Feeding Practices Study	1994–1995	Pre- and postnatal women and their children who participate in WIC	Demographics, rates of breast and formula feeding, factors associated with breast feeding.	FNS/USDA
Knowledge, Attitude, and Behavior Assessments				
DHKS	1994–1996	Adults 20 years and older who participated in CSFII 1994–1996	Demographics, self-perceptions of relative intake, awareness of diet and health relationships, food-label use, perceived importance of following diet and health recommendations, beliefs about food safety, and knowledge of sources of nutrients; data can be linked with intake through CSFII data	ARS/USDA
Infant Feeding Practices Survey	1993–1994	New mothers and healthy infants to 1 year of age	Demographics, prior infant feeding practices, baby's social situation, characteristics associated with breastfeeding, development of allergies	FDA
Consumer Food Handling Practices and Awareness of Microbiological Hazards	1998 1992–1993	Civilian, noninstitutionalized over 18 years with telephones	Demographics, prevalence of unsafe food handling practices, knowledge of food safety principles, use of sources of information about safe food handling, incidence of foodborne illnesses	FDA
Food Composition and Nutrient Databases				
National Nutrient Data Bank[e]	–	–	This is the repository for values of approximately 7,100 foods and up to 80 components. Essentially all food composition databases are derived from this data bank	ARS (USDA)
Food Label and Package Survey	1977–1996, biennially 2000, 2006	All brands of processed foods regulated by the FDA	Prevalence of nutrition labeling, declaration of select nutrients, prevalence of label claims and other descriptors	FDA (HHS)
Food Supply Determinations				
AC Nielsen SCANTRACK	1985, monthly	~3,000 U.S. Supermarkets	Sales and physical volume of specific market items, selling price, percent of stores selling the product	ERS/USDA
U.S. Food and Nutrient Supply Series	1909, annually	U.S. Population	ERS = Amount of food commodities that disappear into the food distribution system; CNPP = nutrient levels of food supply. Results are totaled for each nutrient and converted to per-day basis.	ERS/CNPP/USDA

Nutrition Monitoring Activities in the States

PedNSS	1973, continuous	Low-income, high-risk children, birth to 17 years, emphasis on birth to 5 years	Demographics, anthropometry, birth weight, hematology	NCCDPHP, CDC (HHS)
PNSS	1973, continuous	Convenience sample of low-income, high-risk pregnant women	Demographics, pregravid weight and maternal weight gain, anemia, behavioral risk factors, birth weight, and formula-feeding data	NCCDPHP, CDC (HHS)
YRBBS	Biennial	Civilian, noninstitutionalized adolescents 12 to 18 years	Demographics, diet and weight; drug, alcohol & tobacco use; seat belt and bicycle helmet use; behaviors that contribute to violence; suicidal tendencies[f]	CDC (HHS)/ NCCDPHP
BRFSS	1984, continuous	Adults 18 years and older in households with telephones located in participating states	Demographics, questions that assess risk factors associated with leading causes of death: alcohol and tobacco use, weight, seat belt and helmet use; use of preventative medical care[g]	CDC (HHS)/ NCCDPHP

[a]A complete guide to nutrition monitoring in the United States can be found at: http://www.cdc.gov/nchs/data/misc/nutri98.pdf

[b]Abbreviations: ARS = Agricultural Research Service; BRFSS = Behavioral Risk Factor Surveillance System; CDC = Centers for Disease Control and Prevention; CNPP = Center for Nutrition Policy and Promotion; CSFII = Continuing Survey of Food Intakes by Individuals; DHKS = Diet and Health Knowledge Survey; ERS = Economic Research Service FDA = Food and Drug Administration; HHANES = Hispanic Health and Nutrition Examination Survey; HHS = Health and Human Services; HNIS = Human Nutrition Information Service; NFCS = Nationwide Food Consumption Survey; NCCDPHP = National Center for Chronic Disease Prevention and Health Promotion; NCHS = National Center for Health Statistics; NCI = National Cancer Institute; NHANES = National Health and Nutrition Examination Survey; NHIS = National Health Interview Survey; NIA = National Institute on Aging; NIH= National Institutes of Health; PedNSS = Pediatric Nutrition Surveillance System; PNSS = Pregnancy Nutrition Surveillance System; SNDA = School Nutrition Dietary Assessment Study; TDS = Total Diet Study; USDA = U.S. Department of Agriculture; WIC = Women, Infants, and Children; YRBSS = Youth Risk Behavioral Surveillance System.

[c]http://www.cdc.gov/nchs/data/nhanes/survey_content_99_16.pdf complete survey content of NHANES 1999–2016

[d]CSFII and NHANES were combined into a single survey

[e]Now FoodData Central on the USDA website: https://fdc.nal.usda.gov/

[f]https://www.cdc.gov/healthyyouth/data/yrbs/results.htm - YBRSS report 2019, reports available through CDC Web site

[g]https://www.cdc.gov/brfss/about/index.htm - Behavioral Risk Factor Surveillance System full information

The National Health and Nutrition Examination Survey

The NHANES is a program of studies designed to assess the health and nutritional status of the U.S. population. The survey combines health interviews and physical examinations with dietary information (**Table 1–6**).

Beginning in 1999, the NHANES became a continuous surveillance program with data released to the public biannually. Rather than using a random sample, the NHANES uses a complex, multistage, probability sampling design to select participants representative of the civilian, noninstitutionalized U.S. population. Oversampling of certain population subgroups (i.e., Hispanic Americans, African Americans, and persons 60 and older) increases the reliability and precision of health status indicator estimates for these subgroups. Data collection by the NHANES occurs at three levels: a brief household screener interview, an in-depth household survey interview, and a medical examination. Because detailed interviews, clinical, laboratory, radiological examinations are conducted, the response burden to participants is significant. Interviews and medical examinations take place in a mobile examination center. Because of this sampling design, using appropriate statistical analyses of NHANES data are critical. To assure that NHANES analyses reflect a nationally representative sample, it is important to use the described weighting system and specialty software (e.g., SUDAAN. Stata).[62]

TABLE 1–6
Data Available Through NHANES

Health Exam Tests
Health Measurements by Participant Age and Gender

- Physician's exam—all ages
- Blood pressure—ages ≥8 years
- Bone density—ages ≥8 years
- Condition of teeth—ages ≥5 years
- Vision test—ages ≥12 years
- Hearing test—ages 12–19 and ≥70 years
- Height, weight, and other body measures—all ages
- Ophthalmology exam for eye diseases—ages ≥40 years
- Breathing tests—ages 6–79 years

Lab Tests on Urine (≥6 years)

- Kidney Function tests—ages ≥6 years
- Sexually transmitted diseases (STD), Chlamydia and gonorrhea—ages 14–39 years
- Exposure to environmental chemicals—selected persons ages ≥X years
- Pregnancy test—girls and women ages ≥12 years and girls ages 8–11 years who have periods

Lab Tests on Blood: (≥1 year and older)

- Anemia—all ages
- Total cholesterol and high-density lipoprotein (HDL) —ages ≥6 years
- Glucose measures—ages ≥12 years
- Infectious diseases—ages ≥2 years
- Kidney function tests—ages ≥12 years
- Lead—ages ≥1 years
- Cadmium—ages ≥1 years
- Mercury—ages ≥1 years
- Liver function tests—ages ≥12 years
- Nutrition status—ages ≥1 years
- Thyroid function test—ages ≥12 years
- Prostate-specific antigen (PSA) —men ages ≥40 years
- Sexually transmitted diseases (STD)
  — Genital herpes—ages 14–49 years
  — Human immunodeficiency virus (HIV) —ages 18–49 years
  — Human papillomavirus (HPV) antibody—ages 14–59 years
- Exposure to environmental chemicals—selected persons ages ≥6 years

Lab Tests on Water

- Environmental chemicals—ages ≥12 years in half of households

Other Lab Tests

- Vaginal swabs (self-administered) —girls and women aged 14–59 years
- Human papillomavirus (HPV) —ages 14–59 years

Private Health Interviews

- Health status—ages ≥12 and older
- Questions about drug and alcohol use—ages ≥12 years (no drug testing will be done)
- Reproductive health—girls and women ages ≥12 years
- Questions about sexual experience—aged 14–69 years
- Tobacco use—ages ≥12 years

Anthropometry from the Mobile Examination Center

- Body mass index; for children ages 2–19 years; BMI z-score is also determined
- Waist circumference
- Skinfold measurements and body fat measures through DXA

Dietary Information from the Mobile Examination Center

- 24-hour dietary recalls; parents or guardians report for children 0–5 years of age; children 6–11 years are assisted by an adult; children ≥12 years self-report
- Food frequency questionnaire

After the Visit to the NHANES Examination Center

- Persons asked about the foods they eat will receive a phone call 3–10 days after their exam for a similar interview, all ages.
- Then participants, or an adult for participants 1–15 years old, are asked about food shopping habits.
- Persons who test positive for hepatitis C will be asked to participate in a brief telephone interview 6 months after the exam. Parents will respond for children.

It is difficult to quantify the tremendous impact that NHANES and related programs have had on health policy and health research in the United States.[63] One way to look at this is the number of publications generated using NHANES data. A PubMed search in February of 2021 using the term "NHANES" produced 53,993 publications on topics as diverse as the relationship between lean body mass indices, physical activity, and systolic blood pressure; income-related inequalities in untreated dental caries among young children; number of adults meeting prediabetes criteria; and the association between eating behavior and diet quality when eating alone vs. with others. NHANES data have also shown that there are ethnic/racial and income differences in dietary intake, including food sources for nutrients[64,65] control of cardiovascular risk factors vary according to socioeconomic status;[66] and hypertension morbidity is increased in U.S. immigrant groups but varies by race/ethnicity and gender.[67] These findings have important implications for intervention strategies.

Strategy Tip

Take a guided tour of the mobile examination center at https://www.cdc.gov/nchs/nhanes/participant/information-collected.htm

Study Designs and Uses
Epidemiologic Studies

In addition to the NCHS data, a number of long-term, primarily government funded epidemiologic studies on adults and children/adolescents have provided critical information used to guide the nation's health policies and federal programs. The Bogalusa Heart Study (BHS), the Framingham Heart Study (FHS), and the Coronary Artery Risk Development in Young Adults (CARDIA) are leading examples. Other important U.S. epidemiologic studies that have contributed to our knowledge of risk reduction and disease prevention are The Nurses' Health Study (NHS; N = 170,000 female registered nurses between the ages of 30 and 55 years at the beginning of the study) and the NHS II (NHS II established in 1989, N = ~117,000 female nurses aged between 25 and 42 years); and the all-men Health Professional Follow-up Study (initiated in 1986 with 2-year scheduled follow-ups), which was designed to complement the NHS, relating nutritional factors to the incidence of serious illnesses, such as cancer, heart disease, and other vascular diseases in 51,529 male health professionals. Also of import is the Iowa Women's Health Study with a cohort of 41,837 postmenopausal women who have been followed since 1985. These studies combined have produced more than 2,000 scientific publications and have helped shape medical care, risk reduction and health promotion, and public policy.

The Bogalusa Heart Study was extended and many findings were duplicated in another population through the Young Finns Study. To learn more about the Young Finns Study, go to https:/youngfinnsstudy.utu.fi

The Bogalusa Heart Study (BHS)

The BHS[68-70] was designed initially to examine the early natural history of coronary heart disease and essential hypertension in a biracial (black/white) pediatric population. The BHS population consists of approximately 5,000 individuals who have been studied at various growth phases and have been followed for as long as 15 years. The mixed epidemiologic design of the study has included cross-sectional and longitudinal surveys to provide information on three questions: 1) what are the distribution and prevalence of cardiovascular disease (CVD) risk factors in a defined pediatric population and how are abnormal serum lipid levels, blood pressure, and other risk factors defined in children; 2) do cardiovascular risk factors track and change over time; and 3) what is the interrelationship among these risk factors? Other questions, notably what is the interaction of genetics and the environment in CVD, were also posed.

Data from the BHS have contributed significantly to our knowledge and understanding of cardiovascular risk factors in children as well as the history of CVD in early life. For example, information on children, adolescents, and young adults from birth to 31 years of age has provided the framework to establish desirable cholesterol levels in children, and has led investigators to recommend screening of cardiovascular risk factors for all children, not only those with a parental history of heart disease or dyslipidemia, beginning at elementary school age.

Data have also suggested that risk factors for CVD "track," that is, they remain in a rank relative to peers over time. For example, children with elevated serum total cholesterol or low density lipoprotein cholesterol (LDL-C) levels are likely to become adults with dyslipidemia. Bogalusa Heart Study data have been used to characterize diets of children and secular trends in children's diets for more than 30 years.[71] BHS data were used as the rationale by the American Academy of Pediatrics for their recommendation that the DGA could apply to healthy children 2 years of age and older and to develop the Academy's original position paper on dietary guidance for healthy children 2 to 11 years of age.[72]

One of the major accomplishments of the BHS did not come from epidemiologic data per se, but from autopsy studies of participants,[73] usually those killed in accidents. Data from the BHS confirmed and extended earlier studies[74] that showed fatty streaks in the aorta were evident in the first decade of life and that the extent of these lesions was highly associated with serum total cholesterol and LDL-C levels. These findings provided the rationale for interventions that focused on healthy lifestyles for children.

Framingham Heart Study

The FHS has been described as "one of the most impressive medical works in the 20th century."[75] The Framingham Study has provided information critical to the recognition and management of atherosclerosis and its causes and complications. Initiated under the auspices of the National Heart Institute (now the NHLBI) in 1948, 1,980 males and 2,421 females were enrolled originally in a 3-year observational study in Framingham, Massachusetts, which at the time was a novel idea. Published in 1961, the first report, titled, "Factors of risk in the development of coronary heart disease—six-year follow-up experience; the Framingham Study," identified high blood pressure, smoking, and high cholesterol levels as major factors in heart disease and conceptualized them as risk factors.[76] Continued study of the population has provided health professionals with multifactorial risk profiles for cardiovascular disease that have assisted in identifying individuals at high risk as well as providing the basis for preventative measures. During its more than 70-year history, the FHS has introduced the concept of biologic, genomic, environmental, and behavioral risk factors; identified major risk factors associated with heart disease, stroke, and other diseases; revolutionized preventive medicine; and changed how the medical community and general population regard disease pathogenesis.[77] The National Cholesterol Education Program[78] uses the Framingham risk scoring system to determine the 10-year risk of CHD in adults. New findings from the FHS genomics measures are being used to study how modifiable lifestyle factors may affect the risk of chronic disease.[79]

In 1971, the Framingham Heart Offspring Study began,[80] consisting of 5,124 males and females, 5 to 70 years of age, who were offspring and spouses of the offspring of the original Framingham cohort. The objectives of that study were to determine the incidence and prevalence of CVD and its risk factors, trends in CVD incidence and its risk factors over time, and family

To learn more about working with NHANES data, complete the online tutorial at https://wwwn.cdc.gov/nchs/nhanes/tutorials/default.aspx

patterns of CVD and risk factors. The Offspring Study provided the opportunity to evaluate a second generation of participants, assess new or emerging risk factors and outcomes, and provide a resource for future genetic analyses. In 2020, funding was granted for the development of the FHS Brain Aging Program, which will evaluate FHS participants for dementia and incorporate data from the original and subsequent cohorts of the FHS to further conduct research into genetic and other factors involved with Alzheimer's disease and vascular dementia.[81]

The quality of data from surveys and epidemiologic studies depends on the training of personnel and adherence to rigid protocols. It also depends on the validity and reliability of the test instruments used as well as on the responses of the subjects. Instruments may need to be modified for specific populations. For example, in the BHS, the 24-hour diet recall method had to be adapted for use in children.[82,83] To improve the reliability and validity of the 24-hour diet recall, quality controls included the use of a standardized protocol that specified exact techniques for interviewing, recording, and calculating results; standardized graduated food models to quantify foods and beverages consumed; a product identification notebook for probing of snack consumption, and foods and beverages most commonly forgotten; school lunch assessment to identify all school lunch recipes, preparation methods, and average portion sizes of menu items reflected in each 24-hour diet recall; follow-up telephone calls to parents to obtain information on brand names, recipes, and preparation methods of meals served at home; products researched in the field to obtain updated information on ingredients and preparation, and their weights (primarily snack foods and fast foods).[84] All interviewers participated in rigorous training sessions and pilot studies before the field surveys to minimize interviewer effects. One 24-hour diet recall was collected on each study participant, and duplicate recalls were collected from a 10% random subsample to assess interviewer variability.

Metabolic Diet Studies

Metabolic diet studies are conducted in clinical research centers where study participants are randomized into test or control groups and are fed an experimental diet or "regular" diet, respectively. Different designs are available for metabolic diet studies,[85] but the one that provides the most valid results is a double-blind, placebo-controlled study. In these studies, neither the investigator nor the participant knows whether the test or control diet is offered. Because it is difficult and expensive to do these studies, they are usually short term and have a small sample size; compliance and drop-out rates are problems.

Dietary Approaches to Stop Hypertension (DASH)

The Dietary Approaches to Stop Hypertension (DASH)[86] and DASH sodium[87] trials are classic examples of metabolic diet studies. Epidemiologic, clinical trials, and studies using experimental animals showed that intake of some nutrients, notably low levels of sodium, and high levels of potassium and calcium lowered blood pressure; however, people eat food—not isolated nutrients. To test the impact that combination diets incorporating foods high in these nutrients had on blood pressure, the DASH study was conducted. DASH was a randomized controlled trial conducted at four academic medical centers with 459 adult participants. Inclusion criteria were untreated systolic blood pressure <160 mm Hg and diastolic blood pressure 80 to 95 mm Hg. For 3 weeks, participants ate a control diet. They were then randomized to 8 weeks of a control diet; a diet rich in fruits and vegetables; or a combination diet rich in fruits, vegetables, and low-fat dairy foods, and low in saturated fatty acids, total fat, and cholesterol. Salt intake and weight were held constant, and diets were isoenergic. All food was prepared in a metabolic kitchen and was provided to participants. The combination diet (or "DASH diet") was shown to quickly (within 2 weeks) and substantially lower blood pressure.

In DASH sodium, a subsequent study, 412 participants were assigned to a control diet or a DASH diet; within the assigned diet, participants ate meals with high (3,450 mg/2,100 kcals), intermediate (2,300 mg/2,100 kcals), and low (1,150 mg/2,100 kcals) levels of sodium for 30 consecutive days each, in random order. Reduction of sodium intake to levels below the current recommendation of 100 mmol/day and the DASH diet substantially lowered blood pressure, with the most significant effect seen in lowering blood pressure with the lowest sodium concentration coupled with the DASH diet. The DASH diet has been widely embraced for the treatment of hypertension; nutrition education materials are readily available. As elegant and persuasive as the DASH studies were; one drawback to feeding studies is that participants receive all foods. Therefore, the studies cannot assess how compliant people are after the study ends. The PREMIER study[88] demonstrated that free-living individuals were able to make the lifestyle changes associated with decreased blood pressure.

Clinical Trials

Clinical trials are commonly used to determine the efficacy of drugs or other pharmacologic agents; however, they can also be used to assess diet or dietary interventions. They have many of the same advantages and disadvantages of metabolic studies. Because clinical trials of diet may involve pharmacologic intervention, they carry a risk that is not usually seen with metabolic diet studies. The classical example of this was seen in the Alpha-Tocopherol, Beta-Carotene Cancer Prevention Study (ATBC Study)[89] and the Beta-Carotene and Retinol Efficacy Trial (CARET).[90] Based on epidemiologic data that showed a relationship between dietary intake of fruits and vegetables[91,92] or, specifically, of beta carotene[93] and a reduced risk of developing lung cancer, especially in smokers,[94] the ATBC and CARET studies used high doses of beta-carotene in major cancer chemopreventive trials. Investigators expected to see reductions in lung cancer by as much as 49% in some high-risk groups. In actuality, the opposite was seen and beta-carotene increased the risk of lung cancer, forcing the CARET study to be stopped early.[95] These studies clearly point to the necessity of additional research and have important public health implications.

Animal Studies

Animal studies are important in nutrition research for many reasons. Laboratory animals that are genetically identical and exposed to the same environmental conditions can be fed carefully characterized diets with different combinations of nutrients; thus, the number of variables studied are limited. Special treatments, such as genetic and metabolite alterations to mimic cognitive impairments,[96] can be performed on animals. Because the lifespan of most laboratory animals is short, the effects of dietary manipulation can be followed over several generations. Animals can be sacrificed at the end of the experiment and the effect of the treatment can be examined closely at the organ, tissue, or cellular level. Animal studies can explore molecular mechanisms behind a given observation in humans. For example, ferrets were used to determine that high doses of beta-carotene caused keratinized squamous metaplasia in lung tissues that was exacerbated by exposure to cigarette smoke.[97] This explains the paradoxical relationship between beta-carotene and smoking that is seen in the clinical trials above. It points out another use of animal studies: that the metabolism of natural products should be investigated using animal models *before* beginning intervention trials, particularly if nutrient doses exceed recommended levels.[98]

Animals most commonly used in nutrition research are rats, mice, rabbits, guinea pigs, dogs, sheep, and monkeys. The species selected for a given experiment should be that which is the most similar to human metabolism for a particular nutrient. The importance of this is illustrated in the classic studies of vitamin C metabolism. Guinea pigs are the only laboratory animal that, like humans, have an obligatory requirement for this nutrient; thus, a review of the literature shows only guinea pigs were used for vitamin C research.

Many of the elements that make animal studies so appealing in nutrition research are also drawbacks. With the exception of monozygotic twins, humans are not genetically identical; thus, no matter how carefully a human experiment is controlled, responses to dietary manipulations may be different due to individual genetic backgrounds. Interactions between genetics and the environment are easy to study in animals, but results are difficult to translate to humans.

Community and Public Health Services

There are many programs and services run by the government that serve to create nutrition policies and help the public make healthier choices with regard to overall health and specifically nutrition. All of them draw from the wealth of information created by the surveys, studies, and surveillance systems that report on the health and nutrition status of the U.S. population. *Healthy People 2030* and the **Dietary Reference Intakes** create a framework to guide nutrition policy in the country. All other programs and services use that framework to communicate a unified message for health and nutrition for the nation. Examples of these programs and services include the Dietary Guidelines for Americans, **MyPlate**, the Healthy Eating Index, and food labels and health claims. Public health dietitians/nutritionists can leverage these programs and services in their work with the community.

Healthy People 2030

Individual health is closely linked to community health—the health of the community and environment in which individuals live, work, and play. Community health, in turn, is profoundly affected by the collective beliefs, attitudes, and behaviors of everyone who lives in that community. *Healthy People 2030*, published by the Office of Disease Prevention and Health Promotion (OCPHP) in the Department of Health and Human Services (HHS),[99] is the set of public health priorities designed to guide the health and well-being of the nation; HP goals remain in place for 10 years; the next update will be HP2040. Each new HP iteration is created out of the knowledge gained from the previous decades; HP2030 is the 5th iteration based on the past 4 decades of information. In 1979, *Healthy People: The Surgeon General's Report on Health Promotion and Disease Prevention*[100] provided nutritional goals for reducing premature deaths and preserving independence for older adults. In 1980, *Promoting Health/Preventing Disease: Objectives for the Nation*, targeted 226 health objectives for the nation to achieve over the next 10-year period.[101] These were followed by HP 2000, 2010, 2020, and now 2030 goals.

Dietary Reference Intakes A system of nutrition recommendations from the Institute of Medicine's Food and Nutrition Board (now the Health and Medicine Division of the National Academies of Sciences, Engineering, and Medicine). Introduced in 1997, the DRI's were developed to broaden the Recommended Dietary Allowances.

MyPlate Is the "visual translation" of the Dietary Guidelines for Americans for the public.

The overarching goals for HP2030 are[99]

- Attain healthy, thriving lives and well-being free of preventable disease, disability, injury, and premature death
- Eliminate health disparities, achieve health equity, and attain health literacy to improve the health and well-being of all
- Create social, physical, and economic environments that promote attaining the full potential for health and well-being for all
- Promote health development, healthy behaviors, and well-being across all life stages
- Engage leadership, key constituents, and the public across multiple sectors to take action and design policies that improve the health and well-being of all

Healthy People 2030 Established by the Department of Health and Human Services, this is the comprehensive health promotion and disease prevention agenda for the nation.

Healthy People 2030 has 62 topic areas and tracks 355 core (or measureable) objectives. It also designates some objectives as developmental and research objectives, neither of which are measured in the HP2030 framework (though these objectives have the potential to become core objectives during the course of the decade as more research and data become available). Developmental objectives are high-priority public health issues with evidence-based interventions but lacking reliable baseline data whereas research objectives are public health issues with a high health or economic burden or with significant disparities in the population that do not yet have evidence-based interventions. This represents a change from HP2020, which had approximately 1,200 measurable objectives; fewer core objectives allows HP2030 to prioritize the most pressing public health issues in this country for the next decade while still representing additional public health issues with developmental and research objectives. HP2030 also has 23 Leading Health Indicators (LHIs) (**Table 1–7**) organized to

---

TABLE 1–7
Leading Health Indicators of Healthy People 2030

All Ages
Children, adolescents, and adults who use the oral healthcare system (2+ years)
Consumption of calories from added sugars by persons aged 2 years and over (2+ years)
Drug overdose deaths
Exposure to unhealthy air
Homicides
Household food insecurity and hunger
Persons who are vaccinated annually against seasonal influenza
Persons who know their HIV status (13+ years)
Persons with medical insurance (<65 years)
Suicides

Infants
Infant deaths

Children and Adolescents
Fourth grade students whose reading skills are at or above the proficient achievement level for their grade
Adolescents with major depressive episodes (MDEs) who receive treatment
Children and adolescents with obesity
Current use of any tobacco products among adolescents

Adults and Older Adults
Adults engaging in binge drinking of alcoholic beverages during the past 30 days
Adults who meet current minimum guidelines for aerobic physical activity and muscle-strengthening activity
Adults who receive colorectal cancer screening based on the most recent guidelines
Adults with hypertension whose blood pressure is under control
Cigarette smoking in adults
Employment among the working-age population
Maternal deaths
New cases of diagnosed diabetes in the population

TABLE 1–8

Healthy People 2030 Nutrition andHealthy Eating Objectives

General	NWS-01 Reduce household food insecurity and hunger NWS-02 Eliminate very low food security in children NWS-06 Increase fruit consumption for people aged 2 years and over NWS-07 Increase vegetable consumption for people aged 2 years and older NWS-08 Increase consumption of dark green vegetables, red and orange vegetables, and beans and peas for people aged 2 years and older NWS-09 Increase whole grain consumption for people aged 2 years and over NWS-10 Reduce consumption of added sugars for people aged 2 years and over NWS-11 Reduce consumption of saturated fats for people aged 2 years and over NWS-12 Reduce consumption of sodium for people aged 2 years and over NWS-13 Increase calcium consumption for people aged 2 years and over NWS-14 Increase potassium consumption for people aged 2 years and over NWS-15 Increase vitamin D consumption for people aged 2 years and over NWS-16 Reduce iron deficiency in children aged 1 to 2 years ECBP-D02 Increase the proportion of schools that don't sell less-healthy foods and drinks
Adolescents	AH-04 Increase the proportion of students participating in the School Breakfast Program AH-R03 Increase the proportion of eligible students participating in the Summer Food Service Program
Cancer	C-R01 Increase quality of life for cancer survivors
Diabetes	D-D01 Increase the proportion of eligible people completing CDC-recognized type 2 diabetes prevention programs
Heart Disease and Stroke	HDS-04 Reduce the proportion of adults with high blood pressure HDS-06 Reduce cholesterol in adults
Infants	MICH-15 Increase the proportion of infants who are breastfed exclusively through age 6 months MICH-16 Increase the proportion of infants who are breastfed at 1 year
Overweight and Obesity	NWS-03 Reduce the proportion of adults with obesity NWS-05 Increase the proportion of healthcare visits by adults with obesity that include counseling on weight loss, nutrition, or physical activity
Women	MICH-12 Increase the proportion of women of childbearing age who get enough folic acid NWS-17 Reduce iron deficiency in females aged 12 to 49 years
Workplace	ECBP-D05 Increase the proportion of worksites that offer an employee a nutrition program

Note: The numbering system is categorized by the workgroup assigned to each objective followed by the number of the objective. D indicates a developmental objective; R indicates a research objective.

U.S. Department of Health and Human Services, Healthy People 2030 Nutrition andHealthy Eating objectives. Retrieved from https://health.gov/healthypeople/objectives-and-data/browse-objectives/nutrition-and-healthy-eating/eliminate-very-low-food-security-children-nws-02

address the entire life span. All LHIs are core objectives. **Table 1–8** shows the principal objectives associated with HP2030's Nutrition and Healthy Eating objectives; 22 are core objectives, three are developmental objectives, and two are research objectives. Many of these nutrition objectives are similar to those of the DGA, as discussed below.

The NCHS is responsible for coordinating efforts to monitor progress toward the HP objectives. Data are gathered from over 80 sources, including the NCHS data systems[102] and other Federal Government data systems. Criteria for data sources for HP2030 include nationally representative, publicly available, and known population coverage, response rates, and documentation completeness. Data from HP2030 can be explored by viewing individual objectives or customizable groups of objectives in the Objectives and Data portion of the HP2030 website.[103]

For HP2020, many states developed their own HP plans.[104] Development of state-specific plans allowed states to prioritize health problems, address needs of specific racial or ethnic groups, and develop solutions that were economically feasible for state budgets. States and territories had a Healthy People Coordinator who served as a liaison with the OCPHP.

Pandemic Learning Opportunity

HP2030 includes a COVID-19 custom list of objectives pertaining to the pandemic. ODPHP provided a shareable link for this list, and the list is editable for individuals or groups that wish to use pandemic-related objectives. Take some time to review the list and consider how you might customize it for nutrition programs for the public. https://health.gov/healthypeople/objectives-and-data/browse-objectives/nutrition-and-healthy-eating

Nutrient Requirements

The first Recommended Dietary Allowances (RDAs) were published in 1941 "to serve as a basis for food relief efforts both in the United States and internationally, where war or economic depression had resulted in malnutrition or starvation."[105] The first edition included recommendations only for energy and nine nutrients: protein, thiamine, riboflavin, niacin, ascorbic acid, vitamins A and D, calcium, and iron. In the seventh edition (1968), additional nutrients were included: folate; vitamins E, B_6, and B_{12}; phosphorus; magnesium; and iodine. The last edition of the RDAs (1989) added vitamin K, zinc, and selenium. The RDAs should be geared to groups of healthy people, such as the military or school feeding programs, rather than to individuals. The RDAs are however, often used to assess the adequacy of an individual's diet.

In 1993, the question of whether the RDAs should be changed was posed by the National Academies of Sciences, Engineering, and Medicine's Health and Medicine Division (HMD) (formerly the Institute of Medicine's (IOM) Food and Nutrition Board (FNB)). Support for change included that: 1) sufficient, new scientific information had accumulated to substantiate reassessment of these recommendations; 2) sufficient data for efficacy and safety existed; reduction in the risk of chronic diet-related diseases needed to be considered—previously, the RDA had focused on preventing deficiency diseases; 3) upper levels of intake should be established where there were data concerning risk of adverse effects; and 4) components of food that gave possible health benefits. Components of food, not meeting the traditional concept of a nutrient—such as phytochemicals, should be reviewed, and if adequate data existed, reference intakes should be established.

Between 1994 and 2004, the then IOM's Food and Nutrition Board, Dietary Reference Intakes (FNB DRI) extended and replaced the former RDAs and the Canadian Recommended Nutrient Intakes.[106] The DRIs are available on the website of the Food and Nutrition Information Center of the National Agricultural Library. The DRIs are specified on age, gender, and lifestage (e.g., pregnancy or lactation) and cover more than 40 nutrient substances. Conceptually, the DRIs are the same as the RDAs in that their formulation relies on the best scientific evidence available at the time of issuance, are designed for healthy individuals over time, and can vary depending on life cycle stage or gender. The reference values for heights and weights of adults and children used in the DRIs are from NHANES III. The DRIs differ from the original RDAs in that they incorporate the concepts of disease prevention, upper levels of intake and potential toxicity, and nontraditional nutrients. The latter establishes a precedent; as scientists learn more about the relationship of phytochemicals, herbals, or botanicals and health, these too can be incorporated into the recommendations. Where scientific evidence is available, the DRIs are a set of at least four nutrient-based reference values. Briefly, the four reference values are the estimated average requirement (EAR), RDA, tolerable upper intake level (UL), and adequate intake (AI). The EAR is the median usual intake value estimated to meet the requirements of half of the healthy individuals; it is based on specific criteria of adequacy and is based on careful review of the scientific evidence. Not all nutrients have an EAR since there may not be an acceptable science base upon which to define one. The EAR is used to calculate the RDA (RDA = EAR + 2 standard deviations of the requirement), which is the average daily dietary intake level sufficient to meet the nutrient requirement of approximately 98% of individuals. If there is no EAR for a nutrient, there can be no RDA. If this is the case, an AI for the nutrient is provided. This value is deemed by experts and is intended to meet or to

Phytonutrients are compounds produced by plants that may have different effects on and benefits for the body. Scientists have identified thousands of these compounds, but only a fraction of them have been studied closely. Examples include carotenoids, isoflavones, and flavonoids. To learn more about phytonutrients, go to the USDA's Food and Nutrition Information Center page on phytonutrients: https://www.nal.usda.gov/fnic/phytonutrients. To learn more about dietary supplements, go to the National Institutes of Health's website for the Office of Dietary Supplements: https://ods.od.nih.gov

exceed the needs of a healthy population. The AI can be used as a guide for intake but cannot be used for all of the applications for which the EAR can; it is also an indication that additional research is required for a nutrient. The assumption is that when this research is completed and evaluated, the AI can be replaced by an EAR and RDA. The UL is the highest level of continued daily nutrient intake that is unlikely to pose an adverse health effect. It is important to note that the word "tolerable" was chosen to avoid implying a possible beneficial effect.

The HMD has published DRIs and related information for: electrolytes and water;[107] energy, carbohydrate, fiber, fat, fatty acids, cholesterol, protein, and amino acids;[108] vitamins A and K, arsenic, boron, chromium, copper, iodine, iron, manganese, molybdenum, nickel, silicon, vanadium, and zinc;[109] vitamin C, vitamin E, selenium, and carotenoids;[110] the B vitamins;[111] calcium, phosphorus, magnesium, vitamin D, and fluoride;[112] an updated volume on vitamin D and calcium;[113] and an updated volume on sodium and potassium.[114] A complete set of the DRI books is available online or can be ordered in book form.

Important uses of the DRIs include individual diet planning, dietary guidance, institutional food planning, military food and meal planning, planning for food assistance programs, food labeling and fortification, developing new or modified food products, and guaranteeing food safety. In planning menus/diets for individuals or groups, it is important to meet the RDA or AI without exceeding the UL. The HMD has incorporated the DRIs and other data into a series of reports, including School Meals: Building Blocks for Healthy Children,[115] Local Government Actions to Prevent Childhood Obesity,[116] the Public Effects of Food Deserts[117] (workshop summary), Nutrition Standards and Meal Requirements for National School Lunch and Breakfast Programs: Phase I. Proposed Approach for Recommending Revisions,[118] and the Use of Dietary Supplements by Military Personnel.[119] Summaries of the development of the DRI[113] as well as the uses of the DRI in dietary assessment[120,121] and to plan menus[122] can be found in the literature.

The Center for Nutrition Policy and Promotion

The CNPP, created in December of 1994, is an office of the USDA's Food and Nutrition Service. Its mission is "to improve the health and well-being of Americans by developing and promoting dietary guidance that links scientific research to the nutrition needs of consumers."[123] The CNPP carries out its mission to improve the health of Americans by: 1) serving as the Federal authority on evidence-based food, nutrition, and economic analyses to inform policy and programs; 2) translating science into actionable food and nutrition guidance for all Americans; and 3) leading national communication initiatives that apply science-based messages to advance consumers' dietary and economic knowledge and behaviors.[124]

The major projects of the CNPP are shown in **Table 1–9**.

The National Agricultural Library has an online tool to calculate daily nutrient recommendations called the Interactive DRI for Health Professionals at https://www.nal.usda.gov/fnic/dri-calculator/DRI books are available online at: https://www.nal.usda.gov/fnic/dri-nutrient-reports

TABLE 1–9
Projects of the Center for Nutrition Policy and Promotion

Dietary Guidelines for Americans	Nutrition Evidence Systematic Review
MyPlate/MiPlato	Nutrient Content of the U.S. Food Supply
Healthy Eating Index	Pregnancy and Birth to 24 Months Project
USDA Food Patterns	Health and Medicine Division Study
USDA Food Plans: Cost of Food	Archived Projects
Expenditures on Children by Families	

The CNPP considers MyPlate/MiPlato and the Start Simple with MyPlate App tools to help the public navigate healthy eating; it includes recipes in the MyPlate Kitchen and individualized meal plans with the MyPlate Plan.

Dietary Guidelines for Americans

The DGA[125] are the foundation of federal nutrition policy, nutrition education programs, and information activities. The DGA are evidence-based recommendations for food (and some nutrient) intake and are designed to promote health and reduce the risk of chronic disease for Americans throughout the lifespan, including during pregnancy. The National Nutrition Monitoring and Related Research Act of 1990 (Pubic Law [PL] 101-445) mandates that the DGA are developed and published jointly by the Departments HHS and USDA every 5 years.[60] This relatively quick turnaround time is a result of the changing science as new studies are added to the evidence base. The ninth edition of the DGA (2020–2025) was released in December of 2020 (earlier editions were published in 1980, 1985, 1990, 1995, 2000, 2005, 2010, 2015) and includes a call to action: "Make Every Bite Count with the *Dietary Guidelines*." The 2020–2025 DGA will remain in effect until the 2025–2030 DGA is released. Changes in the DGA must reflect current scientific and medical knowledge that is available at the time of publication. Two important documents demonstrate the necessity of relying on a science base: The 1988 *Surgeon General's Report on Nutrition and Health*[126] and 1989 *National Research Council's Report, Diet and Health: Implications for Reducing Chronic Disease Risk*.[1]

The DGA appears as succinct statements of nutrition recommendations for the general public, as seen in **Table 1–10** and **Table 1–11**. The detailed discussion of the evidence and the initial recommendations are made by the Dietary Guidelines Advisory Committee. Take a moment to learn about the process of how the DGA are developed and what is available on the DGA website. Tools for client education and consumer information can be found on related websites such as Healthfinder.gov, MyPlate.gov, and Foodsafety. gov; these are linked on the DGA website. Additionally, Food Sources of Select Nutrients provides lists of foods that are good sources of calcium, potassium, dietary fiber, vitamin D, and iron. Two lists are provided: standard portions and smaller portions.

MyPlate is the "translation" of the DGA for the public,[127] although it also has information available for nutrition professionals.[128] This information includes Nutrition Communicators Network, Communicator's Guide, Teachers, Health Professionals, and MyPlate Graphic Resources.

The DGA dictates U.S. federal nutrition policies and programs, which directly affect nearly 45 million Americans receiving electronic benefits from the Supplemental Nutrition Assistance Program (SNAP);[130] 22.6 million children participating in the National School Lunch Program;[131] approximately 6.5 million women, infants, and children receiving benefits under the Special Supplemental Nutrition Program for Women, Infants, and Children program;[132,133] and 2.4 million adults over 60 years of age through the Older Americans Act Nutrition Services Program.[133] The DGA also

---

TABLE 1–10
The 2020–2025 Dietary Guidelines for Americans[125]

1. Follow a healthy dietary pattern at every life stage.
2. Customize and enjoy nutrient-dense food and beverage choices to reflect personal preferences, cultural traditions, and budgetary considerations.
3. Focus on matching food group needs with nutrient-dense foods and beverages and stay within calorie limits.
4. Limit foods and beverages higher in added sugars, saturated fat, and sodium, and limit alcoholic beverages.

TABLE 1–11
Key Recommendations that Support the Four Dietary Guidelines[125]

At every stage of life—infancy, toddlerhood, childhood, adolescence, adulthood, pregnancy, lactation, and older adulthood—it is never too early or too late to eat healthfully.

- **For approximately the first 6 months of life**, exclusively feed infants human milk. Continue to feed infants human milk through at least the first year of life, and longer if desired. Feed infants iron-fortified infant formula during the first year of life when human milk is unavailable or insufficient. Provide infants with supplemental vitamin D beginning soon after birth.
- **At approximately 6 months**, introduce infants to nutrient-dense complementary foods. Introduce infants to potentially allergenic foods along with other complementary foods. Encourage infants and toddlers to consume a variety of foods from all food groups. Include foods rich in iron and zinc, particularly for infants fed human milk.
- **From 12 months through older adulthood**, follow a healthy dietary pattern across the lifespan to meet nutrient needs, help achieve a healthy body weight, and reduce the risk of chronic diseases.

A healthy dietary pattern consists of nutrient-dense forms of food and beverages across all food groups, in recommended amounts, and within calorie limits.
The core elements that make up a health dietary pattern include:
- Vegetables of all types—dark green; red and orange; beans, peas, and lentils; starchy; and other vegetables
- Fruits, especially whole fruit
- Grains, at least half of which are whole grain
- Dairy, including fat-free or low-fat milk, yogurt, and cheese, and/or lactose-free versions and fortified soy beverages and yogurt as alternatives
- Protein foods, including lean meats, poultry, and eggs; seafood; beans, peas, and lentils; and nuts, seeds, and soy products
- Oils, including vegetable oils and oils in food, such as seafood and nuts

A small amount of added sugars, saturated fat, or sodium can be added to nutrient-dense foods and beverages to help meet food group recommendations, but foods and beverages high in these components should be limited. Limits include:
- **Added sugars**—Less than 10% of calories per day starting at age 2. Avoid foods and beverages with added sugars for those younger than age 2 years.
- **Saturated fat**—Less than 10% of calories per day starting at age 2 years.
- **Sodium**—Less than 2,300 milligrams per day—and even less for children younger than age 14 years.
- **Alcoholic beverages**—Adults of legal drinking age can choose not to drink or to drink in moderation by limiting intake to two drinks or fewer in a day for men and one drink or fewer in a day for women, when alcohol is consumed. Drinking less is better for health than drinking more. There are some adults who should not drink alcohol, such as women who are pregnant.

Key Dietary Principles are designed to help people meet the Guidelines and Key Recommendations to achieve a healthy dietary pattern:
- **Meet nutritional needs primarily from foods and beverages.** An underlying premise of the *Dietary* Guidelines is that nutritional needs should be met primarily from foods and beverages—specifically nutrient-dense foods and beverages. In some cases, when meeting nutrient needs is not otherwise possible, fortified foods and nutrient-containing dietary supplements are useful.
- **Choose a variety of options from each food group.** Enjoy different foods and beverages within each food group. This can help meet nutrient needs—and also allows for flexibility so that the *Dietary Guidelines* can be tailored to meet cultural and personal preferences.
- **Pay attention to portion size.** *Portion size* is a term often used to describe the amount of a food or beverage served or consumed in one eating occasion. It is important to pay attention to portion size when making food and beverage choices, particularly for foods and beverages that are not nutrient-dense.

In tandem with the recommendations above, Americans aged 2 years and above—children, adolescents, adults, and older adults—should meet the Physical Activity Guidelines for Americans to help promote health and reduce the risk of chronic disease. Americans should strive to achieve and maintain a healthy body weight. The relationship between diet and physical activity contributes to calorie balance and managing body weight. As such, the Dietary Guidelines for ages 3–17, adulthood, and older adulthood include a recommendation for physical activity.[129]*

*The Guidelines recommend that preschool-aged children be active throughout the day through active play in a variety of activity types (light, moderate, or vigorous intensity) for at least 3 hours per day for enhanced growth and development. Children and adolescents aged 6 to 17 year should do at least 60 minutes (1 hour) of moderate-to-vigorous aerobic activity each day. They also need to perform muscle- and bone-strengthening activities such as climbing on playground equipment, playing sports, and jumping rope.
For adults and older adults, do aerobic activity, muscle-strengthening activity, and move more and sit less.
For substantial health benefits, do one of the following for aerobic activity:
- 150–300 minutes (2 hours and 30 minutes to 5 hours) each week of moderate-intensity aerobic physical activity (such as brisk walking or tennis)
Adults of all ages need muscle-strengthening activity (such as lifting weights or doing push-ups) at least 2 days each week.

affects information policy in tools and resources including MyPlate, food labels, and federal nutrition education programs such as the Supplemental Nutrition Assistance Program Education (SNAP-Ed). SNAP-Ed includes resources like the *SNAP-Ed Toolkit: Obesity Prevention Interventions and Evaluation Framework*, which provides evidence-based policy, systems, and environmental changes that support direct educational social marketing and ways to evaluate them across various settings.[134] The reliance on and the consistency of following the DGA assure that nutrition information promulgated by the government is the same for all federal programs. Although not mandated, the DGA also provide the foundation for nutrition recommendations and programs from nonfederal agencies such as the American Heart Association and the American Cancer Society.

MyPlate

In the United States, food group plans have provided dietary guidance based on current scientific knowledge for over 100 years. The USDA published its first recommendations in 1916. Between 1916 and the 1940s, plans had between five and 16 separate food groups and were published by various government agencies. In 1943, as part of the wartime effort, the USDA published the *National Wartime Nutrition Guide. The Basic Seven Food Guide*, derived from the *Wartime Guide*, was issued and was used until 1955 when the Department of Nutrition at the Harvard School of Public Health recommended collapsing the groups to four. This format was accepted by the USDA in 1956 and in 1979 a fifth group—fats, sweets, and alcohol—was added. These plans had two things in common: they were designed to meet nutrient requirements and to prevent nutritional deficiencies. As the relationship between diet and chronic disease risk and the development of the DGA, researchers understood how important it was to develop a food guidance system that included recommendations to prevent the excesses or poor food choices associated with chronic disease. In 1984, these groups were illustrated as a "Food Wheel" and the goals were shifted to a total diet approach for nutrient adequacy and moderation.

These efforts culminated with the Food Guide Pyramid that was released in 1992, MyPyramid in 2005, MyPlate in 2011, and MyPlate, MyWins in 2015. The introduction of MyPlate coincided with the release of the 2010 DGA.[135] With the release of DGA 2020–2025, the guide was changed back to MyPlate with a new *Start Simple with MyPlate* campaign. The MyPlate icon (**Figure 1–1**) depicts the five food groups: fruit, vegetables, grains, protein foods, and dairy foods, but it provides a new, simpler reminder to

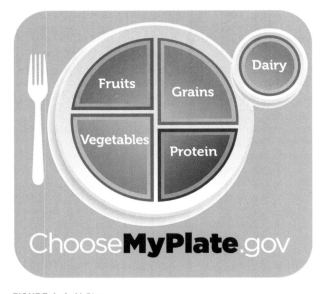

FIGURE 1–1 MyPlate.

Courtesy of USDA. Choose My Plate. http://www.choosemyplate.gov

TABLE 1–12
Consumer Messages for MyPlate

Core Message

- The benefits of healthy eating add up over time, bite by bite. Small changes matter. *Start Simple with MyPlate.*

Food Groups

- Fruits—Make half your plate fruits and vegetables: focus on whole fruits
- Vegetables—Make half your plate fruits and vegetables: vary your veggies
- Grains—Make half your grains whole grains
- Protein Foods—Vary your protein routine
- Dairy—Move to low-fat or fat-free dairy milk or yogurt (or lactose-free dairy or fortified soy versions)

Make every bite count

- Learn how much you need from each food group. Get a personalized MyPlate Plan that's right for you, based on your age, sex, height, weight, and physical activity level.
- Take a look at your current eating routine. Pick one or two ways that you can switch to choices today that are rich in nutrition.
- A healthy eating routine can help boost your health today and in the years to come. Think about how your food choices come together over the course of your day or week to help you create a healthy eating routine.
- It is important to eat a variety of fruits, vegetables, grains, protein foods, and dairy and fortified soy alternatives. Choose options for meals, beverages, and snacks that have limited added sugars, saturated fat, and sodium.

U.S. Department of Agriculture. Accessed January 31, 2021. Retrieved from https://www.myplate.gov/eat-healthy/what-is-myplate

choose healthy foods at mealtimes than either the Food Guide Pyramid or MyPyramid. *Start Simple with MyPlate* is designed to help people meet healthy eating goals one at a time. The *Start Simple with MyPlate* app helps consumers choose simple daily food goals, track progress toward goals, and learn helpful tips and recipes in line with their goals. It uses the five food groups to categorize nutrition goals; the app currently limits goals to three per food group with the option to edit goals at any time. The new MyPlate website contains a core message (*Start Simple with MyPlate*) as well as five consumer messages based on the five main food groups and four additional messages to support the "Make every bite count" call to action from the DGA 2020–2025. (**Table 1–12**[136]) The MyPlate website includes a variety of information about healthy food choices and videos to provide a visual for individuals.

MyPlate is more than simply an icon. The website provides easy-to-understand information on healthy food choices for all ages for both consumers and health professionals. In addition to the *Start Simple with MyPlate* app, tools also include a personalized MyPlate Plan to develop food group targets within a calorie allowance and MyPlate Quiz to help consumers identify gaps in their eating habits as well as resources to address those gaps. Toolkits for professionals are provided on the website as well and are geared toward registered dietitian dietitians/nutritionists, food producers and retailers, community and professional organizations, and communicators and educators.

Pandemic Learning Opportunity

Start Simple with MyPlate provides a tip sheet called Food Planning During the Coronavirus Pandemic that can help consumers navigate healthy eating while they adjust to a new routine with the quarantines and social distancing required during the pandemic. Links to additional information about Coronavirus/COVID-19 as well as additional food planning resources are also included further down the page. https://www.myplate.gov/eat-healthy/healthy-eating-budget/covid-19

Healthy Eating Index Provides a measure of diet quality that assesses how well a set of foods aligns with key recommendations in the Dietary Guidelines for Americans.

Healthy Eating Index

The **Healthy Eating Index (HEI)** provides a measure of diet quality that assesses how well a set of foods aligns with key recommendations in the DGA.[137-139] Originally developed by the CNPP in 1995 using 1989–1990 Continuing Survey of Food Intakes by Individuals (CSFII) data, it is updated every 5 years as new DGA are released using NHANES data. The updates reflect collaboration between the CNPP and the National Cancer Center. Plans to update the HEI to align with the 2020–2025 DGA are underway. The scoring metric for the HEI-2015 is composed of 13 components, each of which is assigned a standard for achieving both a maximum and minimum (zero) score. The components are summed for a total possible score of 100. Of the components, nine: total fruits, whole fruits, total vegetables, greens and beans, whole grains, dairy, total protein foods, seafood and plant proteins, and fatty acid ratios receive "adequacy scores." These are foods to encourage and a higher score indicates higher consumption. The four remaining components: refined grains, sodium, added sugars, and saturated fats, receive a "moderation score" and a higher score indicates lower consumption (**Figure 1–2**).[139] Recently it was shown, using NHANES 2011-2012 data, that the total population ($\geq$2 years of age; n=7,933) had a total score of 59.0±0.95 (standard error); children (2–17 years of age; n=2,857) had a total score of 55.07±0.72; and older adults ($\geq$65 years of

HEI–2015[1] Components & Scoring Standards			
Component	**Maximum points**	**Standard for maximum score**	**Standard for minimum score of zero**
Adequacy:			
Total Fruits[2]	5	$\geq$0.8 cup equiv. per 1,000 kcal	No Fruit
Whole Fruits[3]	5	$\geq$0.4 cup equiv. per 1,000 kcal	No Whole Fruit
Total Vegetables[4]	5	$\geq$1.1 cup equiv. per 1,000 kcal	No Vegetables
Greens and Beans[4]	5	$\geq$0.2 cup equiv. per 1,000 kcal	No Dark Green Vegetables or Legumes
Whole Grains	10	$\geq$1.5 oz equiv. per 1,000 kcal	No Whole Grains
Dairy[5]	10	$\geq$1.3 cup equiv. per 1,000 kcal	No Dairy
Total Protein Foods[6]	5	$\geq$2.5 oz equiv. per 1,000 kcal	No Protein Foods
Seafood and Plant Proteins[6,7]	5	$\geq$0.8 oz equiv. per 1,000 kcal	No Seafood or Plant Proteins
Fatty Acids[8]	10	(PUFAs + MUFAs)/SFAs $\geq$2.5	(PUFAs + MUFAs)/SFAs $\leq$1.2
Moderation:			
Refined Grains	10	$\leq$1.8 oz equiv. per 1,000 kcal	$\geq$4.3 oz equiv. per 1,000 kcal
Sodium	10	$\leq$1.1 gram per 1,000 kcal	$\geq$2.0 grams per 1,000 kcal
Added Sugars	10	$\leq$6.5% of energy	$\geq$26% of energy
Saturated Fats	10	$\leq$8% of energy	$\geq$16% of energy

[1] Intakes between the minimum and maximum standards are scored proportionately.
[2] Includes 100% fruit juice.
[3] Includes all forms except juice.
[4] Includes legumes (beans and peas).
[5] Includes all milk products, such as fluid milk, yogurt, and cheese, and fortified soy beverages.
[6] Includes legumes (beans and peas).
[7] Includes seafood, nuts, seeds, soy products (other than beverages), and legumes (beans and peas).
[8] Ratio of poly- and monounsaturated fatty acids (PUFAs and MUFAs) to saturated fatty acids (SFAs).

FIGURE 1–2 HEI–2015[1] Components & Scoring Standards.

National Institutes of Health. Accessed January 31, 2021. Retrieved from https://epi.grants.cancer.gov/hei/developing.html#2015c

age; n=1,032) had a total score of 68.29±1.76.[139] In addition to age being associated with better diet quality, HEI scores are also higher in individuals with higher incomes and more education.[140] Overall, in the United States, diet quality appears to be slowly improving; it's not clear, however, if improvement will be rapid enough to meet all of the HP 2020 nutrition goals. Only improvements in whole fruit intake and empty calories appear to be on track to meet these goals.[141]

Tools for researchers, including basic steps to calculate HEI scores at different levels: national food supply, food processing, community food environment, and individual food intake, and SAS Macros are available for calculating the HEI-2005, the HEI-2010, and the HEI-2015.[142]

The Food Label

The **Nutrition Labeling and Education Act (NLEA) of 1990 (Public Law [PL] 101-535)** amended the Federal Food, Drug, and Cosmetic Act to provide, among other things, that certain nutrients and food components be included on the label. The regulatory authority for the food label rests with the U.S. Food and Drug Administration (FDA) and the Federal Trade Commission. The Secretary of HHS (and by delegation, the FDA) can add or delete nutrients included in the food label or labeling if this action is necessary to assist consumers in maintaining healthy dietary practices. In response to these provisions, in the Federal Register of November 27, 1991, the FDA published a proposed rule titled, *"Food Labeling: Reference Daily Intakes and Daily Reference Values; Mandatory Status of Nutrition Labeling and Nutrient Content Revision."* In that document, the agency proposed to require that foods bear nutrition labeling listing certain nutrients and the amount of those nutrients in a serving of the food.

Under the NLEA, some foods are exempted from the food labeling laws: food served for immediate consumption (e.g., that served in hospital cafeterias and airplanes), and sold by food service vendors (e.g., mall cookie counters, sidewalk vendors, and vending machines); ready-to-eat food that is not for immediate consumption but is prepared primarily on site (e.g., bakery, deli, and candy store items); food shipped in bulk as long as it is not for sale in that form to consumers; medical foods (e.g., those used to address the nutritional needs of patients with certain diseases); plain coffee and tea, some spices; and other foods with no significant amounts of any nutrients.

Placement of information on the label, type size, manufacturer name and contact information, and other information related to content are also mandated. To accommodate foods sold in small packages, there are special requirements. Furthermore, the USDA regulates poultry in accordance with the Poultry Products Inspection Act and meat under the Federal Meat Inspection Act. Daily values (DV) are one of the key elements of the food label; these are the daily dietary intake standards used for nutrition labeling. The first daily intake standards, referred to as the U.S. Recommended Daily Allowances, for the nutrition label were established in 1973 and were based on the RDAs.[142-144]

Food label criteria continue to change to meet current scientific research and public demand. Another example is the Food Allergen Labeling and Consumer Protection Act of 2004 (Public Law [PL] 108-282, Title II), which mandated that as of January 1, 2006, foods containing or potentially containing any of the eight most common food allergens—milk, eggs, fish, Crustacean shellfish, tree nuts, peanuts, wheat, and soybeans—include the food name on the label in "plain English" (e.g., this product contains EGGS). These foods account for 90% of food allergic reactions in children and adults.

Nutrition Labeling and Education Act of 1990 (Public Law [PL] 101-535) Amended the Federal Food, Drug, and Cosmetic Act to provide certain nutrients, food components, and health claims (among other information) be included on the food labels. The law was amended in 2004 (PL 108-282, Title II) to mandate that foods containing or potentially containing the eight most common food allergens have that allergen included on the label in "plain English," e.g., the food contains EGGS. The law was amended again in 2016 to update labeling regulations for foods and dietary supplements to assist consumers in making healthy food choices using a newly designed Nutrition Facts Label.

The FDA also provides guidance for industry from a standpoint of allergens and potential allergens in the food.[145] Although gluten is not an allergen, in 2013, the FDA set a threshold for gluten of less than 20 parts per million in foods that are labeled "gluten-free," "no gluten," "free of gluten," and "without gluten."[146]

In 2016, the FDA amended the labeling regulations for foods and dietary supplements to assist consumers in making healthy food choices using the Nutrition Facts Label.[147] The new Nutrition Facts Label updated the list of nutrients required (or permitted) to be declared, updated Daily Reference Values and Reference Daily Intake values to align with current dietary recommendations, amended requirements for foods that claim to be specifically for children under age 4 and pregnant and lactating women and established nutrient reference values for these populations, and revised the format of the Nutrition Facts Label. The final rule became effective in July 26, 2016; originally, the compliance date was 2 years later in 2018 for manufacturers with $10 million or more in annual food sales and 3 years later in 2019 for manufacturers with less than $10 million in annual food sales. These compliance dates were extended to 2020 and 2021, respectively, to allow for sufficient time to make the changes. Figure 1–3 shows the difference between the old and new Nutrition Facts Labels. Six Key Changes were made to information

Nutrition Facts

Serving Size 2/3 cup (55g)
servings Per Container About 8

Amount per serving

Calories 230	Calories from Fat 72

	% Daily Value*
Total Fat 8g	**12%**
Saturated Fat 1g	**5%**
Trans Fat 0g	
Cholesterol 0mg	**0%**
Sodium 160mg	**7%**
Total Carbohydrate 37g	**12%**
Dietary Fiber 4g	**16%**
Sugars 1g	
Protein 3g	

Vitamin A	10%
Vitamin C	8%
Calcium	20%
Iron	45%

* Percent Daily Values are based on a 2,000 calorie diet. Your daily value may be higher or lower depending on your calorie needs.

	Calories:	2,000	2,500
Total Fat	Less than	65g	80g
Sat. Fat	Less than	20g	25g
Cholesterol	Less than	300mg	300mg
Sodium	Less than	2,400mg	2,400mg
Total Carbohydrate		300g	375g
Dietary Fiber		25g	30g

Nutrition Facts

8 servings per container

Serving size	**2/3 cup (55g)**

Amount per serving

Calories	**230**

	% Daily Value*
Total Fat 8g	**10%**
Saturated Fat 1g	**5%**
Trans Fat 0g	
Cholesterol 0mg	**0%**
Sodium 160mg	**7%**
Total Carbohydrate 37g	**13%**
Dietary Fiber 4g	**14%**
Total Sugars 12g	
Includes 10g Added Sugars	**20%**
Protein 3g	

Vitamin D 2mcg	10%
Calcium 260mg	20%
Iron 8mg	45%
Potassium 235mg	6%

* The % Daily Value (DV) tells you how much a nutrient in a serving of food contributes to a daily diet. 2,000 calories a day is used for general nutrition advice.

FIGURE 1–3 Comparison of the Original and New Nutrition Facts Labels.

U.S. Food and Drug Administration. Changes to the Nutrition Facts Label. Retrieved from https://www.fda.gov/media/99331/download

TABLE 1–13
The Six Key Changes to the Nutrition Facts Label

1. Servings	- Serving size in larger, bold font - Servings per container in larger font - Serving sizes were updated to "better reflect the amount people typically eat and drink"; food and beverage items in containers that contain 1–2 servings but could be eaten in one sitting require nutrition facts for the entire container; a second column may be added to provide a smaller serving size for part of the container if desired
2. Calories	- Calories in a larger, bold font
3. Fat	- Calories from Fat is removed since research shows that type of fat is more important than amount
4. Added Sugars	- "Added sugars" in grams and as a percent Daily Value (%DV) is now required - This information is added in a line below "Total Sugars" and written as "Includes __g Added Sugars" - Added sugars include sugars added during food processing (such as dextrose or sucrose), foods packaged as sweeteners (such as table sugar or brown sugar), sugars from syrups and honey, and sugars from concentrated fruit or vegetable juice
5. Nutrients	- Vitamin D and potassium are now required - Vitamins A and C are no longer required - Amount in milligrams or micrograms and %DV must be listed for vitamin D, calcium, iron, and potassium - Daily Values for nutrients updated based on newer scientific evidence; these are used to calculate the %DV on the label
6. Footnote	- The footnote at the bottom of the label is adjusted to better explain the meaning of %DV

and/or appearance on the Label: servings, calories, fat, added sugars, nutrients, and footnote (**Table 1–13**).[148-149]

Food and Dietary Supplement Claims

As mandated by the NLEA of 1990, the FDA issued the final food labeling rules for health claims. Updated in 2008, information on the FDA website qualifies and explains claims that can be made for conventional food and dietary supplements. The claims fall into four categories: 1) Nutrient Content Claims; 2) Health Claims; 3) Qualified Health Claims (QHC); and 4) Structure Function Claims.[150] Nutrient Content Claims are fairly straightforward, including words like *free*, *high*, *low*, *more*, *reduced*, or *lite* (e.g., calorie free: <5 kcal per reference amount customarily consumed (RACC) per labeled serving or low calorie: ≤40 kcal per RACC). Furthermore, "when levels exceed: 13 g Total Fat, 4 g Saturated Fat, 60 mg Cholesterol, and 480 mg Sodium per RACC, per labeled serving or, for foods with small RACC, per 50 g, a disclosure statement is required as part of claim (e.g., "See nutrition information for content" with the blank filled in with nutrient(s) that exceed the prescribed levels). Nutrient Content Claims also encompass conditions for the use of "healthy."[151]

Health claims on foods and dietary supplements are more complicated but can be made after such statements have been reviewed and authorized by the FDA. Before industry can place such a claim on a label, stringent requirements must be met; there are also specific criteria that all foods must fulfill to be allowed to bear such health claims.[152] The FDA has provided industry guidance on the *evidence-based review system* that the FDA uses to evaluate the publicly available scientific evidence for significant scientific agreement health claims or qualified health claims (QHC) on the relationship between a substance and a disease or health-related condition. Approved claims must be clearly stated along with the requirements for the food, the claim requirements, and model claim; statements are available on the FDA's website.[153] The FDA has acknowledged that consumers benefit from more information on food labels about diet and health. The FDA thus established interim procedures whereby QHCs can be made for conventional foods and for dietary supplements. Past court decisions have clarified the need to provide for health claims based on less scientific evidence rather than just on the standard of SSA as long as the claims do not mislead the consumers. The FDA began considering QHCs under its interim procedures on September 1, 2003. Table 1–14a-c show the health claims and qualified health claims allowed on food labels.[152,153] Finally, structure/function claims are allowed on labels.

TABLE 1–14A
Health Claims Subject to Enforcement Discretion[152]

- Calcium and Osteoporosis and Calcium, Vitamin D, and Osteoporosis
- Dietary Fat and Cancer
- Sodium and Hypertension
- Dietary Saturated Fat and Cholesterol and the Risk of Coronary Heart Disease
- Fiber-Containing Grain Products, Fruits, and Vegetables and Cancer
- Fruits, Vegetables and Grain Products that contain Fiber, particularly Soluble Fiber, and Risk of Coronary Heart Disease
- Fruits and Vegetables and Cancer
- Folate and Neural Tube Defects
- Dietary Non-Cariogenic Carbohydrate Sweeteners and Dental Caries
- Soluble Fiber from Certain Foods and Risk of Coronary Heart Disease
- Soy Protein and Risk of Coronary Heart Disease
- Plant Sterol/stanol esters and Risk of Coronary Heart Disease

TABLE 1–14B
FDA Modernization Act Health Claims (Health Claims Authorized Based on an Authoritative Statement by Federal Scientific Bodies)[152]

- Whole Grain Foods and Risk of Heart Disease and Certain Cancers
- Whole Grain Foods with Moderate Fat Content and Risk of Heart Disease
- Potassium and the Risk of High Blood Pressure and Stroke
- Fluoridated Water and Reduced Risk of Dental Carries
- Saturated Fat, Cholesterol, and Trans Fat, and Reduced Risk of Heart Disease
- Substitution of Saturated Fat in the Diet with Unsaturated Fatty Acids and Reduced Risk of Heart Disease

TABLE 1–14C
Qualified Health Claims Subject to Enforcement Discretion

- 0.8 mg Folic Acid & Neural Tube Birth Defects
- B Vitamins & Vascular Disease
- Selenium & Cancer
- Antioxidant Vitamins & Cancer
- Phosphatidylserine & Cognitive Dysfunction and Dementia
- Nuts & Heart Disease
- Walnuts & Heart Disease
- Omega-3 Fatty Acids & Coronary Heart Disease
- Monounsaturated Fatty Acids from Olive Oil and Coronary Heart Disease
- Green Tea & Cancer
- Chromium Picolinate & Cancer
- Calcium and Colon/Rectal Cancer & Calcium and Recurrent Colon/Rectal Polyps
- Calcium & Hypertension, Pregnancy-Induced Hypertension, and Preeclampsia
- Tomatoes and/or Tomato Sauce & Prostate, Ovarian, Gastric, and Pancreatic Cancers
- Unsaturated Fatty Acids from Canola Oil and Reduced Risk of Coronary Heart Disease
- Corn Oil and Corn Oil-Containing Products and a Reduced Risk of Heart Disease
- 100% Whey Protein Partially Hydrolyzed Infant Formula & Atopic Dermatitis

These differ from health claims in that structure/function claims describe the role of a substance intended to maintain the structure or function of the body. Structure/function claims do not require preapproval by the FDA. Products with structure/function claims must include this disclaimer: "This statement has not been evaluated by the Food and Drug Administration. This product is not intended to diagnose, treat, cure, or prevent any disease." Examples are "calcium builds strong bones" and "antioxidants maintain cell integrity."[150]

Helping clients understand food labels—including 1) using them to make careful food selections, which may reduce or even prevent chronic disease, 2) providing specific information targeted to individuals with certain disease states, and 3) integrating foods into a total food plan—is clearly within your purview as a nutrition professional. Information on how to read the food label and educating the public on the changes to the Nutrition Facts label is available online.[153]

Summary

Often, there are complaints that nutrition recommendations are conflicting and confusing; however, these recommendations are remarkably similar across agencies, including the **Dietary Guidelines for Americans**, the American Heart Association, the American Cancer Institute, and therapeutic diets like Dietary Approaches to Stop Hypertension. Why? Because the recommendations are based on what the evidence behind the programs dictates. The challenge for all nutrition professionals is to evaluate the scientific evidence critically before it is translated into public health practice. Nutrition professionals need to use this information to design, execute, and evaluate programs and policies so that positive recommendations are communicated to the public in a unified way. Doing so assures that consumers are getting the most accurate and comprehensive information available, which allows them to make positive lifestyle changes. This chapter reviewed the science behind public health policies, programs, nutrition education materials, and legislation.

Dietary Guidelines for Americans These are evidence-based recommendations for food (and some nutrient intake) and are designed to promote health and reduce the risk of chronic disease for healthy Americans across their entire lifespan. They are the foundation of federal nutrition policy, nutrition education programs, and information activities.

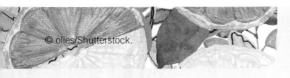

Learning Portfolio

Key Terms

	page
National Health and Nutrition Examination Survey	6
Public health nutritionist	7
Evidence-based practice	8
Nutrigenomics	8
Peer-reviewed literature	8
PubMed	9
Hierarchy of evidence	12
Cross-sectional studies	12
Cohort studies	12
Randomized controlled trials	12
Evidence Analysis Library	12
Nutrition monitoring	12
Center for Nutrition Policy and Promotion	14
National Nutrition Monitoring and Related Research Program	16
Dietary Reference Intakes	25
MyPlate	25
Healthy People 2030	26
Healthy Eating Index	34
Nutrition Labeling and Education Act of 1990 (Public Law [PL] 101-535)	35
Dietary Guidelines for Americans	39

Issues for Discussion

1. Dietary recommendations for the public change as scientific studies discover new information. How can these changes be brought to the public in a way that doesn't confuse them or make them feel resentful?
2. What ethical responsibility, if any, does industry or the media have in assuring the public's health?
3. The Dietary Guidelines for Americans and MyPlate promote healthy dietary patterns, but Americans clearly have difficulty following these recommendations. Why? If people cannot follow them, should we continue to make these recommendations?
4. The changes to the Nutrition Facts Label are designed to help consumers better navigate healthy eating by making nutrition information of food choices more intuitive. Do you think the new Nutrition Facts Label will achieve this? Why or why not?

Case Study: HP 2030 vs. DGA 2020–2025

Both *Healthy People 2030* and the Dietary Guidelines for Americans 2020–2025 reduced the quantity of their objectives and goals in order to focus on the priority of health needs of Americans. Work in pairs to choose 2–3 *HP 2030* objectives or one DGA 2020–2025 goal and follow the evidence to figure out why those objectives or goals were chosen and how they differ from the previous iteration of their respective programs.

Case Study: Using the Evidence-Based Approach

Pick any topic in this chapter and show, step-by-step, how you would go about finding more valid information concerning the issue.

References

1. National Academy of Sciences, National Research Council, Food and Nutrition Board. *Diet and Health: Implications for Reducing Chronic Disease Risk*. Washington, DC: National Academy Press; 1989.
2. U.S. Senate Select Committee on Nutrition and Human Needs. *Dietary Goals for the United States*, 2nd ed. Washington, DC, U.S. Government Printing Office; 1977.
3. Centers for Disease Control and Prevention. National Center for Health Statistics. FastStats. *Deaths and Mortality*. Accessed January 31, 2021. https://www.cdc.gov/nchs/fastats/deaths.htm
4. Benjamin EJ, Virani SS, Callaway CW, et al. Heart Disease and Stroke Statistics—2018 Update: A report from the American Heart Association. *Circulation*. 2018;137(12):e67-e492.

5. National Cancer Institute. *Cancer Prevalence and Cost of Care Projections*. Accessed January 31, 2021. https://costprojections.cancer.gov

6. American Diabetes Association. Economic costs of diabetes in the U.S. in 2017. 2018;41(5):917-928.

7. Trogdon JG, Murphy LB, Khavjou OA, et al. Costs of chronic diseases at the state level: the chronic disease cost calculator. *Prev Chronic Dis*. 2015;12:E140.

8. National Kidney Foundation. *Kidney Disease: The Basics*. Accessed January 31, 2021. https://www.kidney.org/news/newsroom/factsheets/KidneyDiseaseBasics

9. Hales CM, Carroll MD, Fryar CD, Ogden CL. Prevalence of obesity among adults and youth: United States, 2015–2016. *NCHS Data Brief*. 2017;(288):1-8.

10. Centers for Disease Control and Prevention. About Child & Teen BMI. Accessed April 10, 2016. http://www.cdc.gov/healthyweight/assessing/bmi/childrens_bmi/about_childrens_bmi.html

11. Biener A, Cawley J, Meyerhoefer C. The high and rising costs of obesity to the US healthcare system. *J Gen Intern Med*. 2017;32(suppl 1):S6-S8.

12. World Health Organization. *Noncommunicable diseases*. Updated 1 June 2018. Accessed January 31, 2021. https://www.who.int/news-room/fact-sheets/detail/noncommunicable-diseases

13. World Health Organization. Global action plan for the prevention and control of noncommunicable diseases: 2013-2020. 2013.

14. Virani SS, Alonso A, Benjamin EJ, et al. Heart disease and stroke statistics—2020 update: a report from the American Heart Association. *Circulation*. 2020;141(9):e139-e596.

15. Goldman L, Benjamin G, Hernandez S, et al. Advancing the health of communities and populations: a vital direction for health and health care. *NAM Perspectives. Discussion Paper*, National Academy of Medicine, Washington, DC. 2016.

16. Curry L. The Future of the Public's Health in the 21st Century. Institute of Medicine. Board on Health Promotion and Disease Prevention. Washington DC: The National Academies Press; 2003.

17. Dzau VJ, McClellan MB, McGinnis JM, et al. Vital directions for health and health care: priorities from a National Academy of Medicine initiative. *JAMA*. 2017;327(14):1461-1470.

18. Wahl DR, Villinger K, Blumenschein M, et al. Why we eat what we eat: assessing dispositional and in-the-moment eating motives by using ecological momentary assessment. *JMIR mHealth and uHealth*. 2020;8(1):e13191.

19. Dover RV, Lambert EV. "Choice Set" for health behavior in choice-constrained settings to frame research and inform policy: examples of food consumption, obesity and food security. *Int J Equity Health*. 2016;15(48).

20. Cecchini M, Warin L. Impact of food labelling systems on food choices and eating behaviours: a systematic review and meta-analysis of randomized studies. *Obes Rev*. 2016;17(3):201-210.

21. Hardcastle SJ, Thøgersen-Ntoumani C, Chatzisarantis NL. Food choice and nutrition: a social psychological perspective. *Nutrients*. 2015;7(10):8712-8715.

22. VanKim NA, Erickson DJ, Laska MN. Food shopping profiles and their association with dietary patterns: a latent class analysis. *J Acad Nutr Diet*. 2015;115(7):1109-1116.

23. Kamerow D. Why don't people exercise, even a little? *BMJ*. 2015;350:h3024.

24. Côté-Lussier C, Fitzpatrick C, Séguin L, Barnett TA. Poor, unsafe, and overweight: the role of feeling unsafe at school in mediating the association among poverty exposure, youth screen time, physical activity, and weight status. *Am J Epidemiol*. 2015;182(1):67-79.

25. Iso-Ahola SE. Conscious-nonconscious processing explains why some people exercise but most don't. *Journal of Nature and Science (JNSCI)*. 2017;3(6):e384.

26. Jung EH, Walsh-Childers K, Kim HS. Factors influencing the perceived credibility of diet-nutrition information web sites. *Comput Human Behav*. 2016;58:37-47.

27. Mayo Clinic. Healthy lifestyle: nutrition and healthy eating. *Nutrition Claims: How to tell fact from fiction*. Accessed February 7, 2021. https://www.mayoclinic.org/healthy-lifestyle/nutrition-and-healthy-eating/in-depth/nutrition-claims-how-to-tell-fact-from-fiction/art-20300972

28. Adamski M, Truby H, Klassen KM, Cowan S, Gibson S. Using the Internet: nutrition information-seeking behaviours of lay people enrolled in a massive online nutrition course. *Nutrients*. 2020;12(3):1-18.

29. Health Literacy Online. A Guide for Simplifying the User Experience. Accessed April 11, 2016. http://health.gov/healthliteracyonline

30. Center for Evidence-Based Medicine. Levels of evidence: an introduction. Accessed February 7, 2021. https://www.cebm.ox.ac.uk/resources/levels-of-evidence/levels-of-evidence-introductory-document

31. Academy of Nutrition and Dietetics. Evidence Analysis Library. *Evidence-Based Practice*. Accessed February 7, 2021. https://www.andeal.org/evidence-based-practice

32. Agency for Healthcare Research and Quality. Evidence-based Practice Centers (EPC) Program overview. Accessed April 11, 2016. http://www.ahrq.gov/research/findings/evidence-based-reports/overview/index.html

33. Guyatt G, Rennie D, Meade MO, Cook DJ. Users' guides to the medical literature. Essentials of evidence-based clinical practice. *JAMA Evidence*. 3rd ed. 2015. New York. McGraw Hill Education.

34. Mueller C, Compher C, Ellen DM, American Society for Parenteral and Enteral Nutrition (A.S.P.E.N.) Board of Directors. A.S.P.E.N. clinical guidelines: nutrition screening, assessment, and intervention in adults. *JPEN J Parenter Enteral Nutr*. 2011;35(1):16-24.

35. Academy of Nutrition and Dietetics. Evidence Analysis Library. *Nutrition Screening in Adults*. Accessed February 7, 2021. https://andeal.org/topic.cfm?menu=5382

36. Nutrition screening as easy as mana: a guide to completing the Mini Nutritional Assessment (MNA®). Nestlé Nutrition Institute. Accessed April 11, 2016. http://www.mna-elderly.com/forms/mna_guide_english.pdf

37. Dietitian/Dietitians/nutritionists from the Nutrition Education Materials Online. *Validated malnutrition screening and*

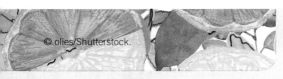
© olies/Shutterstock.

Learning Portfolio

assessment tools: comparison guide. Accessed February 7, 2021. https://www.health.qld.gov.au/__data/assets/pdf_file/0021/152454/hphe_scrn_tools.pdf

38. American Diabetes Association. *About the risk test.* Accessed February 7, 2021. https://diabetes.org/risk-test

39. United States Department of Agriculture, Economic Research Service. *Food security in the United States: survey tools.* Accessed February 7, 2021. https://www.ers.usda.gov/topics/food-nutrition-assistance/food-security-in-the-us/survey-tools

40. Academy of Nutrition and Dietetics. *Nutrition Assessment Snapshot.* 2018. Accessed February 8, 2021. https://www.ncpro.org/nutrition-assessment-snapshot

41. National Cancer Institute. Dietary Assessment Primer. Accessed February 8, 2021. https://dietassessmentprimer.cancer.gov

42. Eldridge AL, Piernas C, Illner A-K, et al. Evaluation of new technology-based tools for dietary intake assessment—an ILSI Europe dietary intake and exposure task force evaluation. *Nutrients.* 2019;11(1):55.

43. McClung HL, Ptomey LT, Shook RP, et al. Dietary intake and physical activity assessment: current tools, techniques, and technologies for use in adult populations. *Am J Prev Med.* 2018;55(4):e93-e104.

44. National Center for Health Statistics. *What We Eat In America, DHHS–USDA Dietary Survey.* Accessed February 8, 2021. https://www.cdc.gov/nchs/nhanes/wweia.htm

45. National Cancer Institute. *Usual Dietary Intakes: The NCI method.* Accessed February 8, 2021. https://epi.grants.cancer.gov/diet/usualintakes/method.html

46. Food and Agriculture Organization of the United Nations. *Dietary Assessment: A Resource Guide to Method Selection and Application in Low Resources Settings.* Rome, Italy; 2018.

47. Molag ML, de Vries JH, Ocké MC, et al. Design characteristics of food frequency questionnaires in relation to their validity. *Am J Epidemiol.* 2007;166(12):1468-1478.

48. Martin CK, Correa JB, Han H, et al. Validity of the Remote Food Photography Method (RFPM) for estimating energy and nutrient intake in near real-time. *Obesity (Silver Spring).* 2012;20(4):891-899.

49. U.S. Department of Agriculture. MyPlate. *Start Simple with MyPlate App.* Accessed January 30, 2021. https://www.myplate.gov/resources/tools/startsimple-myplate-app

50. United States Department of Agriculture. Food patterns equivalents database. Accessed February 8, 2021. https://www.ars.usda.gov/northeast-area/beltsville-md-bhnrc/beltsville-human-nutrition-research-center/food-surveys-research-group/docs/fped-overview/

51. United States Department of Agriculture. FoodData Central. Accessed February 8, 2021. https://fdc.nal.usda.gov

52. United States Department of Agriculture. Agriculture Research Service. Food and nutrient database for dietary studies. Accessed January 30, 2021. https://www.ars.usda.gov/northeast-area/beltsville-md-bhnrc/beltsville-human-nutrition-research-center/food-surveys-research-group/docs/fndds/

53. World Health Organization. *Report of the technical discussions at the twenty first World Health Assembly on "national and global surveillance of communicable diseases."* A2.1. 18-5-1968. Geneva, Switzerland.

54. U.S. Department of Agriculture. Economic Research Service. Guess who's turning 100? Tracking a century of American eating. Accessed February 8, 2021. https://www.ers.usda.gov/amber-waves/2010/march/guess-who-s-turning-100-tracking-a-century-of-american-eating/

55. U.S. Department of Agriculture, Agricultural Research Service. *History of Human Nutrition Research in the U.S. Department of Agriculture, Agricultural Research Service: People, Events, and Accomplishments.* Washington, DC: 2017.

56. National Research Council (US) Coordinating Committee on Evaluation of Food Consumption Surveys. *National Survey Data on Food Consumption: Uses and Recommendations.* Washington (DC): National Academies Press (US); 1984.

57. Centers for Disease Control and Prevention, National Center for Health Sciences. *National Health and Nutrition Examination Survey: History.* Accessed February 8, 2021. www.cdc.gov/nchs/nhanes/history.htm

58. U.S. Department of Health, Education, and Welfare; Health Services and Mental Health Administration; and Centers for Disease Control and Prevention. *Ten-state nutrition survey, 1968-1970. Highlights.* Atlanta, GA: 1972.

59. United States Environmental Protection Agency. Science Inventory. *Pediatric Nutrition Surveillance System (PEDNSS).* Accessed February 8, 2021. https://cfpub.epa.gov/si/si_public_record_Report.cfm?Lab=OEI&dirEntryID=132414

60. Congress.gov. *H.R.1608 – National Nutrition Monitoring and Related Research Act of 1990.* Accessed January 30, 2021. https://www.congress.gov/bill/101st-congress/house-bill/1608/summary/00

61. Centers for Disease Control and Prevention, National Center for Health Statistics. *What we eat in America, dietary survey integration.* Accessed February 7, 2021. https://www.cdc.gov/nchs/nhanes/wweia.htm

62. Centers for Disease Control and Prevention, National Center for Health Statistics. *National Health and Nutrition Examination Survey.* Accessed February 8, 2021. https://www.cdc.gov/nchs/nhanes/index.htm

63. Ahluwalia N, Dwyer J, Terry A, Moshfegh A, Johnson C. Update on NHANES dietary data: focus on collection, release, analytical considerations, and uses to inform public policy. *Adv Nutr.* 2016;7(1):121-134.

64. Eicher-Miller HA, Fulgoni VL 3rd, Keast DR. Energy and nutrient intakes from processed foods differ by sex, income status, and race/ethnicity of US Adults. *J Acad Nutr Diet.* 2015;115(6):907-918.e6.

65. Brooks CJ, Gortmaker SL, Long MW, Cradock AL, Kenney EL. Racial/ethnic and socioeconomic disparities in hydration status among US adults and the role of tap water and other beverage intake. *Am J Public Health.* 2017;107(9):1387-1394.

66. Odutayo A, Gill P, Shepherd S, et al. Income disparities in absolute cardiovascular risk and cardiovascular risk factors in the United States, 1999-2004. *JAMA Cardiol.* 2017;2(7):782-790.

67. Divney AA, Echeverria SE, Thorpe LE, Trinh-Shevrin C, Islam NS. Hypertension prevalence jointly influenced by acculturation and gender in US immigrant groups. *Am J Hypertens.* 2019;32(1):104-111.

68. Berenson GS (ed). *Causation of Cardiovascular Risk Factors in Childhood: Perspectives on Cardiovascular Risk in Early Life.* New York: Raven Press; 1986:408.

69. Berenson GS, McMahan CA, Voors AW, et al. *Cardiovascular Risk Factors in Children–The Early Natural History of Atherosclerosis and Essential Hypertension.* New York: Oxford University Press; 1980:450.

70. Berenson GS, Wattigney WA, Bao W, Srinivasan SR, Radhakrishnamurthy B. Rationale to study the early natural history of heart disease: The Bogalusa Heart Study. *Am J Med Sci.* 1995;310(suppl 1):S22-S28.

71. Nicklas TA, Demory-Luce D, Yang SJ, Baranowski T, Zakeri I, Berenson G. Children's food consumption patterns have changed over two decades (1973–1994): The Bogalusa heart study. *J Am Diet Assoc.* 2004;104(7):1127-1140.

72. Nicklas TA, Hayes D, American Dietetic Association. Position of the American Dietetic Association: nutrition guidance for healthy children ages 2 to 11 years. *J Am Diet Assoc.* 2008;108(6):1038-1044, 1046-1047. doi: 10.1016/j.jada.2008.04.005 . PMID: 18564454

73. Berenson GS, Wattigney WA, Tracy RE, et al. Atherosclerosis of the aorta and coronary arteries and cardiovascular risk factors in persons aged 6 to 30 years and studied at necropsy (The Bogalusa Heart Study). *Am J Cardiol.* 1992;70(9):851-858.

74. Strong JP, McGill HC Jr. The natural history of coronary atherosclerosis. *Am J Pathol* 1962;40(1):37-49.

75. Metha NJ, Khan AI. Cardiology's 10 greatest discoveries of the 20th century. *Tex Heart Inst J.* 2002;29(3):164-171.

76. Kannel WB, Dawber TR, Kagan A, Revotskie N, Stokes J. Factors of risk in the development of coronary heart disease—six year follow-up experience. The Framingham Study. *Ann Intern Med.* 1691;55:33-50.

77. Framingham Heart Study. Research Milestones. Accessed February 8, 2021. https://framinghamheartstudy.org/fhs-about/research-milestones/

78. National Institutes of Health; National Heart, Lung, and Blood Institute. *Third Report of the National Cholesterol Education Program (NCEP) Expert Panel on Detection, Evaluation, and Treatment of High Blood Cholesterol in Adults (Adult Treatment Panel III). Final report.* 2002. Accessed February 4, 2021. https://www.nhlbi.nih.gov/files/docs/resources/heart/atp-3-cholesterol-full-report.pdf

79. Corlin L, Liu C, Lin H, et al. Proteomic signatures of lifestyle risk factors for cardiovascular disease: a cross-sectional analysis of the plasma proteome in the Framingham Heart Study. *J Am Heart Assoc.* 2021;10(1):e018020.

80. Framingham Heart Study. *Offspring Cohort.* Accessed February 8, 2021. https://framinghamheartstudy.org/participants/participant-cohorts/

81. Framingham Heart Study. *Researchers Awarded $26.56 Million NIH Grant for FHS Brain Aging Program (FHS-BAP).* Accessed February 8, 2021. https://framinghamheartstudy.org/2020/09/21/fhs-bap/

82. Farris RP, Nicklas TA. Characterizing children's eating behavior. In: *Textbook of Pediatric Nutrition.* Suskind RM, Suskind LL, eds. New York: Raven Press; 1993:505-516.

83. Nicklas TA, Forcier JE, Webber LS, Berenson GS. School lunch assessment as part of a 24-hour dietary recall for children. *J Am Diet Assoc.* 1991;91(6):711-713.

84. Frank GC, Hollatz AT, Webber LS, Berenson GS. Effect of interviewer recording practices on nutrient intake—Bogalusa Heart Study. *J Am Diet Assoc.* 1984;84(12):1432-1436, 1439.

85. Davy KP, Davy BM. Advances in nutrition science and integrative physiology: insights from controlled feeding studies. *Front Physiol.* 2019;10:3141.

86. Appel LJ, Moore TJ, Obarzanek E, et al. A clinical trial of the effects of dietary patterns on blood pressure. *N Engl J Med.* 1997;336:1117-1124.

87. Sacks FM, Svetkey LP, Vollmer WM, et al. Effects on blood pressure of reduced dietary sodium and the Dietary Approaches to Stop Hypertension (DASH) diet. *N Engl J Med.* 2001;344:3-10.

88. Funk KL, Elmer PJ, Stevens VJ, et al. PREMIER—a trial of lifestyle interventions for blood pressure control: intervention design and rationale. *Health Promot Pract.* 2008;9(3):271-280.

89. Albanes D, Heinonen OP, Taylor PR, et al. α-Tocopherol and β-carotene supplements and lung cancer incidence in the Alpha-Tocopherol, Beta-Carotene Cancer Prevention Study: effects of base-line characteristics and study compliance. *J Natl Cancer Inst.* 1996;88(21):1560-1570.

90. Omenn GS, Goodman G, Thornquist M, et al. The β-Carotene and Retinol Efficacy Trial (CARET) for chemoprevention of lung cancer in high risk populations: smokers and asbestos-exposed workers. *Cancer Res.* 1994;54(suppl 7):2038s-2043s.

91. Block G, Patterson B, Subar A. Fruit, vegetables, and cancer prevention: a review of the epidemiological evidence. *Nutr Cancer.* 1992;18(1):1-29.

92. Steinmetz KA, Potter JD. Vegetables, fruit, and cancer. I. Epidemiology. *Cancer Causes Control.* 1991;2:325-357.

93. Le Marchand L, Hankin JH, Kolonel LN, Beecher GR, Wilkens LR, Zhao LP. Intake of specific carotenoids and lung cancer risk. *Cancer Epidemiol Biomarkers Prev.* 1993;2(3):183-187.

94. Steinmetz KA, Potter JD, Folsom AR. Vegetables, fruit, and lung cancer in the Iowa Women's Health Study. *Cancer Res.* 1993;53(3):536-543.

95. Smigel K. Beta carotene fails to prevent cancer in two major studies; CARET intervention stopped. *J Natl Cancer Inst.* 1996;88(3-4):145.

96. Go J, Chang, DH, Ryu YK, et al. Human gut microbiota *Agathobaculum butyriciproducens* improves cognitive impairment in LPS-induced and APP/PS1 mouse models of Alzheimer's disease. *Nutr Res.* 2021;86:96-108.

97. Wolf G. The effect of low and high doses of beta-carotene and exposure to cigarette smoke on the lungs of ferrets. *Nutr Rev.* 2002;60(3):88-90.

98. Russell RM. The enigma of β-carotene in carcinogenesis: what can be learned from animal studies. *J Nutr.* 2004;134(1):262S-268S.

99. *Healthy People 2030.* Accessed January 30, 2021. https://health.gov/healthypeople

100. US Department of Health and Human Services. *Healthy People: The Surgeon General's Report on Health Promotion and Disease*

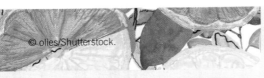
© olies/Shutterstock.

Learning Portfolio

Prevention. Washington, DC: Government Printing Office; 1979: Section 25.

101. Perspectives in Disease Prevention and Health Promotion Implementing the 1990 Prevention Objectives: Summary of CDC's Seminar. *Morbid Mortal Wkly Rep.* 1983;32:21-24.

102. Centers for Disease Control and Prevention. *Surveys and Data Collection Systems.* Accessed April 11, 2016. http://www.cdc.gov/nchs/surveys.htm

103. Healthy People 2030. Objectives and data. Accessed January 30, 2021. https://health.gov/healthypeople/objectives-and-data

104. Healthy People 2020. State and territorial Healthy People plans. Accessed April 11, 2016. https://www.healthypeople.gov/2020/healthy-people-in-action/State-and-Territorial-Healthy-People-Plans

105. Murphy SP, Yates AA, Atkinson SA, Barr SI, Dwyer J. History of nutrition: the long road leading to the dietary reference intakes for the United States and Canada. *Adv Nutr.* 2016;7(1):157-168.

106. United States Department of Agriculture. National Agricultural Library. Dietary Reference Intakes. Accessed January 30, 2021. https://www.nal.usda.gov/fnic/dietary-reference-intakes

107. Institute of Medicine (U.S.). *Dietary Reference Intakes for Water, Potassium, Sodium, Chloride, and Sulfate.* Washington, DC: National Academies Press; 2005.

108. Institute of Medicine (U.S.). *Dietary Reference Intakes for Energy, Carbohydrate, Fiber, Fat, Fatty Acids, Cholesterol, Protein, and Amino Acids (Macronutrients).* Washington, DC: National Academies Press; 2005.

109. Institute of Medicine (U.S.). *Dietary Reference Intakes for Vitamin A, Vitamin K, Arsenic, Boron, Chromium, Copper, Iodine, Iron, Manganese, Molybdenum, Nickel, Silicon, Vanadium, and Zinc.* Washington, DC: National Academies Press; 2001.

110. Institute of Medicine (U.S.). *Dietary Reference Intakes for Vitamin C, Vitamin E, Selenium, and Carotenoids.* Washington, DC: National Academies Press; 2000.

111. Institute of Medicine (U.S.). *Dietary Reference Intakes for Thiamin, Riboflavin, Niacin, Vitamin B_6, Folate, Vitamin B_{12}, Pantothenic Acid, Biotin, and Choline.* Washington, DC: National Academies Press; 1998.

112. Institute of Medicine (U.S.). *Dietary Reference Intakes for Calcium, Phosphorus, Magnesium, Vitamin D, and Fluoride.* Washington, DC: National Academies Press; 1997.

113. Institute of Medicine (U.S.). *Dietary Reference Intakes for Calcium and Vitamin D.* Washington, DC: National Academies Press; 2011.

114. National Academies of Sciences, Engineering, and Medicine (U.S.). *Dietary Reference Intakes for Sodium and Potassium.* Washington, DC: The National Academies Press; 2019.

115. Institute of Medicine. *School Meals: Building Blocks for Healthy Children.* Washington, DC: National Academies Press; 2010. Accessed January 30, 2021. https://www.nap.edu/catalog/12751/school-meals-building-blocks-for-healthy-children

116. Institute of Medicine. *Local Government Actions to Prevent Childhood Obesity.* 2009. Accessed January 30, 2021. https:// www.nap.edu/catalog/12674/local-government-actions-to-prevent-childhood-obesity

117. Institute of Medicine. *The Public Health Effects of Food Deserts. Workshop Summary.* 2009. Washington, DC: National Academies Press. Accessed January 30, 2021. https://www.nap.edu/catalog/12623/the-public-health-effects-of-food-deserts-workshop-summary

118. Institute of Medicine. *Nutrition Standards and Meal Requirements for National School Lunch and Breakfast Programs: Phase I. Proposed Approach for Recommending Revisions.* Washington, DC: National Academies Press; 2008. Accessed January 30, 2021. https://www.nap.edu/catalog/12512/nutrition-standards-and-meal-requirements-for-national-school-lunch-and-breakfast-programs

119. Institute of Medicine. *Use of Dietary Supplements by Military Personnel.* Washington, DC: National Academies Press; 2008. Accessed January 30, 2021. https://www.nap.edu/catalog/12095/use-of-dietary-supplements-by-military-personnel

120. Murphy SP, Poos MI. Dietary Reference Intakes: summary of applications in dietary assessment. *Public Health Nutr.* 2002;5(6a):843-849.

121. Murphy SP, Barr SI, Poos MI. Using the new dietary reference intakes to assess diets: a map to the maze. *Nutr Rev.* 2002;60(9):267-275.

122. Barr SI, Murphy SP, Agurs-Collins TD, Poos MI. Planning diets for individuals using the dietary reference intakes. *Nutr Rev.* 2003;61(10):352-360.

123. United States Department of Agriculture, Food and Nutrition Service. Center for Nutrition Policy and Promotion. Accessed January 30, 2021. https://www.fns.usda.gov/cnpp

124. United States Department of Agriculture, Food and Nutrition Service. Center for Nutrition Policy and Prevention. *About CNPP.* Accessed January 30, 2021. https://www.fns.usda.gov/about-cnpp

125. U.S. Department of Agriculture and U.S. Department of Health and Human Services. *Dietary Guidelines for Americans, 2020-2025.* 9th edition. December 2020. Accessed January 30, 2021. https://www.dietaryguidelines.gov

126. U.S. Department of Health and Human Services, Public Health Service. *The Surgeon General's report on nutrition and health.* DHHS (PHS) Publication No. 88-50215; 1988.

127. United States Department of Agriculture. MyPlate. Accessed January 30, 2021. http://www.myplate.gov

128. United States Department of Agriculture. MyPlate, Professionals. Accessed January 30, 2021. http://www.myplate.gov/professionals

129. U.S. Department of Health and Human Services. *Physical Activity Guidelines for Americans, 2nd edition.* Accessed January 30, 2021. https://health.gov/our-work/physical-activity/current-guidelines

130. United States Department of Agriculture. Food and Nutrition Service. *SNAP Data Tables.* Accessed January 30, 2021. https://www.fns.usda.gov/pd/supplemental-nutrition-assistance-program-snap

131. United States Department of Agriculture. Food and Nutrition Service. National School Lunch Program. *Child Nutrition*

Tables. Accessed January 30, 2021. https://www.fns.usda.gov
/pd/child-nutrition-tables

132. United States Department of Agriculture. Food and Nutrition Service. *WIC Data Tables.* Accessed January 30, 2021. https://www.fns.usda.gov/pd/wic-program

133. United States Department of Agriculture. Older Americans Act Nutrition Services Program. Accessed January 30, 2021. https://agid.acl.gov/Resources/DataOutputs/Data_Story _Nutrition_Services_Program.pdf

134. United States Department of Agriculture. SNAP-Ed Toolkit: Obesity Prevention Interventions and Evaluation Framework. *The Toolkit.* Accessed January 30, 2021. https://snapedtoolkit .org

135. United States Department of Agriculture. MyPlate. *A Brief History of USDA Food Guides.* Accessed January 30, 2021. https://www.myplate.gov/sites/default/files/2020-12 /ABriefHistoryOfUSDAFoodGuides.pdf

136. United States Department of Agriculture. MyPlate. *What is MyPlate?* Accessed January 30, 2021. https://www.myplate .gov/eat-healthy/what-is-myplate

137. Kennedy ET, Ohls J, Carlson S, Fleming K. The Healthy Eating Index: design and applications. *J Am Diet Assoc.* 1995;95:1103-1108.

138. Bowman SA, Lino M, Gerrior SA, Basiotis PP. *The Healthy Eating Index: 1994-96.* U.S. Department of Agriculture, Center for Nutrition Policy and Promotion. Washington, DC: CNPP-5; 1998.

139. United States Department of Agriculture. Center for Nutrition Policy and Promotion. *Healthy Eating Index.* Accessed January 30, 2021. https://www.fns.usda.gov/resource/healthy -eating-index-hei

140. Drewnowski A, Aggarwal A, Cook A, Stewart O, Moudon AV. Geographic disparities in Healthy Eating Index scores (HEI–2005 and 2010) by residential property values: findings from Seattle Obesity Study (SOS). *Prev Med.* 2016;83: 46-55.

141. Wilson MM, Reedy J, Krebs-Smith SM. American diet quality: where it is, where it is heading, and what it could be. *J Acad Nutr Diet.* 2016;116(2):302-310.

142. Pennington JA, Hubbard VS. Derivation of daily values used for nutrition labeling. *J Am Diet Assoc.* 1997;97:1407–1412.

143. Origin and framework of the development of dietary reference intakes. *Nutr Rev.* 1997;55:332-334.

144. U.S. Food & Drug Administration. *Nutrition Labeling and Education Act (NLEA) Requirements-Attachment 1.* Accessed January 31, 2021. https://www.fda.gov/nutrition-labeling -and-education-act-nlea-requirements-attachment-1

145. U.S. Food and Drug Administration. Guidance & Regulation (Food and Dietary Supplements). *Food Allergen Labeling and Consumer Protection Act of 2004 (FALCPA).* Accessed January 31, 2021. https://www.fda.gov/food/food-allergensgluten-free -guidance-documents-regulatory-information/food-allergen -labeling-and-consumer-protection-act-2004-falcpa

146. U.S. Food and Drug Administration. Food Labeling and Nutrition. *Gluten and Food Labeling.* Accessed January 31, 2021. https://www.fda.gov/food/nutrition-education-resources -materials/gluten-and-food-labeling

147. U.S. General Services Administration. eRulemaking Program Management Office. Regulations.gov. *Food Labeling: Revision of the Nutrition and Supplement Facts Labels.* Accessed January 31, 2021. https://beta.regulations.gov/document /FDA-2012-N-1210-0875

148. U.S. Food & Drug Administration. *The New and Improved Nutrition Facts Label—Key Changes.* Accessed January 31, 2021. https://www.fda.gov/media/135302/download

149. U.S. Food & Drug Administration. Food Labeling & Nutrition. *Label Claims for Conventional Foods and Dietary Supplements.* Accessed January 31, 2021. https://www.fda.gov/food/food -labeling-nutrition/label-claims-conventional-foods-and-dietary -supplements

150. U.S. Department of Health and Human Services. Food and Drug Administration, and Center for Food Safety and Applied Nutrition. *A Food Labeling Guide: Guidance for Industry (9. Appendix A: Definitions of Nutrient Content Claims, 10. Appendix B: Additional Requirements for Nutrient Content Claims).* Accessed January 31, 2021. https://www.fda.gov /media/81606/download

151. U.S. Department of Health and Human Services. Food and Drug Administration and Center for Food Safety and Applied Nutrition. *A Food Labeling Guide: Guidance for Industry (11. Appendix C: Health Claims).* Accessed January 31, 2021. https://www.fda.gov/media/81606/download

152. U.S. Department of Health and Human Services. Food and Drug Administration and Center for Food Safety and Applied Nutrition. *A Food Labeling Guide: Guidance for Industry (12. Appendix D: Qualified Health Claims).* Accessed January 31, 2021. https://www.fda.gov/media/81606/download

153. U.S. Food & Drug Administration. Nutrition Education Resources & Materials. *The New Nutrition Facts Label.* Accessed January 31, 2021. https://www.fda.gov/food/nutrition -education-resources-materials/new-nutrition-facts-label

CHAPTER 2

Nutritional Epidemiology: An Introduction

Lisa S. Brown, PhD, RDN, LDN

Elizabeth Newton, MS

(We would like to acknowledge the work of Dolores M. Wolongevicz, PhD, MS, RDN, LDN; Elisabeth Offenberger, MS, RDN, and Stefanie O'Connor, MS, RDN, who contributed to the past editions of Nutrition in Public Health.)

Learning Outcomes

AFTER STUDYING THIS CHAPTER AND REFLECTING ON THE CONTENTS, YOU SHOULD BE ABLE TO:

1. Define nutritional epidemiology and understand its role in health and disease.
2. Identify the various types of study designs commonly used in nutritional epidemiologic research.
   a. Discuss the strengths and weaknesses of each study design.
3. Describe the commonly used dietary assessment methods in nutritional epidemiologic research.
   a. Discuss the strengths and weaknesses of each dietary assessment method.
4. Discuss important methodological issues in dietary data collection and analyses in nutritional epidemiologic research.
5. Discuss how nutritional epidemiology impacts the public health nutritionist.

Epidemiology assesses the occurrence of a disease within a set population. This field also looks at the factors that prevent and hasten the disease's development.

Nutritional epidemiology utilizes the processes of epidemiology to look at the influence of dietary factors on a disease or health condition in the population.

Pandemic Learning Opportunity

If epidemiologists were able to act faster than what occurred in 2021, how would the outcome change? Going further, how important is it to have a fully functioning epidemiology unit working in the United States?

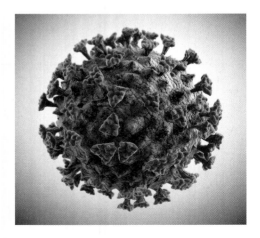

The covid-19 molecule.

© Giovanni Cancemi/Shutterstock.

Introduction

This chapter focuses on the field of nutritional **epidemiology** and its role in the public health setting. To further understand **nutritional epidemiology**, it is important to review the types of research studies as well as the benefits and challenges of each type of study. The most well-known studies within the field of nutritional epidemiology are mentioned throughout the chapter to connect these studies with their designs and data collection methods. As it can be challenging to collect appropriate nutritional data, the collection methods are also discussed by highlighting the advantages and disadvantages of each method. By addressing these components, the role of nutritional epidemiology in the public health arena can be understood better. Application of nutritional epidemiologic research in public health and new frontiers for application of research will be briefly discussed at the end of the chapter.

Overview of Epidemiology

In 2020, a global health pandemic sparked new interest in the field of scientific inquiry known as epidemiology. The world watched as infectious disease epidemiologists took center stage to solve the mysteries of where the virus came from and how we could minimize its spread. Epidemiologists combined observational tools such as counting cases and contact tracing with experimental proof-of-concept studies such as understanding the structure of the virus and testing how long the severe acute respiratory syndrome coronavirus 2 (SARS-CoV-2), which causes coronavirus disease 19 (Covid-19), could remain on surfaces under various conditions.[1] Using a combination of observational and experimental techniques, epidemiologists were quickly able to conclude that Covid-19 spreads primarily through the air in both large and small droplets (aerosols), infecting people as it is inhaled deep into the lungs.[2] This type of investigation changed the official recommendations on safety measures and reinforced mask mandates. It also placed more emphasis on ventilation and less emphasis on enhanced surface cleaning.[3] An epidemiologist uses their observational data in the same way that some might use the picture on the box of a jigsaw puzzle. What an epidemiologist observes playing out in everyday life is the big picture that all of the little pieces must fit. The experimental data help us understand where each piece belongs within the puzzle.

Epidemiology is the study of disease distribution within a population and the factors, both protective and promoting, that influence the occurrence of disease. Epidemiology utilizes both observational and experimental techniques to discover patterns related to disease development. One of the first epidemiologic studies of the modern era occurred in 1854 when John Snow discovered that a water pump on Broad Street in the Soho district of London was the source of a cholera outbreak within the city. His systematic technique of counting the number of cases in each area of London led him to Soho and eventually to the pump on Broad Street.[4] Once he identified the water as the suspected cause, using experimental techniques, he could then test his theory to prove that it was the source of the outbreak. Based on Snow's work, the pump was shuttered and the outbreak ended.

Although this is a very clear demonstration of a disease that could be traced to a single source, the same basic principles are used today to connect more complex diseases with potential causes. First, the cases are tracked to identify potential causes. Causes may be as simple as a single water source or a much more complex interaction between several factors such as exercise and diet. Once potential sources are identified, hypotheses are created and tested using observational techniques. Finally, if possible, the hypostasis is tested using experimental designs (to be expanded in a later section). It is

1. Suspect that a factor (exposure/independent variable/X) influenced disease (outcome/dependent variable/Y) occurrence.
   - Descriptive epidemiology
     - Examining disease patterns
     - Descriptive studies (ecological and cross sectional studies)

2. Form specific hypotheses regarding the exposure-disease association

3. Conduct epidemiologic study to determine relationship between exposure and disease ("analytic epidemiology")

4. Judge whether association may be causal. Need to consider:
   - Chance, bias, confounding
   - Strengths and weaknesses of study design
   - Context of study in other epidemiologic research

5. Create intervention strategies to reduce the burden of disease

FIGURE 2–1 Common Pathway for Epidemiologic Research of Nutrition.

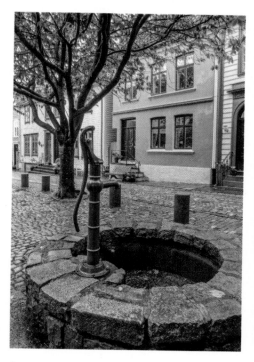

One of the first epidemiologic studies of the modern era occurred in 1854 when John Snow discovered that a water pump on Broad Street in the Soho district of London was the source of a cholera outbreak within the city.

© Rhkamen/Moment/Getty Images.

precisely this set of steps that has led to many health-related discoveries, which allowed for interventions to decrease the spread of disease within a population. **Figure 2–1** illustrates this process. For example, the discovery that exposure to tobacco smoke causes cancer led to labeling and education campaigns, taxation on cigarettes, and finally, limitations in many places regarding where smoking is permitted.[5]

Overview of Nutritional Epidemiology

In nutritional epidemiology, researchers apply epidemiologic methods to specifically study the connection between dietary factors and health outcomes. As with the broader field of epidemiology, its purpose is to identify targets for intervention that could reduce the burden of disease within a population. For example, nutritional epidemiologists have spent decades examining the connection between dietary fat intake and development of cardiovascular disease. The result of these investigations has led to expert guidelines recommending limited total and saturated fat intake, while endorsing the benefits of more liberal consumption of mono- and polyunsaturated fat.[6-8]

Early observations of the role of diet in disease prevention and health promotion are evident in the writings of Hippocrates, who is considered the Father of Medicine. Hippocrates wrote over 2,000 years ago: "A low diet of food and drink is on the whole a surer way to health than violent changes from one diet to another."[9] It was not until the 18th century; however, that one of the first controlled clinical trials into the relationship between food, nutrition, and disease risk was conducted.

In 1747, James Lind divided 12 sailors with scurvy into pairs and assigned five of the pairs to receive one of several treatments accepted as a remedy for the condition at that time.[10] The sixth pair received lemons and oranges, which was considered an experimental treatment. The only sailors to recover from scurvy were those who received the citrus fruits. Not long after this experiment was conducted, the English Navy became the dominant force of the seas, all because they could stay out longer without getting sick. English sailors became known as "Limeys" because of their new association with citrus fruit. It can be said that nutrition conquered the sea! While Lind could not identify the exact compound responsible for the effect, he was among the first to demonstrate that scurvy was the result of a dietary deficiency. As we are now aware, the vitamin in question is vitamin C, which was not isolated until 1928.[11]

Early experiments like Lind's showed that something within certain foods had an essential role in human functioning; however, recognition of the actual vitamins and minerals necessary for human health did not occur until the late 19th and the 20th centuries.[12] Early studies on nutrition focused on identifying deficiency diseases associated with specific vitamins and minerals. As new vitamins were discovered and applied to populations deficient in them, certain diseases almost miraculously disappeared including beriberi, scurvy, and pellagra.

While the single nutrient model remains important today (e.g., the fortification of folic acid in the American food supply in 1998 has greatly reduced the occurrence of neural tube defects in newborns), this model has many limitations as well. Specifically, it does not seem to fit well when applied to complex diseases with multiple interrelated causes. Diseases such as obesity, diabetes, and cardiovascular disease are a result of an interaction between genetics and environmental factors, and the old single-cause model has failed to adequately capture the multifactorial foundation of noncommunicable/chronic disease. In more recent years, the field of nutritional epidemiology has progressed beyond the single nutrient/deficiency disease model to include multifaceted investigations of the nutritional determinants of disease related to excess nutrient consumption.[13,14] The connections between excess nutrition and chronic disease development are generally much more complicated than the single-nutrient model and can only be studied by observing free-living populations on a larger scale over a long time period. These complex models have taken shape primarily in the study of dietary patterns, nutrition indices, and nutrient risk scores. These studies capture multiple dimensions of diet as a single variable to compare the combined impact of the type of dietary pattern that the individual follows against their risk of developing disease.

One of the first large-scale studies of the modern era of nutritional epidemiology is the Framingham Heart Study (FHS), which was initiated in 1948 to identify factors contributing to cardiovascular disease (CVD) development.[15] CVD had become the leading cause of death in the United States by the mid-twentieth century, as chronic diseases superseded infectious disease as the leading cause of death due to improved medical technology and hygeine.[16,17] In response, the U.S. government held a contest to find a "typical" American town that would be followed medically over many years to determine potential causes of cardiovascular disease. Framingham, Massachusetts, was selected as the representative American town and two-thirds of the residents agreed to participate. Early findings included the discovery of a link between blood cholesterol levels and development of heart disease. Although early single-nutrient–driven investigations found no connection between nutrition and cardiovascular disease development, later research used a more complex model of examining dietary patterns and stratified participants by age, gender, and other pertinent factors such as smoking status. These studies have greatly contributed to our knowledge of the connections between diet and several chronic diseases.[18-23]

The Nurses' Health Study (NHS),[24] which was initiated in 1976, has also been an extremely valuable source of information in nutritional epidemiology. The NHS originally included approximately 122,000 female nurses and has been instrumental in advancing our understanding of the effect of

Discussion Prompt

Describe the factors that prevented the recognition of a nutrition link and good health. How did epidemiology change this thinking?

diet and lifestyle factors on health. One of the unique features of both the NHS and its male counterpart, the Health Professionals Follow-Up Study (HPFS),[25] is that the population was defined by professional status instead of physical location. While the result may have been relative socioeconomic and educational homogeneity, it also allowed for much greater diversity in terms of environmental and cultural exposures. Unlike Framingham, which was a geographically homogenous population, the NHS included women from all over the United States. By redefining population, these studies were able to look at many new factors related to chronic disease development that were not possible in geographically and culturally similar populations. Another major strength of having a broader definition of population was the ability to recruit large numbers of subjects. With such a large-scale study, investigations into less common diseases, including many cancers, is made possible, and both the NHS and the HPFS have been invaluable in their contributions to nutritional epidemiology.

Like the Framingham and the Nurses' Health studies described above, many other community-based cohorts have been recruited and followed to help illuminate the complex connections between lifestyle behaviors and health outcomes. Some, like Bogalusa,[26] focus on a younger population and others, such as The Strong Heart Study,[27] focus on a minority population; combined, we are able to observe patterns that help put together the pieces of the multipart puzzle that connects lifestyle and disease.

Types of Study Designs Used in Nutritional Epidemiology

Once a hypothesis is created, the first thing to be decided is how to test most effectively if there is a possible link. The main tool used by the epidemiologist to determine potential connections is study design. A variety of study designs or methodologies is utilized to conduct nutritional epidemiologic investigations. The type of study design that is selected depends on the research question to be investigated, the type of data available to answer the question, time frame (past, present, or future) of data collection, feasibility (cost, time allotted for data collection, staff, and technical resources to carry out the study, etc.), and ethical considerations.

The most common research designs used in nutritional epidemiology are descriptive studies, such as ecological and cross-sectional investigations and analytic studies, including case-control, cohort, and experimental investigations. Descriptive studies are considered less scientifically rigorous than analytic designs. However, it is important to emphasize that all study designs have a place in the **hierarchy** of research methodologies (Figure 2–1). For example, descriptive research often provides valuable information for generating hypotheses (research questions) that can then be tested using analytic research techniques.

Descriptive studies also tell us about the current status of a problem. For example, a cross-sectional study could be conducted to identify what percentage of the population is anemic, vitamin D–deficient, smoking, exercising regularly, etc. This process measures the **prevalence** of a disease. The term prevalence in epidemiology refers to the percentage of the population that has a disease at any given point; for example, the percentage of the population living with diabetes in the United States on a given date. Prevalence numbers can be compared over time to create an ongoing picture of progress toward a public health goal or simply to indicate the severity of a problem at any given time point.

Hierarchy refers to the ability of a type of study to determine causality based on the strengths and weaknesses of its inert design.

Results from epidemiological studies can then be presented in a result map found at http://www.cdc.gov/obesity/data/childhood.html

Prevalence indicates how many individuals within a population have a disease or health condition at one moment in time.

Review of epidemiologic studies is also found in Chapter 1.

Incidence is the development of new cases of a disease over a period of time.

Analytic study designs are considered more effective for determining whether certain factors may be a potential cause or protective factor for a certain disease. With the exception of the case-control study, analytic studies follow populations over time, which is considered a key factor in determining a potential causal link between the exposure and the outcome. Using a time element, **incidence** can be calculated. Incidence is another important concept in epidemiology. It refers to the occurrence of new cases of disease in a specific population within a certain time frame, for example, how many people develop diabetes in the United States within a given year. Incidence and prevalence are discussed in depth later in this chapter.

An understanding of the characteristics, strengths, and limitations of each study design is necessary to determine the most appropriate method to address a particular nutritional concern. **Table 2–1** describes each of the study designs in more detail and gives examples of some landmark studies that represent that study design within nutritional epidemiology. Nutritional epidemiologic investigations take a common path (Figure 2–1).

Strategy Tip

The choice of study design is driven largely by the exact nature of the study question, type of data available to answer the question, and financial resources available. Other issues, such as the ethics of answering that question with certain experimental techniques, is also an issue that every researcher must confront. It would be unethical to expose someone to a factor that you are reasonably sure would do them harm. An example is purposely exposing a group to cigarette smoke after it was suspected to cause cancer. On the other side of the ethical question, it is not considered ethical to withhold a treatment that appears significantly protective. For these important ethical considerations, there are many protections that have been developed for human and animal subjects, including the use of Institutional Review Boards (IRBs), to approve studies and study review panels to assess results for experimental trials during the course of the investigation.

Guidelines for Causality

Causality is the ability of a variable in a study to be so strongly linked to the result that it can be determined that the variable caused the result. This can only be determined in a randomized controlled trial type of study with all other types falling into a hierarchy.

One important goal of epidemiologic investigations is to prove that factor x causes outcome y and subsequently design an intervention to alter that relationship. Some study designs are well suited to prove **causality**, with the randomized controlled trial (RCT) considered the gold standard.[52] **Figure 2–2** shows the "hierarchy of study design." Hierarchy in this context refers to the ability of these study designs to determine causality. Observational techniques are considered less convincing than experimental design, but there are several elements that can raise the validity of the results.

In 1965, Austin Bradford Hill proposed recommendations for evaluating causation. The principles that he created are referred to as the *Bradford-Hill guidelines* and are still used extensively to help researchers determine if there is indeed a causal link between an exposure and an outcome.[53]

1. **Strength**: The larger the effect or strength of association, the more likely it is causal. Caveat: A small association does not mean that there is not a causal effect. The effect may be weak or the sample size may be small.

TABLE 2–1
Descriptive Study Designs

Ecological/Correlational
Examines relationships between a risk factor and a disease outcome at the population level

Strengths: • Relatively quick and inexpensive • Utilizes available data • Takes advantage of large differences in exposure to a given risk factor between different populations • Good for hypothesis generation • Random error is relatively small *Weaknesses:* • Only shows potential association, NOT causation • Cannot be applied directly to individuals • Assumes that exposure to the risk factor is equal across the entire population • Assumes that other factors are the same between the two populations being compared	*Examples:* • Keys, A.—Coronary Heart Disease in Seven Countries[28,29]

Cross-Sectional/Prevalence
Creates a "snapshot" of an existing disease and factors that may be associated
• Data on exposure, disease, and confounders are all collected at the same time

Strengths:
 	
• Relatively quick and inexpensive
• Utilizes available data
• Good for hypothesis generation
• Good for diseases with long latency
• Provides information about a causal relationship when exposure is immutable or unlikely to change (sex, blood type, etc.)
• Measures prevalence
  — Good for assessing burden of disease, targeting the need for intervention programs
  — Comparison of several surveys can indicate the trend of a variable
 	
Weaknesses:
 	
• Lack of temporality between exposure and disease (gathering information about exposure and disease at the same time)
• Difficult to use to assess causation (outcome may have affected "exposure")
• Number of prevalent cases may be affected by incidence and duration
	Examples:
	
	• National Health and Nutrition Examination Survey[30,31]
	• Behavioral Risk Factor Surveillance System (BRFSS)[32]

Analytic Study Designs
Case-Control
Used to determine potential exposures in relation to a disease outcome. A group with the disease is recruited and compared with an equivalent group without disease. Information on the disease and possible exposures are collected at the same time and the two groups are compared for differences in exposure history.

• People with disease are defined as *cases* and those without are *controls*.
• It is often used for rare diseases or diseases that take a long time to develop.

Strengths: • Same method of obtaining exposure history from all respondents • Efficient for diseases that take a long time to develop • Efficient for rare diseases • Effective for diseases where little is known about etiology (can evaluate multiple exposures in relation to disease) • Good for dynamic populations • Less cost and time than prospective cohort studies (because no follow-up is needed and smaller sample) *Weaknesses:* • Recall bias: Information about previous diet is collected from those with and without the disease. Cases may recall exposures differently from controls because they are more motivated to discover what caused their disease.	*Examples:* • Ballestero et al.—Gluten-free diet and nutritional status in kids with and without Celiac[33] • Verlaan et al.—Nutritional status in older adults with and without sarcopenia[34] • Radujkovic et al.—Vitamin D deficiency and Covid outcomes[35] • Leiva-Gea et al.—Microbiome composition and type 1 diabetes[36]

(continues)

TABLE 2–1
Descriptive Study Designs *(continued)*

• Interviewer bias: If interviewers understand status of cases and controls, and also know the hypothesis, they may ask questions differently to cases and controls. They may probe cases for more information on exposures. • Temporality between exposure and disease sometimes uncertain • Inefficient for rare exposures • Control group selection may be difficult • Cannot estimate relative risk directly; must use odds ratio • Only show association NOT causation	

Cohort
Examines relationships between an exposure and a disease outcome at the population level; subjects are followed over time and information on exposures is collected prior to the development of disease.

Prospective Cohort
Subjects are grouped according to exposure and then followed to see who develops the disease.

Strengths: • Estimate risk directly using incidence • Good for assessing causal relationships • Good for minimizing selection bias and confounding • Good for studying rare exposures • Collect exposure data (i.e., current diet) without being biased by already having the disease *Weaknesses:* • Difficult with rare outcomes because even very large cohorts will not accumulate a sufficient number of cases within a reasonable amount of time • Difficult for long latency because too long to follow • Best for studying a particular exposure • Costs • Potential problem with subjects lost to follow-up	*Examples:* • Nurses' Health Study (NHS)[24,37-39] • Framingham Heart Study (FHS)[15,40] • Strong Heart Study[27,41] • Health Professionals Follow-up Study[25] • Honolulu Heart Program[42]

Retrospective Cohort
Investigator evaluates association between exposure and incidence of disease in a sample where exposure and disease have already occurred.

Strengths: • Estimate risk directly using incidence • Excellent for diseases with long latency periods • Good for studying rare exposures • Less expensive than prospective studies *Weaknesses:* • Difficult with rare outcomes • Heavy reliance on data from memory, preexisting records, and quality of recordkeeping • Problem with subjects lost to follow-up • Many inherent problems with internal validity	*Examples:* Nishioka et al.—Nutritional Status Changes and Activities of Daily Living After Hip Fracture[43]

Clinical Controlled Trial
Applies a controlled intervention to test the effect in prevention or treatment of disease, investigators assign who receives treatment, and what treatment is given.
• Subjects are randomized into either a treatment or control group.
• Ideally, neither the subject nor the investigator knows whether the subject receives the treatment or the placebo.

Strengths: • High validity • Can distinguish small and modest effects • Randomization should ensure that both known and unknown associated risk factors are evenly distributed among the treatment and control groups. *Weaknesses:* • Expense • May be unethical if the "treatment" is potentially harmful; potential benefit must outweigh potential harm • Subject compliance with treatment may not be good, especially if the treatment is complicated or difficult	*Examples:* • The Dietary Approaches to Stop Hypertension (DASH)[44,45] • Women's Health Initiative (WHI)[46,47] • The PREDIMED and PREDIMED-PLUS Trials[48,49] • Child & Adolescent Trial for Cardiovascular Health (CATCH)[50] • OMNI-Heart[51]

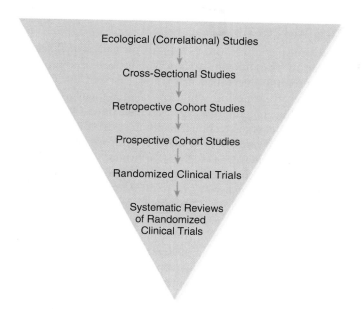

FIGURE 2–2 Hierarchy of Study Designs.

Centers for Disease Control and Prevention (CDC). Nutrition, Physical Activity and Obesity: Data, Trends and Maps. https://www.cdc.gov/nccdphp/dnpao/data-trends-maps/index.html.

2. **Consistency**: Consistent findings observed by different persons in different places with different samples strengthens the likelihood of an effect. For this reason, studies must be replicated multiple times to confirm results.

3. **Specificity**: Causation is likely when a specific population at a specific site shows incidence of a specific disease with no other explanation. The more specific an association between a factor and an effect is, the bigger the probability of a causal relationship.

4. **Temporality**: The effect has to occur after the cause (and if there is an expected delay between the cause and expected effect, the effect must occur after that delay).

5. **Biological gradient**: Greater exposure should generally lead to greater incidence of the effect. However, in some cases, the mere presence of the factor can trigger the effect. In other cases, an inverse proportion is observed: greater exposure leads to lower incidence.

6. **Plausibility**: A plausible mechanism between cause and effect is helpful although it should be kept in mind that knowledge of the mechanism is limited by current knowledge.

7. **Coherence**: Coherence between epidemiologic and laboratory findings increases the likelihood of an effect. However, Hill noted that "… lack of such [laboratory] evidence cannot nullify the epidemiological effect on associations."[53]

8. **Experiment**: "Occasionally it is possible to appeal to experimental evidence."[53]

9. **Analogy**: The effect of similar factors may be considered.

This is not to say that if a hypothesis passes all of the tests the relationship is indisputably causal; it is simply a good way to rule out those who are likely not. Hill himself said, "None of my nine viewpoints can bring indisputable evidence for or against the cause-and-effect hypothesis and none can be required *sine qua non*."[53]

Sine qua non means that without something, something else would not be possible.

Incidence and Prevalence

Incidence and prevalence are the two main measures of disease frequency within a population. They allow us to compare groups or to monitor progress. Incidence measures the development of new cases of disease in a population during a given time period while prevalence measures the proportion of the population that has the disease at a given time. One of the best ways to visualize these concepts is to imagine a faucet dripping water into a sink. Incidence would be measured by the number of drops of water that fall from the faucet in a given time frame (such as an hour). Prevalence would be the total amount of water in the sink at any given time.

Some diseases have a relatively low incidence but a high prevalence. This would occur when a disease is common within a population and people tend to live for a long time after diagnosis. For example, heart disease and diabetes are both very common in the American population and, although they are two of the leading causes of death in the United States, thanks to medical advances over the past half century, numerous people live many years with them. Other diseases may have an incidence that is relatively high compared with a low prevalence. This would happen if people who are diagnosed with the disease are either quickly cured or die. For example, the common cold occurs frequently within a population over a given time span, but a relatively small percentage of the population has it at any one time. Pancreatic cancer is another example of a disease with a high incidence compared with a relatively lower prevalence, based on the high mortality rate of the disease.

Strategy Tip

The Sars-CoV-2 virus that causes Covid-19 presents an interesting opportunity to look at how we can use incidence and prevalence to better understand a disease. For many, Covid-19 was a short-duration illness. Incidence of new cases was high, as would be expected with a novel virus that humans had no innate immunity to. The prevalence, however, was higher than would be expected based on our observations of viral illness such as the common cold or the flu, or even previously identified SARS viruses. This higher-than-expected prevalence was largely due to people with "long-haul Covid," who were not able to clear the virus effectively once they were infected, keeping the number of active cases in the population (the prevalence) at a higher level than expected. Further investigation into those with compromised immunity who were often identified as having long Covid has found that the virus appears to take advantage of those individuals to mutate into variants more suited to the environment. This observation is important for anticipating and potentially heading off new variants.[54]

In nutritional epidemiology, we can also use incidence and prevalence to see how effective treatment is for a given disease by looking at changes over time. For example, for many decades in the middle of the 20th century, cardiovascular disease had a relatively low incidence-to-prevalence ratio because of a relatively high death rate from cardiovascular disease. We had no tools to identify those most at risk to target for early intervention, and once identified, we had few effective treatments.[16,17] With the creation of the Framingham Risk Score and the discovery of many new medications such as statins, we can now identify and treat cardiovascular disease, allowing people to live for long periods of time with the disease.[55] This has shifted the incidence-to-prevalence ratio so that now, cardiovascular disease has a much higher prevalence compared with incidence. Cancer prevention, diagnosis, and treatment is currently going through a similar metamorphosis as new diagnostic and treatment options become available.[56]

Measuring Dietary Exposure: Dietary Assessment Methods

At the core of nutritional epidemiologic investigations is the ability to define nutritional/dietary exposures, including the estimation of population and individual food and nutrient intake and characterization of long-term, habitual dietary intake patterns. Several dietary assessment methods are available to measure diet in nutrition research. These include 24-hour recalls, food records or diaries, and food frequency questionnaires.[57,58] Each method is briefly discussed in subsequent sections. Detailed descriptions of each method can be found elsewhere.[59] All of them rely on self-reported data and each has its own set of strengths and weaknesses[60] that are also discussed below. Like study designs, it is important to be able to distinguish between the characteristics of each technique to determine which dietary assessment tool would be the most appropriate to use for the nutrition question and population under investigation.

Dietary Recalls

The 24-hour recall requires the respondent to retrospectively recall everything they ate and drank during the previous 24-hour period. In standard application, a trained interviewer asks the subject what they consumed and records it. Newer techniques include multiple "passes" and strategic prompting to help the subject recall any drinks, condiments, snacks, etc., that otherwise may be forgotten. Respondents are asked to report portion size, which is usually based on standard sizes (i.e., a cup of milk) and/or using food models to improve accuracy of portion size estimation. A 24-hour recall can be done quickly during a clinic visit; it is then coded and matched to foods in the corresponding nutrient analysis database and analyzed for nutrient content.

A single 24-hour recall is generally thought to be effective at quantifying mean group intake over a large population but it is considered an inaccurate method for estimation of usual intake for an individual.[60,61] Alternatively, multiple 24-hour recalls may be used to estimate usual intake on an individual level. The primary limitation generally cited for the 24-hour recall is that they are dependent on the ability of the subject to comprehensively remember what they consumed and accurately report portion sizes.[62-65] Although this is generally assumed to be true when recall data are interpreted, it has been shown that subjects may not accurately remember and report their intake. Karvetti and Knuts,[63] in a group of 140 subjects who provided recalls one day after their food intake was directly observed and measured, found that the subjects only accurately remembered 58–74% of what they had eaten. Inaccuracy of this type is referred to as **recall bias** and would clearly lead to some level of error when correlating the reported dietary intake with disease outcomes.

Food Records

Food records attempt to avoid recall bias by requiring the respondent to immediately record what they eat and drink during a given time period. A minimum of 3 days of records are collected to estimate typical intake for an individual and/or population, with 1 weekend day and 2 weekdays as a standard protocol, but some studies may collect as many as 7 to 10 days.[59,60]

Read more about 24-hour dietary recall methods at: https://dietassessmentprimer.cancer.gov/learn/recall-record.html

Recall bias is inaccurate reporting by a study subject that leads to less accurate study results.

Dietary intake is recorded by the respondent in real time and is turned in to the research team that manually codes and inputs the information into a nutrient analysis database to create a nutrient profile.

Food records are considered better estimates of an individual's intake compared with recalls and are equally good or better estimates of group intake compared with recalls.[60-62] The primary limitations cited for the dietary record method include a high respondent burden resulting in failure of subjects to comply and fill out the records or fill them out incompletely. Food records are often also criticized for suspected respondent failure to fill them out in real time, subjecting them to the same limitations of the recall. Methods to address portion size are similar to that of the 24-hour recall.

As with the food recall, it has been found that the assumptions upon which the accuracy of the food record are based are not always met. A major limitation of food records is reporting bias in which a subject may not wish to disclose everything they have consumed, may limit what they eat and drink on the days that consumption is recorded, or may selectively report only "healthier" foods. One common form of reporting bias is underreporting of true intake either intentionally or due to poor estimation of portion size. Underreporting is thought to be widespread and has been demonstrated to be a problem. Many studies have quantified underreporting by comparing the food record with a biological marker.[66-68]

Food Frequency Questionnaires

Food frequency questionnaires (FFQs) became popular in the 1980s to facilitate collection of dietary data in large cohort studies. The respondent is asked to estimate frequency of consumption of foods listed on a predetermined food list. The majority of FFQs are designed to be *self-administered*, meaning that the subject fills out the form themself, with a trained professional assigned to review the form for completeness.[58-60]

Unless directed by a specific research question, food items are usually listed using generic names; cooking methods are often not specified, for example, French fries that are baked in the oven versus fried in a fryolator. FFQs generally include several similar foods on the same line (e.g., "potato chips, pretzels, and tortilla chips"), and groups may vary between different FFQs, depending on the decisions made by the investigators. A food frequency questionnaire may contain as many as 200 or more line items or as few as 30 to 40 lines, with longer questionnaires demonstrating a higher validity compared with shorter questionnaires.[69,70] Portion size may be specified for every item on the FFQ (known as *quantitative*), specified for some items but not others (known as *semiquantitative*), or may be left unspecified. Controversy remains regarding the value of including portion size.[71,72] A nutrient analysis database specific to each FFQ is created to analyze nutrient content; forms are generally created to be either scanned directly by the computer or input by hand by a data entry specialist. No literature exists in the public domain documenting the process of creating the FFQ database and there is currently no standard procedure established.

Food frequency questionnaires are generally acknowledged as the least-precise method of estimating nutrient intake, and as such are often validated against other diet assessment methods when biomarkers are not available.[73-75] Error implicit in the FFQ includes the generic nature of the foods listed and the corresponding generic nature of the nutrient values assigned in the database. FFQs may not accurately represent the usual diet if foods commonly consumed by an individual are not listed on the form. Respondents may not understand how to fill out the form correctly and may not accurately account for things such as eating a double portion of a food at the same meal or on the same day. As with recalls, FFQs are not filled out in real time, so recall

Read more about food frequency questionnaires at: https://diet assessmentprimer.cancer.gov/learn /questionnaire-screeners.html

bias may be a problem. Likewise, respondents may not wish to report less healthy foods that they consume making reporting bias a concern, similar to diet records.

Currently, FFQs are widely used despite their limitations; they are well known to be the most cost-effective method of collecting dietary data within a large cohort and are considered *reasonably* valid compared with biomarkers and other dietary collection methods including multiple 24-hour recalls and 3-day food records. It is generally recommended that nutrient profiles derived from FFQs should not be used to characterize an individual's absolute nutrient intake given the generic nature of the assessment. Instead, they are used for relative ranking of individuals within a cohort.[60,64,76]

Validity of Dietary Data

Several potential sources of error have been identified in the collection and analysis of typical dietary intake, and these may contribute to the attenuation between estimated diet and risk of disease development.[59,61] As discussed previously, bias related to the dietary assessment tool is an area of concern when interpreting correlations. Confounding is also a concern to be considered when determining if a relationship truly exists between a dietary variable and disease outcome.

A **confounder** is a variable that is associated with both the outcome and the exposure. Confounding occurs when the effect attributed to the variable of interest is possibly due to another highly correlated, potentially unmeasured factor. Theoretically, statistical modeling will account for such effects, but as Fraser highlights in his commentary, "dietary analyses are peculiarly predisposed to confounding simply because of the complexity of this variable."[77] He goes on to discuss that an investigator may believe they are studying the effect of a particular nutrient of interest; however, in reality, they may be studying the effect of another nutrient or food-based chemical that is highly correlated but is measured or defined poorly. See **Table 2–2**.

> A **confounder** is a variable that is associated with both the exposure and the outcome, which then skews the results of the study.

TABLE 2–2
Strengths and Weaknesses of Dietary Assessment Methods

Method of Dietary Assessment	Strengths	Weaknesses
24-hour Dietary Recall	• Can be completed quickly • Easily gathers intake data for large population	• Does not show common intake of an individual • Recall bias • Underreporting
Multiple 24-hour Dietary Recalls	• Better indicator of common intake of an individual than a single day of recall • Can still be completed relatively quickly	• Recall bias • Underreporting
3-Day Food Record	• Gathers average intake of an individual accounting for differences between weekdays and weekends • Collects data in real time, reducing recall bias	• Underreporting • Reduced compliance due to burden on the individual • May lead to incomplete data or recall bias
Food Frequency Questionnaire	• Cost-effective • Relatively quick data gathering • Good for ranking levels of nutrient intake within a population or large group, making comparisons of high and low intake possible. • Good for deriving dietary patterns based on relative frequency of intake of common foods.	• Least accurate assessment method of nutrient intake • Generic reports of data make intake analysis challenging • Recall bias • Inaccurate completion of questionnaire • May miss unique foods eaten by an individual if not common in the population

General Considerations in Nutritional Epidemiologic Studies

Epidemiologic study techniques can be invaluable tools to identify underlying causes of disease within a population, allowing for intervention to moderate or eliminate disease. There are several limitations of epidemiologic research; however, and a good understanding of these limitations is important to designing and interpreting studies.

One of the biggest obstacles to drawing connections between diet and disease outcomes is that measuring diet is a difficult process. As discussed previously, a self-reported diet usually includes several forms of bias that create error in measurement of dietary variables. Even if diet could be measured without any source of error, there are other challenges, not the least of which is that diet is a complex set of exposures that are strongly inter-correlated. For example, an individual who eats a diet high in saturated fat also may eat a diet high in cholesterol, sodium, and trans-fat, making it hard to tease out the effects of each variable. To make matters worse, people who have these sorts of diets may also exercise less, be more obese, and engage in several other behaviors that make it very hard to isolate the effects of one specific factor.

Another major challenge for the nutritional epidemiologist is that it is almost impossible to compare a truly unexposed group to an exposed group. Unlike with behaviors such as smoking, all individuals are exposed to dietary factors to some degree. For example, it is impossible to completely avoid consumption of saturated fat. The best we can do is compare those who appear to be less exposed with those who have relatively higher exposure. When the range of intake of a certain nutrient is narrow, it is very difficult to see the impact of that nutrient on health outcomes. For example, it is likely that early investigations into whether saturated fat and cholesterol are linked to heart disease failed to find a connection because the American public had a very high intake across the population.

To further complicate the problem, eating patterns evolve over time. It is possible that dietary habits in childhood are a major determinant of future health. Unfortunately, current study techniques either reflect poorly or completely fail to capture dietary habits practiced over a lifetime.

Another obstacle in the way of determining the influence of diet on health is that individuals are biologically different from each other and may process nutrients differently. There are some individuals who may tolerate a high fat or high carbohydrate diet well, while others develop disease on the exact same diet.

Finally, there is the problem that food is not consistent. Vitamin content can vary by the soil where the food is grown, how it is stored, and how it is prepared. Farming techniques also change our food supply on the most basic level. A cow fed a corn-based diet is not nutritionally the same as a cow that grazes on grass. We may think we are comparing the proverbial apples to apples, but in reality, often those apples have very different nutrient contents that make our results incomprehensible.

This is not to say that there is no point to trying to study the connections between diet and disease; it simply explains why it is a much more difficult process than the public expects. Only through the refining of our study techniques and continuing to perform well-designed studies across a variety of populations in a variety of circumstances can we ever answer the important questions of nutritional epidemiology and effectively intervene to help people live longer, healthier lives.

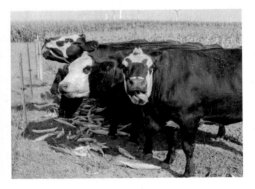

Corn fed cows may not produce nutritionally exact milk of those grass-fed.

© PBouman/Shutterstock.

Strategy Tip

Discuss the many factors that go into calculating one's 24-hour recall or food frequency questionnaire. How will these factors affect the true representation of the nutrient(s) consumed?

The Role of Nutritional Epidemiology in Public Health

Nutritional epidemiology is a key component to understanding how nutrition impacts chronic health conditions commonly targeted by public health efforts. One example of such an effort is the Rethink Your Drink campaign that is implemented across the country. This campaign was created from mounting research that found that sugar-sweetened beverages were linked with increased chance of weight gain, obesity, type 2 diabetes mellitus, and metabolic syndrome.[78] For this reason, billboards, radio advertisements, demonstrations, nutrition education curricula, and other media of communicating this research to the public were created and distributed. In addition to the development of campaigns and programs, public health nutritionists and public health registered dietitians/nutritionists may prepare and implement policy change based on nutritional epidemiology.[79] These positions can be found in departments and offices of public health, state university extension offices, and other organizations focused on community and public health.

More broadly, nutritional epidemiology is at the core of disease prevention through efforts such as the Dietary Guidelines for Americans. Every 5 years, nutrition scientists, including many epidemiologists, review the latest evidence on the relationship between food and development of disease and create an updated set of Dietary Guidelines for Americans.[80] These guidelines are used for things such as setting the standards for Federal Nutrition Programs, including The National School Lunch Program.[81]

Recently, nutritional epidemiology has sought to move public health efforts forward by focusing on very specific applications aimed at clarifying the effect of specific types of foods, nutrients, and dietary patterns on human health and the environment in ways that can inform program creation and public policy. Two examples are the Dietary Inflammatory Index (DII) and the Global Dietary Quality Score (GDQS).

The DII was created by nutritional epidemiologists to measure the impact of specific foods and nutrients on inflammation and how foods in combination affect inflammation. The potential inflammatory effects of diet are an important area of study in preventing chronic diseases, because inflammation can have harmful effects on the body and may promote chronic conditions such as heart disease.[82] The DII is used to measure the inflammatory potential of a person's diet by correlating the effects of 45 foods and nutrients with signs of inflammation in the body.[82-84] Unlike other diet-related indexes such as the Healthy Eating Index, which is based on nutrition recommendations, the DII was designed to provide objective evidence on the inflammatory effect of individual foods to help study relationships between diet, inflammation, and diseases across a wide variety of humans.[83,85]

The Global Diet Quality Score (GDQS) tool was developed to measure diet quality across many different populations in order to better capture and compare nutrition-related health globally.[86] The GDQS is a food-based scoring tool used to determine the healthfulness of a diet. It has 25 food groups, 16 healthy and 9 unhealthy, and points are given based on intake of those food groups using information from food frequency questionnaires or other diet assessments.[86,87] High scores point to a healthier diet, and lower scores indicate a relatively less-healthy diet. It was created using data from cross-sectional and cohort studies from 14 different countries in the Americas, Africa, and Asia. The United States contributed data from the Nurses' Health Study II, the second generation of the Nurses' Health Study, to help create the GDQS.[88-90] The Harvard Global Health Institute initiated and has championed the GDQS with the aim of using information gathered

Read more about the Dietary Inflammatory Index at: https://scholar.google.com/scholar?q=Dietary+inflammatory+index+PDF&hl=en&as_sdt=0&as_vis=1&oi=scholart

Read more about the Global Dietary Quality Score at: https://scholar.google.com/scholar?hl=en&as_sdt=0%2C10&as_vis=1&q=Global+Dietary+Quality+Score&btnG=

by the tool to better share and compare nutrition data across countries. With more comparable information, global policies around health, nutrition, and environmental sustainability can be proposed and evaluated. The GDQS is a big step toward creating a framework to evaluate public health interventions.

Summary

Epidemiology has evolved over the past few centuries to help researchers connect disease with their underlying causes. Although this is not always a straightforward process, it is very valuable in helping direct intervention efforts to minimize the impact of disease. Traditional epidemiologic techniques have been extremely effective in eliminating certain nutrition-related diseases that can be linked to a single cause, such as a vitamin deficiency. More recent applications of epidemiology have become more complex as more diseases with multiple causes are studied.

Chapter 2 focuses on nutritional epidemiology to highlight its place in public health. By reviewing the beginnings of epidemiology, the historical background is set for the development of nutritional epidemiology. From the discovery that citrus fruits could benefit sailors experiencing scurvy to the development of the Nurses' Health Study, nutritional epidemiology has developed to examine the relationships between single nutrients and dietary patterns on various conditions and diseases. To account for the range of topics studied in nutritional epidemiology, various study designs are utilized in the field. Reviewing the types of study designs, their flaws, and their strengths allows for a better understanding of their use throughout the literature. When defining a cause-and-effect response, a randomized controlled trial is the only plausible study design; all other designs fall into a hierarchy that can be better understood through the Bradford-Hill guidelines. Assessing strengths and weaknesses is also relevant to methods of data collection as it can be arduous to gather accurate, appropriate data. Understanding these precepts of nutritional epidemiology allows for a better understanding of the relevance of such studies in the literature as well as how they can be used in the field of public health.

Learning Portfolio

© olies/Shutterstock.

Issues for Discussion

1. Discuss how nutrient recommendations have been affected by epidemiologic studies.
2. Describe the various factors that can be measured for nutritional epidemiologic studies.
3. List and discuss the techniques used to gather information for nutritional epidemiologic studies.
4. Discuss the positives and negatives of the hierarchy of types of studies in research and how to choose the best study for a scenario.

Practical Activities

1. Search for a nutritional epidemiologic study in the literature and consider and/or discuss the following questions. Which study design was used? Was it appropriate? Which method of data collection was implemented? Where does this study fall in the hierarchy of causality?
2. Research another cohort, like the Framingham Heart Study group, which was not discussed in this chapter. What are the focuses of this data collection? Have any studies been conducted yet on the collected data?
3. Think about the nutritional concerns of your community and search for research on this topic. Conceptualize a program or policy change you could implement as a public health professional, based on the scientific evidence, to work toward relieving this issue.

Key Terms

	page
Epidemiology	48
Nutritional epidemiology	48
Hierarchy	51
Prevalence	51
Incidence	52
Causality	52
Recall bias	57
A confounder	59

Case Study: Type 2 Diabetes Epidemiology Study

This case study will provide a scenario in which a nutritional epidemiologic study is warranted. Following the case, there will be questions based upon the scenario presented.

You are a nutritionist working at a community health center providing basic nutrition education through general nutrition group education courses. Prior to the beginning of each course, you ask your clients to fill out a questionnaire that asks about various chronic diseases they have to better tailor your education throughout the course. You notice that over the last year, there has been an increased number of individuals who have reported new onset type 2 diabetes mellitus. You wonder if the increase in this disease is just in the clients whom you are seeing or if this is occurring within the greater community of your health center and that community food and exercise habits may be impacting the trend you have noticed. Your supervisor decides that it would be beneficial for you to look into the trend that you are seeing and conduct a small study using health center resources.

1. What is the purpose of your study?
2. Which type of study design should you choose for your study? What are the strengths and weaknesses of the study design chosen?
3. Which type of dietary assessment method would best fit with your design and purpose? What are the advantages and disadvantages to using this type of method?
4. Would your study result in significant causality? Is that necessary for your purpose?

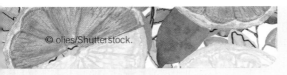

© olies/Shutterstock.

Learning Portfolio

Case Study: Food Frequency Questionnaire

Create an FFQ

1. Which elements would the FFQ contain?

2. What problems in accurate measurement might this instrument have?

3. Why is it more important to use a peer-reviewed FFQ than one an individual might create?

Resources

1. Research Information: http://www.iarc.fr/en/research-groups/NEP/index.php
2. NHANES: http://www.cdc.gov/nchs/nhanes.htm
3. World Health Organization: http://www.who.int/healthinfo/survey/en/

References

1. Editorial. How epidemiology has shaped the COVID pandemic. *Nature.* 2021;589:491-492. https://doi.org/10.1038/d41586-021-00183-z
2. Morawska L, Milton DK. It is time to address airborne transmission of coronavirus disease 2019 (COVID-19). *Clin Infect Dis.* 2020;71(9):2311-2313. https://doi .org/10.1093/cid/ciaa939
3. World Health Organization (WHO). Transmission of SARS-CoV-2: implications for infection prevention precautions. *Scientific Brief.* 2020. Available at: https:// www.who.int/publications/i/item/modes-of-transmission-of-virus-causing-covid-19 -implications-for-ipc-precaution-recommendations
4. Summers J. *Soho—A History of London's Most Colourful Neighborhood.* London, UK: Bloomsbury; 1989:113-117.
5. Teng A, Atkinson J, Disney G, Wilson N, Blakely T. Changing smoking-mortality association over time and across social groups: national census-mortality cohort studies from 1981 to 2011. *Sci Rep.* 2017;7(11465). doi: 10.1038/s41598-017 -11785-x
6. Dietary Guidelines Advisory Committee. *Scientific Report of the 2020 Dietary Guidelines Advisory Committee: Advisory Report to the Secretary of Agriculture and the Secretary of Health and Human Services.* U.S. Department of Agriculture, Agricultural Research Service, Washington, DC: 2020.
7. Van Horn L, Carson JA, Appel LJ, et al. Recommended dietary pattern to achieve adherence to the American Heart Association/American College of Cardiology (AHA/ACC) Guidelines: a scientific statement from the American Heart Association. *Circulation.* 2016;134(22):e505-e529. doi: 10.1161/cir.0000000000000462
8. Grundy SM, Stone NJ, Bailey AL, et al. 2018 AHA/ACC/AACVPR/AAPA/ABC/ ACPM/ADA/AGS/APhA/ASPC/NLA/PCNA Guideline on the Management of Blood Cholesterol: executive summary: a report of the American College of Cardiology/ American Heart Association Task Force on Clinical Practice Guidelines. *J Am Coll Cardiol.* 2019;73(24):3168-3209. doi: 10.1016/j.jacc.2018.11.002. Epub 2018 Nov 10. Erratum in: *J Am Coll Cardiol.* 2019;73(24):3234-3237. PMID: 30423391.
9. Hippocrates. *Hippocratic Writings.* London, UK: Penguin Books; 1983:193.
10. Lind J. *A Treatise on the Scurvy in Three Parts.* London, UK: Millar; 1753.

11. Svirbely JL, Szent-Györgyi AS. The chemical nature of vitamin C. *Biochem J.* 1932;26(3):865-870.

12. Langseth L. *Nutritional Epidemiology: Possibilities and Limitations.* Washington, DC: International Life Sciences Institute; 2000.

13. Satija A, Yu E, Willett WC, Hu FB. Understanding nutritional epidemiology and its role in policy. *Adv Nutr.* 2015;6(1):5-18. doi: 10.3945/an.114.007492. PMID: 25593140; PMCID: PMC4288279.

14. Bhupathiraju SN, Hu FB. Epidemiology of obesity and diabetes and their cardiovascular complications. *Circ Res.* 2016;118(11):1723-1735. doi: 0.1161/CIRCRESAHA.115.306825

15. Long MT, Fox CS. The Framingham Heart Study — 67 years of discovery in metabolic disease. *Nat Rev Endocrinol.* 2016;12(3):177-183. doi: 10.1038/nrendo.2015.226

16. Hinman AR. 1889 to 1989: a century of health and disease. *Public Health Rep.* 1990;105(4):374-380.

17. Mensah GA, Wei GS, Sorlie PD, et al. Decline in cardiovascular mortality. *Cir Res.* 2017;120(2):366-380. doi: 10.1161/circresaha.116.309115

18. Ma J, Jacques PF, Hwang S-J, et al. Dietary Guideline Adherence Index and Kidney Measures in the Framingham Heart Study. *Am J Kidney Dis.* 2016;68(5):703-715. doi: 10.1053/j.ajkd.2016.04.015

19. Mangano KM, Sahni S, Kiel DP, Tucker KL, Dufour AB, Hannan MT. Dietary protein is associated with musculoskeletal health independently of dietary pattern: the Framingham Third Generation Study. *Am J Clin Nutr.* 2017;105(3):714-722. doi: 10.3945/ajcn.116.136762

20. Makarem N, Bandera EV, Lin Y, Jacques PF, Hayes RB, Parekh N. Carbohydrate nutrition and risk of adiposity-related cancers: results from the Framingham Offspring cohort (1991–2013). *Br J Nutr.* 2017;117(11):1603-1614. doi: 10.1017/s0007114517001489

21. Shishtar E, Rogers GT, Blumberg JB, Au R, Jacques PF. Long-term dietary flavonoid intake and risk of Alzheimer disease and related dementias in the Framingham Offspring cohort. *Am J Clin Nutr.* 2020;112(2):343-353. doi: 10.1093/ajcn/nqaa079

22. Foster MC, Hwang S-J, Massaro JM, Jacques PF, Fox CS, Chu AY. Lifestyle factors and indices of kidney function in the Framingham Heart Study. *Am J Nephrol.* 2015;41(4-5):267-274. doi: 10.1159/000430868

23. Walker ME, Xanthakis V, Peterson LR, et al. Dietary patterns, ceramide ratios, and risk of all-cause and cause-specific mortality: the Framingham Offspring Study. *J Nutr.* 2020;150(11):2994-3004. doi: 10.1093/jn/nxaa269

24. Colditz GA, Philpott SE, Hankinson SE. The impact of the Nurses' Health Study on population health: prevention, translation, and control. *Am J Public Health.* 2016;106(9):1540-1545. doi: 10.2105/AJPH.2016.303343. Epub 2016 Jul 26. PMID: 27459441; PMCID: PMC4981811.

25. Li Y, Schoufour J, Wang DD, et al. Healthy lifestyle and life expectancy free of cancer, cardiovascular disease, and type 2 diabetes: prospective cohort study. *BMJ.* 2020;368:l6669. doi: 10.1136/bmj.l6669. PMID: 31915124; PMCID: PMC7190036.

26. Zhang T, Xu J, Li S, et al. Trajectories of childhood BMI and Adult diabetes: the Bogalusa Heart Study. *Diabetologia.* 2018;62(1):70-77. doi: 10.1007/s00125-018-4753-5

27. Muller CJ, Noonan CJ, MacLehose RF, et al. Trends in cardiovascular disease morbidity and mortality in American Indians over 25 Years: the Strong Heart Study. *J Am Heart Assoc.* 2019;8(21). doi: 10.1161/jaha.119.012289

28. Keys AC. *Seven Countries: A Multivariate Analysis of Death and Coronary Heart Disease.* Boston: Harvard University Press; 1980:362-371.

29. Kromhout D, Menotti A, Blackburn H. *Prevention of Coronary Heart Disease: Diet, Lifestyle, and Risk Factors in the Seven Countries Study.* Norwell, MA: Kluwer Academic Publishers; 2002.

30. Centers for Disease Control and Prevention. *National Health and Nutrition Examination Survey.* September 15th, 2017. Accessed February 17, 2021. https://www.cdc.gov/nchs/nhanes/about_nhanes.htm

31. Johnson CL, Dohrmann SM, Burt VL, Mohadjer LK. National health and nutrition examination survey: sample design, 2011–2014. *National Center for Health Statistics. Vital Health Statistics* 2014;2(162).

32. Pickens CM, Pierannunzi C, Garvin W, Town M. Surveillance for certain health behaviors and conditions among states and selected local areas — Behavioral Risk Factor Surveillance System, United States, 2015. *Morbidity and Mortality Weekly Report (MMWR) Surveillance Summaries.* 2018;67(9):1-90. doi: 10.15585/mmwr.ss6709a1

33. Ballestero Fernández C, Varela-Moreiras G, Úbeda N, Alonso-Aperte E. Nutritional status in Spanish children and adolescents with celiac disease on a gluten free diet compared to non-celiac disease controls. *Nutrients.* 2019;11(10):2329. doi: 10.3390/nu11102329. PMID: 31581546; PMCID: PMC6835854.

34. Verlaan S, Aspray TJ, Bauer JM, et al. Nutritional status, body composition, and quality of life in community-dwelling sarcopenic and non-sarcopenic older adults: a case-control study. *Clin Nutr.* 2017;36(1):267-274. doi: 10.1016/j.clnu.2015.11.013. Epub 2015 Nov 27. PMID: 26689868.

35. Radujkovic A, Hippchen T, Tiwari-Heckler S, Dreher S, Boxberger M, Merle U. Vitamin D deficiency and outcome of COVID-19 patients. *Nutrients.* 2020;12(9):2757. doi: 10.3390/nu12092757. PMID: 32927735; PMCID: PMC7551780.

36. Leiva-Gea I, Sánchez-Alcoholado L, Martín-Tejedor B, et al. Gut microbiota differs in composition and functionality between children with type 1 diabetes and MODY2 and healthy control subjects: a case-control study. *Diabet Care.* 2018;41(11):2385-2395. doi: 10.2337/dc18-0253. Epub 2018 Sep 17. PMID: 30224347.

37. Wang T, Heianza Y, Sun D, et al. Improving adherence to healthy dietary patterns, genetic risk, and long term weight gain: gene-diet interaction analysis in two prospective cohort studies. *BMJ.* 2018;360:j5644. doi: 10.1136/bmj.j5644

38. Eckel N, Li Y, Kuxhaus O, Stefan N, Hu FB, Schulze MB. Transition from metabolic healthy to unhealthy phenotypes and association with cardiovascular disease risk across BMI categories in 90 257 women (the Nurses' Health Study): 30 year follow-up from a prospective cohort study. *Lancet*

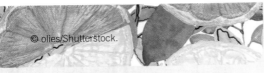

Learning Portfolio

Diabet Endocrinol. 2018;6(9):714-724. doi: 10.1016/s2213-8587(18)30137-2

39. Bao Y, Bertoia ML, Lenart EB, et al. Origin, methods, and evolution of the three Nurses' Health Studies. *Am J Public Health.* 2016;106(9):1573-1581. doi: 10.2105/ajph.2016.303338

40. Andersson C, Johnson AD, Benjamin EJ, Levy D, Vasan RS. 70-year legacy of the Framingham Heart Study. *Nat Rev Cardiol.* 2019;16(11):687-698. doi: 10.1038/s41569-019-0202-5

41. Wang W, Lee ET, Howard BV, Devereux R, Zhang Y, Stoner JA. Large cohort data based cost-effective disease prevention design strategy: Strong Heart Study. *World J Cardiovasc Dis.* 2018;8(12):588-601. PMID: 30687583 PMCID: PMC6343848 doi: 10.4236/wjcd.2018.812058

42. Berg ZK, Rodriguez B, Davis J, Katz AR, Cooney RV, Masaki K. Association between occupational exposure to pesticides and cardiovascular disease incidence: the Kuakini Honolulu Heart Program. *J Am Heart Assoc.* 2019;8(19). doi: 10.1161/jaha.119.012569

43. Nishioka S, Wakabayashi H, Momosaki R. Nutritional status changes and activities of daily living after hip fracture in convalescent rehabilitation units: a retrospective observational cohort study from the Japan Rehabilitation Nutrition Database. *J Acad Nutr Diet.* 2018;118(7):1270-1276. doi: 10.1016/j.jand.2018.02.012. Epub 2018 May 8. PMID: 29752190.

44. Chiavaroli L, Viguiliouk E, Nishi SK, et al. DASH dietary pattern and cardiometabolic outcomes: an umbrella review of systematic reviews and meta-analyses. *Nutrients.* 2019;11(2):338. doi: 10.3390/nu11020338. PMID: 30764511; PMCID: PMC6413235.

45. Filippou CD, Tsioufis CP, Thomopoulos CG, et al. Dietary Approaches to Stop Hypertension (DASH) diet and blood pressure reduction in adults with and without hypertension: a systematic review and meta-analysis of randomized controlled trials. *Adv Nutr.* 2020;11(5):1150-1160. doi: 10.1093/advances/nmaa041. PMID: 32330233; PMCID: PMC7490167.

46. Cauley JA, Crandall C. The Women's Health Initiative: a landmark resource for skeletal research since 1992. *J Bone Miner Res.* 2020;35(5):845-860. doi: 10.1002/jbmr.4026. Epub 2020 Apr 21. PMID: 32286708.

47. Chlebowski RT, Aragaki AK, Anderson GL, et al. Dietary modification and breast cancer mortality: long-term follow-up of the Women's Health Initiative Randomized Trial. *J Clin Oncol.* 2020;38(13):1419-1428. doi: 10.1200/JCO.19.00435. Epub 2020 Feb 7. PMID: 32031879; PMCID: PMC7193750.

48. Martínez-González MA, Salas-Salvadó J, Estruch R, et al. Benefits of the Mediterranean diet: insights from the PREDIMED study. *Prog Cardiovasc Dis.* 2015;58(1):50-60. doi: 10.1016/j.pcad.2015.04.003. Epub 2015 May 1. PMID: 25940230.

49. Salas-Salvadó J, Díaz-López A, Ruiz-Canela M, et al. Effect of a lifestyle intervention program with energy-restricted Mediterranean diet and exercise on weight loss and cardiovascular risk factors: one-year results of the PREDIMED-Plus trial. *Diabet Care.* 2019;42(5):777-788. doi: 10.2337/dc18-0836. Epub 2018 Nov 2. PMID: 30389673.

50. Perry CL, Stone EJ, Parcel GS, et al. School-based cardiovascular health promotion: the Child and Adolescent Trial for Cardiovascular Health (CATCH). *J Sch Health.* 1990;60(8):406-413.

51. Haring B, von Ballmoos MC, Appel LJ, Sacks FM. Healthy dietary interventions and lipoprotein (a) plasma levels: results from the Omni Heart Trial. *PLoS One.* 2014;9(12):e114859. doi: 10.1371/journal.pone.0114859. PMID: 25506933; PMCID: PMC4266632.

52. Bhide A, Shah PS, Acharya G. A simplified guide to randomized controlled trials. *Acta Obstetricia et Gynecologica Scandinavica.* 2018;97(4):380-387. doi: 10.1111/aogs.13309

53. Hill AB. The environment and disease: association or causation? *Proc Royal Soc Med.* 1965;58:295-300.

54. Truong TT, Ryutov A, Pandey U, et al. Persistent SARS-CoV-2 infection and increasing viral variants in children and young adults with impaired humoral immunity. *EBioMedicine.* 2021. doi: 10.1101/2021.02.27.21252099. PMID: 33688673; PMCID: PMC7941650.

55. Rodriguez F, Maron DJ, Knowles JW, Virani SS, Lin S, Heidenreich PA. Association of statin adherence with mortality in patients with atherosclerotic cardiovascular disease. *JAMA Cardiol.* 2019;4(3):206-213. doi: 10.1001/jamacardio.2018.4936. PMID: 30758506; PMCID: PMC6439552.

56. Dunn BK, Kramer BS. Cancer prevention: lessons learned and future directions. *Trends Cancer.* 2016;2(12):713-722. doi: 10.1016/j.trecan.2016.11.003. PMID: 28138568; PMCID: PMC5271581.

57. Naska A, Lagiou A, Lagiou P. Dietary assessment methods in epidemiological research: current state of the art and future prospects. *F1000Res.* 2017;6:926. doi: 10.12688/f1000research.10703.1

58. Walton J. Dietary assessment methodology for nutritional assessment. *Top Clin Nutr.* 2015;30(1):33-46. doi: 10.1097/tin.0000000000000018

59. Friedenreich CM, Slimani N, Riboli E. Measurement of past diet: review of previous and proposed methods. *Epidemiol Rev.* 1992;14(1):177-196.

60. Subar AF, Freedman LS, Tooze JA, et al. Addressing current criticism regarding the value of self-report dietary data. *J Nutr.* 2015;145(12):2639-2645. doi: 10.3945/jn.115.219634

61. Knüppel S, Norman K, Boeing H. Is a single 24-hour dietary recall per person sufficient to estimate the population distribution of usual dietary intake? *J Nutr.* 2019;149(9):1491-1492. doi: 10.1093/jn/nxz118

62. Castell GS, Serra-Majem L, Ribas-Barba L. What and how much do we eat? 24-hour dietary recall method. *Nutrición Hospitalaria.* 2015;31(3):46-48.

63. Karvetti RL, Knuts LR. Validity of the 24-hour dietary recall. *J Am Diet Assoc.* 1985;85(11):1437-1442.

64. Willett W. In: Nutritional Epidemiology. 3rd ed. New York: Oxford University Press; 2013:50-62.

65. Kahn HA, Whelton PK, Appel LJ, et al. Validity of 24-hour dietary recall interviews conducted among volunteers in an adult working community. *Ann Epidemiol.* 1995;5(6):484-489.

66. Burrows TL, Ho YY, Rollo ME, Collins CE. Validity of dietary assessment methods when compared to the method of doubly

labeled water: a systematic review in adults. *Front Endocrinol.* 2019;10. doi: 10.3389/fendo.2019.00850

67. Walker JL, Ardouin S, Burrows T. The validity of dietary assessment methods to accurately measure energy intake in children and adolescents who are overweight or obese: a systematic review. *Eur J Clin Nutr.* 2018;72(2):185-197. doi: 10.1038/s41430-017-0029-2

68. Freedman LS, Commins JM, Moler JE, et al. Pooled results from 5 validation studies of dietary self-report instruments using recovery biomarkers for potassium and sodium intake. *Am J Epidemiol.* 2015;181(7):473-487. doi: 10.1093/aje/kwu325

69. Steinemann N, Grize L, Ziesemer K, Kauf P, Probst-Hensch N, Brombach C. Relative validation of a food frequency questionnaire to estimate food intake in an adult population. *Food Nutr Res.* 2017;61(1):1305193. doi: 10.1080/16546628.2017.1305193

70. Molag ML, de Vries JH, Ocké MC, et al. Design characteristics of food frequency questionnaires in relation to their validity. *Am J Epidemiol.* 2007;166:1468-1478.

71. Noethlings U, Hoffmann K, Bergmann MM, Boeing H. Portion size adds limited information on variance in food intake of participants in the EPIC-Potsdam study. *J Nutr.* 2003;133(2):510-515.

72. Kang M, Park S-Y, Boushey CJ, et al. Portion sizes from 24-hour dietary recalls differed by sex among those who selected the same portion size category on a food frequency questionnaire. *J Acad Nutr Dietet.* 2018;118(9):1711-1718. doi: 10.1016/j.jand.2018.02.014

73. Shim J-S, Oh K, Kim HC. Dietary assessment methods in epidemiologic studies. *Epidemiol Health.* 2014;36:e2014009. doi: 10.4178/epih/e2014009

74. Visser M, Elstgeest LE, Winkens LH, Brouwer IA, Nicolaou M. Relative validity of the HELIUS Food Frequency Questionnaire for measuring dietary intake in older adult participants of the longitudinal aging study Amsterdam. *Nutrients.* 2020;12(7):1998. doi: 10.3390/nu12071998. PMID: 32635636; PMCID: PMC7400819

75. Zheng M, Campbell KJ, Scanlan E, McNaughton SA. Development and evaluation of a food frequency questionnaire for use among young children. *PLoS One.* 2020;15(3):e0230669. doi: 10.1371/journal.pone.0230669. PMID: 32210467; PMCID: PMC7094848.

76. Carroll RJ, Freedman LS, Hartman AM. Use of semiquantitative food frequency questionnaires to estimate the distribution of usual intake. *Am J Epidemiol.* 1996;143(4):392-404.

77. Fraser GE. A search for truth in dietary epidemiology. *Am J Clin Nutr.* 2003;78(suppl 3):521S-525S.

78. Malik VS, Hu FB. Sugar-sweetened beverages and cardio-metabolic health: an update of the evidence. *Nutrients.* 2019;11(8):1840. doi: 10.3390/nu11081840

79. Bruening M, Udarbe AZ, Jimenez EY, Crowley PS, Fredericks DC, Edwards Hall, LA. Academy of nutrition and dietetics: standards of practice and standards of professional performance for registered dietitian nutritionists (competent, proficient, and expert) in public health and community nutrition. *J Acad Nutr Diet.* 2015;115(10):1699-1709.

80. History of the *Dietary Guidelines.* Accessed March 19, 2021. https://www.dietaryguidelines.gov/about-dietary-guidelines/history-dietary-guidelines#:~:text=diet%20and%20health.-,USDA%20and%20HHS%20Collaborate%20to%20develop%20the%20Dietary%20Guidelines,in%20making%20daily%20food%20choices

81. The National Academies of Sciences, Engineering, and Medicine; Health and Medicine Division; Food and Nutrition Board; Committee to Review the Process to Update the Dietary Guidelines for Americans. Redesigning the process for establishing the *Dietary Guidelines for Americans.* Washington (DC): *Nat Acad Press* (US). 2017; PMID: 29232083.

82. Cavicchia PP, Steck SE, Hurley TG, et al. A new dietary inflammatory index predicts interval changes in serum high-sensitivity C-reactive protein. *J Nutr.* 2009;139(12):2365-2372. doi: 10.3945/jn.109.114025

83. Shivappa N, Steck SE, Hussey JR, Ma Y, Hebert JR. Inflammatory potential of diet and all-cause, cardiovascular, and cancer mortality in National Health and Nutrition Examination Survey III Study. *Eur J Nutr.* 2017;56(2):683-692. doi: 10.1007/s00394-015-1112-x

84. King DE, Xiang J. The dietary inflammatory index is associated with diabetes severity. *J Am Board Fam Med.* 2019;32(6):801-806. doi: 10.3122/jabfm.2019.06.190092

85. Hébert JR, Shivappa N, Wirth MD, Hussey JR, Hurley TG. Perspective: the Dietary Inflammatory Index (DII)—lessons learned, improvements made, and future directions. *Adv Nutr.* 2019;10(2):185-195. doi: 10.1093/advances/nmy071

86. Fung T, Bromage S, Li Y, et al. A global diet quality index and risk of type 2 diabetes in U.S. women. *Curr Dev Nutr* 2020;4(suppl 2):1401-1401. doi: 10.1093/cdn/nzaa061_029

87. Bromage S, Zhang Y, Holmes M, et al. A novel food-based diet quality score is associated with nutrient adequacy and reduced anemia among rural adults in ten African countries. *Curr Dev Nutr.* 2020;4(suppl 2):1381. doi: 10.1093/cdn/nzaa061_009

88. Global Diet Quality Score (GDQS). Bromage S. https://scholar.harvard.edu/sabri/save-date. 2021.

89. Belanger CF, Hennekens CH, Rosner B, Speizer FE. The Nurses' Health Study. *Am J Nurs.* 1978;78:1039-1040.

90. Fung T, Bromage S, Li Y, et al. A global diet quality index and weight gain in U.S. women. *J Acad Nutr Diet.* 2020;120(9):A73. doi: 10.1016/j.jand.2020.06.045

PART II

Shaping the Policies that Affect the Public's Health

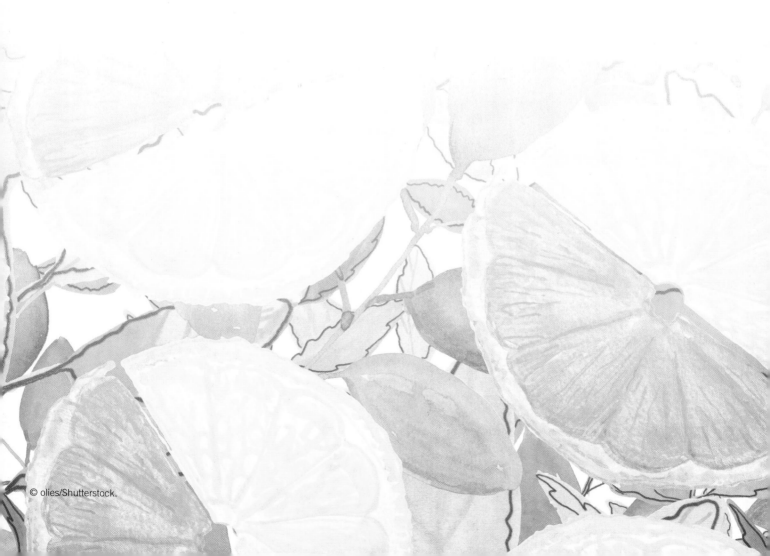

CHAPTER 3

Creating and Influencing Public and Nutrition Policy

Jody L. Vogelzang, PhD, RDN, FAND, CHES
(We would like to acknowledge the work of Bruce Rengers, PhD, RDN, in past editions of Nutrition in Public Health.)

Learning Outcomes

AFTER STUDYING THIS CHAPTER AND REFLECTING ON THE CONTENTS, YOU SHOULD BE ABLE TO:

1. Define public policy.
2. Explain the characteristics and importance of public policy.
3. Evaluate the ethical tensions that exist in public health policy.
4. Discuss the evolution of nutrition policy in the United States.
5. Describe the role various levels of government play in creating public health policy.
6. Explore the role of the individual nutrition professional in advocating for health policy.

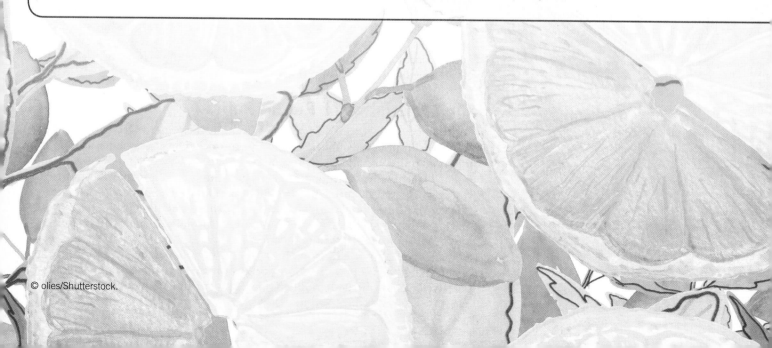

Introduction

To accomplish something in an organized and efficient manner, you must have a goal and a plan of action. This is the reason for creating policy. In a general sense, a policy is a set of rules to solve a problem, real or perceived. Most policies consist of two parts 1) a statement or goal of what is to be accomplished, and 2) a set of practical rules, guidelines, programs, or regulations to accomplish the stated goal.

This chapter is about public policy, specifically public health policy as it relates to nutrition. Policy is labeled **public policy** when it is created by federal, state, or local government. The government creates policies to regulate its own actions and to govern the actions of citizens, businesses, and other entities under its control. Ultimately, what a government does is a reflection of its public policy. Some would say that what the government does is public policy, regardless of what may be written or stated.

Birkland describes public policy as having several attributes, including being made in the public's interest, that it is interpreted and implemented by public and private actors, that it is a reflection of what the government intends to do, and what the government chooses not to do. Policy is also more than simply the sum total of all of the government's laws and regulation. Policy is also created daily by people as they implement policy.[3]

At the federal level, public policy may be created by the legislative, executive, or judicial branch of government. Generally, policy is created by legislation that is introduced and passed by the legislative branch. This legislation or policy is then translated into a set of practical rules by the executive branch to accomplish the intent of the legislation. Policy, however, also may be informal, indirect, and even unwritten. For example, a governing political party may have a philosophical belief of government involvement in food regulation. This philosophy becomes the government's guiding public policy. **Special interest groups**, professional organizations, trade groups, and influential individuals may also play an important role in determining public policy.

Government policy is reflected as much in what the government won't do as in what it will do. Many unwritten and informal policies are more about what the government will not be involved in. If the government identifies a problem, such as advertising directed at children, and then takes no action to regulate such advertising, this is a reflection of government policy. The decision not to become involved may be based on philosophies of downsizing government, reducing spending, decreasing regulation, responding to special interest groups, or even a distrust of the evidence that says such advertising may be harmful. Because these philosophies direct the actions of the government, they become part of public policy.

Characteristics of Public Policy

Policy is generally created in response to a problem, perceived or real. In an ideal world, policy would be created from objective assessments to identify potential problems and then prevent them. This, however, is rarely how public policy is created. Government officials generally create policy in response to emerging or existing problems that are important to the public, special interest groups, or professional or scientific groups. These emerging problems may be real or only perceived problems. Sometimes, popular belief or philosophies may result in identification of a concept as a symptom of a problem or as a root cause of a problem, when in fact there is little evidence to support the belief. It has been stated that more public policies fail from working to solve a perceived, yet invalidated, problem than from creating the wrong plan to solve

Public policy[2] The principles, often unwritten, on which social laws are based.

Special interest group May convince policy makers to create or avoid legislation that would affect their interests. Food and nutrition issues are frequently brought forward by professional associations such as the Academy of Nutrition and Dietetics, The American Public Health Association, and the Society of Nutrition Education and Behavior. These organizations may disseminate policy in a document called a "White Paper" which advocate for a certain position or solution.

a real problem. Many policy issues are emotionally or financially driven, and solutions are created based on philosophical beliefs rather than an objective understanding of the facts.

Public policy is often controversial. Because it generally affects a great number and variety of people and interests, it tends to be more controversial than less expansive private policies. Public policy generally results in some form of control that limits the **autonomy** of individuals so that the majority may experience a greater benefit. This ethical theory of looking at the greater good is referred to as utilitarianism and is a foundational consideration in much of public health policy. There are those who believe the government should limit its role and allow society to function with minimal interference. Under this philosophy of limited involvement, economics and the free market create an environment where individuals have responsibility for their own actions and situations.

This is in contrast to a social justice philosophy, which acknowledges that society may share in the responsibility for a person's health. Although it may be true that a person who overeats is responsible for their diet, there also may be societal determinants that strongly influence a person's diet. For example, a person working for low wages in a decaying neighborhood without grocery stores or public transportation may have few options other than to buy calorie-dense foods from a local convenience store.

Public policy may be needed to alter environmental conditions in order for a person to have a reasonable ability to choose a healthy diet and lifestyle. This may include advocating for a fair living wage, improved public transportation or improved food shopping options. Some argue that it is the role of the government to create or at least support, conditions that make healthy choices easier and unhealthy choices harder. Through the changing of the food landscape, healthy, affordable, and accessible foods provide choice and promote autonomy.

The mission of community and public health is to assure conditions in which people can be healthy. To assure these conditions requires policies that result in government intervention. The decision to limit personal choices and freedoms cannot be taken for granted; however, the benefit from such public policies must be balanced against economic costs and losses of individual freedom.

In the United States, we are conflicted with these two philosophies of public policy. For example, we want the government to ensure that our food supply is healthy, yet we also want the personal freedom to purchase unhealthy food. This tension presents an ethical dilemma as we balance autonomy and beneficence in all issues related to community and public health. We want it both ways—freedom to make harmful choices, yet protection from harm when we do make those choices.[4-6]

While many argue for less government, public policy is necessary in a complex society, especially to safeguard health. To use a simple example, in a nation with little population and only a few cars, no significant public policy may be necessary with respect to automobiles. In a nation with millions of automobiles crowded into a dense area, public policies are needed with respect to driving, parking, passenger safety, road building and maintenance, car manufacturing, auto emissions, and even car disposal.

The same idea can easily be applied to other health issues in a society. For example, as societies become larger, it becomes more important that a family not dump its sewage and other waste into a commonly used local water supply. Or, as our food supply changes and becomes more processed, policies are needed to ensure a nutritious and safe food supply; and develop a system by which consumers are informed of these changes, such as the Nutrition Facts

Autonomy The ability to make uncoerced, informed choices.

Community and Public Health Strategy

Communities should consider adding grocery stores for fresh food accessibility through public policy.

Discussion Prompt

Have a class discussion on a person's right to eat unhealthy food if they choose. What steps can be taken to persuade people to want to be healthy?

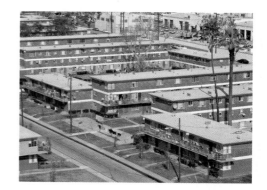

Inner cities can become food deserts, without a grocery store providing fresh food.

© Trekandshoot/Shutterstock.

Code of Federal Regulations (CFR)
The codification of the general and permanent rules published in the Federal Register by the executive departments and agencies of the federal government. It is divided into 50 titles that represent broad areas subject to federal regulation. (www.ecfr.gov This is not the legal version of the CFR but is updated electronically on a daily basis. www.gpo.gov This is the annual legal version of the CFR)

Discussion Prompt

How does public policy affect societal rights? Is this good or bad?

label. In a democratic society, there must be a balance between the need to create a healthier society and the need to maintain personal freedoms.

As a result of a need for public policy in a complex society, public policy touches almost every aspect of our lives. One only need visit the government documents section of a library or peruse the **Code of Federal Regulations (CFR)** to see that there are numerous public policies that affect our daily lives. Public policy is a reality. Life in a complex society without policies would be difficult and disorderly. Policy development for community living is a universal requirement.

U.S. Public Health Policy

Government has many reasons for being interested in the health of its citizens. A democratic government is elected by its citizens, and, therefore, has an interest in the welfare of the citizens who have created it. Beyond the needs of individual health, the collective health of a country's citizens is vital to a country's economic health and independence as a nation. Health is a social as well as individual responsibility.

Many of the major improvements in the health of the American people have come about because of changes in public health policy. By one estimate, 25 of the last 30 years added to the U.S. life expectancy rate have been a result of changes brought about by public health policy. Since 1990, 44% of the improved life expectancy was related to community and public health interventions, supported by public policy.[7]

The successes of public health are frequently taken for granted and only noticed when they fail. Health policy is determined more by crises, hot issues, politics, and the concerns of organized interest groups than careful analysis of objective data and technical knowledge about health.

Pandemic Learning Opportunity

In the COVID-19 pandemic, mask wearing became a politically charged public health issue. Instead of relying on technical and evidence-based information regarding mask wearing as one of the essential steps in preventing the spread of the virus, millions of Americans refused to comply. Those who masked and those refusing became a political lightning rod. What did we learn from this instance?

Nutrition Policy: A Brief History

As with the national health policy in general, there is no single or unifying public policy that guides the activities of government agencies with respect to nutrition in the United States. Nutrition policy is fragmented among numerous laws, agencies, programs, and branches of the government. Nutrition policy is often conflicting and inconsistent. Much of it is antiquated, having been created in the past when different nutritional problems affected the public.

At the beginning of the 20th century, little was known about nutrition. The main nutritional concerns of most people and the government were related to getting enough food to eat and avoiding foods that would make people sick. Early nutrition policy was, therefore, primarily agricultural policy. The government created policies to provide the population with a consistent and plentiful food supply at low cost. Because getting adequate calories was a major concern, emphasis was placed on providing foods that were a dense source of calories. These agricultural policies of the past had a major impact on shaping food supply that continues to this day.

With the discovery of vitamins in the early part of the twentieth century, nutrition experts began to create guidelines providing direction on food choices based on science. In 1917, the USDA created the Five Food Groups to encourage people to eat food that provided all of the then-known nutrients. This guide was modified over time into a variety of forms to ensure that people were eating well-balanced diets. It wouldn't be until much later that nutrition guidelines from the government would start mentioning moderating, or limiting, intakes of certain types of foods, such as those high in fat or sodium.

During the first half of the twentieth century, other nutrition policies were enacted, including fortification of salt with iodine, food distribution programs to feed children and other hungry people during the depression of the 1930s, the first Nationwide Food Consumption Survey, and establishment of the National School Lunch Program. In 1941, the first set of Recommended Dietary Allowances (RDAs) was published, making recommendations for levels of certain nutrients in the diet. The emphasis was still on getting an adequate diet and avoiding nutrient deficiencies.

During the 1960s, the attention of the public health community started to change from an emphasis on infectious diseases to one on chronic diseases. Many accomplishments had been made in controlling communicable disease, and chronic diseases had become the main causes of death in the United States. Public interest in nutrition, environment, and its effects on long-term health was heightened by the publication of books in the popular press by Adelle Davis, Rachel Carson, and others, which stirred interest and controversy in the long-term effects of food, food additives, and environmental pollutants on health. Continued interest in ensuring that people got enough food led to the establishment of the Food Stamp Program (now called Supplemental Nutrition Assistance Program [SNAP]), School Breakfast Program, and the Special Supplemental Food Program for Women, Infants and Children (WIC) during the 1960s and 1970s.

In 1977, the Senate Select Committee on Nutrition and Human Needs issued the first edition of the Dietary Goals for the United States. It was one of the first governmental attempts at making nutritional recommendations, based on theories about the effects of diet on chronic disease. This started a change in dietary recommendations that addressed moderation of certain foods and making choices between foods within a food group. The focus of recommendations and policy was changing from just getting an adequate diet to making qualitative choices related to diet. Moderation and choosing one type of food over another because of its effects on chronic disease became important.

Since the Dietary Goals for the United States were released, many government documents have been created that make recommendations about diet with respect to chronic diseases. The Surgeon General Report on Nutrition and Health presented the first comprehensive review of the scientific evidence associating diet with chronic disease. Nutrition and Your Health: Dietary Guidelines for Americans, created by DHHS and USDA and jointly published every 5 years since 1980, recommended dietary changes to help people avoid certain chronic diseases. The Dietary Guidelines were intended to be the foundation of all federal nutrition policies and programs and a vehicle for the government to speak with one voice on nutrition and health. Unfortunately, many federal policies, such as agricultural policies, do not follow the Dietary Guidelines and promote foods high in components such as saturated fat and sodium that are overconsumed by the public.

The Farm Bill was passed in 1933 when Franklin Roosevelt was president. It was written in the midst of the Great Depression when farmers needed financial stability and the government was committed to having an adequate food supply. These same issues continue to be included in the Farm Bill almost 90 years later.

Discussion Prompt

Were rights violated in forming these food assistance programs?

The Healthy People initiative led by the DHHS Office of Disease Prevention and Health Promotion has become the latest model for policy development, including nutrition policy. For the past 4 decades, Healthy People has been committed to improving the quality of United States health by producing a framework for community and public health prevention priorities and actions. The most recent version, Healthy People 2030, was developed by DHHS with input from all of its operating divisions, state and local government partners, national membership organizations, nongovernmental organizations, corporate sponsors, and public input. Going beyond just federal government involvement, the meeting of the 355 measurable health objectives requires collaboration between all levels of governmental and nongovernmental health organizations. It has been suggested that Healthy People 2030 may be DHHS's most effective nonlegislative policy vehicle for improving public health.

Nutrition Policy: Goals and Methods

If the goal of community public health policy is "fulfilling society's interest in assuring conditions in which people can be healthy," then nutrition policy would have the goal of assuring conditions in which people can be healthy through diet. There are two broad ways that are used to try to influence what people eat: through health promotion and health education, and through modification of the food supply. For example, if a group of people were found to have a nutritional problem with inadequate amounts of vitamin A in the diet, the approach would be to teach them about the need for and sources of vitamin A and assure that they have culturally acceptable, inexpensive, and appealing sources of vitamin A available. Another approach to finding a culturally acceptable and appealing source of vitamin A would be to create a new source for the vitamin through fortification of food, as has been done with some nutrients in the United States. This approach only works; however, when the lacking substances are known nutrients that can be easily added to common foods that are readily available.[7]

The problem becomes more complicated when the major nutritional problems being encountered are ones of excess, as with calories, sodium, and certain types of fat, or when whole food groups need to be increased, such as with fruits and vegetables. How does government create policies to discourage the consumption of certain foods and encourage the consumption of others?

The preferred policy method by many is education: training the public on which foods should be consumed and which foods should be avoided or eaten in moderation. This may be accomplished through social media campaigns, mandated nutrition education in food assistance programs, and community and public health programming. However, using education to influence food choices is effective only if nutritious food is the easiest and cheapest choice. Some may argue that a more powerful way to influence dietary choices is through modifying the food supply. Foods that are healthful should be more readily available and less expensive than those that would be considered less healthful or that are currently eaten in excess. Some have argued that the current obesity epidemic is due to a toxic environment in which the wrong types of foods are readily available in supersized amounts.[8] Portion sizes of foods in restaurants have increased, the number of convenience foods has multiplied, and vending machines make low-nutrient foods readily available almost everywhere. A change in the food supply, coupled with education, is generally considered a more successful strategy for dietary change.

Discussion Prompt

We use influencers online today. What do they influence?

Government policies have a great impact on what foods are available to the public and at what price. Many of the current food policies come from a time when providing adequate food at a cheap price was the goal of U.S. agricultural and nutrition policy. The conditions and health issues that existed when those policies were created are not the same as what exists now. From a nutrition policy point of view, these policies need to be reevaluated to create food policies that support the sustainable production, equitable and transparent marketing, and affordability and accessibility of foods that are associated with a healthier diet. This is not a readily acceptable option to many; however, because it means dramatic changes in economic realities for those whose livelihoods depend on current government food and agricultural policy.[9-11] Beyond agricultural policy, there are ways to control the food supply that have been tried or suggested. Some of these suggestions include altering school lunch menus to meet the Dietary Guidelines, offering low-cost or free fruits and vegetables to schools, free doubling of fruits and vegetables purchased at farmer's markets, adding fruits and vegetables and limiting the fat content in WIC food packages, limiting vending machines and pouring rights for soft drinks in schools, taxing soda, making water available throughout the day in child and adult food programs, removing candy from the checkout stands of supermarkets, and providing nutrition information on menus and/or menu boards.[12-15]

Another way the government attempts to modify the food supply, at least for a select part of the population, is through redistribution. The government purchases foods for those who lack resources to purchase healthy or adequate amounts of food. The Supplemental Nutrition Assistance Program (SNAP), WIC, and commodities programs are examples of these types of programs.[16] Nutrition policy is also required for nutrition monitoring and surveillance, research, food assistance, licensure, and food safety and quality.

Policy Formulation

Policy formation is a complex, dynamic, and sometimes difficult process. In an ideal world, nutrition policy would be formed using an accurate community assessment focused on community values, nutritional needs, the latest scientific information about nutrition, and information about effective strategies. Policy evaluations would be formative and summative, revised as needed, and would be created proactively to prevent as well as to solve problems. Nutrition policy would be integrated with other public policies, and all public policies would be supportive of the same goals. This is the thinking behind the initiative of the Centers for Disease Control and Prevention's "Health in All Policies" (HiAP). The goal of this initiative is to meld national health strategies with the Healthy People objectives so that collaboration can occur across various sectors in both the recommendation and implementation of health policy.

Public policy is created in a political environment. Although community and public health officials prefer to look at problems and solutions in an objective manner, valuing technical expertise and scientific data, most policymakers work in a political environment where public values, popular opinions, and organized special interest groups have considerable influence. There are many players in the public policy development process, and some are considered more important than others. There are special interest groups, social media influencers, congressional committees and subcommittees, agencies of the executive branch of government, professional organizations,

Discussion Prompt

Is removing candy from check-out stands a good policy? Why? Does this violate rights? What should we do?

political parties, private and nonprofit organizations, economic and religious groups, individuals, and the traditional media outlets. Each of these has its own perspectives and philosophies that influence what is perceived as problems and what solutions should be created to solve problems. Scientific evidence may or may not coincide with the views of these groups. In the political process, all views become important, and public health officials must work to put forward solutions to problems that are objective and consistent with scientific evidence. To many politicians, the opinion of public health officials may be just another opinion, and not necessarily an important, informed opinion.[11,12]

Policy is generally created to solve a specific problem—often an emerging problem—that has generated public concern. As stated earlier in this chapter, the problem may be real or it may simply be something that is perceived to be a problem. The more severe the problem is perceived to be and the more public interest the problem generates, the more likely it will result in new policy.[17]

Most policies are created in an incremental fashion. Public officials prefer **incrementalism** because it allows them to draw on past experience, work within an existing framework, and avoid major changes that could create large, unforeseen problems and political fallout. On the other hand, incrementalism stifles innovation and may add to the complexity of existing policy. If multiple small changes are made to a policy to solve immediate problems, sometimes the overall integrity of the original policy starts to break down. This is often observed in federal food programs, where incremental policy changes continue to add policy requirements without making changes to the overall program to accommodate these changes.

Once policies are created, there is a reluctance to change them, especially as they become accepted practice. Old policies, which become ineffective because the conditions for which they were created have changed, often stay in force because of resistance to change. Changing old policies is especially difficult when economic interests are dependent on the old policy. As noted by the Institutes of Medicine (IOM) and others, much of U.S. public health policy was created at a time when conditions were quite different from what they are today, i.e., the Farm Bill, which began in 1933 in the middle of the Great Depression.

Most political scientists identify at least four steps for creating public policy:

1. Agenda setting
2. Policy formulation
3. Policy implementation
4. Policy evaluation

Agenda Setting

The first steps in creating new policy are to identify the problem to be solved, create broad goals to resolve the problem, and then position the issue on the policymaker's agenda. A number of potential problems may make it difficult or impossible to move beyond these steps in policy creation, however.

Identify the Real Problem and Create Goals

Identifying the real problem may be easier than it sounds. For example, one of the goals of Healthy People 2030 is to reduce foodborne illnesses in the United States by improving food safety-related behaviors and practices. There are many theories about why food safety continues to be a problem in

Incrementalism Policy making in small steps, rather than with large comprehensive reforms.

the United States, but which reason (production, processing, packing, distribution/transportation, or storage) may be the real reason(s) and, therefore, most important for further policy development?

Changes to which of them would have the greatest impact on foodborne illness rates? Public opinion, people's belief structures, and special interest groups may be passionate about their views on what prevents foodborne illness rates from decreasing, but the real reasons may not be readily apparent. Creating policy to solve the wrong problem would have a limited impact on food safety outcomes.

Promoting Policymaker Initiatives

Once problems have been identified and policy goals set, public health officials need to create a plan to get their recommended policy on the policymaker's agenda. Although the value of creating a policy to deal with a nutrition issue may be obvious to community and public health officials, it may not be to policymakers. In addition, getting a policy issue on the political agenda may be difficult and time-consuming. In general, policy issues are more likely to get on the political agenda when a great number of people believe the problem is real, and when people believe the consequences of the problem are likely to be severe, immediate, and affect them personally.

Even when a problem is perceived by many people to be a threat, it still may not get on the political agenda. Policymakers must believe that the problem is something that warrants government intervention. There must also be room on the political agenda, and the issue must have enough priority over other issues. In a year when there are many significant problems facing policymakers, even an important issue may not make the political agenda. Special interest groups that are opposed to a policy may also have enough clout to prevent a worthy policy issue from making the political agenda.[18,19]

Lawmakers and the public must believe that a new policy is actually a legitimate policy for the government to make. What the public believes is legitimate for policymakers to tackle changes over time. One only has to look at how nonsmoking policies have changed over the past 40 years. In the 1980s, the notion of smoke-free bars and restaurants would have been unthinkable, but today 43 states and the District of Columbia have local laws in effect that require nonhospitality workplaces and/or restaurants and/or bars to be 100% smoke free.[20]

Policy Formulation

Once an agenda has been set and a public health problem is placed on that agenda, the next step is formulation of an actual policy to address the issue. Alternative proposals are created. Information is collected about each of the proposals, and then a case is made for the proposal that seems to be the best solution for the problem.

Policy formation is about compromising and bargaining. Generally, one solution to a problem will not be accepted and championed to succeed without substantial changes and compromises. More likely, many different solutions and versions will be presented and debated. The solution that is eventually successful will often be modified before it reaches its final form. These modifications may weaken or strengthen the policy. Modifications are generally based on the ideologies and interests of various players in the political process, who have an interest in the outcome and effects of the proposal.

Discussion Prompt

Is food safety a food industry problem or is it a consumer problem?

Discussion Prompt

Making establishments smoke-free has allowed better consumer health. However, was the government overstepping? Why or why not?

Nutrition policy[1] A set of concerted actions, based on a governmental mandate, intended to ensure good health in the population through informed access to safe, healthy, and adequate food.

Policy Implementation

After a new policy has been created, it must be implemented. New policies are rarely written with adequate detail to allow their implementation. The policy must be interpreted with rules and regulations written to spell out how a policy will be implemented. Responsibility and financial resources must be assigned so that the policy can be instituted.

The usual process for policy creation at the federal level is for Congress to pass legislation that then goes to various government cabinets, usually the USDA or DHHS for **nutrition policy**, where the new law is interpreted through creation of rules and regulations that reflect practical application of the law.

It may be tempting to believe that once a law has been passed, public health officials should feel confident that the policy is now in place and will be effective. The implementation phase is very critical for the success of public policy. Sometimes, laws are passed establishing a new policy, but no funding is given for implementation, or those who write the rules and regulations do so in such a way as to make the policy weak or ineffective. This is referred to as an "unfunded mandate," which dates back to post-world war two (WW II,). These mandates are legislatively approved federal programs that are sent to the states and local level governments for implementation. An example of this is the Medicaid program where the federal government only provides partial funding, with the remaining costs covered by the states. It is possible for states to have different participation guidelines as seen in April of 2020 when 35 states expanded income guidelines that allowed more Americans to obtain healthcare coverage (See **Figure 3–1**). How a policy is implemented is critical to its success and must be guided by those who have the knowledge and expertise to create rules to make the policy successful.[21,22]

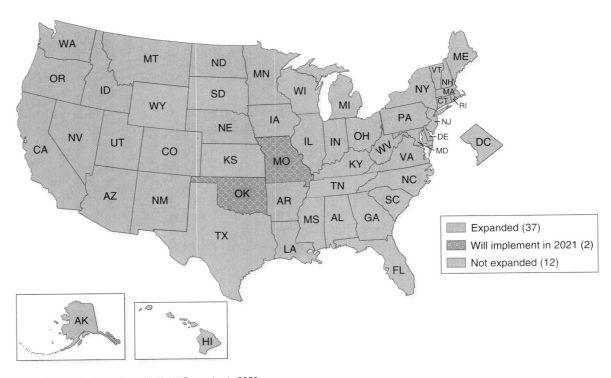

FIGURE 3–1 Status of State Medicaid Expansion in 2020.
© Center on Budget and Policy Priorities.

Policy Evaluation

The final stage in policy development is policy evaluation. Despite the best efforts of everyone involved in policy development, new policies are rarely perfect. Once a policy has been implemented, it needs to be evaluated for success. If the policy is successful, it should be evaluated to see how it can be changed to make it more successful. Few policies retain the same level of value, simply because the environment and conditions for which they were created change with time.[23] Sometimes a sound nutrition policy is formulated that later becomes a policy that promotes poor nutrition. As an example, when the WIC program was originally created, its policies regarding the amount of juice in the food package made sense. In 2007 (implemented in 2009), as obesity became a more urgent problem in the United States, the amount of juice in the WIC food package was considered a nutritional problem related to childhood obesity and was cut by approximately 50%. Policies need to be continuously evaluated so that they may be modified or discontinued as new health issues emerge.

Policy Creation at the Federal Level

The federal government was created to have a separation of powers. There are three branches of the federal government, each with its own responsibility and power. The legislative branch (Congress) is responsible for creating laws, the executive branch (the President) for enforcing laws, and the judicial branch (the courts) for interpreting laws.

In the United States, most public policy is created by legislation. Congress has the authority to pass laws that initiate, modify, and authorize, and appropriate funding for all programs and services administered by the federal government. The legislative process is started when a member of Congress introduces a bill for consideration. If the bill is introduced in the Senate, it is given a designation starting with S., followed by an identifying number; if the bill is introduced in the House of Representatives, it is given a designation starting with H.R., followed by an identifying number. The leadership of the Senate or House then assigns the bill to a subcommittee or committee that will consider the bill. Because of the numerous bills that are introduced to Congress each year, many die from low priority in subcommittees and committees.

Congressional committees have considerable power in determining what will move forward to possibly become law and what will be tabled. If the bill is of interest to the members of the assigned committee, is of sufficient priority, and the political climate is right, the committee may hold hearings on the bill. The committee may decide to amend the bill by adding or deleting parts. The clean bill (amended version) is voted on and is reported out either to a committee if it was in a subcommittee or to the entire Senate or House if the bill was in a committee. If the bill was started in the Senate, it will be debated by the Senate, possibly amended, and then voted on. The bill would then go to a committee in the House for consideration. The House committee would then consider the bill, possibly amend it, and send it to the House for amendments and a vote. To save time, versions of the same bill may be introduced into both the Senate and House at the same time. These are referred to as companion bills.

If a bill is successfully voted on and passed by both the Senate and the House, the bill is often sent to a conference committee made up of members of both the Senate and House. This is necessary when there are differences in versions of a bill passed by the Senate and House. The conference committee

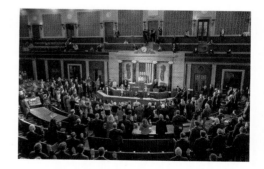

Congressional committees meet to hear legislation on a bill.

Courtesy of the White House.

attempts to resolve any differences between the two versions of the bill. The conference version of a bill must be sent back to both the Senate and House for a final vote before the bill is sent to the President.

The President has three choices when receiving a bill: First, he may sign the bill within 10 days and it becomes law. Second, he may veto the bill and send it back to Congress. This effectively kills the bill unless two-thirds of the members of both the Senate and House vote in favor of the bill to override the veto. Third, the President may do nothing with the bill when it is received.

If the President does nothing with the bill after it has been sent to him by Congress, there are two possibilities. If Congress is in session, the bill will become law in 10 days (excluding Sundays) even without the President's signature. If Congress is not in session, the bill does not become law. This is known as a pocket veto.

Although most public policy in the United States is created by legislation through Congress, the other two branches of government can and do create public policy. Legislation passed by Congress must be turned into practical rules and regulations so that they may be carried out. This is the duty of federal employees in the executive branch of government. The rules and regulations created to implement policy will have a great impact on whether the original intent of a policy can be accomplished. These employees have considerable policymaking power, because they create the rules and regulations of policy implementation.

The executive branch of government also is responsible for the enforcement of legislation. Decisions about how forcefully or even whether to enforce legislation have significant impact on policy. Public policy is what the government actually does or does not do. If enforcement is lax, the intended outcome of legislation or policy will be lost.

The agenda of a U.S. president and his political party can have a significant impact on how legislation is turned into practical policies and how they are enforced and funded. Members of the executive branch of government, including the President, have a large role in advocating for budget allocations, enforcing policy, and acting as advisors to members of Congress on technical issues.

The President may also create public policy through executive orders. Executive orders are sometimes used to avoid public debate and opposition on an issue. Executive orders are usually considered equivalent to federal statutes and do not require the approval of Congress. In 2000, President Clinton created policy just before leaving office by making an executive order that the WIC program would screen children under age 2 for immunizations.

The judicial branch of the federal government makes public policy through court decisions that decide the intent and meaning of laws, whether a public health agency is operating within its scope of legislative authority, and whether public health statutes and regulations are constitutionally permissible. The U.S. Supreme Court has made many decisions of importance to public health, including upholding the power of the government to protect the public's health.[24-26] As early as 1905, the Supreme Court, by a 7-2 majority, said in Jacobson v. Massachusetts that the city of Cambridge, Massachusetts, could fine residents who refused to receive smallpox injections. Fast forward to the present, in 2020, the Supreme Court also considered many public health mandates related to COVID-19.

See **Figure 3–2** on how a bill becomes a law.

Pandemic Learning Opportunity

Was it a good idea to have the Supreme Court decide some public mandates to Covid-19? Why or why not?

HOW DOES A BILL BECOME A LAW?

① EVERY LAW STARTS WITH AN IDEA

That idea can come from anyone, even you! Contact your elected officials to share your idea. If they want to try to make it a law, they will write a bill.

② THE BILL IS INTRODUCED

A bill can start in either house of Congress when it's introduced by its primary sponsor, a Senator or a Representative. In the House of Representatives, bills are placed in a wooden box called "the hopper."

③ THE BILL GOES TO COMMITTEE

Representatives or Senators meet in a small group to research, talk about, and make changes to the bill. They vote to accept or reject the bill and its changes before sending it to:

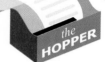

Here, the bill is assigned a legislative number before the Speaker of the House sends it to a committee.

the House or Senate floor for debate or to a subcommittee for further research.

④ CONGRESS DEBATES AND VOTES

Members of the House or Senate can now debate the bill and propose changes or amendments before voting. If the majority vote for and pass the bill, it moves to the other house to go through a similar process of committees, debate, and voting. Both houses have to agree on the same version of the final bill before it goes to the President.

DID YOU KNOW?

The House uses an electronic voting system while the Senate typically votes by voice, saying "yay" or "nay."

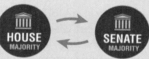

⑤ PRESIDENTIAL ACTION

When the bill reaches the President, he or she can:

✓ **APPROVE and PASS**
The President signs and approves the bill. The bill is law.

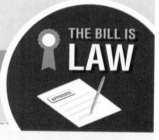
THE BILL IS LAW

The President can also:

Veto
The President rejects the bill and returns it to Congress with the reasons for the veto. Congress can override the veto with 2/3 vote of those present in both the House and the Senate and the bill will become law.

Choose no action
The President can decide to do nothing. If Congress is in session, after 10 days of no answer from the President, the bill then automatically becomes law.

Pocket veto
If Congress adjourns (goes out of session) within the 10 day period after giving the President the bill, the President can choose not to sign it and the bill will not become law.

FIGURE 3–2 How a bill becomes a law.

USA.gov, How Laws Are Made and How to Research Them. Retrieved from https://www.usa.gov/how-laws-are-made#item-213608

Policy Development at All Levels of Government: Federal, State, and Local

Policy development is important at all levels of government in order for public health agencies to fulfill their role in ensuring health. Each level of government has its own unique contributions to make in policy development and in providing community public health services. From a historical and constitutional perspective, states have the primary responsibility for the health of citizens of the United States. Local governments, in turn, receive their authority from state governments. The federal government has, over time, developed a larger role in the promotion of health and now has many technical and leadership roles that influence state and local health policies.

It is important that all levels of government work together to create effective health and nutrition policy. By the very nature of having so many divisions of government, policies can become fragmented, overlapping, redundant, and at times contradictory. To deliver a convincing policy message in an organized and efficient way, all levels of government must work together.

Health problems, including nutritional problems, are seldom confined to one set of boundaries in the United States. For example, obesity rates may be higher in some parts of the nation, but overall, it is a problem in all parts of the nation. Food is grown in various parts of the country but is then distributed to the entire country. Most processed foods are universally distributed across the nation. Media advertising and the lifestyle effects of media are universal throughout the United States. Food franchises, food labeling, and the effects of federal nutrition programs are nearly the same everywhere in the nation. The factors that improve or detract from our nutritional health are generally widespread and not confined to a single state, county, or city. To make changes in policy that affect nutritional health requires a concerted policy effort by all levels of government giving a unified message. [16,24,27,28]

The Role of the Federal Government in Policy Development

The federal government plays a vital role in health and nutrition policy development. Many nutrition problems, such as obesity, increased prevalence of certain cancers, and heart disease, are faced by everyone in our nation, and they are affected by behaviors and conditions that exist throughout the country. These problems require national policy attention as well as state and local attention, if they are to be solved (See **Figure 3–3**).

The federal government's policies affect the nutritional health of U.S. citizens in several ways:

1. Federal policies greatly affect the food supply in the United States, including the quantity, types, and pricing of available foods. Because the food supply affects nutritional health, any changes in agricultural policy would need to come from the federal level.
2. Because most food production, processing, packaging, labeling, and marketing are done at the national level, federal policies are necessary to bring about any changes.
3. The major food and nutrition programs in the United States are all administered and funded by the federal government. These programs impact a significant portion of the public. The policies of these programs determine what foods are given and what nutritional information are provided. For most states, the majority of the nutritionists and dietitians working in public health are employed by these programs. For some states, these programs constitute almost their entire public nutrition policy. Because federal programs, such as WIC, purchase such large quantities of foods such as cereals and infant formulas, program regulations affect manufacturing and marketing practices of the foods to the entire population.
4. The federal government plays an important role in assessing nutritional health of the population of the United States. The National Health and Nutrition Examination Survey, Behavioral

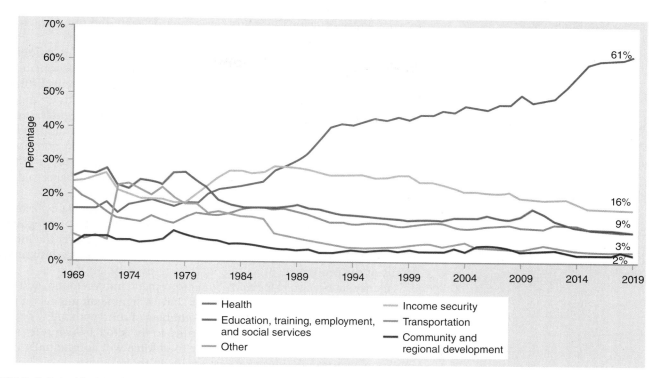

FIGURE 3–3 Federal Grants to States and Local Governments.

Reproduced from Tax Policy Center. Retrieved from https://www.taxpolicycenter.org/briefing-book/what-types-federal-grants-are-made-state-and-local-governments
-and-how-do-they-work

Risk Factor Surveillance System, and other surveys give the
nutrition public health community the nutritional data upon which
to base policy decisions.

5. The federal government has built up a resource of scientific and
technical assistance that may be used by states to identify nutrition
and health issues and to help create effective policies for solving
the problems. Outward facing endeavors include the Nutrition
Facts label (FDA) and My Plate (USDA).

6. Because most nutritional problems are national, the federal
government must play a role in policy leadership to identify,
monitor, and resolve nutritional issues.

7. The federal government has the technical and financial resources
for research to understand and solve nutrition problems.

8. Finally, the federal government has financial resources to assist
states with public policies to solve public health nutrition
problems. These funds become available to states and researchers
in the form of grant money.

> Are grants a good use of taxpayer dollars?
> Why?

The Role of Public Agencies in Policy Development

In the context of this chapter, agencies are governmental units that oversee
nutrition programs. These agencies can exist at all levels of government, from
the federal to the local level. At the federal level, the USDA is the agency that
has been given the primary responsibility for nutrition programs and policy.
Nutrition programs such as SNAP, the Commodity Supplemental Food Program (CSFP), WIC, and the National School Lunch Program are administered
at the federal level by the USDA. Operation of these programs is delegated

to state agencies, which in many cases then delegate the programs to local agencies where services are actually provided.

Nutrition programs are created through legislation that is written with broad goals and a basic design for a program. It is the responsibility of agencies to translate these broad goals and designs into practical rules and regulations that allow for the actual operation of programs. This arrangement permits legislatures to create broad policies to accomplish goals and then allows agency staff to use their expertise to create the rules that provide for actual delivery of services. Agency staff has more expertise in nutrition and in techniques to improve nutrition behavior than legislative staff, so this is a good arrangement. Agency staff can work out details in programs that allow them to be effective and to work in an efficient manner.

If rules and regulations are written poorly, programs will be ineffective and the goals of legislated policy will not be achieved. If the rules and regulations are well written, the program may have great success. Whatever the intent by legislators, the end result depends in great measure on those designing the details of the programs.

Agency staff is also responsible for enforcement, interpretation, and prioritization of rules and regulations. This can have a significant impact on policy. Most government programs have large numbers of rules with many details. It is virtually impossible to follow all the rules to the letter. Which rules agency staff decide to focus their energy on or to enforce will substantially impact public policy through the accomplishments of the program.

Agency staff members also have a role in advising policymakers at various levels of government. Agency staff can make recommendations for legislation and budgets. Because many agency staff are experts in their subject areas, such as nutrition, they can advise policymakers about proposed policies and proposed budgets and can recommend new policies. For example, if agency staff monitoring health statistics finds that fruit and vegetable consumption in school-age children is lacking, they can make recommendations for legislation to encourage fruit and vegetable consumption. Likewise, if a legislator decides that a new program is needed to address obesity, agency staff can help develop the legislation and make recommendations for how the legislation is written, methods for decreasing obesity, and how much money should be allocated. Agency staff often makes recommendations for policy when new legislation is being created and when programs are being reauthorized by Congress.[29]

The Role of State Government in Policy Development

State governments are responsible for the health of their citizens. This responsibility was given to the states by the U.S. Constitution. States may delegate some of this responsibility to local governments, but the ultimate responsibility rests with the states. Since the 1960s, the federal government has been playing a larger role, providing resources and expertise to help state governments fulfill their responsibility for the health of their citizens. States have a responsibility to collect and analyze information on the health of their citizens, to set policies and standards, to carry out national and state mandates, and to respond to health issues. The IOM recommended that each state has a health council that reports on health issues in the state and makes policy recommendations to the governor and legislature for policy development.[30]

Policy does not just happen, and legislatures are generally not looking for new public health policies to create. Because many states do not have a single lead nutritionist responsible for policy development, it is the responsibility of all nutrition professionals in a state to assess their state's nutritional health and determine what legislation is needed. This includes nutritionists at the state-agency level and their professional associations. Nutritionists also need to monitor all legislative activities for policy changes that could affect the nutrition of the public.

State personnel are sometimes restricted in their government positions from advocating for legislation, at least while functioning as a government employee. Local dietetic associations and nutrition alliances, such as antihunger groups or nutrition networks, may be effective in proposing and advocating for nutrition policy changes.

State governments offer an advantage in policy development in that most state legislators are more accessible than federal legislators. Legislators may be more responsive to small groups of advocates. Nutritionists at the state level have been successful at getting legislation introduced and passed regarding licensure of dietitians, pro-breastfeeding policies, issues affecting school nutrition, and reimbursement for certain types of nutrition counseling.

The Role of Local Government in Policy Development

Local governments vary considerably in their form and configuration as well as how they deal with health issues. There are a great many units of local government with a wide range of structures, functions, and size. Some local governments are larger than some state governments, and others are so small that they have few resources and staff for health functions.

Local government is where nutrition services are implemented. State governments often delegate portions of their responsibility for health to local government units because it is local governments that are able to actually provide health services. Many nutrition programs, while administered at the state level, provide services through units of local governments. In some communities, nutrition needs are deeper and more prevalent than what the local government is able to cover with state or local funds. Not-for-profits often step into these gaps and augment services. For instance, local food security work frequently complements national programs like SNAP, WIC, and CSFP through the establishment of neighborhood food pantries.

Policy development needs to occur at the local level, as at all levels of government. Local governments may be the most accessible of all when trying to create policy.[31] A passionate nutritionist with a strong social network, and good organizational and people skills, can do great things with respect to nutrition policy while working with the school board, local health department, physicians, and city government. It may be possible to get legislation created and passed around nutrition education or vending machines in the school, breastfeeding issues, or senior nutrition programs. Policies created at the local level can become models and open doors to get similar policies passed at the state level. It is always important that local policies target goals similar to national nutrition policies and faithfully collect outcome data to further promote and sustain model programs.

Much like agency personnel, local nutrition professionals have a great impact on actual nutrition policy as it is administered. A nutritionist working for a federal nutrition program at the local level can determine how well that program functions and interacts with other health programs. Local nutritionists working for WIC, who reach out to the community and build a quality WIC program, helps create effective nutrition policy. Likewise, a nutritionist who builds coalitions with Head Start, preschools, daycare programs, nurse partnerships, and other programs can create an environment where nutrition issues are addressed and the nutritional health of the community benefits. A nutritionist in the same community who creates barriers to WIC services and builds walls with other programs will have the opposite effect on nutrition in the community.

Discussion Prompt

Name some governmental agencies in your community where dietitians work. What are their roles? Should those roles be expanded?

Leadership Roles for Nutritionists

The purpose of a community public health policy is to create conditions in which people can be healthy. Public policy should create conditions where it is easier to be healthy and harder to make decisions that contribute to a person being less healthy. Policymakers at all levels of government are responsible for policy development.

Good nutrition policy does not just happen. Policy development is a long and complex process, affected by many players and filled with compromises. There is no "nutrition czar" in the United States to watch out for needed nutrition policy legislation. It is the role of every nutritionist to be involved and to work for good nutrition policy.[32] Nutritionists need to be informed and work together to bring about changes for better nutrition. This is especially true as the United States faces one of its most challenging nutritional epidemics, that of obesity.

Strategy Tip

Associations Advocating for Nutrition Legislation

The Academy of Nutrition and Dietetics provides comments regularly on nutrition-related legislation. (https://www.eatrightpro.org/news-center/on-the-pulse-of-public-policy/regulatory-comments)

Members of the Society for Nutrition Education and Behavior also participate in policy activities as it relates to their mission and vision. (https://www.sneb.org/index.php?submenu=PolicyStatements&src=directory&view=Public_Documents&srctype=Public_Documents_Policies)

The American Public Health Association has a very active advocacy branch and addresses a wide range of public health issues by providing formal comments to regulators. (https://www.apha.org/policies-and-advocacy/advocacy-for-public-health/testimony-and-comments)

Advocating and Influencing Health and Nutrition Policies

Advocacy Public support for or recommendation of a particular cause or policy.

Advocacy is the act of supporting or promoting a cause. Public health and nutrition professionals must advocate for nutrition policy. Nutrition policy does not just happen. We tend to take for granted nutrition policies from the past and to allow market forces and special interest groups to determine nutrition policies for the future. For nutrition and public health professionals, it is a primary responsibility to advocate for effective public policies that will improve the nutritional health of people in the United States. Although those employed in leadership roles in community and public health nutrition have specialized roles for leading in policy development, it is the responsibility of all nutritionists to advocate for effective nutrition policy.[31]

A local, close-to-home place to start a collaborative nutrition agenda is through the establishment of a Food Policy Council (FPS). These groups bring together interested stakeholders from the community in order to network, share resources, write, and advocate for implementation of food policy. Examples of their work include urban land use, food waste, and healthy food access.

Advocacy for new policies often starts at the local level since this is where politicians are elected. Visits to the local offices of politicians are a good way to start building relationships and support for a new or proposed policy. When local policies are put in place to improve nutrition, they can serve as models for state or **federal policy**. Many nutrition initiatives had their start in local government. For example, the HiAP movement started as a collaboration between the American Public Health Association and the California Department of Public Health and has been used as a model in states, counties, and cities throughout the United States.[33]

Federal policy Of, relating to, or denoting the central government of the US.

Influencing Legislation

The first step in creating new public policy is to get the proposed policy on the agenda of lawmakers. This may be the most difficult part of the policy-making process. Legislators have many issues, many individuals, and many interest groups vying to capture their attention. Organized interest groups whose purpose is to create legislation have proliferated. In a given year, far more bills are proposed than can possibly be turned into policies. Also, nutrition issues must compete with policy issues unrelated to health, as well with other health issues.

A number of factors help determine which bills are likely to get put on the policy agenda and successfully move on to become law. Bills are more likely to be successful at being placed on the policy agenda if:

- A greater number of people perceive the policy issue to be a problem (i.e., rising rates of obesity).
- The problem is perceived to have greater severity (i.e., impacts mortality rates).
- The problem is more immediate and novel (i.e., COVID-19).
- More people are affected by the problem personally (i.e., food security).
- The political atmosphere is supportive of the policy (i.e., Democrat majorities in the House and Senate).
- The policy appeals to the public (i.e., those that are least punitive and preserve individual autonomy are usually better accepted).

In democracies, public opinion and special interest groups have a substantial impact on whether a bill for new policy will be put on the legislative agenda. It is, therefore, important for public health officials to know how to influence public opinion and to obtain the support of organized interest groups. Working effectively with the media to form public opinion is an important relationship and skill to cultivate. Well-organized and financed special interest groups can also sway policymakers away from following public opinion in some situations. This is especially true when the policy only affects a small number of people, large economic interests are involved, or the issue is very technical in nature. Even if public opinion can get legislation passed, influential interest groups can have a substantial impact on the fine print of legislation that substantially changes the actual intent or effectiveness of a new policy.

Building Support for New Policies

1. The Policy
   The first step in building support for a new policy is to create a defensible, sound policy. Community and public health leaders must know the scientific literature and be able to present a strong case in favor of the policy. Is there sufficient scientific information

Pandemic Learning Opportunities

Food banks were a necessity for handling the Covid-19 pandemic. Food banks should be managed to include timely safeguards and provisions for community and public health.

to justify the policy? The potential risk of creating policy with inadequate information needs to be weighed against the need for the policy.

Public health leaders must also be able to assess the feasibility of the new policy, the costs and benefits of having the policy, the costs and benefits of not having the policy, and the compatibility of the policy with public values. The human rights burden, the effects of the new policy on personal freedoms, fairness of cost distribution, and reasonableness between means and end must also be considered. It is the responsibility of the policy developer to justify the costs and burdens of new policy against its benefits.

2. Public Opinion
Since public policy tends to follow public opinion, it is very important to build public support for new policies. Finding the right community champion(s) is extremely important. This champion can help navigate the political waters and an essential part of a successful policy campaign. Building public support for an issue can be done through the media, public officials, celebrities, and public awareness campaigns. Public opinion can also be developed by building coalitions or alliances, citizen participation in policy development, communication with the public at large, and communication with elected officials. The community, as well as elected officials, must see public health personnel as technical experts and as advocates for the community and supportive of community values. Both technical knowledge and public values determine how public health is practiced. Rather than having a paternalistic approach to communication, public health needs to encourage debate and empower communities to create solutions to their own health issues.

3. Timing of Policy Proposals
Timing is critical. Policy agendas may be filled with other issues that are considered high priorities; therefore, a new policy may not become part of the political agenda even when it is well supported. It is important to judge the political climate when introducing new policy. Reintroduction of the health policy in a different legislative session, when fewer priority items are on the agenda, may increase the likelihood of getting the proposed policy on the political agenda.

Sometimes, it takes many attempts to get a new policy on the legislative agenda. Once it is on the agenda, it may also take multiple tries to get the legislation passed. Repeated attempts help gather support and decrease opposition in many cases. To get legislation for dietetic licensure in one state, the sponsors of the legislation had to agree to exempt dietitians employed in certain practice settings. This wasn't the intent of the original policy, but it allowed a licensure bill to become law. In the following years, the legislation was amended to include some of the dietitians originally excluded. Through incremental change over time, the original intent of the policy was eventually accomplished.

4. Lobbying
Lobbying is the process of trying to influence the members of a legislature. Lobbying is an art, not a science. It can be done by professional lobbyists or it can be done by individuals or groups trying to advance their cause. There are almost 12,000 active professional lobbyists in Washington, D.C., which makes for a lot of people trying to influence policymakers' decisions.

Lobbyists serve several functions in their roles. They attempt to educate legislators on issues that are important to their cause, stimulate public debate on issues, and encourage participation in the political process while trying to gather public support for their legislative issues. "Lobby" has also come to have a negative connotation, referring to pressure groups that run sophisticated and heavily moneyed campaigns to influence legislators by a variety of persuasive methods.[30]

Public health professionals, health professionals, and consumer advocate groups have taken up lobbying as a way to influence legislation on public policy. In general, public health lobbyists are fewer in number and are less well-financed than those from commercial interests. It is a challenge to overcome the influence of lobbyists from well-funded groups that may not favor certain policy changes that are important for health. Government programs are generally prohibited from lobbying, as are government employees under many circumstances. Because government programs need the benefits of lobbying, they sometimes form private groups that will lobby for them. For example, many state and local WIC programs are members of the National WIC Association (NWA). NWA is a private, nonprofit organization that advocates for WIC and issues related to the WIC program. NWA provides information to legislators, makes recommendations on funding and policy changes related to WIC, and works to build community support for the program.

5. Groups That Are Part of the Political Process
Political Action Committees (PACs) are organized for the purpose of raising and spending money to elect or defeat political candidates. Most PACs have specific legislative agendas and work to elect political candidates who are sympathetic to their cause. Health-related groups have created PACs so that their members can contribute money to help elect candidates that support their issues. In 2020, 112 professional leadership PACs gave away over 20 million dollars to support political candidates. As an example, the Academy of Nutrition and Dietetics has an active PAC and in funding year 2019–2020 gave out about $125,000 to political candidates (See https://www.opensecrets.org/political-action-committees-pacs /C00143560/summary/2020 for more information).

A coalition is a group of people and organizations that have common interests and come together to influence outcomes. For example, a coalition of interested citizens, social service organizations, and religious groups may come together to find ways to increase food security in a community. Coalitions can be an excellent way for public health officials to broaden input, reduce overlapping services, and tear down silos. They bring together community and health-related groups as well as public and private organizations for community public health issues.

Alliances are groups of healthcare and public health organizations that combine forces to address public health issues in a specific geographic area. Alliances can also bring together public and private groups to work on a common issue. Coalitions and alliances allow for synergism in solving problems. Collectively, the group can do more than all of the partners separately. For example, The National Alliance for Nutrition and Activity is composed of over 500 members and advocates within the legislative and executive branches of government, a better understanding of the importance of healthy eating, physical activity, and obesity control to the nation's health and healthcare costs. (See http://www .cspinet.org/nutritionpolicy/nana.html for more information.)

Professional organizations of health professionals, such as the Academy of Nutrition and Dietetics (AND), the Society for Nutrition Education and Behavior (SNEB), Society for Public Health Education (SOPHE), or the American Public Health Association (APHA), have a strong role in advocating for public health issues. These organizations can create policy statements that support legislation. They can hire lobbyists, and they have the ability to mobilize members to lobby legislators on specific legislation. They can be technical resources when legislation is being created and provide expert testimony. Belonging to a professional organization that advocates for nutrition and community public health is an important responsibility every nutritionist has to the nation's health.

Health advocacy organizations generally focus on a specific health issue. They help advocate for public health in the same way as professional organizations. For example, the American Diabetes Association (ADA) would be active in advocating for health issues related to diabetes. They can be an important partner in an alliance or coalition working for public policy change.

Consumer advocacy groups can have a very powerful influence on legislatures. The American Association of Retired People (AARP) is one of the largest advocacy groups in the United States, and as such has tremendous influence with legislatures. It represents a very large and growing block of voting citizens.

The Center for Science in the Public Interest (CSPI) is another consumer advocacy group that has had considerable impact on nutrition policy in the United States. CSPI's goals include providing useful, objective information to the public and policymakers on food and nutrition; representing citizens' interests before government units; and ensuring that science and technology are used for the public good. CSPI has brought significant attention to nutrition issues, especially in controversial areas, through use of the media.

Political parties have a major role in determining public policy. This is done by formal party manifestos prior to elections, or in an informal way through the philosophical beliefs under which the political parties operate. A political party that is supportive of health policy can be indispensable in helping to draft health legislation and to get it on the policy agenda. A political party opposed to health legislation can be a formidable hurdle.

The National Academy of Science (NAS) is a private, nonprofit society that was given a charter by Congress in 1863. NAS has a mandate to advise the federal government on scientific and technical matters. IOM was established under the charter of the NAS in 1970 to provide independent, objective, evidence-based advice to policymakers, health professionals, the private sector, and the public. The IOM conducts policy studies on health issues as part of the National Academies composed of the National Academy of Sciences, National Academy of Engineering, and the National Research Council. Congress often refers health issues to the IOM when a nonpartisan, impartial review and recommendation are needed. Documents from the IOM are invaluable in advocating for change in public health and nutrition policy.[30]

The media helps shape the public's view of reality and can have strong effects on public opinion. Anyone who has ever worked with the media is aware of how important it is to develop a positive and mutually beneficial relationship with the media. How the media "frames" an issue can make a major difference in whether the public will support or reject proposed policy. The media needs news stories of interest to entice the public, and public health officials need the media to educate the public. In addition to the traditional media, social media has become a widely used and influential way to shape opinion. According to the Pew Research Center, about ⅓ of Americans say they often or sometimes comment about political issues on social media. The majority cite using Facebook for their comments and about 20% prefer that Twitter Public health officials must stay engaged in both social and traditional media and become dependable sources of accurate information for the media so that the media may frame them as knowledgeable experts when health issues arise.

Discussion Prompt

In which groups do readers belong? What benefits do they offer for membership?

Importance of Building an Infrastructure of Support

For public health officials to be effective advocates for policy change, they need to have the support of the community, other health professionals, and politicians. The IOM has made several recommendations for building a base of political support:

- Public health officials should develop relationships with legislatures and other public officials and educate them on community and public health issues.
- Public health agencies should train staff in community relations and citizen participation.
- Public health agencies should develop relationships with physicians and other private sector representatives, including professional societies and academic medical centers.
- Public health agencies should seek stronger relationships and common goals with other professional and citizen groups involved with health issues.
- Agencies should undertake education of the public on health issues.
- Agencies should review the quality of contacts among employees and clients to ensure the public is treated with cordiality and respect.

The IOM noted that these relationships need to be cultivated and fostered on an ongoing basis. Building these relationships is part of the political process necessary to accomplish goals. It has been suggested that political skills must be consistently used in order to maintain them.

Advocacy Activities and Skills for Individuals

Many professional organizations provide member training on advocacy skills. It is the actions of members and other individuals that make these groups effective. For example, the Academy of Nutrition and Dietetics sponsors an Advocacy Summit annually for their members. It is important not to underestimate the power of the trained individual advocate when confronting major health or nutrition problems. Passionate, persistent individuals have made remarkable differences in the face of poor odds.

There are many ways that an individual can advocate for nutrition policy, either as a private individual or as a professional. The following suggestions apply to individuals advocating on their own or as part of groups made up of individuals:

- Know your elected officials and develop professional relationships with them.
- Attend town hall meetings and make your opinions heard. Be assertive, but polite, friendly, and tactful. Write letters, email, telephone, and visit your elected officials telling them your views on public health and nutrition issues. Even when it is unlikely that the official will be swayed to change their mind on an issue, it is still good to let them know your views. It may soften his or her opposition.

Strategy Tip

Read about your elected officials from more than one source and their voting records. Get to know their philosophies and voting records related to health issues.

Strategy Tips

Contacting elected officials

Vote in elections to influence who will represent your views in government.

- Join a professional association or advocacy group(s) that advocates for public health. Many voices are generally louder than one. Be active in the group and encourage policy involvement.
- Conflicts arise. Don't take them personally. Learn from your opponent's position; it may strengthen your own position. Accept that some people may reject you for your position on an issue.
- Write letters to the editor of the newspaper when you have a strong position on a health or nutrition issue.
- Identify and know your audience. Adjust your message to better target their concerns and needs.
- Be persistent. Learn from your own mistakes and move on with that knowledge to do a better job next time.
- Take the time to comment on policy proposals and changes. The government often requests written comments on new policies and policy changes. These requests for comments are printed in the Federal Register for comment periods of 30 to 90 days. This is one of those unusual times when someone is required to read your letter and comments. Federal employees are required to read and compile all comments received during a comment period. These compiled comments are then used to support approval, change, or rejection of proposed policies.

The Future of Public Health

The future of public health will be determined by those with the greatest influence on public policy development. It is critical that public health officials work to become effective advocates of public health. Good public policy does not happen on its own. Without effective leadership from public health officials, public health will be determined by those with the greatest economic interest or political need. Effective skills and strategies in policy development must be developed by public health professionals.

These skills require development of a broad base of support in the community and credibility as technical experts. As individuals, those with concerns for public health must remember that it is the actions of many individuals that result in positive changes for public health. Each public health professional as an individual and as part of organized groups must advocate for optimal health for all.

Summary

To accomplish something in an organized and efficient manner you must have a goal and a plan of action. This is the reason for creating policy. Public policy may be created by the legislative, executive, or judicial branch of government. Generally, policy is created by legislation that is introduced and passed by the legislative branch. This legislation or policy is then translated into a set of practical rules by the executive branch to accomplish the intent of the legislation. Policy, however, also may be informal, indirect, and even unwritten.

As a result of a need for public policy in a complex society, public policy touches almost every aspect of our lives. The successes of community public health are frequently taken for granted and only noticed when they fail. Health policy is determined more by crises, hot issues, and the concerns of organized interest groups than careful analysis of objective data and technical knowledge about health.

Government policies have a great impact on which foods are available to the public and at what price. Many of the current food policies come from a time when providing adequate food at a cheap price was the goal of U.S. agricultural and nutrition policy. The conditions and health issues that existed when those policies were created are not the same as exist now. From a nutrition policy point of view, these policies need to be reevaluated to create food policies that support the production, marketing, and low price of foods that are associated with a healthier diet rather than support the production of less-healthy foods.

Good nutrition policy does not just happen. Policy development is a long and complex process, affected by many players and filled with compromises. It is the role of every nutritionist to be involved and to work for good nutrition policy. Nutritionists need to be informed and work together to bring about changes for better nutrition.

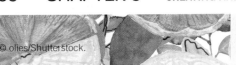

© olies/Shutterstock.

Learning Portfolio

Key Terms

	page
Public policy	72
Special interest group	72
Autonomy	73
Code of Federal Regulations (CFR)	74
Incrementalism	78
Nutrition policy	80
Advocacy	88
Federal policy	89

Issues for Discussion

1. Why is public policy important to health issues?
2. Discuss the barriers to effective public policy.
3. What types of tensions are evident in public policy setting? Illustrate your answer with a nutrition example.
4. Building a base of public support is important to get a public health policy through the legislature. Explain how to develop public support in respect to a policy on child obesity.
5. Research a nutrition advocacy group. What issues are they advocating for? How successful have they been in their past advocacy efforts?
6. Why is advocacy a professional practice issue?

Case Study 1: Food Desert

Alisha has been interested in food ever since she can remember. Some of her favorite memories include cooking with her auntie and grandma, and she still makes those favorite dishes in her college apartment when she has the time. Alisha is now a registered dietitian/nutritionist and graduate student in public health. She is amazed that her peers have very few cooking skills and relies on convenience foods from the neighborhood store, the fast food outlet across the street from the University, or foods from vending machines.

Alisha sees educational opportunities with her fellow students but also sees many barriers to healthy eating. She is interested in making the best food choice the easiest food choice in order to change her friends' eating behaviors but needs a community champion to assist her in an advocacy campaign for a healthier food landscape.

1. What are the assets of Alisha's peer group?
2. What are the barriers to healthy eating among this group of university students?
3. How could Alisha build support for healthier eating?
4. What policy options might assist her advocacy campaign?

Case Study 2: Urban Evening Food Desert

Sam is a Registered Dietitian/Nutrition and a new graduate student in public health. His classes are primarily in the evenings from 6:00–9:00 pm on an urban campus. Most of his fellow students come directly from work to the classroom and frequently bring in their fast food supper to eat in class. Sam is a bit of an outlier since he brings his own meals from home. His friends are always interested in what he has in his tote and complain that no healthy food exists around campus or on their way from work to campus, forcing them to make the best choice of the many not so good choices on the menu. The one university food outlet on the urban campus closes at 4:00 pm.

Sam has almost 40 students in his class; how could he be the impetus and advocate for food system and policy change on his campus?

Resources

1. Story MT, Duffy E. Supporting healthy eating: synergistic effects of nutrition education paired with policy, systems, and environmental changes. *Nestle Nutr Inst Workshop Ser.* 2019;92:69-82. doi: 10.1159/000499549. Epub 2019 Nov 28. PMID: 31779013.

2. McIsaac JD, Spencer R, Chiasson K, Kontak J, Kirk SFL. Factors influencing the implementation of nutrition policies in schools: a scoping review. *Health Educ Behav.* 2019;46(2):224-250. doi: 10.1177/1090198118796891. Epub 2018 Sep 3. PMID: 30173576.

3. Crawford PB. nutrition policies designed to change the food environment to improve diet and health of the population. *Nestle Nutr Inst Workshop Ser.* 2019;92:107-118. doi: 10.1159/000499552. Epub 2019 Nov 28. PMID: 31779015.

4. Wetherill MS, White KC, Seligman HK. Nutrition-focused food banking in the United States: a qualitative study of healthy food distribution initiatives. *J Acad Nutr Diet.* 2019;119(10):1653-1665. doi: 10.1016/j.jand.2019.04.023. Epub 2019 Jun 28. PMID: 31262694; PMCID: PMC6765436.

5. Bleich SN, Moran AJ, Vercammen KA, et al. Strengthening the public health impacts of the supplemental nutrition assistance program through policy. *Annu Rev Public Health.* 2020;41:453-480. doi: 10.1146/annurev-publhealth -040119-094143. PMID: 32237988.

See PubMed.gov for more research articles.

References

1. Nutrition policy. A Dictionary of Food and Nutrition. Retrieved January 2, 2021, from Encyclopedia.com: https://www.encyclopedia.com/education/dictionaries-thesauruses -pictures-and-press-releases/nutrition-policy

2. The New Oxford Dictionary of English. Oxford University Press; 2020.

3. Birkland TA. An introduction to the policy process: theories, concepts, and models of public policy making, 5th ed. Routledge; 2019.

4. Block LE. Health policy: What it is and how it works. In: Harrington C, Estes CL, Eds. *Health Policy: Crisis and Reform in the U.S. Health Care Delivery System*, 6th Ed. Jones and Bartlett; 2012:4-16.

5. Kawauchi I, Lang I, Ricciardi W, Nutbeam D. Developing healthy public policy. In: Oxford Handbook of Public Health Practice. 4th ed. Oxford University Press; 2020:304-311.

6. Pomeranz, J., Zellers, L., Bare, M. and Pertschuk, M. State pre-emption of food and nutrition policies and litigation: undermining government's role in public health. *Am J Prevent Med.* 2019;56(1):47-57.

7. Buxbaum JD, Chernew ME, Fendrick AM, Cutler DM. Contributions of public health, pharmaceuticals, and other medical care to US life expectancy changes, 1990-2015. *Health Aff.* 2020;39:1546-1556.

8. Gostin L, Wiley L. Public health law: power, duty, restraint. 3rd ed. University of California Press; 2016.

9. Hirsch IB, Evert A, Fleming A, et al. Culinary medicine: advancing a framework for healthier eating to improve chronic disease management and prevention. *Clin Ther.* 2019;41(10):2184-2198.

10. Institute of Medicine, Committee for the Study of the Future of Public Health. The Future of Public Health.: National Academy Press; 1988.

11. Leadership and policy development. In: Rowitz L, ed. *Public Health Leadership: Putting Principles into Practice.* Aspen; 20081:211-232.

12. Institute of Medicine, Committee on Assuring the Health of the Public in the 21st Century. The Future of the Public Health in the 21st Century: National Academy Press; 2002.

13. Nestle M. Soda Politics: Taking on Big Soda (and Winning). Oxford University Press, 2015.

14. U.S. Department of Agriculture and U.S. Department of Health and Human Services. Dietary Guidelines for Americans, 2020-2025. 9th Edition. 2020. Retrieved January 2, 2021. https://www.dietaryguidelines.gov/sites/default/files /2020-12/Dietary_Guidelines_for_Americans_2020-2025 .pdf

15. Botterill J. Mobile eating: a cultural perspective. *Int Rev Soc Res.* 2017;7(2):71-79. doi: 10.1515/irsr-2017-0009

16. Charvet A, Huffman FG. Beverage intake and its effect on body weight status among WIC preschool-age children. *J Obes.* 2019:1-8. doi: 10.1155/2019/3032457

17. Institute of Medicine of the National Academies. Local government actions to prevent childhood obesity. Washington, DC: National Academy Press; 2009.

18. Koh YM. Shaping your organizations policy. In: Pencheon D, Guest C, Melzer D, Muir Gray JA, eds. *Oxford Handbook of Public Health Practice.* Oxford: Oxford University Press; 2001:128-135.

19. Hart S, Jackson N. Primer on policy: the legislative process at the federal level. In: Harrington C, Estes CL, eds. Health Policy: Crisis and Reform in the U.S. Health Care Delivery System, 3rd ed. Sudbury, MA: Jones and Bartlett; 2008:370-372.

20. McGowan AK. Kramer KT, and Teitelbaum JB. Healthy People: the role of law and policy in the nation's public health agenda. *J Law Med Ethics.* 2019;(suppl);47:63-67.

21. Wall P. Influencing government policy: a national review. In: Pencheon D, Guest C, Melzer D, Muir Gray JA, eds. Oxford Handbook of Public Health Practice. Oxford, UK: Oxford University Press; 2001:156-161.

22. Rowitz L. Public health leadership: putting principles into practice. Gaithersburg, MD: Jones and Bartlett; 2013.

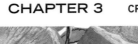
© olies/Shutterstock.

Learning Portfolio

23. Dodd CJ. Can meaningful health policy be developed in a political system? In: Harrington C, 26. Estes CL, eds. *Health policy: Crisis and Reform in the U.S. Healthcare Delivery System*, 3rd ed. Sudbury, MA: Jones and Bartlett; 2008:373-382.

24. Anderson G, Hussey PS. Influencing government policy: a framework. In: Pencheon D, Guest C, Melzer D, Muir Gray JA, eds. *Oxford Handbook of Public Health Practice*: Oxford University Press; 2001:146-154.

25. Frommer M, Leeder S, Rubin G, Tjhin M. Translating goals and targets into public health action. In: Pencheon D, Guest C, Melzer D, Muir Gray JA, eds. *Oxford Handbook of Public Health Practice*. Oxford University Press; 2001:136-144.

26. Misiroglu G. The Handy Politics Answer Book. Visible Ink Press; 2003.

27. Muir Gray JA. The public health professional as political activist. In: Pencheon D, Guest C, Melzer D, Muir Gray JA, Eds. *Oxford Handbook of Public Health Practice*. Oxford University Press; 2001:262-267.

28. Poole MK, Mundorf AM, Englar NK, Rose D. From nutrition to public policy: improving healthy food access by enhancing farm-to-table legislation in Louisiana. *J Acad Nutr Diet*. 2015;115(6):871-875.

29. National Academies of Sciences, Engineering, and Medicine. 2017. Review of WIC food packages: Improving balance and choice: Final report. Washington, DC: The National Academies Press. https://doi.org/10.17226/23655

30. Stein K. Fighting for the profession: the recent history of legislative and public policy efforts at the academy. *J Acad Nutr Diet*. 2017;117(suppl 10):S19-S36.

31. Wright, LE, Doby C. The Academy of Nutrition and Dietetics Political Action Committee: shaping the future of the profession. *J Acad Nutr Diet*. 2020;120(7):1220-1222.

32. USDA National Agriculture Library; Food and nutrition information center: Retrieved on January 5, 2021. https://www.nal.usda.gov/fnic

33. Rudolph L, Caplan J, Ben-Moshe K, Dillon L. Health in all policies: a guide for state and local governments. 2013. American Public Health Association and Public Health Institute.

CHAPTER 4

The Role of the Federal Agencies in Community and Public Health Nutrition

Juliana Ross Gilenberg, RDN, CSO, CNSC, LDN

(We would like to acknowledge the work of Sari Edelstein, PhD, RDN; Beverly J. McCabe-Sellers, PhD, RDN; and Margaret L. Bogle, PhD, RDN, in past editions of Nutrition and Public Health.)

Learning Outcomes

AFTER STUDYING THIS CHAPTER AND REFLECTING ON THE CONTENTS, YOU SHOULD BE ABLE TO:

1. List the major federal agencies within the United States that contribute to the practice of community and public health nutrition.
2. Identify the primary programs that provide food assistance and nutrition education.
3. Discuss the agencies whose roles are to provide research data to support human nutrition in community and public health.
4. Discuss the major vehicles by which agencies contribute to nutrition policy and promotion of health.
5. Discuss the perspective of nutrition education within federal agencies.

Introduction

The United States Department of Agriculture (USDA), Food and Drug Administration (FDA), Centers for Disease Control and Prevention (CDC), and the Environmental Protection Agency (EPA) are large, complex federal organizations that administer a diverse set of agencies and programs for the welfare of the American public. Since the USDA is perhaps the largest of these agencies that administers food and nutrition policy and programs, this chapter will lean heavily on their role on nutrition in community and public health.

Since the 1994 reorganization of the federal government, the USDA has had three major programs that impact public health nutrition: 1) Food, Nutrition, and Consumer Services (FNCS); 2) Food Safety; and 3) Research, Education, and Economics (REE). These agencies will be discussed for their individual major roles but, in reality, a large amount of interdependence and collaboration are needed to achieve their mutual mission and their goals of meeting the food and nutritional needs of Americans.

Overview of Food, Nutrition, and Consumer Services

The Food, Nutrition, and Consumer Services (FNCS) has two major agencies: the Food and Nutrition Service (FNS) and the Center for Nutrition Policy and Promotion (CNPP). FNCS's ongoing goal is:

> "…to leverage our nation's agricultural abundance to ensure every American has access to wholesome, nutritious food, even when they face challenging circumstances. FNCS continued its focus on customer service and integrity, with an eye toward helping more Americans move toward self-sufficiency."[1]

This extra emphasis on self-sufficiency was introduced by the last administration when they tightened rules and regulations for the programs like the Supplemental Nutrition Assistance Program (SNAP), which help alleviate food insecurity for millions of Americans.[2]

Food and Nutrition Service

The Food and Nutrition Service (FNS) increases food security and reduces hunger in partnership with cooperating organizations by providing children and low-income people access to food, a healthy diet, and nutrition education in a manner that supports U.S. agriculture and inspires public action.

FNS administers some 15 domestic food service programs that serve about one in four Americans at some point during the year.[3] The programs work individually and in concert, alongside state and tribal programs, to increase food security and provide a nutrition safety net for children and low-income adults.[3] The most recent USDA budget for fiscal year 2021 allocates 65% of its total planned expenditure toward nutrition assistance programs including the Supplemental Nutrition Assistance Program, the National School Lunch Program, the Special Supplemental Nutrition Program for Women, Infants and Children (WIC), the School Breakfast Program, and the Child and Adult Care Food Program.[4]

Supplemental Nutrition Assistance Program

The first Food Stamp Program (FSP) was created in 1939 and since 1980, SNAP has been the largest federal food assistance program and a mainstay of the federal safety net. The program's intent is to enable people with low

Strategy Tip

To learn the full extent about each of the food assistance programs online at the USDA's Food and Nutrition Services website at http://www.fns.usda.gov/fns/

income to obtain a nutritionally adequate diet by providing assistance to allow for the purchase of food and nonalcoholic beverages in authorized community stores. In 1988 and 1990, the introduction of Electronic Benefit Transfer (EBT) payments streamlined the process and reduced fraud by creating a debit card system for the transfer of government benefits directly to the retailer account for products purchased. In 1992, a SNAP education program (SNAP-ed) was implemented to provide education to recipients regarding making healthy food choices within a limited budget. The 2008 Farm Bill saw the FSP name changed officially to SNAP to reduce associated stigma.[5] SNAP is currently performing a 2-year test pilot for online grocery shopping in order to enhance food access similar to the rest of the American populace's access to order and pay for groceries online.[6] (You can read more about food/grocery deserts in Chapters 3, 5, and 13.)

To qualify for SNAP benefits, a household without an aged or disabled member must have a gross income less than 130% of the official poverty guidelines. The household's net income must fall below the poverty line and must meet asset limits. In determining the benefit level, FNS assumes that a household will contribute 30% of its countable income toward food purchases.[7] In addition, the Thrifty Food Plan for a family of four is determined by FNS to calculate the basic expenditure by which a family of four could purchase a nutritionally adequate diet with minimum costs.[8]

Most people who receive food stamps rely on the program for support over a relatively long period of time because of high re-entry rates. Individuals' economic circumstances, such as employment status (job instability) and income level, are an important determination of participation patterns. Children, older people, and people with disabilities comprise two-thirds of SNAP participation.[9] (Read more about food insecurity in the United States in Chapter 13.)

Among nondisabled adults, recent research shows that SNAP participants are more likely to use the program during periods of joblessness (62% of use during months not working vs. 44% of use during months working). However, this research demonstrated that regardless of length of participation, nondisabled adults do work for >50% of the time in which they received SNAP benefits.[9]

Nevertheless, and despite welfare reform legislation of 1996, the new rule for SNAP eligibility requires able-bodied adults without dependents to work or participate in an employment program for at least 20 hours per week to continue to receive benefits for more than 3 months over a 36-month period.[9,2] Notably, a Disaster SNAP Policy, revised in 2014 to aid families with "disaster-related expenses," was implemented during the COVID-19 pandemic of 2020.[10] Under the Families First Coronavirus Response Act, the time limit for able-bodied adults without dependents was suspended.[11]

A major goal of the Supplemental Nutrition Assistance Program is to protect against food insecurity and hunger. The latest data report from 2017 suggests an ongoing decrease in food-insecure households. However, there were still an estimated 15 million food insecure households reported including nearly one-third of these with very low food security. Food insecurity varies considerably by state and is greater than the national average in minority populations including Black- and Hispanic-headed households, households near or below the federal poverty line, and families with single parents. In the month prior to the 2017 report, about 58% of food insecure families reported participating in SNAP, WIC, or the National School Lunch Program.[12] Read more about the federal poverty levels and their impact in Chapter 7.

Discussion Prompt

See and discuss the ethics of the current eligibility criteria as they appear on the Food and Nutrition Service's website at http://www.fns.usda.gov.

Pandemic Tip

During the Covid-19 pandemic, describe and discuss how these programs helped individuals? Where did new programs develop, even if they were temporary? What were some of the programs?

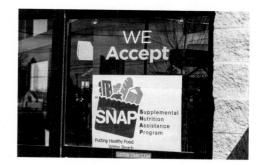

Food stamps.
© Jeff Bukowski/Shutterstock.

Pandemic Tip

Research the Families First Coronavirus Response Act to find out more extensive details.

Special Supplemental Nutrition Program for Women, Infants, and Children

The WIC program, administered by the USDA's Food and Nutrition Service, was established as a pilot program in 1972 and made permanent in 1974. By the end of 1974, WIC sites were operating in 45 states.[13] WIC currently serves nearly half of all infants born in the United States at any given time.[14] Current programs are funded by federal grants and administered by some 90 state agencies in all 50 States, 34 Indian Tribal Organizations, American Samoa, District of Columbia, Guam, Commonwealth of the Northern Mariana Islands, Puerto Rico, and the Virgin Islands.[15] The program eligibility is based on two premises: 1) inadequate nutritional patterns and health behaviors of low-income women and children mean they are more vulnerable to adverse health outcomes; and 2) food interventions during critical times of growth and development can help prevent future medical and developmental problems.[15,16] Data from the WIC Infant and Toddler Feeding Practices Study 2: Fourth Year Report suggest that 46% of WIC participants continue to receive care and education until their child's 4th year of life. The top three reasons why caregivers continued participating in WIC at 42 months were: the education, information, and advice they receive from WIC, the WIC food package, and WIC staff listen to their thoughts about their child's health. The Healthy Eating Index 2015 (HEI-2015) scores for children with ongoing WIC participation at 48 months were comparable to a national sample of 2-to-5 year olds and 3 points higher on average compared with children who had left WIC after their first year. Data also suggest that approximately 90% of surveyed WIC children consumed the WIC package including fruits, vegetables, grains, milk, meats, and proteins on any given day. However, data also showed that 82% of these same children consumed desserts, candies, and sugar-sweetened beverages and median intake of vitamins K and D were below the recommended levels. Positively, 70% of WIC caregivers reported changing their eating habits due to the education received during their participation in WIC.[17]

The WIC program is a broad-based and comprehensive food and nutrition program providing three main benefits to participants: 1) supplemental foods, 2) nutrition education, and 3) referrals to healthcare and social service providers. Improved outcomes include reduced infant mortality and birthing outcomes including longer gestation and reduced preterm birth, improved diet and nutrient intakes, increased breastfeeding rates, improved cognitive development, and increased likelihood of children having regular access to medical care.[18]

Supplemental Foods

WIC food supplements are designed to target nutrition needs by setting guidelines for specific foods and beverages to be purchased monthly by its participants. The supplemental foods for pregnant women are designed to improve nutritional status during pregnancy, improve pregnancy outcomes, and promote a better nutritional status for mothers and infants. Supplements for lactating women are designed to provide special nutrients needed for lactation, improve lactation performance, and promote a better nutritional status for the mother and infant. WIC food supplements for postpartum mothers who are not breastfeeding are intended to improve nutritional status during the postpartum period to better meet the physical demands of postnatal care and improve nutritional status and health for any future pregnancy.[19] The WIC package was updated in 2009 to provide increased amounts of fruit, vegetables, whole grains, lower fat dairy, and expand culturally appropriate

Some of the allowable WIC foods.

© Jonathan Weiss/Shutterstock.

Discussion Prompt

Locate online the current WIC food package at https://fns-prod.azureedge .net/sites/default/files/wic/SNAPSHOT-of -WIC-Child-Women-Food-Pkgs.pdf and discuss the merits of the included foods.

options for the women and children the program serves. Outcomes measured after the new food package was implemented to include increased availability of healthy foods in WIC authorized stores, increased HEI-2015 scores among mothers and children, and a reversal in the increasing prevalence of obesity among 2 to 4 year olds participating in WIC.

With the COVID-19 pandemic, the previously mentioned Families First Coronavirus Response Bill appropriated extra funds to support the WIC program and waved some of the regulatory requirements to allow greater participation due to the increase in unemployment and subsequent increased food insecurity. The pandemic has also led to an increase in online ordering, curbside pick-up, or home delivery of groceries provided by the food package.[20]

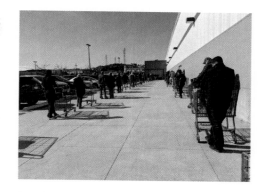

Long food lines during the COVID-19 pandemic.

© Greenseas/iStock Editorial/Getty Images Plus/Getty Images.

Nutrition Education

The WIC program also provides nutrition education to improve the nutritional status of participants. WIC State agencies are responsible for creating easy-to-understand and practical education plans. WIC continues to promote and emphasize breastfeeding for its mothers and improve the nutritional status of infants.[15] WIC also works with farmers markets to provide participants greater access to produce while supporting the local community's economy.[21] The creation of the Revitalizing Quality Nutrition Services (RQNS) was prompted by two studies, which found that WIC needed to become more client oriented in their education approach, adopt a more "behavioral approach" to their education, and focus on healthy nutrition for life. The RQNS is a continuous improvement project designed to enhance the effectiveness of WIC education programs.[22] Special grants awarded emphasize an ongoing recognition and promotion of the value of breastfeeding by Vermont WIC in 2009, a "texting for retention program" in 2014 developed by Colorado WIC, and the 2011 Massachusetts WIC Enhanced Referral and Family Support project to help high-need families navigate and find community resources for complex situations.[23] Another RQNS project is an online program called "WIC Works Resource System," an online repository of education and training materials for state and local clinics administration and use.[24] WICSmart is an application for participant use and includes education modules for self-teaching, of which all lessons can be customized by the local WIC agency.[25]

Referrals for Health Care

Referrals to healthcare providers are intended to promote good health care by increasing the use of prenatal and postpartum care, and by improving access to routine preventive services such as immunization, smoking cessation, and family planning. Social service referrals to substance abuse treatment, housing assistance, **Medicaid**, and food stamps assistance are intended to meet a full range of health and nutrition needs of low-income women and their children.

Center for Nutrition Policy and Promotion

The second major agency within FNCS is the Center for Nutrition Policy and Promotion (CNPP). It was created in 1994 as the focal point within the USDA where scientific research is linked with the nutritional needs of the public. CNPP works to improve the health and well-being of Americans by developing and promoting dietary guidance that links scientific research to the nutrition needs of consumers. Center staff help to define and coordinate nutrition education policy within the USDA and translate nutrition

Discussion Prompt

See http://www.Medicaid.gov/ to learn about those who qualify for Medicaid. Discuss the qualification guidelines. Are these guidelines fair and ethical?

Strategy Tip

Why is a behavioral approach necessary?

Medicaid A federal system of health insurance for those requiring financial assistance.

Strategy Tip

How do registered dietitians promote good nutrition and health in communities? How can we make sure there is access to dietitians in communities?

research into information and materials for consumers, policymakers, and professionals in health, education, industry, and the media. Under its two major offices, the CNPP leads Dietary Guidelines development, conducts research and analysis of certain USDA food programs and the Healthy Eating Index. The office of Marketing and Communication is responsible for the creation of MyPlate and also develops and promotes actionable nutrition and health messages.[26]

Healthy Eating Index

The Healthy Eating Index (HEI) was developed by CNPP in 1995 to assess and monitor the quality of the U.S. diet.[26] The tool uses a scoring system from 0–100 to evaluate a set of foods.[27] The HEI is revised every 5 years following the updated Dietary Guidelines for Americans (DGA) to reflect evolving research and evidence regarding healthy eating.[28] The most current HEI-2015 reflects key recommendations from the 2015–2020 Dietary Guidelines for Americans. The mean score for Americans is 59 of 100 on the HEI-2015, indicating that diet quality does not conform to recommendations and in fact is a grade F. The mean score among separate age groups is similar.[27] This mean score has remained stable compared with data from HEI-2010, demonstrating a plateau in the prior improvements over time from a prior low HEI mean score of 49 in 1999–2000.[29,30]

Dietary Guidelines for Americans, MyPlate, and Thrifty Food Plan

In conjunction with the Department of Health and Human Services, CNPP participates in the review and update of the nutrition science underlying revisions of the Dietary Guidelines for Americans (DGA).[26] The process for updating the Dietary Guidelines includes an evidence-based review of the latest science, which results in recommendations of the Dietary Guidelines Advisory Committee (DGAC). The committee is composed of leading health and nutrition experts from across the country. The process is open, and minutes of meetings of the DGA Committee are posted online through a federal website.[31] Written and oral public comments and feedback about the proposed guidelines are solicited and available online. The Dietary Guidelines for Americans are discussed in Chapter 1. A revision of the food guidance system resulted in the creation of MyPlate (also discussed in detail in Chapter 1) and has been carried out by CNPP in conjunction with the revision of the Dietary Guidelines. The Nutrition Evidence Library was established in 2008 to conduct systematic literature reviews and assist the DGA Committees in 2010 and 2015. The name was changed to Nutrition Evidence Systematic Review (NESR) in 2019 to illustrate that this is a team of professionals, rather than a repository or database of information.[32] The 2020–2025 Dietary Guidelines were revised using data analysis, food pattern modeling, and NESR systematic reviews and were recently released in early 2021.[33,34]

CNPP also maintains and updates the Thrifty Food Plan, which serves as the nutritional basis for determination of benefits in the Supplemental Nutrition Assistance Program. The Low-Cost, Moderate-Cost, and Liberal Food Plans were created in 2003 and are revised along with the Thrifty Food Plan to take into account inflation and reflect updated nutrition guidelines. Each food plan is designed to represent a nutritious diet at various costs. Each has 15 market baskets for each of 15 age-gender groups. The plans are used for a variety of purposes; from determining basic allowance for service members to alimony payments in divorce court.[35] All of CNPP's projects are available on the Internet at https://www.fns.usda.gov/cnpp.

Discussion Prompt

Discuss the cost of food at home at four levels at: https://fns-prod.azureedge.net/sites/default/files/media/file/CostofFoodNov2020.pdf

Overview of the Food Safety and Inspection Service

The Food Safety and Inspection Service (FSIS) is the public health agency within the USDA responsible for ensuring that the nation's commercial supply of meat, poultry, and egg products is safe, wholesome, and correctly labeled and packaged.[36] It provides both education and inspection services. The USDA is responsible for nutrition labeling and inspection of foods not covered by the U.S. Food and Drug Administration. Although not a direct research agency, research does play an important role in FSIS's ability to fulfill its public health mission and to guarantee that the foods it regulates continue to be safe. The agency funds research in food safety and food safety education at various universities and institutes around the country.[37] FSIS is now an important element in homeland security. (Read more about food safety in Chapter 14.)

Overview of Research, Education, and Economics

The USDA-Research, Education, and Economics (REE) agency was created to provide federal leadership in creating and disseminating knowledge spanning the biological, physical, and social sciences related to agricultural research, economic analysis, statistics, extension, and higher education.[38] REE has four major service areas: 1) Agricultural Research Service (ARS); 2) Economics Research Service (ERS); 3) National Agricultural Statistics Service (NASS); and 4) National Institute of Food and Agriculture (NIFA). NIFA is the renamed Cooperative State Research, Education, and Extension Service (CSREES). The Office of the Chief Scientist provides leadership to the four service areas and ensures USDA-funded research is held to the highest standard.[39,40]

Agroecosystems The inclusive agricultural environment with its organisms.

Agricultural Research Service

The Agricultural Research Service remains the principal research arm of the USDA and of human nutrition research. ARS is currently supporting nearly 700 research projects within its 15 national programs all to sustain the nation's **agroecosystems** and to support the nourishment of the American people.[41,42] The Human Nutrition National Program is one of the 15 programs. Its mission statement is:

> "... to define the role of food and its components in optimizing health throughout the life cycle for all Americans by conducting high national priority research."[43]

Program components include:

1. Linking Agricultural Practices and Beneficial Health Outcomes
2. Monitoring Food Composition and Nutrient Intake of the Nation
3. Scientific Basis for Dietary Guidance
4. Prevention of Obesity and Obesity-related Diseases
5. Life Stage Nutrition and Metabolism[43]

Recent projects of the ARS Human Nutrition National program include researching the microbiome in infants, healthy snacking patterns, brain activation and health in obese children, and the launch of FoodData Central in conjunction with the National Agricultural Library, which provides access to all USDA food composition data in one location.[44]

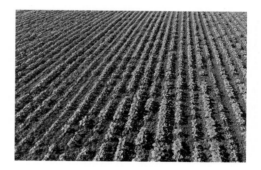

The ARS is responsible for saving agricultural practices.

© AlexandrMusuc/Shutterstock.

Discussion Prompt

The online National Agricultural Library is at http://www.nal.usda.gov. Why is it important to have good recordkeeping in this expertise area for future endeavors?

National Agricultural Library

The NAL is also housed within the ARS.[45] Beyond the traditional functions of a national library of agriculture, the NAL now provides eight online information centers, one of which is the Food and Nutrition Information Center (FNIC). Founded in 1971, FNIC's mission is to collect and disseminate information about food and human nutrition. In 1977, the Food and Agriculture Act (Farm Bill) established FNIC as a permanent entity within the National Agricultural Library. Their target audience are the professional community including educators, clinicians, and researchers. Their website provides wide access to reliable food and nutrition resources. Searchable topics include:

1. Dietary Guidelines
2. Lifecycle Nutrition
3. Diet and Health
4. Food Composition
5. Nutrition Assistance Programs
6. Dietary Supplements
7. Food Labeling
8. Food Safety
9. Professional and Career Resources

The Nutrient Data Library, discussed in detail below, is housed in the FNIC as well.[46]

National Programs in Human Nutrition

The mission of the ARS National Programs in Human Nutrition is carried out in seven locations that serve as major centers for human nutrition research. Each location has special research interests and extensive collaborations and partnerships with universities.[43] A previous eighth location was the Lower Mississippi Delta Nutrition Intervention Research Initiative (NIRI) (Little Rock, AR; founded in 1995). It focused on community intervention research through community-based participatory research in rural communities in Arkansas, Louisiana, and Mississippi.

1. Arkansas Children's Nutrition Center (Little Rock, AR; founded in 1995) has primary studies in brain development and function, dietary factors affecting development, and bone development.
2. Beltsville Human Nutrition Research Center (Beltsville, MD; founded in 1941) focuses on defining the role of food and its components in optimizing human health and reducing the risk of nutrition-related diseases. It also houses the Food Surveys Research Group, discussed below, which have a long history of important contributions to public health nutrition research.
3. Children's Nutrition Research Center at Baylor College of Medicine (Houston, TX; founded in 1979) studies the role of maternal, infant, and child nutrition in optimal health, development, and growth, including childhood dietary habits.
4. Grand Forks Human Nutrition Research Center (Grand Forks, ND; founded in 1977) has long served as the world's leading research center in basic and applied mineral nutrition, including bone health. Other research areas include obesity prevention and health roles of food.
5. Western Human Nutrition Research Center (Davis, CA; founded in 1980) strives to improve health through the study of diet, genetics, and environmental interactions. Specific research areas

include immunity and disease protection via diet to maintain health; obesity; and metabolism.

6. Jean Mayer Human Nutrition Research Center on Aging at Tufts University (Boston, MA; founded in 1980) was founded to study the relationship between nutrition and aging.

7. Plant, Soil, and Nutrition Laboratory at Cornell University (Ithaca, NY; founded in 1940) was established to study the influence of soils on nutritional quality of plant foods and has a proud history of outstanding research, including the award of a Nobel Prize to one of its scientists.[47]

Food Surveys Research Group

Housed within the Beltsville Human Nutrition Research Center, the Food Surveys Research Group (FSRG) has conducted food surveys on Americans since the 1930s. These surveys have summarized nutrient intakes and monitored trends in food intakes. The Continuing Survey of Food Intakes by Individuals (CSFII) was conducted by the USDA in 1977–1978, 1985–1986, 1989–1991, and 1994–1996 before being combined with the National Health and Nutrition Evaluation Survey (NHANES) in 2000. "What We Eat in America" is the dietary interview component of NHANES. Combining the two surveys has allowed data to be collected on an annual basis, rather than sporadically, depending on the availability of monies.[48]

The FSRG has continued to develop, evaluate, and create new dietary assessment tools. In prior data collection, the Multiple Pass Method was used with pencil and paper using a five-step system to obtain free-flowing recall, remember forgotten foods, assign eating occasion, obtain more details, and allow one last opportunity to recall foods. Over a 7-year period, the original method was transferred to a computer-assisted interviewing instrument. The Automated Multiple Pass Method (AMPM) is the cornerstone of a Dietary Intake Data System consisting of three computer systems and an extensive food and nutrient database. Data are collected over 2 days, day 1 in person by the U.S. Department of Health and Human Services (DHHS), and day 2 by phone, 3 to 10 days following the first interview and funded by the USDA. Currently, the food composition data are sourced from the USDA FoodData Central and the Food and Nutrient Database for Dietary Studies (FNDDS) is utilized to process and analyze the collected data from What We Eat in America, NHANES. The FNDDS includes food descriptions, food portions, and their weights and nutrients; a listserv provides emailed alerts when new data or instruments become available.[48]

Effective, efficient, and validated dietary methodology allows the collection of accurate information on what people eat in research studies and over time as free-living individuals. Study of specific nutrients requires accurate and available food composition data of each nutrient in a sufficient number of foods. For large surveys, the food composition data need to include all the foods that the participants are likely to be consuming. The nutrient databases thus need continuous updating as new food products come on the market, new food varieties are developed, and new technologies for nutrient analysis are developed.[49] (Read more about food intake surveys in Chapters 1 and 5.)

Food Composition Databases

The USDA Food Composition Database of the ARS Nutrient Data Lab can now be accessed at FoodData Central. Food Composition data was first published in 1927 with the release of vitamin content of foods in print. Subsequent data were released in print until 2003 when the first

---

Strategy Tip

To be knowledgeable in community nutrition, join the Food Survey Research Group listserv at https://www.ars.usda.gov/northeast-area/beltsville-md-bhnrc/beltsville-human-nutrition-research-center/food-surveys-research-group/docs/listserv/

online data were made available with the release of the Dietary Supplement Database. The Dietary Supplement Databases are now developed by the National Institutes of Health (NIH) in conjunction with the USDA. The original online Food Compositions Database was discontinued in March of 2020 with the launch of FoodData Central. With FoodData Central, all of the USDA's major sources of food and nutrition data are accessible from one website. The goal of this project has been to meet the diverse needs of its users including the lay public, researchers, and health professionals by providing transparent and easily accessible information.[50] The website includes five types of data including the FNDDS for 2017–2018; the Standard Reference Legacy Release (SR Legacy); USDA Global Branded Food Products Database.

1. **Standard Reference Legacy Release (SR Legacy)** has been the primary food composition data type in the United States for decades. Its final update was in April of 2018 and more recent data will be available on the four other data types.

2. **Food and Nutrient Database for Dietary Studies 2017–2018 (FNDDS 2017–2018)** is the most recent data used in the What We Eat in America, NHANES dietary intakes, and report. It was made available to the public in October of 2020 via FoodData Central and has not only been used to facilitate analyses of dietary intakes reported in NHANES but also many other dietary research studies.

3. The **USDA Global Branded Food Products Database (Branded Foods)** are data from a public-private partnership to augment the sharing of nutrient data that appear on branded and private label foods and are provided by the food industry.[51]

The two newer databases provide information that was not previously available to the public. The first is called Foundation Foods, and it provides values for a diverse range of nutrients and food components including extensive underlying metadata regarding sampling and analytic approaches used to obtain the data itself.[51,52] The Experimental foods database, launched in October of 2020, includes foods produced, acquired, or studied under unique conditions including experimental **genotypes** and research protocols.[52]

Genotypes The genetic constitution of an organism.

Underlying human nutrition research and, subsequently, public health nutrition policymaking and practice are quality food composition data. Public health applications include assessing food and nutrient availability and intakes in populations, evaluation of programs to protect and improve nutritional status, research on diet and disease interrelationships, health education and promotion activities, assessment of risk from foodborne contamination, and preserving information on traditional foods. None of these applications can occur without a national nutrient database. Development and maintenance of a high-quality nutrient database continues under the leadership of USDA research scientists.[50]

ARS Publications

ARS continues to provide a bimonthly update regarding the cutting-edge research performed by more than 2,000 scientists across the United States. Previously called Agricultural Research, now Telus, is the ARS digital publication whose highlights include human nutrition, food safety, product innovation, and quality. Recent topics include investigating alternative grains, data sharing to help solve food-manufacturing dilemmas, and finding ways to preserve nutrients during food processing.[53]

National Institute of Food and Agriculture (NIFA)

Formerly known as the Cooperative State Research, Education, and Extension Service (CSREES), the second agency of the USDA-Research, Education, and Economics is the National Institute of Food and Agriculture (NIFA). NIFA was established as part of the 2008 Farm Bill to take the place of CSREES and provides leadership and funding for agriculture related initiatives.[54] Under this new name, the agency continues to allocate federal funding to advance innovation in agriculture, the environment, human health and well-being, and communities by supporting research, education, and extension programs in the land-grant university system and other partner organizations. NIFA is also addressing 21st century concerns such as food security, childhood obesity, and food safety.[54-56] One such program that NIFA continues to fund are the 4-H programs, which affect over 6 million American youths annually. Through 4-H programs, kids and teens have the opportunity to complete hands-on projects under the guidance of staff and volunteers in areas such as health, science, agriculture, and civic engagement.[57]

NIFA's Institute of Food Safety and Nutrition provides practical, science-based education to the public about affordable and accessible food, food resource management, food recovery and food rescue, gleaning, and food donations. They train staff and volunteers at emergency food assistance sites and other locations. Created in 1996 and re-authorized in 2002, the Community Food Projects Competitive Grant Program (CFPCGP) funds projects with the mission to:

- Meet the needs of low-income people by increasing their access to fresher, more nutritious food supplies.
- Increase the self-reliance of communities in providing for their own food needs.
- Promote comprehensive responses to local food, farm, and nutrition issues.
- Meet specific state, local, or neighborhood food and agricultural needs for infrastructure improvement and development.
- Plan for long-term solutions.
- Create innovative marketing activities that mutually benefit agricultural producers and low-income consumers.[58]

To read more about the emphasis areas of the NIFA, visit https://nifa .usda.gov/sites/default/files/resource/NIFA-Fact-Sheet-2019.pdf

Nutrition Programs

NIFA sponsors nutrition-related research including Dietary Practices, serving on National Nutrition Committees, and programs for Minority-Serving Institutions (MSIs). Current Dietary Practice research includes cognitive interviewing using behavior change to affect fruit and vegetable intake in young adults; researching the effect of sodium, soy protein, and iron status and immune function on the health of older women; improving dietary standards by determining the optimal copper requirement for human development, for example; and funding a bilingual nutrition education program to help educate low income, Hispanic, migrant workers, regardless of literacy level.[59]

NIFA is also involved with three national-level, nutrition-related committees including the Nutrition and Health Committee for Planning and Guidance; Nutrition Multistate Regional Committees, and the USDA Human Nutrition Coordinating Committees, which coordinates National Nutrition Month activities at the USDA each March.[60,61] With increased rates of diabetes, obesity, and related heart diseases nationwide and in minority groups, NIFA's

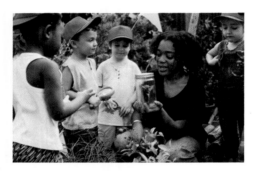

Agro-education programs in minority communities.

© Rawpixel.com/Shutterstock.

Nutrition Program also includes funding programs to enhance Minority Serving Institutes (MSIs). Such research includes multiple healthy living education and agro-education programs in Hawaii, American Samoa, Alaska with the Inupiaq, and various programs with American Indian Arts to promote dietary health and the importance of native foods and culinary traditions.[62]

Food Safety Programs

Through its Food Safety Institute, NIFA seeks to provide a healthier food supply and reduce the risk and prevalence of foodborne illness. Their website contains a multitude of Food Safety Education and Extension materials and the Food Safety Outreach program from 2015 was recently expanded upon in 2019 to deliver customized training on food safety to small and mid-range sized farms including socially disadvantaged farmers. The Improving Food Safety program focuses on enhancing the microbial, chemical, and physical safety of foods through research aimed at improving control strategies and detection methods for foodborne pathogens. Finally, the National Integrated Food Safety Initiative provides grants for projects that include research and education components aimed at applied food safety with a special emphasis on multifunctional activities. Recently funded projects and priority issues have looked at:

- Qualitative and Quantitative Risk Assessments
- Control Measures for Foodborne Microbial Pathogens
- Sources and Incidence of Microbial Pathogens
- Antibiotic-Resistant Microbial Pathogens
- Improving the Safety of Fresh Fruits and Vegetables
- National Coordination of Integrated Food Safety Programs and Resources
- Food Handler Education and Training for Consumers and Youth
- Food Handler Education for High-risk and Hard-to-reach Audiences
- Food Handler Education for Commercial and Noncommercial Audiences, Including Food Handler Certification Training and Other Train-the-Trainer Programs
- Hazard Analysis and Critical Control Points (HACCP) Model Development, Testing, and Implementation
- Home Food Processing and Preservation
- Integrating Food Safety into Related Agricultural Programs
- Alternative Food Processing Technologies that Improve the Safety of Food
- Food Security[63]

Economic Research Service

The Economic Research Service (ERS) is the third service area of the Research, Education, and Economics (REE) agency of the USDA. ERS studies the economics of food, farming, natural resources, and rural America. Their research and data are targeted toward key decision makers at the White House and USDA to help drive public policy by anticipating trends and emerging issues. Research and analysis areas include:

1. Agricultural economy including analyzing data and projections on commodity supply, demand, and prices
2. Food and nutrition including nutrition assistance programs, food choices, and related health outcomes
3. Food safety and the societal benefits and outcomes of regulation vs. industry decisions

4. Global and market trade and economic impacts of imports, exports, and trade barriers
5. Resources and environment, including conservation programs and agricultural competitiveness through technology
6. Rural economy to assess investments made and drivers or economic performance in these communities

Food and Nutrition and Food Safety research areas are housed under the Food Economics Division of the ERS.[64]

Food Economics Division (FED)

Although the ERS does not administer food assistance programs, it carries out research on these programs to ascertain economic evaluation and outcomes under its FED. The FED also studies Food Safety, Food Prices and Markets, and Consumer Behavior.[65]

Ongoing research includes Child Nutrition Programs, WIC, and SNAP. The USDA's Child Nutrition Programs ensure that children receive healthy meals to promote educational readiness and overall well-being. ERS-sponsored research explores the cost constraints to serving nutritious meals through the National School Lunch Program and School Breakfast Program in addition to health outcomes in participating children. In FY2019, ERS research demonstrated that children from food insecure households were more likely to eat school meals and received more of their nutrient intake from school meals than did other children.[66] The ERS and previously discussed FNS have a joint program called the Census-FNS-ERS Joint Project to acquire state census data to collaborate and better understand the success of SNAP and WIC. These programs otherwise have no national data so this effort will provide better insight into program successes across the country and inform improvement projects.[67]

Other areas of research include Food Assistance Data and Collaborative Research Programs to provide data regarding USDA's other food assistance programs; Food Security in the United States, including interactive charts and about food security and insecurity across the country; and Poverty and Income Volatility examining the economic well-being of low-income participants and households in the food and nutrition assistance programs.[66]

Food choices and health represents another research arm of the FED under the ERS. Studies include examining factors driving food choices and the economic impacts of health outcomes; consumer information and labeling; obesity; food access and barriers to affordable nutritious food; and an economic analysis of food consumption and demand.[68] The Food Access group provides publicly available mapping tools including the Food Environment Atlas, which aims to present an overview of a community's access to healthy food and its success in doing so.[69]

ERS-FED research also includes Food Safety including how consumers react to foodborne pathogen outbreaks and recalls and analyzes the economic costs of these illnesses. The ERS also conducts research examining how private markets and government regulation have intersected to provide meat and poultry food safety. This includes minimum food safety quality and innovation in enhancing meat and poultry food safety.[70]

ERS Publications

ERS digitally publishes research and analyses throughout the year including a lay magazine, Amber Waves, weekly email reports, a webinar series/forum ERS insights, and Twitter updates. Amber Waves showcase ERS research ranging from Food Safety and recalls, Food Insecurity data and trends, and management of financial risk for farmers.

Strategy Tip

Pinpoint on a map the locations of the WIC and SNAP programs in your community. What is the reasoning for their locations? Are the programs placed effectively for ease in visits?

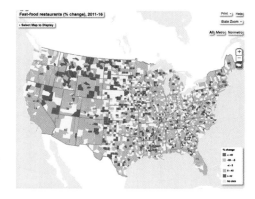

Go live online to the Food Atlas to see how your community is faring at https://www.ers.usda.gov/data -products/food-environment-atlas/go-to-the-atlas/

© USDA United States Dept of Agriculture.

The Food and Nutrition Assistance Research Reports Database makes available all ERS and ERS-sponsored research for both technical and non-technical audiences. Also available are the project summaries reviewing all awards granted through ERS's Research Innovation and Development Grants in Economics (RIDGE).[71]

Important publications include The WIC Program: Background, Trends, and Economic Issues, 2015 edition and The Economic Impacts of Breast-feeding: A Focus on USDA's Special Supplemental Nutrition Program for Women, Infants, and Children (WIC). The most recent publication of The Food Assistance Landscape: Fiscal Year 2019 Report examines most recent trends of the USDA's food assistance programs.[72] Recent publications during the COVID-19 pandemic explore the adverse economic effects of the pandemic on agriculture, food, and rural America. Research includes agricultural imports and exports and effect on food availability and change in price, Outlook Reports on various crops, and higher death rate rationale and outcomes in the rural sector.[73]

History of Nutrition Education at the USDA

The USDA has a rich history of providing science-based nutrition information and education to the public. The Organic Act of 1862 directed the newly formed Department of Agriculture to "acquire and diffuse among the people of the United States useful information on subjects connected to agriculture and rural development." In the 1930s, the USDA's focus was on providing "common-sense knowledge of nutrition," followed by the RDAs in the early 1940s, which emphasized maintaining health for the war effort. In the 1950s, nutrient adequacy was emphasized, and the USDA focused on providing the right kind of information for an adequate diet.[34] In 1969, the White House Conference on Food, Nutrition, and Health was held, and the focus became linking nutrition education to the promotion of optimal health with food. The president of the Academy of Nutrition and Dietetics (former name was The American Dietetic Association) testified in favor of the amendment of the Food Stamp Act in 1969 and the expansion and improvement of the National School Lunch Act in 1969.[74]

In the 1970s, the Food and Agriculture Act of 1977 named the USDA the "lead government agency for nutrition research, extension, and teaching." A call for the development of more effective systems for delivering nutrition information to the public was linked to the growing evidence relating some food components to risks for chronic disease. Increased public interest in diet and disease risks led to the first set of USDA Dietary Guidelines for Americans. **Table 4–1** outlines three USDA Nutrition Education Programs with Legislative Authorization that began in the 1970s: 1) Nutrition Education and Training Programs (NET), 2) WIC, and 3) EFNEP.

The 1980s brought increased interest in nutrition education research for the development of improved materials and methods to better inform the general public about good nutrition. Evaluation of nutrition education tools was increased to measure comprehension and perceived usefulness by the targeted audiences.

In the 1990s, a revised Dietary Guidelines for Americans was released. A greater coordination of nutrition education efforts and survey efforts was called for by the Nutrition Monitoring and Related Research Act.[74] The focus shifted from a simple nutrition information provision to promoting behavioral change and motivating consumers to adopt eating practices to promote optimal health. This focus continues to shape Nutrition Assistance Programs, Research, Education, and Economics all to improve the health and well-being

TABLE 4–1
USDA Nutrition Education Programs with Legislative Authorization

Program	Target Population	Agency Responsible	State Collaborators	Delivery
Nutrition Education and Training Program (NET)	Children, all incomes	CS	State education departments	Training of school food service and teachers, school nutrition education curricula, training for childcare providers and parents
Special Supplemental Nutrition Program for Women, Infants and Children (WIC)	Low-income pregnant and breastfeeding women, infants, and children up to age 5	CS	State health departments and WIC clinics	Individual counseling or group lessons along with WIC food package or vouchers for supplemental foods; two contacts per 6-month certification period
Expanded Food and Nutrition Education Program (EFNEP)	Limited-resource families with young children; low-income youth	SREES	State land-grant universities; county cooperative extension offices	One-on-one home visits or group classes by trained paraprofessional aides; in-depth 6-month program
Education Program (EFNEP)	Limited-resource families with young children; low-income youth	CSREES	State land-grant universities; county cooperative extension offices	One-on-one home visits or group classes by trained paraprofessional aides; in-depth 6-month program

of the American populace. Goals for FY2018–2022 include continuing to efficiently and effectively disseminate USDA programs while maximizing the ability of American agricultural producers all while providing a safe food supply.[75] The latest revision of the Dietary Guidelines for Americans was released for 2020–2025 with a focus on nutrition guidelines by age.[34]

Nutrition, Agriculture, and Health of Americans

The health of rural populations is essential to the production and maintenance of an adequate and safe food supply. The USDA thus has long been committed to improving the nutritional health of Americans through a program of research and education to maintain a food supply of high nutritional quality and to encourage consumption of a healthful diet.

Nutrition is a bridge between agriculture and the health of American consumers in a two-way process. Science-based nutrition messages can motivate Americans to make healthful changes in their diets that will create new demands in the kinds and amounts of food people buy in the marketplace.[76] Market responses to consumer demands can lead, in turn, to the creation of new products and other changes in the food system. Examples include the development of low-fat and reduced-calorie foods, leaner meats, and calcium-enriched orange juice and other beverages.[76] More recent examples include the evolution from the Food Pyramid to MyPlate in 2010. Well-targeted nutrition education and health promotion activities can encourage Americans to adopt new agricultural products into healthy eating habits and eventually lead to positive health outcomes and reduced healthcare costs.

History of the USDA's Research Role in Public Health Nutrition

The founding of food and nutrition science policy was nurtured by the establishment of the Land-Grant College System by the Hatch Act of 1887, shortly after the creation of the Department of Agriculture in 1862.[74] The first federal funding of human nutrition research occurred in 1893–1894. An early beneficiary of the USDA Land Grant program at the University of Connecticut at

Discussion Prompt

Why did the Food Pyramid have to be replaced? Discuss MyPlate as a replacement.

Storrs was Dr. Wilbur O. Atwater, whose "Atwater values for carbohydrates, protein, and fat" are among the first nutrition facts taught in introductory nutrition courses and are used on a daily basis by dietitians and nutritionists. Dr. Atwater, credited as the father of American food science, was appointed the Director of the Office of Experiment Stations, which was funded by the USDA.[77] The contributions of Atwater and other pioneers of the 19th century are the cornerstone of current nutrition science and policy. These principles of rigorous quantitative analysis, using appropriate standard reference materials, are still applied today in the USDA nutrient data laboratory in Beltsville and in collaborating universities' laboratories.[78-80]

The first tables of average nutrient values of foods were published in 1896 as The Chemical Composition of American Food Materials, USDA Bulletin 28. The third version, by Atwater and Bryant in 1906 included analysis of more than 4,000 food items and served as a standard reference for dietitians and nutritionists for more than 4 decades. Within the newer FoodData Central, the Nutrient Data Laboratory and the Food Survey Group of the Agricultural Research Service continue collaboration to plan, develop, and monitor nutrient databanks and methodology that underlie all nutrition surveys and nutrition intervention research in the United States.[50-52] Since 2004, Nutrition.gov has provided a centralized location for the lay public to find credible nutrition and healthy eating information. It was launched as part of the USDA's Obesity Intervention Plan and is funded by the REE mission area.[81]

The USDA has focused largely on promotion of health through supporting food production, food technology, nutrition research, and nutrition education.

Figure 4–1 shows the organizational chart of the USDA.

U.S. Food and Drug Administration

The U.S. Food and Drug Administration (FDA) is a division of the U.S. Department of Health and Human Services (DHHS). The DHHS has a responsibility to protect the health of Americans with the FDA more specifically overseeing food and drugs.[82] Historically, the FDA was established after the passing of the Pure Food and Drugs Act of 1906, which landmarked a consumer protection law. The Pure Food and Drugs Act made mislabeled and adulterated foods, drinks, and drugs illegal. The FDA provides legal protection to the public health by establishing safety standards to all domestic and imported foods.[83] Food additives are also in the jurisdiction of the FDA, where each must be approved prior to use.[84] (Read more about food additives in Chapter 14.)

The FDA established The Hazard Analysis Critical Control Point (HACCP) system, which dictates a safety procedure for handling all food in the United States in the 1990s and early 2000s. The FDA also assisted establishing the Department of Homeland Security (DHS) to protect against bioterrorism in the wake of the 9/11/2001 terrorist attacks. (See Chapter 13 for more about the FDA, food safety, and bioterrorism.) The passage of the Food Allergy Labeling and Consumer Protection Act in 2004 mandated labeling of any food containing any of the eight major food allergens. In 2011, the FDA Food Safety and Modernization Act (FSMA) led to FDA enforcement of imported foods held to the same standards as domestic foods.[85] Most recently, the FDA implemented an agency reorganization in March 2019 that is aimed at modernizing its structure to advance its mission and meet challenges of innovation across industries regulated by the FDA. The Center for Food Safety and Applied Nutrition (CFSAN) is one of six

Strategy Tip

Where in Figure 4–1 should registered dietitians be placed? Why?

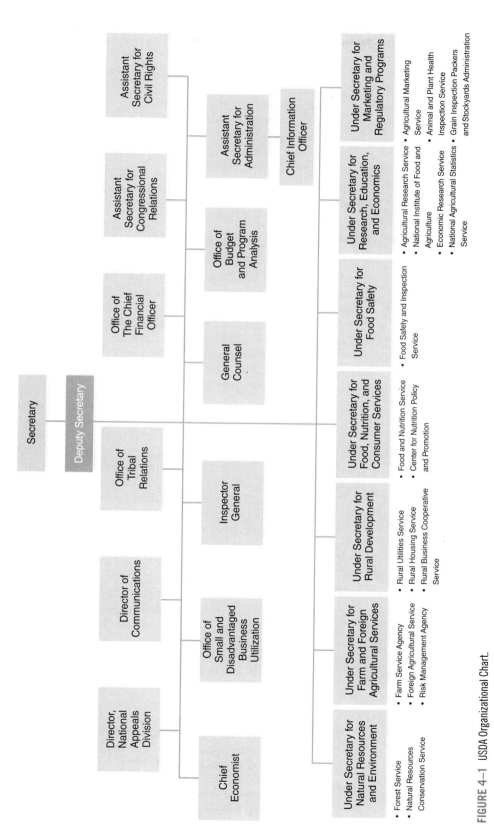

FIGURE 4-1 USDA Organizational Chart.

U. S. Department of Agriculture. USDA Organization Chart. Available at http://www.usda.gov/documents/usda-organization-chart.pdf

product-oriented centers. Its services include safeguarding food, cosmetics, and dietary supplements. This includes:

- Modernize methods to find, track, and eliminate harmful germs and other hazards
- Evaluate the safety of new ingredients for food and the safety of new color additives
- Strengthen manufacturing practices
- Ensure properly labeled food, dietary supplements, and cosmetics
- Foster good nutrition and effective food safety practices
- Investigate causes of foodborne illness outbreaks
- Target unsafe products[86]

Figure 4–2 shows the organizational chart of the CFSAN of the FDA, where many of these products are listed.

Centers for Disease Control and Prevention

Another division of DHHS is the Centers for Disease Control and Prevention (CDC), which was established in 1946, for the main purpose of disease protection. The CDC, under the Division of Nutrition, Physical Activity, and Obesity (DNPAO) is involved in many nutrition initiatives and strategies, which include input in the Dietary Guidelines, healthy and safe food environments, school health and nutrition, physical activity, obesity, breastfeeding, supermarkets with healthy food choice availability, and more consumption of fruits and vegetables. The list below summarizes some of these strategies and current and ongoing initiatives.[87]

- Dietary guidelines and public health approaches to improve population nutrition. A recent initiative includes the Active People, Healthy Nation was created in 2017 with the goal to engage 27 million Americans in becoming more physically active by 2027.[88]
- Racial and Ethnic Approaches to Community Health (REACH) is a CDC-administered program funding and supporting local programs for over 20 years. It is culturally tailored to reduce chronic diseases and risk behaviors.[89]
- Dietary Guidelines encourage individuals to eat a healthful diet— one that focuses on foods and beverages that help achieve and maintain a healthy weight, promote health, and prevent chronic disease.[34]
- Healthy Food Service Guidelines are used to create a food environment in which healthier choices are made easier for consumers. These guidelines are used to increase the availability of healthier food and beverages to increase the likelihood that healthier options are selected by customers.[90]
- The CDC provides funding, training, and technical assistance to Early Care and Education (ECE) programs including obesity prevention education.
- School Health Guidelines to Promote Healthy Eating and Physical Activity serve as the foundation for developing, implementing, and evaluating school-based healthy eating and physical activity policies and practices for students in grades K–12.
- State Public Health Actions to Prevent and Control Diabetes, Heart Disease, Obesity, and Associated Risk Factors and School Health is an initiative funding state health departments to use evidence-based approaches to implement strategies to increase access to and help the populace to achieve good health.

Strategy Tip

Where could a registered dietitian be placed in the FDA Organizational Chart? Why are dietitians excluded? What can be done about including a dietitian in the FDA hierarchy?

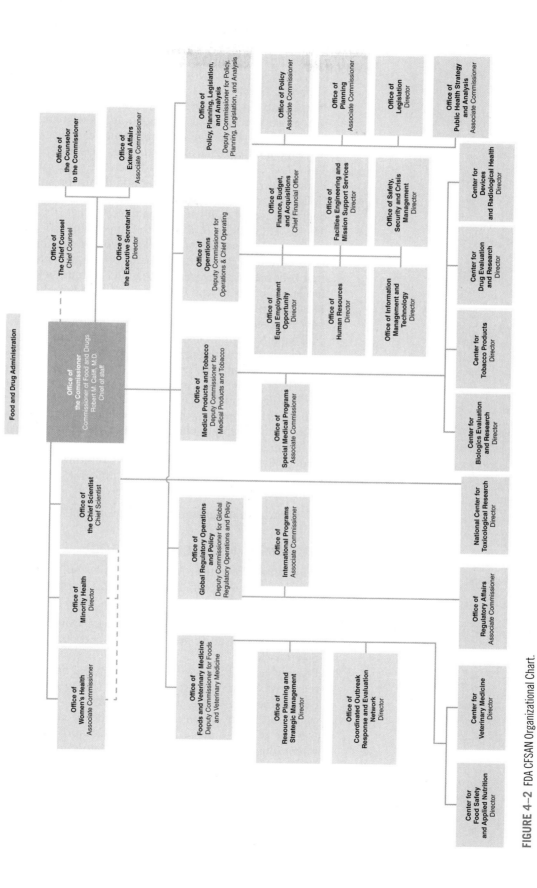

FIGURE 4–2 FDA CFSAN Organizational Chart.

FDA. Food and Drug Administration Organizational Chart. Available at http://www.fda.gov/downloads/AboutFDA/CentersOffices/OrganizationCharts/UCM432556.pdf

- The International Micronutrient Malnutrition Prevention and Control (IMMPaCt) program was established in 2000 to improve micronutrient intakes in vulnerable populations globally. Emphasis is on iron, vitamin A, iodine, folate, zinc, and vitamin D.
- State and Local Program: Nutrition Strategies Initiatives to increase access to healthier foods and beverages in retail venues can improve existing stores, encourage placement of new stores, improve transportation access to healthier food retailers, and/or implement comprehensive in-store markets and promotion.[89]
- The CDC Guide to Strategies to Increase the Consumption of Fruits and Vegetables provides guidance for program managers, policymakers, and others on how to select strategies to increase the consumption of fruits and vegetables.[90]
- The CDC Guide to Strategies to Support Breastfeeding Mothers and Babies provides state and local community members with information to choose the breastfeeding intervention strategy that best meets their needs. The CDC currently monitors and funds programs to improve practices including the Baby Friendly Hospital Initiative (BFHI) to support successful breastfeeding for new moms and infants.[91]
- The New Nutrition Facts Label was updated in 2016 with mandatory use of the new format by 2021. It is the first major change since the label was introduced in 1994 in order to help the American public choose healthier foods. The new label abides by the Dietary Guidelines for 2015–2020 and highlights saturated and trans-fat content, changing serving size quantity to better reflect how much people actually eat, percentage of calories from added sugars, and updated nutrient data for vitamin D.[92]
- The CDC established the Food Safety Initiative Activity focused upon the prevention of food-borne illness. (See Chapter 14 for more about the CDC and food safety.)

Figure 4–3 shows the organizational chart for the CDC.

Environmental Protection Agency

The Environmental Protection Agency (EPA), established in 1970, participates in several goals to protect human health. Their top goals for fiscal year 2018–2022 include:

1. Deliver a cleaner, safer, and healthier environment for all Americans and future generations by carrying out the Agency's core mission
2. Provide certainty to states, localities, tribal nations, and the regulated community in carrying out shared responsibilities and communicating results to all Americans
3. Increase certainty, compliance, and effectiveness by applying the rule of law to achieve more efficient and effective agency operations, service delivery, and regulatory relief

Goal number 1, "A Cleaner, Healthier Environment" most actively affects the nutritional concerns of human health, although each of the others has an indirect cause as well. Their stated goal is to "modernize and update aging drinking water, wastewater and storm water infrastructure which the American public depends on.[93]" To provide for water safety, the EPA has established The Office of Water (OW), which ensures that drinking water is safe, and restores and maintains oceans, watersheds, and their aquatic ecosystems to protect

Strategy Tip

Where could a registered dietitian be placed in the CDC Organizational Chart? Why are dietitians excluded? What can be done about including a dietitian in the CDC hierarchy?

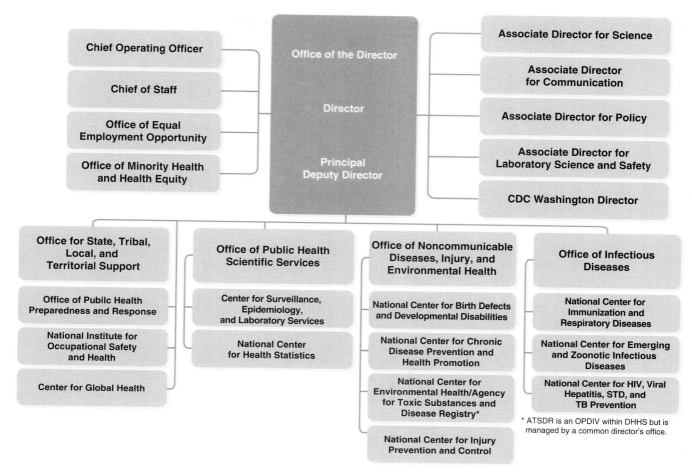

FIGURE 4-3 CDC Organizational Chart.

CDC. CDC Organizational Chart. Available at http://www.cdc.gov/about/pdf/organization/cdc-photo-org-chart.pdf

human health, support economic and recreational activities, and provide a healthy habitat for fish, plants and wildlife.

OW is responsible for implementation[94]:

- Clean Water Act and Safe Drinking Water Act
- Coastal Zone Act Reauthorization Amendments of 1990
- Resource Conservation and Recovery Act
- Ocean Dumping Ban Act
- Marine Protection, Research and Sanctuaries Act
- Shore Protection Act
- Marine Plastics Pollution Research and Control Act
- London Dumping Convention
- International Convention for the Prevention of Pollution from Ships and several other statutes

The OW, headquartered in Washington, D.C., the Office of Water works with the many EPA regional offices, other federal agencies, state and local community governments. (See the EPA's organizational chart in **Figure 4-4**). They also work closely with American Indian tribes, organized professional and interest groups, landowners and managers, corporations, and the public-at-large.[94] (See Chapters 13 and 14 for more about the EPA.)

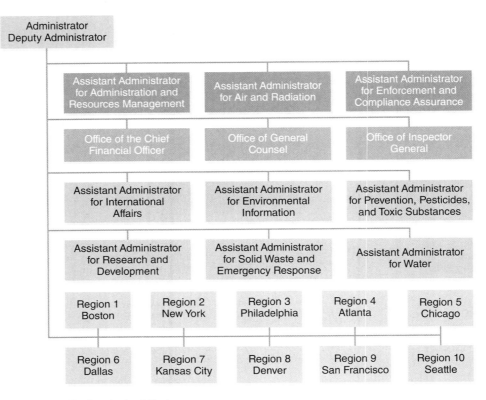

FIGURE 4–4 EPA Organizational Chart.

EPA. EPA Organizational Structure. Available at http://www.4uth.gov.ua/usa/english/politics/agencies/epaorg.htm

Summary

The USDA, FDA, CDC, and EPA are among the large federal organizations who administer a diverse set of nutritional agencies and programs for the welfare of the American public. The USDA is the largest of these agencies that administers food and nutrition policy and programs. The USDA has three major programs that impact on public health nutrition, which are FNCS, Food Safety, and REE. The FDA is a division of the DHHS, which has a responsibility to protect the health of Americans. The FDA more specifically oversees mislabeled and adulterated foods, drinks, and drugs. Food additives are also in the jurisdiction of the FDA, where each must be approved prior to use. The FDA established HACCP, which dictates a safety procedure for handling all food in the United States. Another division of DHHS is the CDC, which was established for the main purpose of disease protection. One of these areas of disease protection is foodborne illness. The EPA participates in the regulation of pesticides, wildlife, water quality standards, and environmental protection. The EPA has been instrumental in supporting research, education, and public awareness programs on these issues.

Learning Portfolio

© olies/Shutterstock.

Issues for Discussion

1. Discuss the pros and cons of having governmental agencies intervene on the public's health?
2. Differentiate what agency covers which areas of nutritional health? Is there any overlap and why?
3. Determine how the USDA and FDA are both similar and different.
4. Determine how the CDC and the EPA are both similar and different.
5. Discuss the worth of these agencies in the lives of the American people. Who benefits?

Practical Activities

1. Search the current news for headlines concerning areas that the USDA covers. Discuss these issues and how the USDA is involved.
2. Search the current news for headlines concerning areas that the FDA covers. Discuss these issues and how the FDA is involved.
3. Search the current news for headlines concerning areas that the CDC covers. Discuss these issues and how the CDC is involved.
4. Search the current news for headlines concerning areas that the EPA covers. Discuss these issues and how the EPA is involved.

Key Terms

	page
Medicaid	103
Agroecosystems	105
Genotypes	108

Case Study: Flint, Michigan, Lead in the Drinking Water

Data from http://www.epa.gov/flint

In 2016, it was discovered that Flint, Michigan, had a dangerous level of lead in the drinking water. Then, President Obama signed an emergency declaration ordering federal assistance to support state and local response efforts in Flint, Michigan. The DHHS has been designated the lead federal agency responsible for coordinating federal government response and recovery efforts in collaboration with other federal agencies including the EPA. What would be the advice and actions of these federal agencies in response to nonsafe drinking water?

Case Study: COVID-19 Pandemic and Government Assistance

Data from United States Department of Agriculture (USDA), Food and Nutrition Service (FNS) Month-To-Month Contingent Approval to Continue Issuing Supplemental Nutrition Assistance Program (SNAP) Emergency Allotments (EA) Benefits under the Families First Coronavirus Response Act of 2020. Retrieved from https://fns-prod.azureedge.net/sites/default/files/resource-files/MA-SNAP-COV -EmergencyAllotmentsExtension9-Acknowledged.pdf

In late 2019, early 2020, the new novel Coronavirus spread to the United States, leading to most states to put their citizens on lockdown, close restaurants and schools, and switch the remote schooling, and halt other activities involving public gatherings all in an effort to stop the spread and rising death toll. The USDA, FNS started issuing emergency allotments (EA) benefits under the Coronavirus Families First Act of 2020. These funds must be requested by the state and then approved by the federal government on a month-to-month basis. How might month-to-month approval of EA affect those participating in SNAP? How might remote schooling affect a family and their children's ability to obtain adequate nutrition?

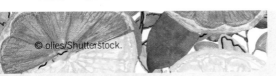
© olies/Shutterstock.

Learning Portfolio

Resources

1. Visit the USDA at https://www.usda.gov/
2. The Food and Nutrition Information Center: https://www.nal.usda.gov/fnic
3. FoodData Central databases: https://fdc.nal.usda.gov/
4. The Dietary Guidelines for Americans including MyPlate resources: https://www.nal.usda.gov/fnic/dietary-guidance-0
5. Agricultural Research Service digital publication Tellus (formerly AgReseach Magazine): https://tellus.ars.usda.gov/
6. FDA Food resources including labeling, dietary supplements, ingredient information at https://www.fda.gov/food
7. CDC Food Safety resources: https://www.cdc.gov/foodsafety/

References

1. FNSC Highlights 2019 Accomplishments. Accessed December 22, 2020. https://www.fns.usda.gov/pressrelease/fns-001719
2. USDA to restore original intent of SNAP: a second chance, not a way of life. Accessed December 22, 2020. https://www.fns.usda.gov/news-item/usda-restore-original-intent-snap-second-chance-not-way-life
3. About FNS. Accessed December 22, 2020. https://www.fns.usda.gov/about-fns
4. USDA FY 2021 Budget Summary. Accessed December 22, 2020. https://www.usda.gov/sites/default/files/documents/usda-fy2021-budget-summary.pdf
5. A Short history of SNAP. Accessed December 22, 2020. https://www.fns.usda.gov/snap/short-history-snap
6. USDA Proposes to close SNAP automatic eligibility loophole. Accessed December 22, 2020. https://www.fns.usda.gov/pressrelease/usda-011319
7. SNAP Eligibility. Accessed December 22, 2020. https://www.fns.usda.gov/snap/recipient/eligibility
8. Carlson A, Lino M, Gerrior SA, Basiotis PP. The low-cost, moderate-cost, and liberal food plans: 2003 administrative report. Center for Nutrition Policy and Promotion, U.S. Department of Agriculture. CNPP-13. Available at: https://fns-prod.azureedge.net/sites/default/files/usda_food_plans_cost_of_food/FoodPlans2003AdminReport.pdf
9. Keith-Jennings, B and Chaudhry, R. Most Working-Age SNAP Participants Work, But Often in Unstable Jobs. Available at: https://www.cbpp.org/research/food-assistance/most-working-age-snap-participants-work-but-often-in-unstable-jobs
10. Disaster SNAP Guidance. Accessed December 22, 2020. https://fns-prod.azureedge.net/sites/default/files/D-SNAP_handbook_0.pdf
11. SNAP – Families first coronavirus response act and impact on time limit for able-bodied adults without dependents (ABAWDs). Accessed December 23, 2020. https://www.fns.usda.gov/snap/ffcra-impact-time-limit-abawds
12. Coleman-Jensen A, Rabbitt MP, Gregory CA, Singh A. Household food security in the United States in 2017. Accessed December 23, 2020. https://www.ers.usda.gov/webdocs/publications/90023/err-256.pdf?v=9775.8
13. History of the WIC program. Accessed December 23, 2020. https://www.ers.usda.gov/webdocs/publications/46648/15834_fanrr27c_1_.pdf?v=41063
14. Special supplemental nutrition program for Women, Infants, and Children (WIC). Accessed December 23, 2020. https://www.fns.usda.gov/wic
15. WIC Fact Sheet. Accessed December 24, 2020. https://fns-prod.azureedge.net/sites/default/files/wic/wic-fact-sheet.pdf
16. About WIC-WIC's mission. Accessed December 24, 2020. https://www.fns.usda.gov/wic/about-wic-wics-mission
17. Special supplemental nutrition program for women, infants, and children (WIC) infant and toddler feeding practices study 2: fourth year report (summary). Accessed December 24, 2020. https://fns-prod.azureedge.net/sites/default/files/resource-files/WIC-ITFPS2-Year4Report-Summary-update.pdf
18. About WIC: how WIC helps. Accessed December 24, 2020. https://www.fns.usda.gov/wic/about-wic-how-wic-helps
19. Navigating supplemental food resources. Accessed December 24, 2020. https://www.hsph.harvard.edu/nutritionsource/navigating-supplemental-food-resources/
20. Dunn C, Kenney E, Bleich S, Fleischhacker S. Strengthening WIC's impact during and after the COVID-19 pandemic. Durham, NC: Healthy Eating Research; 2020. Accessed December 24, 2020. http://healthyeatingresearch.org
21. Farmers market nutrition program. Accessed December 24, 2020. https://www.fns.usda.gov/fmnp/wic-farmers-market-nutrition-program
22. Revitalizing quality nutrition services. Accessed December 24, 2020. https://www.fns.usda.gov/wic/revitalizing-quality-nutrition-services-rqns
23. WIC Works Resource System, explore resources. Available at: https://wicworks.fns.usda.gov/explore-resources?f[0]=topic:526
24. About WIC Works. Accessed December 24, 2020. https://wicworks.fns.usda.gov/about
25. Mobile WIC Education. Accessed December 24, 2020. http://www.wicsmart.com/
26. About CNPP. Accessed December 28, 2020. https://www.fns.usda.gov/about-cnpp
27. Healthy Eating Index (HEI). Accessed December 28, 2020. https://www.fns.usda.gov/resource/healthy-eating-index-hei
28. Krebs-Smith SM, Pannucci TE, Subar AF, et al. Update of the healthy eating index: HEI-2015. *J Acad Nutr Diet*. 2018;118(9):1591-1602. doi: 10.1016/j.jand.2018.05.021. Erratum in: *J Acad Nutr Diet*. 2019. PMID: 30146071; PMCID: PMC6719291.
29. Wilson MM, Reedy J, Krebs-Smith SM. American diet quality: where it is, where it is heading, and what it could be. *J Acad Nutr Diet*, 2016;116(2):302-310.
30. How healthy is the American diet? The Healthy Eating Index helps determine the answer. Accessed December 28, 2020. https://www.elsevier.com/about/press-releases/research

-and-journals/how-healthy-is-the-american-diet-the-healthy-eating-index-helps-determine-the-answer

31. Who's involved in updating the dietary guidelines? Accessed January 21, 2021. https://www.dietaryguidelines.gov/about-dietary-guidelines/process

32. About NESR (formerly NEL). Accessed December 28, 2020. https://nesr.usda.gov/about

33. Scientific Report of the 2020 Dietary Guidelines Advisory Committee. Accessed January 21, 2021. https://www.dietaryguidelines.gov/2020-advisory-committee-report

34. U.S. Department of Agriculture and U.S. Department of Health and Human Services. Dietary Guidelines for Americans, 2020-2025. 9th Edition. December 2020. Available at: https://dietaryguidelines.gov/

35. Carlson A, Lino M, Fungwe T.. The low-cost, moderate-cost, and liberal food plans, 2007 (CNPP-20). 2007. U.S. Department of Agriculture, Center for Nutrition Policy and Promotion.

36. USDA Food safety and inspection service strategic plan 2017-2021. Accessed December 29, 2020. https://www.3tres3.com/3tres3_common/art/3tres3/43390/fitxers/Strategic-Plan-2017-2021.pdf

37. Food safety research priorities. Accessed December 29, 2020. https://www.fsis.usda.gov/wps/portal/fsis/topics/science/food-safety-research-priorities

38. Research, education, economics. Accessed December 29, 2020. https://www.ree.usda.gov/

39. USDA Research, Education, and Economics. Mission statement. Accessed December 29, 2020. https://www.ree.usda.gov/about-ree/mission-statement

40. Agencies and offices. Accessed December 29, 2020. https://www.ree.usda.gov/agencies-and-offices

41. About ARS. Accessed December 29, 2020. https://www.ars.usda.gov/about-ars/

42. National programs. Accessed December 29, 2020. https://www.ars.usda.gov/research/programs/

43. National Program 107: Human nutrition strategic vision. Accessed December 29, 2020. https://www.ars.usda.gov/nutrition-food-safetyquality/human-nutrition/

44. Advancing Human Nutrition Research. Accessed December 29, 2020. https://www.ars.usda.gov/ARSUserFiles/00000000/NPS/OAA/Annual%20Report%20on%20Science/FY2019/onepagers/AdvancingHumanNutritionResearch.pdf

45. ARS organizational chart. Accessed December 30, 2020. https://www.ars.usda.gov/people-locations/organizational-chart/

46. Food and Nutrition Information Center. Accessed December 30, 2020. https://www.nal.usda.gov/fnic#quicktabs-fnic_quick_tabs=1

47. Human Nutrition Research. Accessed December 30, 2020. https://www.ars.usda.gov/oc/human-nutrition-research/

48. Food Surveys Research Group: Beltsville, MD. What we eat in America. Available at: https://www.ars.usda.gov/northeast-area/beltsville-md-bhnrc/beltsville-human-nutrition-research-center/food-surveys-research-group/docs/wweianhanes-related-links/

49. Food Surveys Research Group: Beltsville, MD. Dietary methods research. Accessed December 30, 2020. https://www.ars.usda.gov/northeast-area/beltsville-md-bhnrc/beltsville-human-nutrition-research-center/food-surveys-research-group/docs/dmr-food-categories/

50. FoodData Central FAQ. Accessed December 30, 2020. https://fdc.nal.usda.gov/faq.html

51. FoodData Central About Us. Accessed December 30, 2020. https://fdc.nal.usda.gov/about-us.html

52. U.S. Department of Agriculture (USDA), Agricultural Research Service. FoodData Central: Foundation Foods. Version Current: October 2020. Internet: fdc.nal.usda.gov

53. Tellus Article Archive. Accessed December 30, 2020. https://tellus.ars.usda.gov/stories/

54. USDA National Institutes of Food and Agriculture, History. Accessed December 30, 2020. https://nifa.usda.gov/history

55. USDA National Institutes of Food and Agriculture, About NIFA. Accessed December 30, 2020. https://nifa.usda.gov/about-nifa

56. NIFA Fact Sheet. Accessed December 30, 2020. https://nifa.usda.gov/sites/default/files/resource/NIFA-Fact-Sheet-2019.pdf

57. What is 4-H? Accessed December 30, 2020. https://4-h.org/about/what-is-4-h/

58. Community Food Projects Competitive Grant Program (CFPCGP). Accessed December 30, 2020. https://nifa.usda.gov/program/community-food-projects-competitive-grant-program-cfpcgp

59. NIFA-Funded Research on Dietary Practices. Accessed December 30, 2020. https://nifa.usda.gov/nifa-funded-research-dietary-practice

60. National Nutrition Committees. Accessed December 31, 2020. https://nifa.usda.gov/national-nutrition-committees

61. USDA Human Nutrition Coordinating Committee. Accessed December 31, 2020. https://nifa.usda.gov/usda-human-nutrition-coordinating-committee

62. Nutrition and health-enhancing projects for minority-serving institutions. Accessed December 31, 2020. https://nifa.usda.gov/nutrition-and-health-enhancing-projects-minority-serving-institutions

63. Food safety. Accessed December 31, 2020. https://nifa.usda.gov/topic/food-safety

64. About ERS. Accessed December 31, 2020. https://www.ers.usda.gov/about-ers/

65. Food Economics Division. Accessed December 31, 2020. https://www.ers.usda.gov/about-ers/agency-structure/food-economics-division-fed/

66. Food & Nutrition Assistance. Accessed December 31, 2020. https://www.ers.usda.gov/topics/food-nutrition-assistance.aspx

67. Census-FNS-ERS Joint Project. Accessed December 31, 2020. https://www.ers.usda.gov/topics/food-nutrition-assistance/food-assistance-data-collaborative-research-programs/census-fns-ers-joint-project/#goals

68. Food Choices & Health. Accessed December 31, 2020. https://www.ers.usda.gov/topics/food-choices-health/

69. Food Environment Atlas. Accessed December 31, 2020. https://www.ers.usda.gov/data-products/food-environment-atlas/

70. ERS Food Safety. Accessed December 31, 2020. https://www.ers.usda.gov/topics/food-safety/

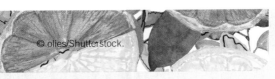
© olies/Shutterstock.

Learning Portfolio

71. Food and Nutrition Assistance Research Reports Database. Accessed December 31, 2020. https://www.ers.usda.gov/data-products/food-and-nutrition-assistance-research-reports-database/

72. Tiehen, L. The food assistance landscape: Fiscal Year 2019 annual report, EIB-218, U.S. Department of Agriculture, Economic Research Service, July 2020.

73. COVID-19 Economic Implications for Agriculture, Food, and Rural America. Accessed December 31, 2020. https://www.ers.usda.gov/covid-19/

74. Cassell JA. Carry the Flame: The history of the american dietetic association. Chicago, IL: American Dietetic Association; 1990.

75. USDA Strategic Goals. Accessed January 11, 2021. https://www.usda.gov/our-agency/about-usda/strategic-goals

76. Kennedy E. The state of nutrition education in USDA: A Report to the Secretary by the State of Nutrition Education in USDA Working Group. Washington, DC: USDA Center for Nutrition Policy and Promotion; 1996.

77. McBride J, Wilbur O. Atwater: father of American nutrition science. *Agric Res*. 1993;41:5-11.

78. Harnly JM, Doherty RF, Beecher GR, et al. Analytical determination of flavonoids (S Aglycones) in foods. In: Proceedings of the 28th National Nutrient Databank Conference, From Farm to Fork-Practical Applications for Food Composition Data. June 23-26. Iowa City, IA: University of Iowa; 2004.

79. Holden JM, Andrews K, Ahao C, et al. Development of the dietary supplement ingredient database, phase II progress. Proceedings of the 28th National Nutrient Databank Conference, From Farm to Fork-Practical Applications for Food Composition Data. June 23-27. Iowa City, IA: University of Iowa; 2004.

80. Teague AM, Sealey WM, McCabe-Sellers BJ, Mock DM. Biotin is stable in frozen foods. *FASEB J*. 2004;18:A118.

81. About Us. Accessed January 27, 2021. https://www.nutrition.gov/about-us

82. History of FDA's Internal Organization. Accessed January 5, 2021. https://www.fda.gov/about-fda/history-fdas-fight-consumer-protection-and-public-health/history-fdas-internal-organization

83. The history of FDA's fight for consumer protection and public health. Accessed January 5, 2021. https://www.fda.gov/about-fda/history-fdas-fight-consumer-protection-and-public-health

84. Regulatory Agencies. Accessed January 5, 2021. http://www.faqs.org/nutrition/Pre-Sma/Regulatory-Agencies.html#ixzz42PyAFhZN

85. Milestones in U.S. Food and Drug Law History. Accessed January 6, 2021. https://www.fda.gov/about-fda/fdas-evolving-regulatory-powers/milestones-us-food-and-drug-law-history

86. What We Do at CFSAN. Accessed January 6, 2021. https://www.fda.gov/about-fda/center-food-safety-and-applied-nutrition-cfsan/what-we-do-cfsan

87. Division of Nutrition, Physical Activity, and Obesity. Accessed January 6, 2021. https://www.cdc.gov/nccdphp/dnpao/index.html

88. Active People, Healthy Nation. Role of public health. Accessed January 6, 2021. https://www.cdc.gov/physicalactivity/activepeoplehealthynation/pdf/Active-People-Healthy-Nation-Role-of-Public-Health-508.pdf

89. Centers for Disease Control and Prevention. What CDC is doing. CDC's work to make health eating easier. Accessed January 6, 2021. https://www.cdc.gov/nutrition/about-nutrition/what-cdc-is-doing.html

90. Healthy Food Environments. Accessed January 27, 2021. https://www.cdc.gov/nutrition/healthy-food-environments/index.html

91. What CDC is doing. CDC's work to support and promote breastfeeding. Accessed January 27, 2021. https://www.cdc.gov/breastfeeding/about-breastfeeding/what-is-cdc-doing.html

92. Learn how the NEW nutrition facts label can help you improve your health. Accessed January 6, 2021. https://www.cdc.gov/nutrition/strategies-guidelines/nutrition-facts-label.html

93. Environmental Protection Agency. Working Together. FY 2018-2022 U.S. EPA Strategic Plan. Accessed January 27, 2021. https://www.epa.gov/sites/production/files/2019-09/documents/fy-2018-2022-epa-strategic-plan.pdf

94. United States Environmental Protection Agency (EPA). About the Office of Water. Accessed January 27, 2021. https://www.epa.gov/aboutepa/about-office-water

PART III

Assessing and Intervening in the Community's Nutrition Needs

CHAPTER 5

Community Needs-Assessment

Melinda Boyd, DCN, MPH, MHR, RDN, FAND

(We would like to acknowledge Elizabeth Metallinos-Katsaras, PhD, RDN, and Katherine Deren, MS, RDN, LDN, for their work on previous editions of Nutrition in Public Health.)

Learning Outcomes

AFTER STUDYING THIS CHAPTER AND REFLECTING ON THE CONTENTS, YOU SHOULD BE ABLE TO:

1. Define community and other needs-assessment terms in the context of public health nutrition.
2. Explain the rationale for community needs-assessment.
3. Describe the steps to follow when conducting a community needs-assessment.
4. Describe the types of data that can be collected about a community and how these data can be obtained (including utilization of existing data sources).
5. Compare assessed needs with the capacity of existing services to meet these needs and identify unmet needs.

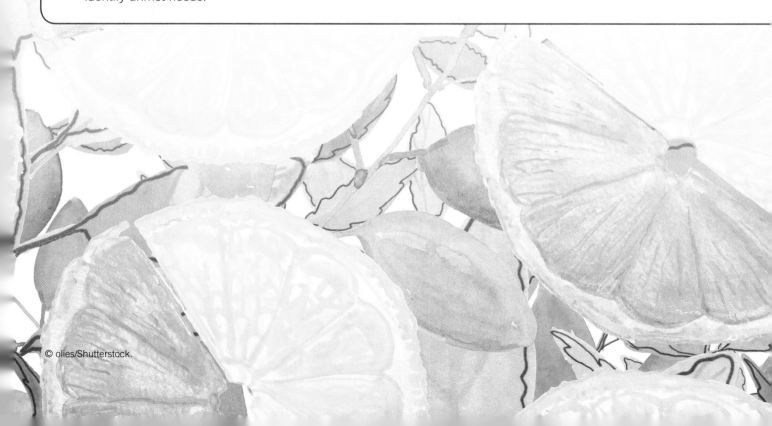

Community A group of people with common characteristics. These can include a location or region; sociodemographic characteristics such as ethnicity, age, education, or occupation; a nutritional problem (e.g., obesity); or a common bond (e.g., members of an organization).

Goal A desired outcome that an entity hopes to achieve. Should be measurable.

Target population A group that is the focus of an assessment, a study, an intervention, or a program.

Discussion Prompt

Describe the players of a needs-assessment problem that could take place in your hometown. Who is the target population? In which city? What is the health concern? Who would conduct the needs-assessment?

Introduction

The commissioner of public health in your town has come to you with the following question: "What are the major nutritional problems of our **community** that are currently not being addressed effectively?" Embedded within this question are several additional queries, including "Who is most affected by the nutritional problems? What are some of the barriers to their improvement? What is the healthcare system doing about them? What resources currently exist to address these problems?" The overarching **goal** of the task you have been handed is to develop new programs or to identify ways in which existing public health nutrition programs can address the most pressing nutritional needs of a community. Such a request from a high-ranking official may sound a bit far-fetched; however, in an era in which the obesity epidemic is at the forefront of not only scientific inquiry but also the media, there is a renewed interest in disease prevention. After all, prevention is the hallmark of public health nutrition.

How would you go about responding to this inquiry? What would you do first? What information or data would you need and where would you get it? This chapter describes the process you can use to determine the unmet nutrition-related needs of a community. Both hypothetical and actual needs-assessment examples are used to exemplify both nutritional status and community resource data.

Community Needs-Assessment: Definition and Overview

An integral step in the public health process is determining the nutritional needs of the community and population with which you are working. Conducting an accurate and focused needs-assessment is an essential step in the planning, implementation, and evaluation of public health programs for several reasons.

First, public health departments and agencies must know about the primary problems and unmet needs of the community prior to developing a new program, modifying existing programs, or distributing resources. Second, in order to allocate resources toward program development and implementation, it is essential to determine the most important and pressing needs of the community. Although we as a community and public health nutritionists are committed to improving all aspects of nutrition-related community health, resource allocation constrains most programmatic decisions. One thus needs to identify the most pressing nutrition-related problems, the underlying causes in the specific group in question, and which problems are not being met by existing resources in order to prioritize and distribute resources.

Equally important in the description of the nutrition problems is who will be affected in order to address their issues. A community can be defined broadly as a group of people with common characteristics. The individuals within the community, who are the focus of the needs-assessment, comprise the **target population**. For example, Baltimore City, Maryland, has many low-income neighborhoods where childhood overweight and obesity is a significant concern in the African American community.[3] In recognition of the importance of obesity prevention, you as the public health dietitian/nutritionist would like to conduct a community needs-assessment of school-age children living in Baltimore City, Maryland. Therefore, the community is Baltimore City, while the target population is school-age children.

Community needs-assessment includes both an assessment of the existing community resources and an assessment of the nutritional status/concerns of the target population. The scope of the community needs-assessment can be large (e.g., a nationwide maternal and child nutrition needs-assessment) or small (e.g., determining the need for breastfeeding support among Laotian-American participants of a specific Special Supplemental Nutrition Program for Women, Infants and Children [WIC] program).

The types of data and methods of obtaining data vary greatly as well. The foundation of some needs-assessments is the identification, compilation, and interpretation of existing (i.e., secondary) data, whereas others incorporate a primary data collection component. Which data collection route should be taken depends on the purpose of the needs-assessment, but it is important to note that numerous existing data sources are publicly available to the public health dietitian/nutritionist (**Table 5–1**). These can be a great resource and should not be underestimated in their usefulness. Some public health nutritionists may embark on primary data collection prematurely, unknowingly ignoring existing data pertinent to their needs-assessment. This can waste precious resources; therefore, we cannot overstate the importance of investigating existing data sources and research in the published literature that may be relevant to your specific needs-assessment.

Who will conduct the community needs-assessment? You might envision a lonely community and public health dietitian/nutritionist setting out to complete all of the phases of the assessment. In reality, in most cases, a team

TABLE 5–1

Examples of Secondary Datasets Available for a Community Needs-Assessment

Dataset and Source	Description
National Center for Health Statistics https://www.cdc.gov/nchs /data_access/ftp_data.htm	Data warehouse for public use data files for: • National Health and Nutrition Examination Survey • National Health Care Survey • National Health Interview Survey • National Immunization Survey • National Survey of Family Growth • National Vital Statistics System • Longitudinal Studies of Aging • State and Local Area Integrated Telephone Survey
Youth Risk Behavior Surveillance System https://www.cdc.gov/healthy youth/data/yrbs/index.htm	Monitors priority health risk behaviors that contribute markedly to the leading causes of death and disability among youth and adults in the United States. Contains public access to data files and documentation. The six categories include: • Behaviors contributing to unintentional injuries and violence • Sexual behaviors related to unplanned pregnancy • and sexually transmitted diseases • Alcohol and drug use • Tobacco use • Unhealthy dietary behaviors • Inadequate physical activity
Economic Research Service, United States Department of Agriculture https://www.ers.usda.gov /topics/food-nutrition-assistance /food-security-in-the-us/	Provides data on food security and agriculture in the United States

is assembled to conduct the assessment. The desirability of this approach is underscored by the fact that numerous and varied skills are needed to effectively conduct a community needs-assessment. While the community public health dietitian/nutritionist is the nutrition expert, they may not be a data or survey development expert. Nor can dietitian/nutritionists alone represent all of the key stakeholders and diverse individuals of the community. Others on the team will complement the public health nutritionist with their expertise in qualitative or quantitative research methods, data analysis, and interpretation.

The needs of a community are in the eye of the beholder. Many decisions can be based on value judgments about the problems that exist in a target population. For example, most consider obesity to be a serious public health problem costing the US $1.72 trillion in healthcare costs in 2016 associated with chronic diseases linked to obesity and overweight,[4] but not every community may find that to be their most pressing health concern. The fact that a public health nutritionist's perceived need may not be met with unanimous agreement by the public makes it important to engender community support for the methods and the findings of the needs-assessment. The needs-assessment process thus not only includes a scientific and analytic component but also a political one. Therefore, it is important to include those individuals or groups in the needs-assessment process who will be affected by the findings.[5] These stakeholders may include individuals from the following groups:

- Consumers/program recipients
- Policymakers
- Members of the target population in that community
- Nutrition program providers
- Nutrition program funders

The individuals represented within each of these groups provide a unique perspective that not only informs the development of the needs-assessment process but also how the nutrition problem in question should be addressed.

Steps to Conduct a Community Needs-Assessment

The community needs-assessment includes a preassessment phase in which the public health nutritionist explores the needs of a community; an assessment, or data-gathering phase; and a postassessment, or utilization phase.[6] The following describes one set of steps to conduct a community needs-assessment. Other valuable resources on conducting community needs-assessment, program planning, and evaluation have been developed by the Association of State and Territorial Public Health Nutrition Directors (http://www.asphn .org/; **Table 5–2**). Another useful tool is Moving to the Future (https://movingtothe future.org), offering both free resources and tools for purchase that can be adapted to meet your needs at all steps of the needs-assessment process.

Phase 1: Needs-Assessment Planning

In the first phase of the needs-assessment, the community or public health dietitian/nutritionist not only must make a case for the needs-assessment in a specific community but must also lay out the organizational framework that will guide the process. The following sections describe the steps necessary to achieve this end.

Step 1: Identify the Community of Interest

At this initial stage of the needs-assessment, you need to articulate which community is of concern. This community can include the group of people who are the focus of your needs-assessment (i.e., the target population) or a

TABLE 5–2

Sources for Demographic and Health Statistics for the Community Needs-Assessment

Source	Description
U.S. Census Bureau Census Data	Data from 2010 Census available. Data from 2020 Census will be available as early as Spring of 2021. Includes state and county data.
Health, United States	2018 National Health statistics produced in report format by the National Center for Health Statistics (NCHS). Comprehensive report drawing from a variety of data sources.
FastStatsAtoZ	Provides state and territorial-specific natality and mortality statistics as well as health and health risk behavior data.
National Health and Nutrition Examination Survey (NHANES)	Reports and study results.
NCHS surveys related to health and health care	
National Vital Statistics	Annual reports present detailed vital statistics data, including natality, mortality, marriage, and divorce.
The Behavioral Risk Factor Surveillance System (BRFSS)	World's largest telephone survey; tracks health risks in the United States; includes national and state statistics as well as statistics on selected metropolitan areas.
Youth Risk Behavior Surveillance System (YRBSS)	Developed in 1990 to monitor priority health risk behaviors that contribute markedly to the leading causes of death, disability, and social problems among youth and adults in the United States.
The Pediatric Nutrition Surveillance System (PedNSS) and the Pregnancy Nutrition Surveillance System (PNSS)	Program-based surveillance systems that monitor the nutritional status of low-income infants, children, and women in federally funded maternal and child health programs.
Data Warehouse for NCHS data	Includes links to detailed statistical tables on a variety of health topics.
United States Department of Agriculture (USDA)	International food consumption patterns Economic Research Service Food Stamp Program statistics WIC Program statistics Food security in the United States links to a variety of data sources on food security.
Association of State and Territorial Public Health Nutrition Directors (ASTPHND)	Provides tools for planning nutrition and physical activity programs.
Food Access Research Atlas	Food access indicators for low-income areas where supermarkets are not available.

Websites with links to statistical information
http://www.census.gov/acs/www/
http://www.cdc.gov/nchs/hus.htm
http://www.cdc.gov/nchs/fastats/state-and-territorial-data.htm
http://www.cdc.gov/nchs/nhanes/nhanes_products.htm
http://www.cdc.gov/nchs
http://www.cdc.gov/nchs/products/vsus.htm
http://www.cdc.gov/brfss/
http://www.cdc.gov/HealthyYouth/yrbs
https://www.ers.usda.gov/data-products/international-food-consumption-patterns/
http://www.ers.usda.gov
http://www.fns.usda.gov/pd/snapmain.htm
https://www.fns.usda.gov/data-research
https://www.ers.usda.gov/topics/food-nutrition-assistance/food-security-in-the-us/
http://www.movingtothefuture.org
http://www.ers.usda.gov/data-products/food-access-research-atlas.aspx

specific region or neighborhood in which they live (e.g., Baltimore City, MD), the nutritional problem of concern (e.g., obesity), or all of the above (e.g., overweight children living in Baltimore City, MD). It is important to be as specific as possible in order to focus your needs-assessment efforts because the initial data may cause the community of interest to shift.

Step 2: Describe the Problem, Research Its Underlying Causes, and State Why a Needs-Assessment Is Necessary

At this point in the process, make sure you've identified a gap in the identified community between what is desired in the community and what they currently have in the community.[6] This makes the case for a true need in the community of interest. Once you've identified the problem, you as the nutrition professional, can prepare a brief, but compelling, statement of the problem. This is especially important if you are applying for funding.[7] It should include a description of the nutritional problem of concern, who is affected, the magnitude of the problem, what is known about its causes, and why there is justification for the needs-assessment. An essential component of the exploration step is to comprehensively review the research in the published literature in terms of both underlying causes and clarify the public health impact to trigger the assessment.[7] Fortunately, resources such as PubMed on the Internet can be used to identify relevant research articles; in many cases, full text articles are available online. In order to minimize the possibility that you are missing important research in this area, you should utilize a reference librarian to guide you in your use of key words and key phrases and in finding the best databases for your topic. Public health nutritionists often are not in a position to conduct scientific research into the underlying causes of nutrition-related problems; however, the wealth of published research available precludes the need for them to do so.

To return to the former example regarding the nutrition-related problem of overweight children in Baltimore City, one needs to examine the literature regarding:

- *Magnitude of the problem.* This includes determining the percentage of children who are overweight or at risk of becoming overweight and identifying which specific groups of children are most at risk.
- *Importance of addressing this problem in children.* This includes the tracking of overweight people from childhood to adulthood; chronic disease consequences, both in childhood and adulthood; and cost to the healthcare system.
- *Define the known causes of children being overweight.* What is known about how overweight indices have increased among children in general? These include increases in sedentary behavior (e.g., TV watching), reductions in physical activity, and increased consumption of specific types of food (e.g., fast food, processed foods, sugar-sweetened beverages).
- *Gaps in the scope of influence.* This refers to those individuals living in a community in whom there are gaps in nutrition knowledge relevant to the identification and resolution of the nutritional problem in the target population. In this case, these would include parents, teachers, school administrators, religious community leaders, and other community members who can influence children's macro- or microenvironment.

Step 3: Define the Target Population

At this point, you have research and data that identify which groups are most at risk for a specific nutritional problem or overall poor nutritional status, and the groups in which the nutritional problem has the greatest effect on public health. This knowledge will guide you to define more clearly the target population for your needs-assessment. For example, in the case of overweight children in Baltimore city, from your review of the published literature, you may have found that the **prevalence** of obesity increases substantially during adolescence. This could provide the justification for choosing preteens living in Baltimore City as the target population, if your needs-assessment is for obesity-prevention programs.

Step 4: Determine the Purpose, Goals, and Objectives of the Community Needs-Assessment

The purpose is a general description of the intent of the needs-assessment. A community needs-assessment may be conducted for any of the following reasons.[8,9]

- To identify groups of people in the community who are at nutritional risk
- To determine which factors are underlying contributors to the nutritional problem in that particular community
- To discover the community's or target population's most critical unmet nutritional needs and prioritize them
- To assess the degree to which existing programs and services meet the needs of the target population
- To distribute resources either within a program (regionally) or between different types of programs based on nutrition needs in the community

It is important to note that the underlying contributors to the problem (second bullet above) must be distinguished from the research question, which is often epidemiological in nature regarding what causes a disease or condition. Although, for example, in the case of the community needs-assessment, there is evidence that TV watching may contribute to the development of obesity in children, a nutrition needs-assessment will ascertain: a) whether TV watching is high among children in that community, and b) the factors in the community that may contribute to the behavior of TV watching. As part of the community needs-assessment, factors such as unsafe neighborhoods, lack of parks, and lack of affordable after-school and summer youth programs may all contribute to high TV watching among children in this community and subsequently contribute to childhood obesity in that community.

Goals and objectives lay the foundation for all activities subsequently conducted for the needs-assessment, including data gathering, analysis, and utilization. Goals drive the type of data that will be needed and how it will be used.[9] There may be more than one goal for the needs-assessment. Objectives, on the other hand, are statements that describe the specific result or outcome that will be achieved or activity accomplished (one result or activity per statement).[9] While we typically think of the acronym SMART (Specific, Measurable, Achievable, Relevant, Time) to develop goals, this can be applied to objectives as well.[9] What is described in each objective should be measurable in some way; thus, by collecting data, you should be able to assess the degree to which you were successful at achieving each specific objective. There are usually two or more objectives per goal.

Step 5: Establish your Team for the Needs-Assessment

This step includes identifying who will direct the needs-assessment and all agency and nonagency members of the needs-assessment team. Which resources will be assigned to this activity, including dedicated staff? How will community members be involved? The composition of the team

Prevalence also called prevalence proportion: Is the proportion of people in a population who have a disease. Whereas, incidence refers to frequency of new cases of a disease in a population over a defined period of time.[2]

responsible for conducting the needs-assessment depends on the goals and objectives of the needs-assessment. It is important to construct a diverse team of individuals.[9] Some important members of the needs-assessment team include a nutrition professional, staff responsible for nutrition program service delivery and program administration, and an expert in quantitative or qualitative data collection/management/analysis methods (depending on the data needed, expertise will vary). Furthermore, relevant community leaders will also need to be included in order to have representation from within the community.

In order for the needs-assessment to be conducted thoroughly and effectively, resources need to be allocated consistent with the scope of the needs-assessment. This can be a challenge for public health agencies at times, and this is one of the underlying reasons for determining resource allocation at the outset. If adequate resources cannot be allocated, the scope of the needs-assessment may need to be narrowed.

Phase 2: Methodology Development

In this phase of the community needs-assessment process, the team will lay out in detail which data will be needed to meet each objective of the needs-assessment and how they will obtain these data. Although time-consuming, this type of planning in advance will facilitate all activities related to the needs-assessment. As with the literature review, careful and systematic attention to completeness and detail will minimize surprises and ensure that all needed data can be obtained. It is important to explore if data may already exist or which data will need to be collected.[9,10]

Step 6: Specify the Data Needed and Design a Plan for Acquiring the Data

The data that may be needed for a nutrition needs-assessment likely will fall under one or more of the following four categories:

- Community data
- Community organizational structure and authorities: Data related to how the community is organized politically and socially
  - Community services and usage: Data related to nutrition-related programs, services, and usage in the community
  - Community demographics and health: The overall health of the community
  - Community environment: Includes local, state, and national policies and systems as well as the specific community's physical environment that can affect the nutritional status of the target population, including access to health care
- Target population data
  - Data related to the nutritional status of the target population
  - Lifestyle factors affecting nutritional status
  - Sociodemographic factors; living and working conditions
  - Data related to attitudes, perceptions, and opinions of the target population

There are pros and cons to having significant amounts of data available for this process.[10] Having numerous indicators implies that the degree to which nutrition-related needs/status is measured is better than having only a few indicators available. Conversely, having too many indicators available can be overwhelming for data management, and tabulation can become unmanageable. Thus, it is important to carefully choose the indicators that relate best to the objectives of your nutrition needs-assessment. The following criteria can be used to assess the potential advantages and disadvantages of selecting indicators:

- *Simplicity:* An indicator needs to be conceptually straightforward, well defined, and a valid and reliable measure of what it purports to represent. Both the public and policymakers should be able to understand it.
- *Stability:* Estimates derived from these indicators should be based on large enough numbers so that they do not fluctuate dramatically due to a small sample size.
- *Availability:* Ideally, the indicator is available at national, state, and local levels, so that even if your needs-assessment is conducted on a local community, it is possible to examine relative health compared with state and national status.
- *Broad representation:* An indicator should reflect the potential nutrition-related concerns of most of the target population as well as higher-risk groups within the target population.
- *Political feasibility:* Although the public health impact of the nutrition-related problem is one of the most important considerations, one must also consider whether the political environment will facilitate or hinder an intervention to deal with this problem.

The types of data that will be obtained for the needs-assessment fall under two general categories: qualitative data and quantitative data. In addition, there are two types of data acquisition: data already collected and in a database or report (i.e., *secondary data sources*) and data that must be collected directly from the community or target population as part of the needs-assessment (i.e., *primary data collection*).

Plan to Obtain Community Data

1. **Community data, including the organizational structure and authorities.** How the community's governmental agencies and healthcare organizations are organized and who is in power can affect the healthcare as well as the preventative service delivery for the target population. Community leaders are also important to identify because not only will they be invaluable sources of information about the unmet needs in the community, but also they will be essential to any successful strategy to address the unmet need identified by the needs-assessment. One method that can be used to identify such individuals is obtaining organizational charts of local government offices and healthcare organizations. This can be done through an Internet search or visiting the offices. In addition, reading the local newspapers and listening to local radio stations will provide information on both community and business leaders as well as influential media groups. Be sure to sample a variety of media outlets to ensure a well-rounded exploration of local politics. Finally, those who have particular influence on, involvement with, or a vested interest in the well-being of the target population (i.e., *stakeholders*) should be identified and included in this process.
2. **Community services and usage.** Information on which nutrition-related services and programs are available in the community can be obtained from the Internet (i.e., government and nonprofit organizations' websites as well as online library

Strategy Tip

Brainstorm on how you would collect primary and secondary data about your college foodservice choices.

American Heart Association is available at http://www.heart.org/

American Red Cross is available at www.redcross.org. The American Diabetes Association is available at www.diabetes.org. The United Way is available at http://www.unitedway.org

sources), local health organizations, existing community nutrition programs, government agencies and civic groups, and voluntary health organizations such as the American Heart Association, the American Red Cross, the American Diabetes Association, and the United Way directories. Usage data includes the number of people using services as well as segments of the target population that are more or less likely to use specific services. This type of information can be obtained from the agencies and programs delivering the services; however, some of this information may not be available to the public. Involving key personnel who are involved in delivering programs relevant to the specific goals of the nutrition needs-assessment, which facilitates access to such data.

3. **Community demographics and health.** Demographic data and health data can be obtained from a variety of sources (as shown in Table 5–2). Some important demographic data include ethnicity, age distribution, gender, marital status, income, and poverty statistics. These all provide a description of who lives in the community. A variety of health statistics reflect the overall health of the community, and these can point to segments of the population that are at risk for malnutrition or chronic diseases linked to obesity. The following are some health statistics that are available at the national and state level through the Centers for Disease Control and Prevention (https://www.cdc.gov/datastatistics/index.html); some may be available for the local level as well:

   - Mortality: These include overall death rates, both in general and from specific diseases.
   - Natality: These statistics include the percentage of mothers with adequate prenatal care, the infant mortality rate, average birth weights, and the percentage of unmarried mothers.
   - Leading causes of death: This is a rank order list of those causes to which deaths are most frequently attributable.
   - Morbidity: These statistics include rates of nutrition-related diseases such as obesity, heart disease, cancer, and diabetes (as well as complications from diabetes).
   - Health risk behaviors: These include sedentary activities, smoking, alcohol use, serum cholesterol concentration, breastfeeding practices, and sexually transmitted diseases (STDs).

   Some of these statistics are also stratified by demographic characteristics, which can then be more accurately compared with the target population demographics. This is particularly useful if local data on a particular health outcome is not available for the specific community. For example, if your community has a large proportion of members who are of Vietnamese descent, but you do not have health statistics on this segment of the population in your specific community, searching on statistics from national data sources or research publications can give you this important information.

4. **Environmental conditions within the community.** This includes access to medical care and access to preventative services. Also included is the availability of food, transportation, parks, walkways, and bicycle paths. All of these factors comprise the environment of the community that can affect the nutritional

status of the target population. Availability of food, for example, is determined by variety, cost, and quality of the food that community grocery stores, supermarkets, co-ops, farmer's markets, restaurants, or fast-food establishments in the area provide. Transportation and road systems are important because this influences the accessibility of available food in a community. Some community members may have to walk to access food, while others may be able to take public transportation, and others may be able to drive themselves. The safety of these methods will also impact the ability to obtain food. Walking on unsafe streets to get to a grocery store will likely hinder access to food even if it is available in a community.

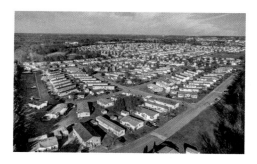

Grocery stores may be miles away in some neighborhoods, limiting accessibility.

© Tokar/Shutterstock.

For many community residents, food availability within the specific community determines what they can buy and have in their homes. How can we ascertain food availability? One of the best ways, if logistically possible, is to walk around the community and visit supermarkets and grocery stores, also noting types of restaurants and transportation availability. Visiting stores and noting food quality, availability, and cost provides valuable qualitative information on what the target population faces in their food procurement on a day-to-day basis. In addition, it also provides an opportunity for you to get a true feel of the community, the ethnic groups represented, and the physical surroundings that can affect opportunities for physical activity. In communities with larger populations of different ethnicities, be sure to explore food markets that meet their cultural dietary needs. Note if these are lacking, it may be a contributor to risk for nutrition-related conditions, including malnutrition. Although food may be available in a community, if these are not the foods the community members are likely to consume, there is another barrier to their access. It may also be helpful to explore the foods the community members are consuming to help you better understand the nutritional value of those traditional foods.

Pandemic Learning Opportunity

How did people get groceries during the Covid-19 pandemic? Wasn't there a markup on foods that were delivered?

Plan to Obtain Data on the Target Population

Data on the nutritional status of the target population can be obtained through either secondary data sources or primary data collection. The former is desirable, if it is appropriate for the needs-assessment, because it requires many fewer resources and can be obtained much more quickly. The Centers for Disease Control and Prevention (CDC) maintains nutrition datasets. You can obtain some of these and conduct further analyses as part of the needs-assessment. For example, it may be that your target population is Puerto Rican, but the statistics you identify are described for those of Hispanic descent as a whole. If the dataset is available, the member of your team who is responsible for data management and analysis can analyze the specific data for Puerto Ricans.

Existing datasets, if they include the indicators pertinent to the nutrition needs-assessment, thus can be used to describe the target population's health and nutritional status. These can also be used as a basis to compare the target population's nutritional status with national and state statistics.

Nutritional status indicators fall under one of the following four assessment categories:

- Anthropometric
- Biochemical (or laboratory)
- Clinical
- Dietary

Body mass index (BMI) = mass (kg)
mass (lb) (height (m))^2 or (height (in))^2 x 703

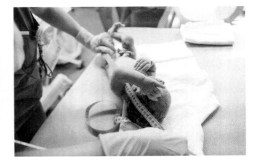

Follow industry standards in taking anthropometric measurements.

© Natalia Deriabina/Shutterstock.

The Pennsylvania Division of Women, Infants and Children has produced a manual that describes how to accurately measure height and weight in children and adolescents. It is available online at https://wicworks.fns.usda.gov/wicworks/Sharing_Center/PA/Anthro/lib/pdf/Anthropometric_Training_Manual.pdf

Anthropometric Assessment

This type of nutritional assessment includes all measures of physical dimensions and body composition.[11,12] Two general objectives of anthropometric assessments are to assess growth and body composition.[11,12] The most commonly used indices of linear growth are recumbent length (in those under 2 years of age) and standing height (in those 2 years of age or older). Head circumference in children under 3 years of age is related to brain size. Weight along with height is used to calculate **body mass index (BMI)**, which is used as an indirect measure of obesity. Other anthropometric measurements used to assess body composition are skinfold thickness (e.g., tricep skinfolds) and circumferences (waist and mid-arm). Note that interpretation of these data requires a comparison to reference data and/or prediction equations to calculate body composition from the data. The CDC has reference growth charts for infants and children (2000 CDC Growth Charts, see below) available and a module for using the BMI for age growth charts. In 2006, the World Health Organization also released growth standards for infants and children up to 71 months of age that were based on an international sample of well-nourished children who have been breastfed and whose mothers have followed the WHO guidelines for breastfeeding support and infant feeding (https://www.who.int/toolkits/child-growth-standards/standards). Both CDC (https://www.cdc.gov/nccdphp/dnpao/growthcharts/resources/sas.htm) and WHO (https://www.who.int/tools/child-growth-standards/software) have software that can be used to convert raw weights, heights into percentiles, and z scores.

Whether you use secondary or primary data, it is essential for the needs-assessment that you use standardized protocols to collect these data (usually height/length or weight). If you use reference data to convert raw data into either percentiles or z-scores, these must be based on the CDC 2000 growth curves.

Biochemical/Laboratory Assessment

This is an objective measure of subclinical nutrient deficiency; it involves a measurement of the nutrient level, a nutrient's metabolite, or functional tests that measure nutrient-dependent enzyme activity or concentrations.[12,13] The aforementioned may be measured in blood, urine, hair, fingernails, or toenails. Many other functional tests exist as well but are likely beyond the scope of a public health nutrition needs-assessment. One of the most common laboratory tests used in nutritional surveillance and in programs such as WIC is hemoglobin or hematocrit, which is used as an indicator of iron deficiency anemia. Note, however, that hemoglobin is a relatively insensitive indicator and is nonspecific; this means that a significant proportion of people may truly have iron deficiency anemia but be classified as having normal hemoglobin (insensitivity), while others may be diagnosed with iron deficiency anemia based on their hemoglobin levels but are not truly anemic (nonspecific). Part of the problem is that hemoglobin (and hematocrit) is affected by many factors other than iron, including inflammation, infections, protein energy malnutrition, thalassemia minor, vitamin B_{12}, or folate deficiencies, to name a few. In order to more accurately identify those who have iron deficiency anemia, other indicators of iron status (e.g., transferrin saturation, serum ferritin) should also be collected.

Clinical Assessment

Clinical assessment occurs via a physical examination and medical history in order to detect physical signs and symptoms of under- or overnutrition.[12] This requires expertise and training on the part of the examiner in order to accurately associate these signs with a nutritional deficiency. Be sure to interpret all physical findings in the context of all other nutrition data collected as some signs and symptoms may be the same for multiple nutrient deficiencies and conditions. Note that by the time clinical signs develop, there will already be a manifestation of an advanced stage of nutrient deficiency, because clinical signs occur when malnutrition is chronic in nature. An example of a clinical sign of vitamin C deficiency is swollen red gums; however, swollen red gums could also be due to various non-nutritional problems (e.g., periodontal disease). Combined with other information (such as a dietary assessment showing a low intake of vitamin C–containing foods), the accurate attribution of this clinical sign to vitamin C deficiency may be made.

Dietary Assessment

Dietary assessment methods are used to collect data on usual food and nutrient intake of individuals. Some frequently used dietary assessment methods are 24-hour recalls (single or repeated), estimated or weighed food records, dietary history, and food frequency questionnaires.[12,14] All of the aforementioned methods have systematic errors.[14] The goal is to minimize these errors as much as possible. There is extensive literature in the area of dietary assessment, including discussion on **validity** and **reliability** of the common tools in various populations. The following is simply a summary of the most important points to consider when using these traditional methods.

There are various challenges to obtaining dietary data that reflect usual diet, not the least of which is that among free-living individuals, dietary intake exhibits variation from day to day. This variation is superimposed on a consistent pattern.[15] What the researcher is attempting to ascertain is that consistent pattern. Depending on the dietary assessment method used, the accuracy of intake data often reflects a person's literacy and educational level (for all methods, but especially food records), memory (24-hour recall and food frequency questionnaire), and ability to accurately quantify foods (24-hour recall and food frequency questionnaire). Another source of error is that individuals often alter their dietary intake while undergoing the assessment, thus reducing the accuracy with which the foods reflect what is usually eaten.

If you are considering collecting dietary data, you need to review several factors. First, who is your population and what method is most

For a copy of the 2000 CDC Growth Charts, along with a comprehensive description, see: http://www.cdc.gov/growthcharts/

For a module on using the BMI-for-age growth charts for infants and children, see: https://www.cdc.gov/nccdphp/dnpa/growthcharts/training/modules/module1/text/module1print.pdf

For training on accurate measurement in children and adolescents, see the HRSA training module: http://depts.washington.edu/growth/module5/text/page7b.htm

Validity When a test is designed to measure what it set out to measure.

Reliability The extent in which when tested, the same result will occur consistently.

appropriate? If your population is a well-educated one, using food records may be a good choice. On the other hand, if the population has limited literacy, repeated 24-hour recalls or a food frequency questionnaire may be a better choice.

Second, the number of days of dietary intake affects the validity with which the data reflects the individual's usual intake. A single day, whether it be a 24-hour recall or a food record, is not adequate to estimate a person's true usual intake for any macro- or micronutrient; a single day, however, can provide an estimate of the average usual nutrient intake of a large population group if all of the days of the week are represented. The degree of day-to-day variability affects the number of days needed, and this also depends on the nutrient under examination. For example, it has been stated that in order to obtain an estimate of an individual's vitamin A intake, such that 95% of observed values are within 10% of the true mean, one needs 105 days of dietary intake data.[15] This may seem absurd, but this example illustrates that it is virtually impossible to estimate an individual's intake based on one 24-hour recall. However, by administering repeated 24-hour recalls, you can improve the validity with which they represent the individual's usual diet.

The third issue is how the data will be analyzed. For 24-hour recalls and food records, you need to use a nutrient analysis program to assess the macro- or micronutrient content of the diet. If using a validated Food Frequency Questionnaire, such as the National Cancer Institute's semiquantitative Block Food Frequency Questionnaire (FFQ), often, the nutrient analysis is provided for a fee by the institution that sponsors that FFQ.

A variety of toolkits and technology-based methods now exist.[14] Smart phone apps and websites allow for more options of data collection. Individuals may be more familiar with how to log their food intake, having done this task previously using an app for personal knowledge. A photography-based collection may also be a viable method of determining intake.[16] At the very least, this can complement traditional forms of data by allowing the researcher to see what was consumed while reviewing the information shared during a 24-hour recall or food diary.

The following are generally recommended methods based on the objective of the dietary assessment:

- Average usual intakes of a population group: Can use a single 24-hour recall or food record, although repeated measures are always better.
- Proportion of the population "at risk" for a nutrient deficiency or excess: Repeated 24-hour recalls or food records. The number of days depends on the nutrient(s) that are the focus of the needs assessment.
- Usual nutrient intakes of individuals: Repeated 24-hour recalls or food records.[7] The number of days depends on the nutrient(s) that are the focus of the needs-assessment.
- A pattern of food use for a group or individual or ranking of individuals: Food frequency questionnaires.

To summarize, if a dietary assessment is needed as a part of the needs-assessment, you should choose the method that will produce the most valid and reliable data for the target population that will meet the objectives of the needs-assessment in the most succinct manner. Ideally, someone on the needs-assessment team should have expertise in the area of dietary assessment, and a review of the literature should be conducted prior to choosing a method.

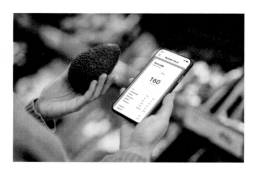

Food diary recordkeeping is available now in an array of apps.

© Oscar Wong/Moment/Getty Images.

For a description of the semiquantitative food frequency questionnaire developed at the National Cancer Institute (NCI) under the leadership of Dr. Gladys Block, visit https://nutritionquest.com/assessment/

Other Types of Data

There are many determinants of food and nutrient intake, nutritional status, and health. Many of the following interact with one another to affect actual food intake, health beliefs, and practices.

- Health risk behaviors: This includes tobacco or alcohol use and drug abuse.
- Availability and accessibility to health care: health insurance, disease screening, annual physical exams, and frequency of visits to a healthcare professional.
- Lifestyle practices: These include time spent engaging in physical activity and sedentary behavior (leisure time and nonleisure time).
- Income: Income distribution and percentage of population living below the poverty level.
- Cultural factors: ethnic group, availability of culturally acceptable food choices, degree of acculturation.
- Religion: Acceptability of the religion in the community, food laws and ability to obtain foods that meet those requirements, and degree of adherence to religious beliefs.
- Educational level: Distribution and percentage attaining specific levels of education.
- Household composition and size: Who lives in the household (e.g., mother, father, grandmother, three children) and how many people live in the household.
- Occupation: Can refer to the occupation of any or all of the adults living in the household.
- Working conditions: Hours of work, job benefits, and job stress.
- Living conditions: Potential health risks associated with the housing (e.g., lead paint).
- Primary social groups: Family, friends, and work groups.
- Technology: Use of social media, including influences from people followed on various platforms and ability to obtain and interpret information from the Internet.

In addition, data on attitudes, perceptions, and opinions can be a critical component of the needs-assessment data collection plan because it is often the lack of insight into the target population's attitudes and perceptions about a nutrition or health problem, the contributing factors, and workable solutions that hinder the successful implementation of an effective plan of action. This type of data can be qualitative in nature.

Methods for Obtaining Data on the Target Populations (Primary Data Collection)

Surveys can be used to obtain data about health risk behaviors, such as use of health care; physical activity and sedentary behaviors; socioeconomic factors; working and living conditions; and attitudes, perceptions, and opinions. Although many set out to develop their own surveys, this is not recommended unless there are survey development experts on the needs-assessment team. Using an already validated survey tool may be a better use of time and resources.

This section is not intended to guide a novice in their quest to develop a survey; there are numerous survey development books that the reader should avail themselves of if they intend to develop a survey. However, this is not recommended. Although it may seem simple enough, survey development is complicated and time-consuming, and if it is not done correctly, the derived data may be unusable. If you are going to use a survey to collect primary data for the needs-assessment, it is recommended that you use the following series of steps that prioritize validated and extensively used surveys over survey development.

1. Identify surveys in the research literature that address the question of interest.
2. Give preference to those surveys that have strong evidence of validity (i.e., construct and predictive validity) and reliability.
3. If there is no strong evidence of survey validity (i.e., no validation or only face or content validity assessed), give preference to those existing surveys used in national nutrition surveillance or monitoring. Although formal validation may not have been done, the questions have been used on large population groups and the data have been analyzed and utilized; this implies that the data were usable for the purpose intended. In addition, this will enable comparison of your local or regional needs-assessment data to national statistics.
4. If a set of survey questions comprise a scale (e.g., body image), it is important to use the entire set of questions that form that scale. Leaving off content or modifying the existing survey may impact the ability to properly interpret the results.

Again, detailed guidance for survey development is beyond the scope of this chapter; however, there are several excellent reference books that provide guidance in developing surveys.[17,18] Drafting questions for a survey seems deceptively simple but, in fact, writing questions that are straightforward, universally understood by all respondents, and truly answer the question the researcher sets out to answer is complicated.

The final wording (and formatting) of the question and response categories evolve from a process of obtaining input from experts, pretesting, and reliability and validity testing. For many, resource constraints preclude such survey development. Unfortunately, what results from hurried attempts at drafting questions are data of questionable quality that may not prove to have been worthwhile to collect using such a survey. **Exhibit 5–1** is a compilation of some important points to consider when drafting your own survey. In addition, if the instrument that you select has been used in samples that are sociodemographically or ethnically different from your target population, you need to test it with your target population prior to its use for the needs-assessment.

Exhibit 5–1 Survey Checklist

This checklist is intended to be a guide for you in the development of your survey. However, following all of these recommendations cannot replace extensive pretesting of your survey instrument to determine what is working and what isn't. In addition to wording and formatting, pretesting can help you determine optimal question and response order. This list combines and summarizes Fowler's guidelines[17] for conducting survey research and improving survey questions along with other observations regarding common errors made when nonsurvey experts attempt to draft surveys for use in research. It is not intended to be an exhaustive list, nor can it be used in lieu of the guidance of survey development experts and a good reference on survey development such as those noted herein. It also does not address other aspects such as mode of administration, training of interviewers, and other facets of collecting high-quality survey data. In addition, because many surveys are now computer assisted, the aforementioned reference books[17,18] also address newer issues of computer-assisted administration.

Questions: Wording, Content, and Order

- Use full sentences with adequate wording to form a complete question.[17]
- Ask all respondents the same questions.
- To ensure consistent meaning for all respondents, define all words that people may potentially interpret differently.[17]
- Be as specific as possible. For example, if asking about smoking, you need to specify the type, and what you are defining as a person who smokes. Consider if vaping will be included as well.
- Language level should match respondent ability.
- Avoid asking multiple questions within a single question.[17] For example, in the last 30 days, how many times did you eat at least five servings of fruits and vegetables per day? This needs better wording to accurately obtain the correct information needed.
- Avoid hypothetical questions and asking about causality.
- Include all of the domains laid out in your conceptual framework in your survey.
- Avoid words like typical, usually, and on average. Define time frames whenever possible.
- If using a self-administered survey, it is very important that you place the most critical information needed for your research near the beginning. This is also important in an interviewer-administered survey, but less so.
- Place sensitive questions appropriately. For an interviewer-administered survey, these need to be near the end. For a self-administered survey, they can be closer to the beginning.
- Avoid derogatory or negative terms/words that may cause bias in response. If there is something threatening or negative in your survey, attempt to neutralize it by inserting an introductory sentence acknowledging that some people do this behavior or have this problem.

Response Categories

- List all possible responses, but only once. Possible responses should be listed after the question.
- If you determine that a respondent can provide a relatively accurate quantitative response, ask for the actual number instead of selecting categories. This is desirable as long as it doesn't make completing the survey more difficult for the respondent. For example, if you want to know how many siblings a person has, simply leave a space or two (depending on the range of sibling number in the population) and let them supply the actual number.
- Specify the response format and unit of measurement (e.g., if you want years, include that in the response).
- If only one answer is required, make response categories mutually exclusive.
- Ensure that the number of response categories captures the full range of possible responses, including adequate variability (e.g., if most people are going to check the last category, you need to break down that category further so that you can differentiate better among people).
- Make the order of responses consistent throughout the survey. For example, if numerical categories are listed, they all need to be listed in the same order (lowest to highest is most common).
- Make sure there is a space for the respondent to respond. For example, if you say "check off one answer," then you need a space (__) or check-off box.

Introductions and Transition Statements and Instructions

- Provide an introduction to the survey itself. Here you will provide a general description of the purpose of the survey, what you expect the respondent to do, and what they should do if they don't understand something or have questions. Also, this is where you should assure the respondent of confidentiality or anonymity (whichever applies in your case).
- If the survey is broken up into sections (which it should be if the survey is longer than a few pages), number and label the sections with section headings, and have a brief introduction to each section.
- Although you may have instructed the respondent at the beginning of a section or at the beginning of the survey, you still need to provide instructions to tell the respondent exactly what to do for every question. Be as clear as possible. The instructions should

(continues)

Exhibit 5–1 Survey Checklist *(continued)*

be in a different font than the question (they can be italicized, bolded, or capitalized). Be consistent throughout in terms of how you want the person to respond (e.g., circle or check off responses). In the instructions, also include how many they can choose (i.e., all that apply or one).

- If you have an "other" option, ask respondents to specify or describe what that is.

Survey Format and Layout

- General rule: Avoid crowding and maximize white space.
- There should be space between questions as well as between questions and response categories.
- Provide plenty of space for the responses (whether it be a number written in or room for them to check something off).
- If you have contingency questions (i.e., questions that depend on a response to another question) and it is a self-administered questionnaire, it is best to use arrows to actually lead the person to the next question. The arrow normally stems from the response. If it is an interviewer-administered survey, it is OK to say "Go to question ___," but these instructions should also be adjacent to the response category.
- However you decide to lay out your response categories, be consistent (in columns or in rows).
- If you have a series of questions with the same response categories and decide to lay them out in a tabular format, shade every other row so that people won't lose their place.
- Make sure that the question and the response categories are on the same page.

General

- Number all pages.
- Each page should have a place for an ID number.
- At the end of each page, note that there are more pages to the survey. You can say "Next page" with an arrow or something else that will tell the respondent that there is more to complete. On the next to the last page of the survey, note "only one more page left." This is essential for any survey that is more than two pages long.

See Chapter 13 for food insecurity questionnaires.

Stakeholders An entity that has an interest in something or something to gain/lose as a result of the outcomes.

Focus Groups

A focus group usually consists of seven to 10 people who are relatively homogeneous and whose input or opinion is sought through broad, open-ended questions about a research topic.[19] These may also be called group discussions.[19] Focus group participants are selected because they are considered knowledgeable about the topic. Focus groups are often used to obtain qualitative data on perceptions, attitudes, or opinions about a specific issue or product. This can be an extremely important tool in the needs-assessment process because it can provide a method for eliciting opinions from the target population on their perceived needs, barriers to preventing disease, or even why certain programs are not working. Key **stakeholders** can be important individuals to include in the focus group process as well. The somewhat spontaneous nature of a focus group discussion allows for unanticipated findings that may not arise in a more structured setting.[19] This type of data can be highly useful for gaining a deeper, more holistic understanding of the problem. For example, in the case of the nutrition problem of childhood obesity in Baltimore City, a focus group of teenagers may provide insight as to why they choose what they do after school, why they don't use certain after-school programs, and what kinds of activities they would participate in that would get them moving.

Although spontaneity is an important quality of this data collection method, it is still necessary to develop a framework for your focus group in advance of its implementation.[19] Key components to address during the planning phase include:

- Focus group implementation team should include the following
  - *Moderator* – facilitates the discussion by asking questions and maintains the focus of the discussion on the topics of interest in addition to maintaining the group dynamics[8,19]
  - *Note taker* – has strictly observational duties; takes detailed notes on what was said, how responses were said, and notes when changes in topics occurred
  - *Audio recorder* – records the discussion so that a transcript may be created afterward
- Participants – who will they be and how will you recruit them.
  - Be specific about exactly who you want information from. Consider characteristics such as age, gender, occupation, and culture.
  - Recruitment strategies include, but are not limited to:
    - Pre-existing lists of people from your target population (quick and inexpensive)
    - "Piggyback" focus groups, during which the focus group is added to another event that was scheduled (convenient)
    - Recruiting in a place where participants do normal activities (e.g., grocery store, museum) and holding the focus group in that location after recruitment
    - Phone calls, during which responders are screened for eligibility
    - Public advertising
    - If possible, selection of participants should be random and systematic[19]
- Location and time of implementation
  - For face-to-face interviews, location should be convenient and comfortable for the participants (i.e., choose a place where the discussion would naturally occur in real life)[19]
  - Timing should also be convenient, so consider your target population[19] (e.g., schedule a focus group for teachers during the summer break and not when school is in session)
- Discussion template
  - Determine major discussion topics
  - Craft specific questions for each topic. Make questions as simple, clear, and easy to understand as possible. Open-ended questions are preferable, as they encourage more detailed, informative responses.
  - The same questions and topics should be asked in all groups if conducting more than one[19]

To minimize the risk of future obstacles, these elements must be determined early in the planning phase. Furthermore, if you plan to implement multiple focus groups, being specific in your intentions will enhance the consistency of your results.

Focus groups can be advantageous for various reasons. Planning and implementing a focus group is reasonably straightforward, and the session typically lasts about an hour. Although it is desirable to hold a focus group in person, it is acceptable to do so over the phone or by video conference for convenience purposes.[19] As previously mentioned, the major advantage of conducting a focus group is the comprehensive information that can be collected in this setting (in contrast to the more simplistic data collected from, say, a survey). The qualitative data give a unique insight to researchers about the personal experiences of individuals in the target population.

As with any data collection method, there are several limitations to this particular method of which one should be aware. Facilitator bias is a major risk when conducting a focus group. Thus, the facilitator must be able to guide the conversation in a neutral manner. For example, instead of asking the question, "As you know, eating five servings of fruits and vegetables is highly beneficial for your health – how important do feel this is?" It is better to ask, "To you, how important is it to meet the recommended five servings of fruits and vegetables daily?" The facilitator must also be able to establish a safe, welcoming environment that encourages the participants to share as much information as possible. It is important to leave out personal emotions or indications of personal feelings. The moderator must be good at establishing rapport so that all participants feel comfortable sharing their experiences and responding to questions in an honest manner.[19] Other limitations include the domination of one or more participants in the discussion, the lengthy data analysis process, and the lack of individual data due to the group dynamic.[19]

These limitations should not overshadow the fact that focus groups can be an extremely appropriate and efficient method of data collection. Certain situations, such as research that requires more in-depth information beyond the scope of quantitative data, can significantly benefit from gathering data from a focus group.

Key Informant Interviews

Key informant interviews represent another method of collecting data that are similar to focus groups in that it is open ended; the major difference is that it queries individuals, as opposed to groups. Key informant interviews consist of structured or unstructured interviews (phone or face-to-face) of individuals (i.e., **key informants**) who have been identified as having specific knowledge about the topic of interest.[8] In this case it would be someone who has knowledge about the community, target populations, services, or other efforts (past or present) to address health- or nutrition-related problems, or stakeholders who may have important insights about the needs of the community or target population.

Similar to focus groups, key informant interviews produce qualitative data that can provide a more comprehensive understanding of a problem. This is also an ideal strategy for quickly acquiring information to inform a survey design and to obtain recommendations for an action plan.[20] In our Baltimore City example, local health professionals (i.e., physicians, school nurses) may be interviewed on an individual basis to assess their knowledge and perceptions of the childhood obesity problem. This information obtained in the interviews would then be used to inform specific questions on a survey that the parents of Baltimore City are expected to complete.

In many ways, planning for key informant interviews is just like planning for a focus group. Team members for implementation, participants (key informants), setting, and discussion questions must be established in advance. When developing a list of questions, it can be helpful to first generate (or refer back to) a list of primary research questions (i.e., *what do you want to know?*). Use these "big picture" questions to inform the more specific questions that will be asked during the interview.

There are several elements to be conscious of when conducting a key informant interview. Just like a focus group, establishing a safe environment to encourage information sharing is essential for successful data collection. By maintaining neutrality and withholding personal opinions, the facilitator can establish a safe environment, as well as reduce the risk of facilitator bias, which

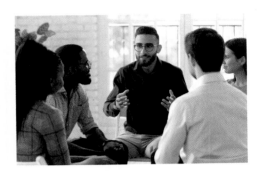

Focus group structure follows a known standard to be considered credible.

© Fizkes/Shutterstock.

Key informants People that provide information about events.

can hinder the validity of the results. During the interviews, notes should be taken for future analysis. Recording the audio may also be helpful to ensure accuracy when analyzing the data later on. If a recording will be used, ensure all interviewees have provided consent. Like focus groups, the analysis process may take longer than simpler forms of data collection. In brief, analyzing data from interviews and focus groups involves sorting through all of the data from each interview and developing themes based on the comments that occurred most frequently. This process is known as thematic analysis and there are special software programs that can assist with this task.[19]

Key informant interviews have similar advantages to focus groups. They are relatively inexpensive, quick, and useful in obtaining more qualitative data. These are a good way to help give the community a sense of ownership in the process.[21] These interviews are also susceptible to similar disadvantages, however, including risk of facilitator bias and a lengthy analysis process. It is also important to note that this method may not be useful or necessary in certain situations, such as when simple quantitative data would suffice.[20] As always, it is important to be as efficient as possible in public health research. Therefore, you should always consider the specific nature of your research and only choose to use methods of data collection that are absolutely necessary.[21]

Phase 3: Data Collection and Analysis

By the time this phase is reached, all of the methods for the needs-assessment, including indicators, existing datasets that will be used, or the methods for primary data analysis, will have been determined. This is the phase in which data will be collected, either directly from participants or from existing reports, or additional analysis will be completed from secondary data sets.

Step 7: Collect Data on the Community and the Target Population

Irrespective of the methods used for the needs-assessment data collection, it is imperative that someone be responsible for overseeing the following:

- Data collection progress and troubleshooting
- Data entry and cleaning (if primary data collection)
- Data management in terms of how databases will be designed and what software will be used
- Quality or limitations of the data

Step 8: Analyze and Interpret Data

In this stage, the pertinent data will be analyzed and summarized for the community and target population. This will allow the community needs-assessment team to describe the unmet needs in the community by:

- Interpreting the health status of the target population that lives in the community.
- Interpreting the pattern of health care, health services, and nutrition- or health-related programs that are designed to reach the target population.
- Assessing the relationship between the health/nutrition needs of the target population and the pattern of services available in the community.

Data analysis is typically completed using computer-based software. It is useful to have a trained statistician on your team for analyzing quantitative data; however, this is not necessary unless you plan to run more complex

Strategy Tip

Who would be the key informants of your college? Are you sure?

Qualitative research Any method of data collecting that generates narrative data or words rather than numerical data or numbers. Typically designed based on a theoretical framework. Commonly used for research focusing on human behavior and to describe social phenomena.[1]

statistical tests and lack someone on the team familiar with statistics. The most common program for analyzing quantitative data, like your surveys, is the Statistical Package for Social Sciences (SPSS). You will want to research which product will work best for you. Cost and user familiarity with the program may influence your decision. The most common program used to analyze qualitative data, like your focus groups and key informant interviews, is called NVivo. This comes with multiple tutorials to assist in learning the coding process. This is helpful if you don't have a seasoned **qualitative researcher** on your team.

The results of the needs-assessment should then be summarized in a report. It is important to tailor the report to the target audience.[8] This summary should include the needs-assessment methods used, a description of the nutritional problems being addressed, the severity and prevalence of those problems, the distribution across the community and target population (e.g., is it worse in urban areas or in specific age or ethnic groups?) of those problems, causes of those that are specific to that target population and community, and the consequences in terms of morbidity and mortality. In addition, you should prepare an executive summary, no longer than one to two pages, that highlights the key points of the needs-assessment.

Phase 4: Using the Needs-Assessment Results

Step 9: Share the Findings of the Assessment

The findings of the needs-assessment must not only be shared with others in the agency who undertook the lead for the needs-assessment and participating agencies and organizations but also with the stakeholders who either provided advice and key information or work with the target population.

Step 10: Prioritize the Needs of the Community and Target Population

Many unmet needs may be identified as a result of the needs-assessment; however, resource limitations often constrain the degree to which all unmet needs can be addressed. Thus, it is essential that needs be prioritized. Various methods of prioritization have been proposed[22]; two will be reviewed here.

In their seminal book, *Community Nutritional Assessment*, Jelliffe and Jelliffe[23] laid out five principles that can be used to set priorities. First, priority should be given to what the community identifies as its priorities, preferences, or concerns. Second, common problems should be given priority over rare ones. Third, serious problems should be prioritized over less critical ones. Fourth, easily preventable problems should have higher priority than those for which prevention is more difficult. Finally, those health problems that have exhibited increases over time should be given preference over those whose frequencies are decreasing or have stabilized.

Another simple method of prioritization is to use members of the target population and program providers who may have been included on the needs-assessment team to rank the top five needs. The series of rankings assigned to each need is assigned the corresponding number (i.e., if a need is ranked as 1, it is given a score of 1); scores are then summed, and those with the lowest numbers are given priority.[22] This is known as forced ranking.

Step 11: Develop a Plan of Action to Use the Needs-Assessment Findings to Improve the Nutritional Status of the Target Population

Once the needs-assessment is completed and unmet needs are identified and prioritized, a plan of action to address the priority needs must be developed. This may involve modifying an existing program or programs to better meet the need or developing new programs, or advocating for funding to address the unmet need, utilizing the needs-assessment results as ammunition. The team needs to include stakeholders in the process of developing this plan of action.

The CDC has developed a useful tool for this process called the CHANGE (Community Health Assessment and Group Evaluation) tool.[24] Using the priorities identified through the analysis of your needs-assessment, the CHANGE tool recommends developing a Community Action Plan. This plan of action uses the needs-assessment priorities to inform specific goals and objectives for either developing new resources or modifying existing ones. The CHANGE tool encourages its users to develop SMART (specific, measurable, achievable, realistic, and time-sensitive) objectives.[24] Furthermore, two specific types of objectives should be developed: project period **objectives** and annual objectives. The project period objectives will provide a framework for achievements over the entire duration of the project, while the annual objectives will be useful in making the project seem more manageable by outlining the work in 1-year increments.[24] As a novice public health professional, it may be useful to use a tool such as the CHANGE tool to guide your process and ensure completeness.

> **Objective** A named task that is hoped to be gained.

> Read more about SMART in Chapter 17.

Needs-Assessment in Practice: Baltimore City

In 2018, Johns Hopkins Hospital & Johns Hopkins Bayview Medical Center conducted a community health needs-assessment to help improve their delivery of benefits to the surrounding community as part of maintaining their tax-exempt status under the Patient Protection and Affordable Care Act.[25] The methodology is composed of both quantitative and qualitative means of data collection. Surveys were used to collect primary data from local residents and staff from the local health network. Focus groups and interviews were used to collect first-hand accounts of the healthcare landscape from a variety of individuals. This included members with an interest in the community, those from populations in need, and those with special knowledge in public health. A total of 131 community members took part in the qualitative methods and 1,331 participants responded to the survey.[25] A total of nine Baltimore City zip codes were included in defining the local community. Target populations were identified, including elderly, at-risk children, and both under and uninsured families and individuals.

Health Indicators Evaluated

Socioeconomic factors were a major contributor to assessing health needs in this community. Other factors included education, individual behaviors, and the physical environment, although these are noted to be components over the communities overall socioeconomic status.

Socioeconomic Indicators

The following socioeconomic indicators were among those used:

- County Health Ranking and Roadmaps data with a focus on socioeconomic factor scoring. Baltimore City ranked the lowest out of all counties in Maryland. Factors that influenced this ranking include unemployment, children living in single-parent homes, violent crime, and high school graduation rates.
- Livable environment-safe, affordable, and clean housing options; low crime rate, availability of healthy foods. FBI crime data was utilized.
- Household income data

The food environment was also assessed.[25] Low-income areas are often disadvantaged when it comes to access of affordable, healthy food choices. The unavailability of grocery stores in these neighborhoods plays a role in health disparities. Data from the 2018 edition of Baltimore City's Food Environment Report on food priority areas were included in the community needs-assessment. U.S. Census Bureau data showed that 29.5% of Baltimore City residents were receiving Supplement Nutrition Assistance Program (SNAP) benefits. Results from this assessment supported the need of community leaders to address access to healthy foods.

At completion of the community needs-assessment, the identified needs of the community were prioritized before starting the implementation planning phase. Socioeconomic needs were identified with the highest priority. One of the action steps identified was to inventory the available resources in the community to seek out possible partnerships. SMART goals were established.

In summary, the Johns Hopkins Hospital & Johns Hopkins Bayview Medical Center 2018 Community Health needs-assessment is the result of a well thought out, complex methodology developed by the hospital system. It provided a clear understanding of factors influencing the health of the community, identified available resources, and helped community leaders and health professionals prioritize interventions for improving the health of the local community. This included access to healthy food and healthcare services. This process is carried out every 3 years as part of the Patient Protection and Affordable Care Act tax-exemption program. It exemplifies the best of public health needs-assessment efforts.

An overview of community needs-assessment, an integral component of the public health process in general, and public health nutrition in particular, has been shown. This overview is intended to act as a starting point for those planning to undertake a community needs-assessment. The aspiring public health dietitian/nutritionist is encouraged to use the more detailed references noted in this chapter at the early stages of the needs-assessment planning process in order to obtain more thorough information about the many steps involved in this process. **Figure 5–1** shows the steps.

Unmet need should be at the forefront of public health consciousness and designing the strategy and obtaining the tools to identify this need in a

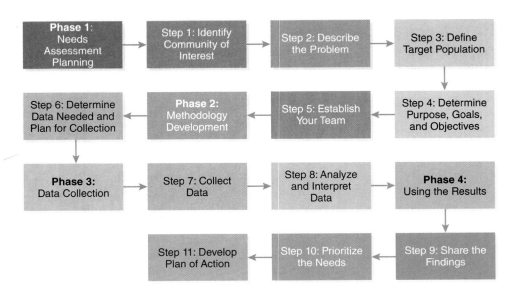

FIGURE 5–1 Summary of Steps for Completing a Community Needs-Assessment.

specific community and target population lay the foundation for its identification. The scope of a community needs-assessment can be broad or limited in nature. Its success doesn't lie in its breadth but rather in its ability to meet its objectives, identify unmet need within the scope defined, and design effective action plans that are inclusive of the public health program personnel, community, and stakeholders. After all, effective teamwork is both the challenge and reward of public health.

Summary

The aim of this chapter is to provide the reader with an introductory-level understanding of community needs-assessments in the realm of public health nutrition. This chapter will discuss the rationale for a needs-assessment and describe the necessary steps in order to complete a valid and useful assessment. Specifically, this chapter will address concepts such as identifying a population of interest, choosing appropriate data collection methods, and using needs-assessment results to develop a plan of action. The reader will be provided with sufficient information to answer important questions like, "What do I intend to learn through my needs-assessment?" "What are the best ways to obtain this information?" and "How can I use this information to benefit the community?" This chapter will also provide suggestions for resources, including sources of existing data and tools that may prove useful in the needs-assessment process. By the end of this chapter, the reader should have a general understanding of how to successfully plan and implement a thorough nutrition-focused community needs-assessment.

Learning Portfolio

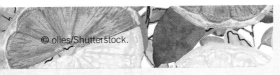
© olies/Shutterstock.

Key Terms

	page
Community	128
Goal	128
Target population	128
Prevalence	133
Body mass index (BMI)	138
Validity	139
Reliability	139
Stakeholders	144
Key informants	146
Qualitative research	148
Objective	149

Issues for Discussion

1. Why would it be important to include program providers as part of your needs-assessment team?
2. What is the rationale for examining the leading causes of death as a measure of the community's health? In relation to mortality, what else could you examine?
3. If the purpose of the Baltimore City example provided in this chapter is to identify the causes of the high prevalence of obesity among children living in Baltimore City, lay out one goal and at least two objectives for such a needs-assessment. Don't forget the acronym SMART.

Practical Activities

1. You need to conduct a focus group with the goal of obtaining information on the attitudes of parents of middle schoolers toward school lunch offerings in your local county. Develop a framework for your focus group. Consider components such as recruitment, time and location, and topics of discussion. Finally, develop at least five discussion questions that you believe would truly ask your question and help you obtain the information you need.
2. Develop a paper survey with at least six questions about any nutrition-related public health topic. Hand it to a friend and ask them to complete the survey. Upon completion, examine the responses and ask the friend to give you feedback. Did your questions ask what you wanted them to ask? Were they clear or confusing? If using multiple response questions, did the choices capture all possible responses?
3. Think about your own community in which you live in. From observation, what is a possible nutrition-related problem that you think needs to be examined? Describe how you might go about developing a rationale for a potential needs-assessment on the problem you are interested in. Consider what kind of information you might want to include in your rationale and where you would look to obtain this information.

Case Study: SNAP Participation in Norwich, MD

The following is the beginning of a needs-assessment case study. Please complete the items that are blank as if you were designing a needs-assessment in the town on Norwich, MD.*

Case Characteristic	Description
Director of Needs-assessment	Feeding Norwich*, a local agency that aims to connect people in the community with access to healthy food
Nutrition Problem	This town experiences a consistently high prevalence of poverty, with 20% of its population below the poverty line. Food insecurity was previously reported as a problem of interest in the local community. Multiple food banks exist in the area, but those are reporting underutilization of their resources.
Community of Interest	City of Norwich, MD*
Needs-Assessment Purpose	To gather information on the awareness of and attitudes toward food bank utilization by those living below 130% of the poverty level.
Target Population	Adults (18 and older) living in poverty in Norwich, MD.

Case Study: SNAP Participation in Norwich, MD

Case Characteristic	Description
Overarching Goal	To evaluate the awareness of and attitudes toward using local food bank resources to minimize food insecurity in order to gain an understanding of the reasons for such low use of existing food bank services.
Assessment Objectives	1. 2. 3.
Type of Data: Target Population	1.
Type of Data: Awareness and Attitudes	1. 2. 3. 4.
To address Objective 1	Type of data: Method of data collection:
To address Objective 2	Type of data: Method of data collection:
To address Objective 3	Type of data:

*Not an actual place or organization.

Case Study: Conducting a Needs Assessment to Develop a Heart Healthy Nutrition Program

You are currently working with your local health department in their Office of Health Promotion. In the last 2 years, the department has noticed an increase in the prevalence of heart disease. Since you have a background in nutrition you have been asked to help develop a program where nutrition will be the focus. They'd like to use some of their budget for the coming year to implement a program that will help decrease heart disease risk among community members. Although the focus will be primary prevention, they've asked that you also consider how to provide secondary and tertiary prevention efforts.

You need to assemble a team and get started with a community needs-assessment in order to best develop and implement the desired program. Start off by identifying the following:

1. Who are your stakeholders?

2. Identify your community of interest

3. Describe your problem

4. Why is a needs assessment necessary?

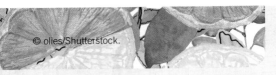

© olies/Shutterstock.

Learning Portfolio

5. Define your target population

6. Identify one goal and one supporting objective for this needs assessment

Now that you have defined your problem and presented to your colleagues why a needs-assessment needs to be conducted, start to think about your team and data collection. Does your community have the data you will need or will you need to develop your own data collection methods?

1. Who will you include on your team?

2. What types of data will you collect?

3. How will you collect each type of data?

Great job collecting your data! Now it's time for the analysis. After the data has been analyzed, what comes next? Describe briefly what you will do with these data and how you will share this information with your colleagues.

Resources

1. Community Action Partnership Community Needs Assessment Resource Guide: https://communityactionpartnership.com/publication_toolkit /community-needs-assessment-resource-guide/

2. Community Tool Box, University of Kansas: https://ctb.ku.edu/en/table-of -contents/assessment

3. Indian Health Service, Community Health Tools: https://www.ihs.gov/hpdp /communityhealth/tools/

4. Moving to the Future: https://movingtothefuture.org

5. Centers for Disease Control and Prevention, Community Needs Assessment Workbook: https://www.cdc.gov/globalhealth/healthprotection/fetp/training _modules/15/community-needs_pw_final_9252013.pdf

6. Assessment and Evaluation Resources for Food Insecure Populations: https:// eatrightfoundation.org/wp-content/uploads/2016/10/Assessmentand EvaluationsResources.pdf

7. Community Food Assessment Tools: https://www.cdc.gov/healthyplaces /healthtopics/healthyfood/community_assessment.htm

8. NHANES Food Frequency Questionnaire: https://epi.grants.cancer.gov/diet /usualintakes/ffq.html

Sample Community Needs Assessments

- https://sirc.asu.edu/sites/default/files/%5Bterm%3Aname%5D/%5 Bnode%3Acreate%3Acustom%3AYm%5D/coordinated_community _health_needs_assessment_focus_group_results_final_fall_2016.pdf

- http://www.rileycountycommunityneedsassessment.org/uploads/4/1 /4/2/41422627/final_riley_county_community_needs_assessment _january_2015.pdf

- https://ncapwv.org/wp-content/uploads/2019/02/NCAP-2018 _Community-Needs-Assessment-Report.pdf

- https://www.changeinc.org/changewp/wp-content/uploads/2019 -Community-Needs-Assessment-1.pdf

- https://www.hospitalcouncil.org/sites/main/files/file-attachments /hospital_council_of_northern_and_central_california_final.pdf

References

1. Isaacs AN. An overview of qualitative research methodology for public health researchers. *Int J Med Public Health*. 2014;4(4): 318-323. Accessed December 25, 2020. doi: 10.4103/2230 -8598.144055.

2. Principles of epidemiology in public health practice. Centers for Disease Control and Prevention. Updated July 2, 2014. Accessed December 25, 2020. https://www.cdc.gov/csels/dsepd/ss1978 /glossary.html

3. Silveira A. Prevalence of overweight and obesity in African American adolescents in Baltimore, Maryland. Accessed December 30, 2020. https://www.jhsph.edu/offices-and -services/student-assembly/student-groups/SPHI/Prevalence _of_Overweight_and_Obesity_in_African_American _Adolescents_in_Baltimore_Maryland_Silveira.pdf

4. Walters H, Graf M. America's obesity crisis: the health and economic costs of excess weight. Milken Institute. Updated October 2018. Accessed December 25, 2020. https://milk eninstitute.org/sites/default/files/reports-pdf/Mi-Americas -Obesity-Crisis-WEB.pdf

5. Needs-assessment: Gathering stakeholder input. North Dakota State University. Accessed December 25, 2020. https://www .ag.ndsu.edu/programplanning/needs-assessment

6. Benge M, Harder A, Warner L. Conducting the needs assessment #1: introduction. *EDIS* 2019;2019(5):4. https://doi .org/10.32473/edis-wc340-2019

7. Guide to grantwriting: conducting a needs assessment. DataHaven website. Accessed December 30, 2020. https:// www.ctdatahaven.org/articles/guide-grantwriting-conducting -needs-assessment

8. Donaldson JL, Franck KL. Needs assessment guidebook for extension professionals. 2016. Accessessed December 30, 2020. https://extension.tennessee.edu/publications/Documents /PB1839.pdf

9. Centers for Disease Control and Prevention (CDC). Community needs assessment. Atlanta, GA: 2013. Accessed January 31, 2021. https://www.cdc.gov/globalhealth/healthprotection/fetp /training_modules/15/community-needs_pw_final_9252013.pdf

10. Community tool box. Chapter 3, Section 4: Collecting information about the problem. University of Kansas. Accessed January 31, 2021. https://ctb.ku.edu/en/table-of-contents /assessment/assessing-community-needs-and-resources/collect -information/main

11. Casadei K, Kiel J. Anthropometric measurement. StatPearls. Last Update April 2020. Accessed February 6, 2021. https:// www.ncbi.nlm.nih.gov/books/NBK537315/

12. Food and Nutrition Technical Assistance III Project (FANTA). 2016. *Nutrition assessment, counseling, and support (NACS): a user's guide—Module 2: nutrition assessment and classification, Version 2.* Washington, DC: FHI 360/FANTA.

13. The University of Hawai'i. Types of scientific studies and nutrition assessment methods. Last Update August 2020. Accessed February 6, 2021. https://med.libretexts.org /Under_Construction/Purgatory/Book%3A_Human_Nutrition _(University_of_Hawaii)_1st_Ed/01%3A_Basic_Concepts_in _Nutrition/1.07%3A_Types_of_Scientific_Studies_and_Nutrition _Assessment_Methods

14. Dao MC, Subar AF, Warthon-Medina M, et al. Dietary assessment toolkits: an overview. *Public Health Nutr*. 2019, 22(3): 404-418. Published October 15, 2018. doi: 10.1017 /S1368980018002951.

15. Willett W. Nature of variation in diet. In: Willett W, ed. *Nutritional Epidemiology*. 3rd ed. United States of America: Oxford University Press; 2013:503.

16. Norman Å, Kjellenberg K, Torres Aréchiga D, et al. "Everyone can take photos." Feasibility and relative validity of phone photography-based assessment of children's diets – a mixed methods study. *Nutr J*. 2020;19(50). https://doi.org/10.1186 /s12937-020-00558-4

17. Fowler, FJ. *Survey Research Methods (5th ed.).* Sage Publications; 2013.

18. Ruel E, Wagner III WE, Gillespie BJ. *The practice of survey research*. Sage Publications; 2015.

19. Roller MR, Lavrakas PJ. Applied qualitative research design: a total quality framework approach. The Guilford Press; 2015.

20. USAID Center for Development Information and Evaluation. Performance monitoring and evaluation tips: conducting focus group interviews. 1996. Accessed February 13, 202. https:// pdf.usaid.gov/pdf_docs/PNABS541.pdf

21. Community Tool Box. Chapter 3, Section 15: Qualitative methods to assess community issues. University of Kansas. Accessed February 13, 2021. https://ctb.ku.edu/en/table-of-contents /assessment/assessing-community-needs-and-resources /qualitative-methods/main

22. Community tool box. Chapter 3, Section 23: Developing and using criteria and processes to set priorities; Tool #1: Some decision-making processes. University of Kansas. Accessed February 15, 2021. https://ctb.ku.edu/en/table-of-contents /assessment/assessing-community-needs-and-resources/criteria -and-processes-to-set-priorities/tools

23. Jelliffe DB, Jelliffe EFP. *Community nutritional assessment: with special reference to less technically developed countries*. Oxford Medical Publications; 1989.

24. Centers for Disease Control and Prevention. Community Health Assessment and Group Evaluation (CHANGE) tool. March 2018. Accessed February 15, 2021. https://www.cdc.gov/nccdphp /dnpao/state-local-programs/change-tool/index.html

25. The Johns Hopkins Hospital & Johns Hopkins Bayview Medical Center 2018 Community Health Needs-assessment. Accessed February 15, 2021. PDF document Available at: https://www .hopkinsmedicine.org/about/community_health/johns-hopkins -hospital/community_health_needs_assessment.html

CHAPTER 6

Planning and Evaluating Nutrition Services for the Community

Julie M. Moreschi, MS, RDN, LDN

Learning Outcomes

AFTER STUDYING THIS CHAPTER AND REFLECTING ON THE CONTENTS, YOU SHOULD BE ABLE TO:

1. Define and list the types of planning.
2. Discuss the need for and advantages of planning.
3. Learn strategies for choosing a planning model for a project.
4. Identify a variety of existing planning models.
5. List the types of program evaluation.

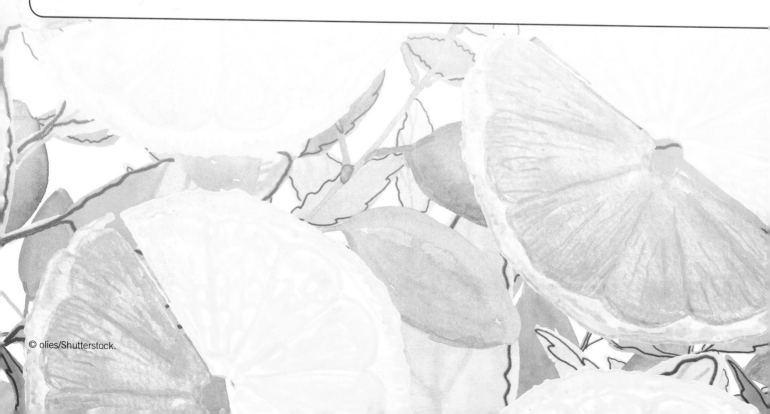

Introduction

What is planning? Why is planning of tremendous relevance to a community and public health dietitian's/nutritionist's success? This chapter will help expand the reader's ability to answer these questions and to apply the concepts toward enhanced work performance in this essential management function.

Planning refers to the management function that involves setting goals and deciding the best route for achieving them. In essence, planning deals with the what, where, when, and how of management. It focuses on solving problems and planning for events in the future. Planning is continuous. It involves following certain steps and progressing through these steps in a logical, preset manner. The Generalized Model for Program Planning, in **Figure 6–1**, outlines these common steps: assessing need, setting goals and objectives, developing an intervention, implementing the intervention, and evaluating the results.[1]

Types of Planning

There are three main types of planning in public health: *strategic*, *long-term* (planning that addresses an organization's overall goals and usually encompasses 3–5 years), and *operational* (short-term and deals with the activities required to meet the organization's goals).

A community or public health dietitian/nutritionist is involved in all three of these types of planning. The nutrition professional in public health is most often involved in program/project management. Program/project management can occur in any of the three types of planning listed above. The majority of this chapter thus focuses on the planning, implementation, and evaluation aspects of program/project management.

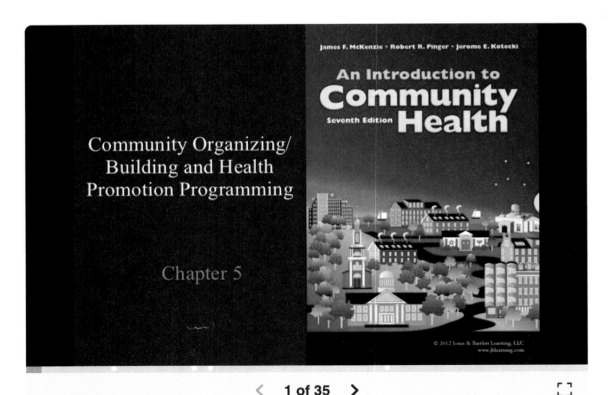

< **1 of 35** >

FIGURE 6–1 Generalized Model for Program Planning.

The Need for and Benefits of Planning

A large amount of data are available regarding the health status of the U.S. population. Many of the health issues affecting the population can be significantly improved by nutrition and lifestyle changes. It follows that the community or public health dietitian/nutritionist may find themselves creating and implementing programs to impact these relevant and profound health concerns.

For example, in 2019, the three leading causes of death in the United States, as reported by the Centers for Disease Control and Prevention's (CDC) National Vital Statistics System,[2] were diseases of the heart, malignant neoplasm, and accidents (unintentional death), as discussed in previous chapters. Smoking and obesity, which both have effective interventions, are responsible for the largest number of deaths in the United States.[3] Other dietary, lifestyle, and metabolic risk factors for chronic diseases also cause a substantial number of deaths in the United States.[3] Health promotion and disease prevention activities focused on the reduction of these risk factors could help to decrease levels of unnecessary illness and death. In addition, a community or public health dietitian/nutritionist could be involved in implementing programs relevant to achieving the objectives of *Healthy People 2030*.[4] Planning is essential in the implementation of health promotion programs that answer the call to reduce or eliminate community, group, and/or individual health issues.

Health is determined by influences at multiple levels, and due to this complexity, it can be helpful to consider program development in terms of a socio-ecological perspective. This concept was introduced by McLeroy, Bibeau, Steckler & Glanz in 1988.[5] The socio-ecological approach causes community and public health dietitians/nutritionists to recognize the interwoven relationships that exist between individuals and their environment. A health prevention program may focus on the individual, interpersonal, organizational, community, or public policy level of influence, and/or a combination of some or all of the levels of influence on health that are depicted in the socio-ecological approach. Depending on the levels of focus of a health promotion program, the choice of a program planning model should consider which specific model can best help the program to reach its goals and objectives.

It is important when program planning for health behavior change to consider not only intervention at the individual level but also to consider multilevel approaches. This concept is illustrated and supported in a position paper that is focused on prevention of childhood obesity, which was developed by the Global Federation of International Societies of Paediatric Gastroenterology, Hepatology and Nutrition (FISPGHAN).[6] The paper notes that obesity prevention will not occur as the result of single-level interventions but rather must be a multicomponent approach that includes individual, family, and societal standards.

Application of a **socio-ecological model** is often seen in public health programs through the combination of efforts focused on improvement of individual-level health behavior combined with policy, system, and environmental (PSE) change. PSE initiatives help communities to make the healthy choice the easy choice. Policy change includes the passing of laws, ordinances, resolutions, mandates, regulations, or rules. Policies greatly influence the choices we make in our lives. Laws that are passed (like workplace policies, school policies) greatly influence the daily decisions we make about our health. System change involves change made to the rules within an organization. Systems change and policy change often work hand-in-hand. Often, systems change focuses on changing

Discussion Prompt

What other cause of overwhelming death in the United States occurred in 2020 that community and public health programs had to plan? What was the role of the dietitian/nutritionist?

Strategy Tip

It is important to learn from mistakes of the past in program planning. Can the reader recall any health programs that disappeared in their community due to not meeting the goals and objectives? What was the reason for the shortfall?

Socio-ecological model A model considers the complex interplay between individual, relationship, community, and societal factors with an emphasis on determining a framework for prevention.

infrastructure within a school, park, worksite, or health setting that focus on supporting healthier habits of the individuals in these systems. Environmental change is a change made to the physical environment.[7]

When working on planning to use a PSE approach, it is also important to consider the concepts of reach, strength, layering, and dose. Reach refers to the number of people touched by an intervention. Strength is the impact of the intervention on each person reached by the intervention. Dose looks at how the reach and strength work together. Layering refers to having several types of interventions in a program, which helps to enhance the reach and dose.[8]

The process of program planning can provide several advantages to an organization. Some of these advantages include consensus and prioritization of organizational goals; establishment of goals and specific, measurable objectives, implementing efficient utilization of manpower and finances; and setting a defined timeframe for project completion.

In summary, planning focuses on approaching work in an organized and defined manner. When planning models are used skillfully, it can help to improve the health of the communities that are being served and provide a structured work environment for employees and managers that will help them to work efficiently and effectively.

Choosing a Program Planning Model

Most community and public health dietitians/nutritionists find it helpful to have a variety of planning models to choose from when organizing and implementing public health programs. A variety of models may be needed due to the nature of the project, or a dietitian/nutritionist and/or the project team may embrace the concepts of one model over another. When choosing a model, the project team should keep in mind that any chosen model serves as a frame from which to build and provide structure and organization for the planning process. No model is perfect. The community and public health dietitian/nutritionist can decide to use a model in its entirety, in parts, or by combining elements from a variety of models. Doing so assures a good fit to meet the demands of the project's mission and goals.

There are many things that a program manager and their team may consider when choosing a planning model. Some of these considerations include: the preferences of stakeholders (e.g., decision makers, program partners, consumers); how much time is available for planning purposes; how many resources are available for data collection and analysis; the degree to which clients are actually involved as partners in the planning process or the degree to which your planning efforts will be consumer-oriented (i.e., planning is based on the wants and needs of consumers); and the preferences of a funding agency (in the case of a grant or contract award).

How and when a **needs assessment** is conducted can influence the choice of a program planning model. As discussed in Chapter 5, when conducting a needs-assessment in the community, a dietitian/nutritionist may discover certain nutritional issues that trigger the need for program planning. There are times when a needs-assessment will be completed, and then choosing a planning model in which to implement corrective actions based on the data from the needs-assessment may occur as separate, sequential steps. In other situations, a broad health problem may be loosely identified in a community, and the needs-assessment will need to be as a more-intricate part of the program planning model. Thus, the nature of the health problem needs-assessment can influence which models are a good fit for a particular project.

Planning teams can consider the planning models in terms of their fluidity, flexibility, and functionality. In terms of fluidity, the planning model is best

Needs assessment A process used by organizations to determine priorities, make organizational improvements, or allocate resources. It involves determining the needs, or gaps, between where the organization envisions itself in the future and the organization's current state.

Strategy Tip

Remember too that program planning models do not have to be used in their entirety, and if a needs-assessment is part of a model that fits the project well, the needs assessment step can be surpassed.

when the steps are sequential or they build upon one another. The planning model should be flexible enough that it can adapt to the needs of the program planning team and any key stakeholders for the program. Finally, in terms of functionality, the model should focus on improving health and not on creating of the program plan itself.

Project Models

The following section acquaints the reader with a variety of program planning models and serves as a reference when selecting models to use in tackling their organization or community public health issues. Each program planning model description is general in nature, and when available, supplemental materials are provided to the reader in order to assist them in using the model for a specific health promotion project.

Project models are often in one of two categories: **ecological models** and **consumer-based models**. An *ecological model* strives to explain health-related behaviors and environments, and to design and evaluate the interventions needed to influence both the behaviors and the living conditions that influence them and their consequences. Ecological models are often used in large public health programs that have a national, state, or span broadly throughout a community. *Consumer-based models* are based on consumer input, are designed with consumers in mind and tend to be used in smaller community-based health promotion programs.

Ecological model Approach focuses on both population-level and individual-level determinants of health and interventions.

Consumer-based model A model that seeks to understand consumer needs and wants and utilizes this information to plan organizational strategies.

Ecological Models

Logic Model

During the 1960s, a planning approach called the Logic Model was developed. **Logic Models** are often used for managing projects for the U.S. government, and a community or public health dietitian/nutritionist most likely will be exposed to an application of this model when working on large collaborative projects. A *Logic Model* is a framework for building a common language for accountability and evaluation across the organization. Logic Models are often referred to as a "roadmap," and they serve to display the sequence of actions that describe what the program is and what it will do. It is a simple linear model that includes elements related to inputs, outputs, and outcomes. Logic models have a variety of advantages

Logic model A logic model is a graphic depiction (road map) that presents the shared relationships among the resources, activities, outputs, outcomes, and impact for your program.

The Community Toolbox is a great source of information for program planning. There are toolkits related to various planning models, intervention planning, evaluation, and much more. http://ctb.ku.edu/en.

Another great resource for logic models can be found at:

The Centers for Disease Control and Prevention's Workplace Health Promotion provides great information related to program needs-assessment, planning, implementation, evaluation, and much more.

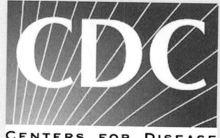

CENTERS FOR DISEASE CONTROL AND PREVENTION

http://www.cdc.gov/workplacehealthpromotion/index.html

Courtesy of Centers for Disease Control and Prevention.

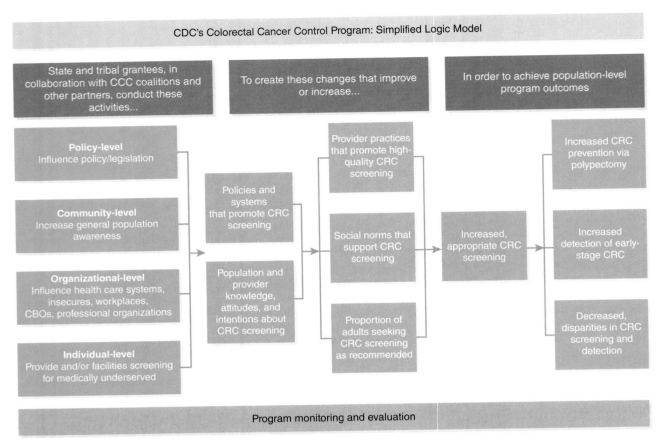

FIGURE 6–2 Simplified Logic Model.

CDC. Colorectal Cancer Control Program (CRCCP): Simplified Logic Model. Available at http://www.cdc.gov/cancer/crccp/logic.htm

to a project team. They keep everyone moving in the same direction, provide a common language and common points of reference for the project team, and create a map of action. **Figure 6–2** and **6–3** provides an example of a logic model.

PATCH and APEX-PH

Planned Approach To Community Health (PATCH) and Assessment Protocol for Excellence in Public Health (APEX-PH) are two planning processes developed by the CDC.

PATCH is a model intended for use in implementing chronic disease prevention and health promotion programs. PATCH was originally established in the mid-1980s with good results; APEXPH was introduced in 1993 to enhance the existing PATCH model. The model begins with the individual in mind. PATCH incorporates five phases:

Phase I: Mobilize the community. A group is formed to define the community, address health issues, and create working groups.

Phase II: Collect and analyze data. Data are collected and used to determine health priorities and program planning.

Phase III: Choose health priorities and target groups. Program objectives and goals are established using data from Phase II.

Phase IV: Choose and conduct interventions. Health interventions are designed and implemented.

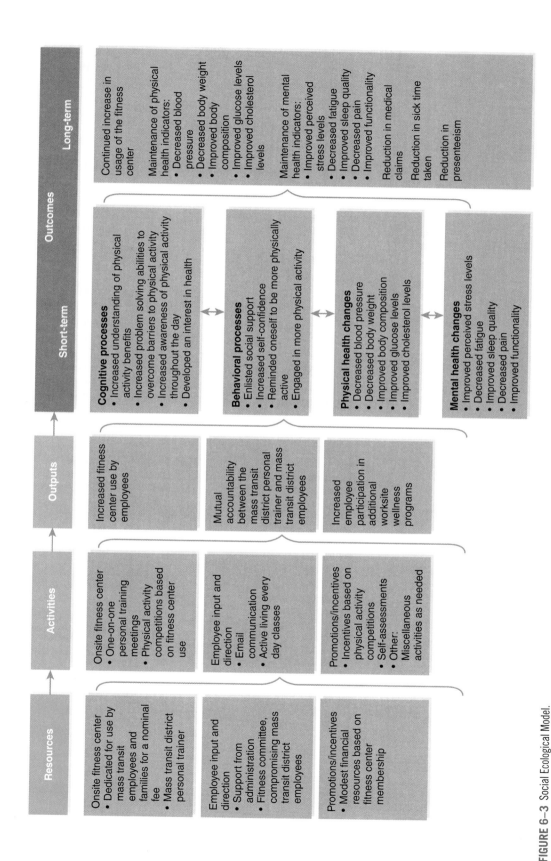

FIGURE 6–3 Social Ecological Model.

Das BM, Petruzzello SJ, Ryan KE. Development of a Logic Model for a Physical Activity–Based Employee Wellness Program for Mass Transit Workers. *Prev Chronic Dis* 2014;11:140124. DOI: http://dx.doi .org/10.5888/pcd11.140124

Phase V: Evaluate PATCH process and interventions. Programs and the PATCH process are evaluated.

APEX-PH was designed for use by local public health departments, and a workbook is available to assist in implementing the program. The program consists of three major parts:

Part I: Organizational capacity assessment

Part II: The community process

Part III: Completing the cycle

In Part I, the community or public health department conducts a self-assessment and determines the strengths and weaknesses of the organization in meeting the community's health needs. In Part II, the community health needs are assessed, and health status goals and program objectives are defined. Part III establishes the basic monitoring and evaluation tools.

PRECEDE-PROCEED

Predisposing, Reinforcing, and Enabling Constructs in Educational/Environmental Diagnosis-Policy, Regulatory, and Organizational Constructs in Educational and Environmental Development (PRECEDE-PROCEED) is a nine-phase planning model (Figure 6–4). Gold, Green, and Kreuter's overarching principle in this model is that most lasting health behavior change is voluntary in nature and must include input from the individual.[9] This principle is reflected in a methodical planning process, which empowers individuals with understanding, motivation, skills, and active engagement in community affairs to improve their quality of life. The model begins with

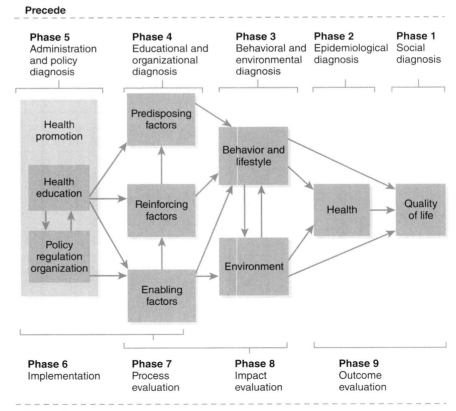

FIGURE 6–4 PRECEDE-PROCEED Planning Model.

the end or final consequence and works back to the causes. PRECEDE is the diagnostic and needs assessment phase. The PROCEED element of this model refers to the developmental stage of planning and begins the implementation and evaluation process.

MATCH

The Multilevel Approach to Community Health (MATCH) planning model was developed in the late 1980s by Simons-Morton and colleagues.[10] The planning model includes five phases: goal selection, intervention planning, program development, implementation, and evaluation. This model emphasizes that intervention approaches can and should be aimed at a variety of objectives and individuals. The MATCH Diagram is pictured in **Figure 6–5**.

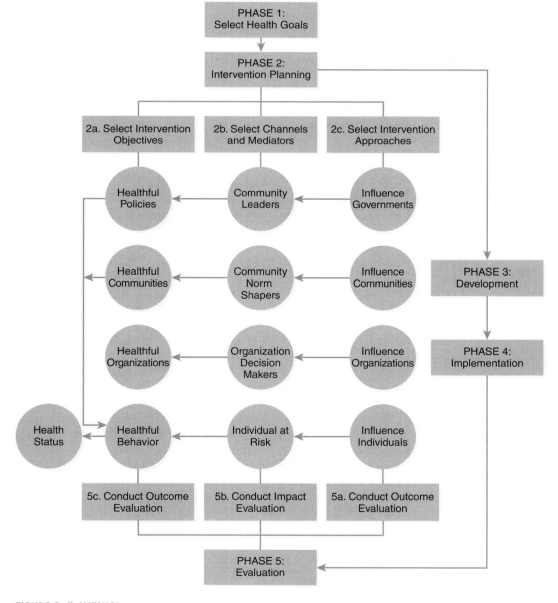

FIGURE 6–5 MATCH Diagram.

Simons-Morton B. G., Greene W. H., Gottlieb N. H. Introduction to health education and health promotion. Prospect Heights, IL: Waveland Press; 1995.

Consumer-based Model

CDCynergy Lite

CDCynergy Lite is an updated version based on the original Social Marketing Edition of CDCynergy. This CDCynergy tool is based on best practice social marketing principles and assists in developing, implementing, and evaluating an effective social marketing plan. The tool is intended for those who have previous social marketing experience and, in particular, those who are familiar with the original version of CDCynergy that was developed in 1998.[11]

CDCynergy Lite uses a five-phase planning model as follows:

1. Problem Description
2. Market Research
3. Market Strategy
4. Interventions
5. Evaluation

The website provides a guide with information to guide them through each step of the planning model. Each stage of the model is accompanied by information about "What It Is" and "How It is Done" plus additional materials such as tools and templates, as shown in **Figure 6–6**.

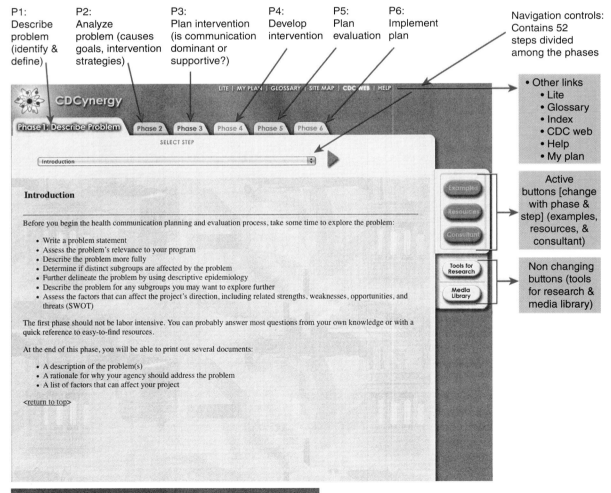

FIGURE 6–6 The CDCynergy Model System.

CDCynergy. How To Use - CDCynergy. Available at http://www.orau.gov/cdcynergy/web/BA/Content/activeinformation/howtouse/howtouse01.htm

The P Process Model

Another planning model is Johns Hopkins University Center for Communication Program's P Process.[12] The P Process provides a framework for the development of strategic health communication programs. The process was developed in 1982 and was used to help design effective communication projects for behavior change. The P Process can be used when developing:

- Project and program design
- Workshops and classes
- Brochures, reports, manuals, posters, presentations, and publications

The five steps in the P Process are described in further detail in the following sections.

Step 1: Analysis

Two types of analyses should be considered: situation and audience/communication. *Situation analysis* refers to determining the severity and causes of problems, identifying factors inhibiting or facilitating desired changes, developing a problem statement, and carrying out formation research that takes the learners' needs and priorities into consideration. *Audience/communication analysis* focuses on conducting a participation analysis to identify partners, audiences, and field workers for the project, carrying out a social and behavioral analysis at the community and individual level, and assessing communication and training needs.

Step 2: Strategic Design

Step 2 deals with developing a strategic design for the project. Elements of this step include establishing clear objectives, developing program approaches, determining marketing channels, and creating implementation and evaluation plans.

Step 3: Development and Testing

The development and testing phase is where the actual program or project is developed. It is then revised as needed before full implementation. This step should not only consider the technical and scientific accuracy of the products but must also include an element of creativity in order to better reach and engage the participants.

Step 4: Implementation and Monitoring

Implementation and monitoring deals with taking the product and disseminating it throughout the target population's community. This phase may incorporate some training or development of personnel delivering the program. The program must be monitored and changes made as necessary to ensure a high-quality product.

Step 5: Evaluation and Replanning

The final step in the P Process is the evaluation and replanning phase. During this step, outcomes are measured, and future needs are assessed. Programs are redesigned and revised as needed based on data collected during this phase. Outcomes during this phase may warrant that the project begin again at Step 1, the analysis phase.

The Health Communication Process

The Health Communication Process is a planning model developed by the U.S. Department of Health & Human Services, the National Institutes for Health (NIH), and the National Cancer Institute (NCI).[13] This model was first designed in 1985, and for almost 25 years, an ongoing evaluation of the communication programs has confirmed the value of using specific communication strategies to promote health and prevent disease.

A manual describing how to use the P Process Model can be downloaded at http://www.thehealthcompass.org/sbcc-tools/p-process

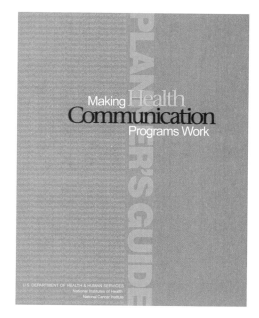

Cover page of Making Health Communication Programs Work.

A copy of *Making Health Communication Programs Work* can be found on the Internet at http://cancer.gov/pinkbook/

TABLE 6–1
Health Communication Process Stages

What Will Be Accomplished?
- Identify how the organization can use communication effectively to address a health problem.
- Identify intended audiences.
- Use consumer research to create a communication strategy and objectives.
- Draft communication plans, including activities, partnerships, and baseline survey for outcome evaluation.
- Develop relevant, meaningful messages.
- Plan activities and draft materials.
- Pretest the messages and materials with intended audience members.
- Begin program implementation, maintaining promotion, distribution, and other activities through all channels.
- Conduct process evaluation via tracking intended audience exposure and reaction to the program. Determine whether adjustments are needed.
- Periodically review all program elements and make revisions as needed.
- Assess your health communication program.
- Identify refinements that would increase the effectiveness of future programs.

The Health Communication Process has four stages:

1. Planning and strategic development
2. Developing and pretesting concepts, messages, and materials
3. Implementing the program
4. Assessing effectiveness and making refinements

Upon completion of each stage, the planners can expect to accomplish the goals shown in **Table 6–1**.

Mobilizing for Action Through Planning & Partnerships

The Mobilizing for Action Through Planning & Partnership (MAPP) planning model was developed by the National Association of County and City Health Officials (NACCHO), in collaboration with the CDC.[14]

MAPP's purpose is to assist communities in developing frameworks to improve public health by helping them to prioritize their public health issues, identify the resources needed to address them, and to implement strategies to fit each community's unique needs.

The MAPP process consists of six phases:

Phase 1: Organization for success and partnership development
Phase 2: Visioning for future planning
Phase 3: Assessment phase including identifying community themes and strengths, a local public health system assessment, a community health status assessment, and a forces-of-change assessment
Phase 4: Identification of strategic issues
Phase 5: Formulation of goals and strategies
Phase 6: Action cycle, which includes planning, implementing, and evaluating the community's strategic plan

NACCHO provides a variety of tools to help communities in using and implementing programs using the MAPP model program managers can access a blueprint executive summary and webinar to assist them in using the MAPP approach (**Figure 6–7**) to tackling the public health issues of their organization or community.[15]

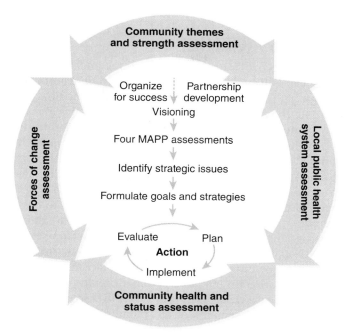

FIGURE 6–7 MAPP Model.

Reproduced from NACCHO. MAPP Basics - Introduction to the MAPP Process. Available at http://archived
.naccho.org/topics/infrastructure/mapp/framework/mappbasics.cfm

MAP-IT

The Department of Health and Human Services has a **program implementation** guide called Healthy People in Healthy Communities, which is focused on helping communities to implement *Healthy People* initiatives. The program management model used for this program is called MAP-IT.[15]
  MAP-IT's acronym is:

Mobilize individuals and organizations that care about the health of your community into a coalition.

Assess the areas of greatest need in your community, as well as the resources and other strengths that you can tap into to address those areas.

Plan your approach: start with a vision of where you want to be as a community; then add strategies and action steps to help you achieve that vision.

Implement your plan using concrete action steps that can be monitored and will make a difference.

Track your progress over time.

  The MAP-IT technique is a strategy that can be applied by communities to help them to "map out" the changes they want to see in their community. By using the MAP-IT approach, a planning team can devise a structured, step-by-step plan focused on a particular community's specific needs and goals. See **Figure 6–8**.

Program implementation Refers to how well a proposed program or intervention is put into practice and is fundamental to establishing the internal, external, construct, and statistical conclusion validity of outcome evaluations.

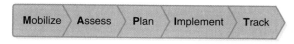

FIGURE 6–8 MAP-IT.

Healthy People, Program Planning. Available at http://www.healthypeople.gov/2020/tools-and-resources
/Program-Planning

Guide for Effective Nutrition Interventions and Education (GENIE)

The Guide for Effective Nutrition Interventions and Education (GENIE) is simple, practical, and evidence-based tool to help nutrition education practitioners design high-quality and effective programs. The program is provided for your use by the Academy of Nutrition and Dietetics and its Foundation with funding support from the ConAgra Foods Foundation. Program planners can benefit from GENIE during the designed process to build effective outcome-based nutrition education programs, to efficiently compare various nutrition education program proposals, and inform funding decisions.[16]

A program planner can use GENIE through the web by completing the system's self-assessment tool. This checklist can be used to begin a new program, improve or modify an existing program, or compare different nutrition education programs. The self-assessment tool contains nine categories including program description and importance; program goal; program framework; program setting, recruitment, and retention plan; instructional methods; program content; program materials; evaluation; and sustainability.

Throughout the checklist, users may hover over icons to be provided with descriptions of certain elements of the planning tool. Program developers are encouraged to ask other colleagues to complete the checklist in order to get an outsider's perspective on the planning or existing program. Once the assessment is completed, an automated summary is created and is available for download. This planning tool is somewhat general in nature and may require the program planner to utilize other planning model tools in order to fully complete a program plan that is ready for implementation.

Intervention Mapping

Intervention mapping is a protocol for developing effective behavior-change interventions. Intervention Mapping was first developed and introduced in 1998 by L. Kay Bartholomew, Guy S. Parcel & Gerjo Kok,-in an article in Health Education & Behavior.[17] In 2001, the concept was developed into the book titled "Planning Health Promotion Programs: An Intervention Mapping Approach" and is now in its 4th edition.[18]

Through use of this model, program planners are brought through a series of steps that help them to develop theory and evidence-based intervention program for the purpose of health prevention. This planning technique incorporates aspects of the Precede-Proceed model when conducting the needs assessment and uses a logic model planning framework. The steps in the protocol include:

1. Logic Model of the Problem
2. Program Outcomes and Objectives (Logic Model of Change)
3. Program Plan
4. Program Production
5. Implementation Plan
6. Evaluation Plan

Community Health Assessment and Group Evaluation (Change)

Community Health Assessment and Group Evaluation (CHANGE) is a data-collection tool and planning resource for community members who want to make their community a healthier one. The Healthy Communities Program (www.cdc.gov/HealthyCommunitiesProgram) within the Division of Adult

Strategy Tip

If a community or public health dietitian/ nutritionist wishes to utilize this model, they may use the book as a guide or attend an annual seminar that is offered by the Applied Social Psychology section of the department of Work & Social Psychology, Faculty of Psychology and Neuroscience, at Maastricht University found at: https:// interventionmapping.com/http://heb .sagepub.com/content/25/5/545.long

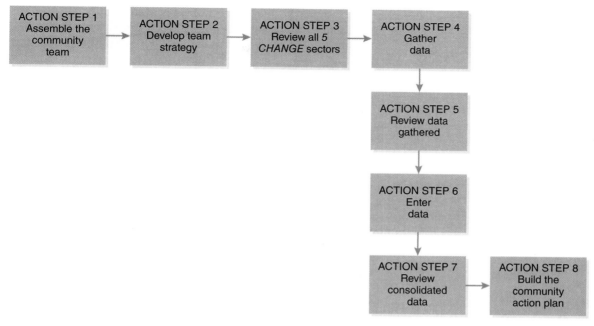

FIGURE 6–9 Action Steps to Complete the CHANGE Tool.

CDC's Healthy Communities Program: Community Health Assessment and Group Evaluation (CHANGE): Building a Foundation of Knowledge to Prioritize Community Needs, An Action Guide. Available at http://www.cdc.gov/nccdphp/dch/programs/healthycommunitiesprogram/tools/change/pdf/changeactionguide.pdf

and Community Health, at the National Center for Chronic Disease Prevention and Health Promotion of the CDC developed the *CHANGE* tool. The CDC's Healthy Communities Program designed the CHANGE tool for all communities interested in creating social and built environments that support healthy living.[19]

Development of the CHANGE tool began in the fall of 2007, and the first draft was piloted with a set of CDC-funded communities. The tool comprises a set of easy-to-use Microsoft Office Excel spreadsheets for collection of local-level data from schools, worksites, community organizations, and healthcare facilities. CHANGE helps communities to assess potential approaches that are innovative as well as approaches that show strong evidence of effectiveness. The steps in the model can be viewed in **Figure 6–9**. Although the CDC is no longer funding this project, the archived website does provide a program planner with the action guide, as well as many templates and examples that can be very helpful.

Protocol for Assessing Community Excellence in Environmental Health (PACE-EH)

Community and public health nutrition professionals are increasingly faced with how to address the impact that the environment is having on community health. NACCHO developed the Protocol for Assessing Community Excellence in Environmental Health (PACE EH), a methodology to guide local communities in identifying and addressing environmental health priorities. PACE EH was developed by a work group of local health officials, under the guidance of a multidisciplinary steering committee and with funding from NACCHO and the National Center for Environmental Health (NCEH) of the CDC, and a guidebook to help communities to use this framework was disseminated in 2000.[20] PACE EH is a 13-task model, and the tasks are available at: https://www.cdc.gov/nceh/ehs/ceha/pace_eh.htm

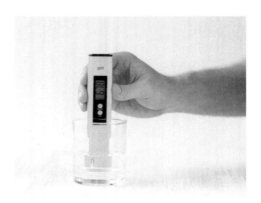

Environmental health includes the safety level for drinking water.

© Dmytro Tyshchenko/Shutterstock.

PACE EH is designed to help communities systematically conduct and act on an assessment of environmental health status in city or county. The tools and instructions in the guidebook are intended to strengthen a collective understanding of and appreciation for the critical role that environmental health plays in the overall health of a community. This model is useful in a community group that is focused on improving the understanding of how the environment may be impacting health and well-being of the people who live there, if there is any disparity in terms of which individuals in the community are being impacted by the environment to a greater extent, how the environment can be protected from further harm, if there is a need to summarize environmental protection measures that are already in place, or determining the key resources in the community that need to be preserved and protected.

The PACE EH website provided a community or public health dietitian/nutritionist with many tools to help in implementing environmental change programming. Resources include access to the toolkit, online training, as well as access to a networking map of users of the PACE EH model.

Program Implementation

Program implementation can be defined as the process of putting a project, service, or program into full effect. It is the management of the execution of the project. Program implementation is a critical part of the planning process and requires the creation of an implementation action plan.

Eight factors to consider when developing an implementation plan are:

1. *Why:* The effect of the objectives to be achieved
2. *What:* The activities required to achieve the objectives
3. *Who:* The individuals responsible for each activity?
4. *When:* A chronological sequence of activities and timing in relation to project implementation activities or organization events
5. *How:* The materials, supplies, technology, devices, methods, media approaches, flow of activities, or techniques to be used. Also, consideration regarding consents, medical clearances, and program safety should be addressed as appropriate.
6. *Where:* Which activities will take place at what locations in the community—at the health promotion site, facility, office, clinic, and center
7. *Cost:* An estimate of expenses for materials, personnel, facilities, and time
8. *Feedback:* When and how to tell if the activities are happening as they should be and if adjustments are needed; use timelines

With all of these elements to consider, a written implementation plan is essential. An easy method to apply when writing an implementation process is to create action plans or timetables. If a dietitian/nutritionist is managing a project, they can take elements from the eight implementation factors listed above and create a detailed timetable.

There are several types of timetables or action planning formats that can be used by program managers. Some examples of such tools include Task Development Timelines, Gantt charts, and PERT charts.

Task Development Timelines and Gantt charts are very similar approaches. They are both a table format, which indicates the timeline in the columns, and the tasks to be completed in the rows. A sample of the Gantt chart can be found in **Figure 6–10**.

The PERT acronym is Program Evaluation and Review Technique. There are three elements in a PERT chart. A program manager begins the process of creating it by listing all activities involved in implementation of the program.

Example: The Gantt chart below shows part of one team's test implementation. Notice the sheer volume of information you can easily absorb simply by looking at this chart. Consider its value as a tracking tool once implementation is under way.

Schedule		Week Number:								
Task	Assigned to	1	2	3	4	5	6	7	8	9
Submit draft for review	Team leader	■								
Review draft	Review comm.		■	■						
Submit comments	Review comm.			■	■					
Revise manual based upon feedback	Team				■	■	■			
Create camera-ready materials	Team leader						■	■		
Print 100 copies of manual	Print shop								■	
Circulate 100 copies to employees	Team leader									■

FIGURE 6–10 Gantt Chart.

Centers for Disease Control and Prevention. Accessed February 25, 2010. Available at http://www.cdc.gov

To create the PERT diagram, each activity would be placed in a circle. Lines are then used to indicate the sequence of events for each task. Solid lines indicate activities that begin with one task and end with another task. Dotted lines are used to show events that are dependent on one another but for which no work is involved. **Figure 6–11** shows an example of a PERT chart.

Example: The PERT chart below is mapping out the critical path for printing and distributing a new form.

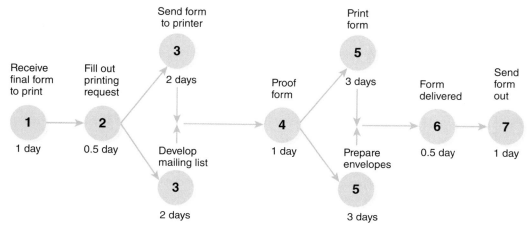

FIGURE 6–11 PERT Chart.

CDC. PERT Chart. Accessed February 25, 2010. Available at http://www.cdc.gov

Determining Team Membership

An important component of any planning project is working effectively through joint efforts. Working together as a team has many benefits, such as providing the group with a variety of viewpoints and backgrounds, pooling resources to get work accomplished, satisfying personal and professional needs of the team members, and gaining community support for your initiative. Development of team membership procedures, however, often is not easy or without cause for concern. Difficult situations can arise when coordinating teams; these can be managing a large group with slow progress on action plans or decision making; difficulty in obtaining volunteer membership due to busy or conflicting schedules; and conflicts of interest of membership, particularly for those working in for-profit venues.

The *Making Health Communication Programs Work* textbook[13] provides several tools to assist planning groups to establish their membership. A partnership planning worksheet is supplied that asks questions regarding potential partners, partners' roles and tasks, benefits to partners when they participate on the team, as well as many other considerations. This guide also provides an excellent resource titled, "Steps for Involving Partners in the Program" **(Table 6–2)**.

Once the project team has been assembled, it can be important to establish guidelines as to how the group will work together. One approach to the development of such a structure is called Terms of Reference (TOR). A TOR template can assist a project manager in communicating effectively and establishing "buy in" with all team members and stakeholders. Information that can be addressed in a project TOR includes the project vision and objectives, a list of the key project deliverables and/or outcomes, a list of the team members and stakeholders along with information of their key roles and responsibilities, and an organizational structure by which the program will operate.

TABLE 6–2
Steps for Involving Partners in the Program

1. Choose organizations, agencies, or individuals (e.g., physicians) that can bring the resources, expertise, or credibility that your program needs.
2. Consider which roles partners might play to best support the program.
3. Involve representatives of the organizations you want to work with as early as appropriate in program planning.
4. Give partners the program rationale, strategies, and messages (in a ready-to-use form). Remember that strategic planning, creative messages, and quality production are the most difficult aspects of a communication program to develop and may be the most valuable product you can offer to a community organization.
5. Give partners advance notice so that they can build their part of the program into their schedule and negotiate what will be expected of them.
6. Allow partners to personalize and adapt program materials to fit their circumstances and give them a feeling of ownership, but don't let them stray from the strategy.
7. Ask partners what they need to implement their part of the program. Beyond the question of funding, consider other assistance, training, information, or tools that would enable them to function successfully.
8. Provide partners with new local/regional/national contacts or linkages that they will perceive as valuable for their ongoing activities.
9. Give partners an appropriate amount of work. Give them a series of small, tangible, short-term responsibilities as well as a feedback/tracking mechanism.
10. Gently remind partners that they are responsible for their activities; help them complete tasks but do not complete tasks for them.
11. Assess progress through the feedback/tracking mechanism and help make adjustments to respond to the organization's needs and to keep the program on track.
12. Provide moral support by frequently saying "thank you" and by providing other rewards (e.g., letter or certificate of appreciation).
13. Give partners a final report of what was accomplished and meet to discuss follow-up activities and resources they might find useful. Make sure that they feel they are a part of the program's success.
14. Share one final tremendous "Thank you for a job well done."

U.S. Department of Health and Human Services, National Institutes of Health, National Cancer Institute, *Pink Book—Making Health Communication Programs Work*. Accessed April 25, 2021. Available at: http://www.cancer.gov/publications/health-communication/pink-book.pdf

Health Program Evaluation

Benefits of Evaluation

Evaluation of health programs is essential to assure that objectives are being met. Health programs aim to result in efficient, effective, and quality outcomes, and the goal of an evaluation process is to prove that these aims are being realized. Evaluations focus on proving that programs are cost-effective, that managerial practices are accountable, and that the programs are contributing to improvements in the community's health.

Types of Evaluations

Several types of evaluation can be conducted, and definitions for some of them are provided here. A *formative evaluation* assesses whether a problem is occurring in a program, the extent of the problem, and if corrective action is necessary. *Summative evaluation* focuses on program impact and program effectiveness. *Program impact* assesses if interventions are producing desired outcomes, and *program effectiveness* determines if outcomes could be achieved at a lower cost and deals specifically with cost-benefit and cost-effectiveness analysis. *Process evaluation* assesses the effectiveness of administrative activities and program implementation. It may be helpful to visualize the interrelationships that exist between the program outcomes, types of evaluations, and evaluation objectives. In his book, *The Practice of Health Program Evaluation*, David Grembowksi[21] describes program evaluation as a three-act play. In the second act of his model, Grembowski discusses program **impact** and **cost-effectiveness evaluation** in great detail. Several designs can be used to measure the impact of programs, each having its own strengths and weaknesses. Designs can be preexperimental, experimental, or quasiexperimental. The design that is chosen to measure program impact should be feasible; fit well with logistical, political, budgetary, and other constraints of the program; and be able to produce reliable results. (See **Table 6–3**.)

PRECEDE-PROCEED Evaluation Model

Impact outcomes look at outcomes correlated with resources and cost. The PRECEDE-PROCEED model presented earlier in this chapter includes an element of impact outcome. This model also includes evaluation elements through the use of intermediate objectives applied to each phase of the model.

Formative evaluation Occurs during program development and implementation. It provides information on achieving program goals or improving your program.

Summative evaluation Intended to provide a package of results used to assess whether a program works or not.

Process evaluation Measures effort and the direct outputs of programs/interventions—what and how much was accomplished (i.e., exposure, reach, knowledge, attitudes, etc.). Examines the process of implementing the communication program/intervention and determines whether it is operating as planned.

Impact evaluation Assesses a program's effect on participants. Appropriate measures include changes in awareness, knowledge, attitudes, behaviors, and/or skills.

Cost-effectiveness evaluation Analysis is a way to examine both the costs and health outcomes of one or more interventions. It compares an intervention with another intervention (or the status quo) by estimating how much it costs to gain a unit of a health outcome, like a life year gained or a death prevented.

TABLE 6–3
Types of Program Designs[1]

Design Type	Subtypes
Pre-experimental	One-group posttest-only design One-group pretest-posttest design Posttest-only comparison group design
Experimental	Pretest-posttest control group design Posttest-only control group design
Quasiexperimental	Single-time series design Multiple-time series design Repeated treatment design Pretest-posttest nonequivalent comparison group design Recurrent institutional cycle design Regression discontinuity design

[1]Refer to statistical resources for detailed explanations of these designs.

Program intervention models look at the impact of outcomes. An example of such a model is based on the acronym RASOGO, an acronym for:

R – Resources lead to activities.
A – Activities lead to sub-objectives.
S – Sub-objectives lead to objectives.
O – Objectives lead to goals.
G – Goals produce outcomes.
O – Outcomes.

CDC's Evaluation Process

The CDC's program evaluation process (Figure 6–12) is laid out in a wheel shape. This can help an organization to summarize and organize the essential elements of program evaluation, provide a common frame of reference for conducting evaluations, clarify the steps in program evaluation, review the standards of effective program evaluation, and address misconceptions about the purposes and methods of the program evaluation. A summary of the CDC evaluation model's steps follows:

Steps in Evaluation Practice

1. Engage stakeholders: Those involved, those affected, primary intended users
2. Describe the program: Need, expected effects, activities, resources, stage, context, logic model
3. Focus the evaluation design: Purpose, users, uses, questions, methods, agreements
4. Gather credible evidence: Indicators, sources, quality, quantity, and logistics
5. Justify conclusions: Standards, analysis/synthesis, interpretation, judgment, recommendations
6. Ensure use and share lessons learned: Design, preparation, feedback, follow-up, and dissemination

Standards of Effective Evaluation

1. Utility: Serve the information needs of intended users.
2. Feasibility: Be realistic, prudent, diplomatic, and frugal.

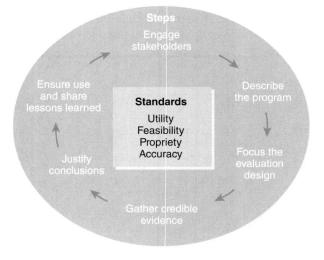

FIGURE 6–12 CDC Evaluation Wheel.

Centers for Disease Control, Framework for Program Evaluation in Public Health. Accessed February 25, 2010. Available at http://www.cdc.gov/epo/mmwr/preview/mmwrhtml/rr4811a1.htm

3. Propriety: Behave legally, ethically, and with due regard for the welfare of those involved and those affected.
4. Accuracy: Reveal and convey technically accurate information.

The Health Communication Planning Guide's Outcome Evaluation Process

The *Health Communication Planning Guide* does provide an outcome evaluation process component. Results of the evaluation should be used to help identify areas of the program that should be changed, deleted, or augmented. The outcome evaluation process has nine steps, as follows:

1. Determine what information the evaluation must provide.
2. Define the data to collect.
3. Decide on data collection methods.
4. Develop and pretest data collection instruments.
5. Collect data.
6. Process data.
7. Analyze data to answer the evaluation questions.
8. Write an evaluation report.
9. Disseminate the evaluation report.

Cost-Effectiveness Analysis

There are three types of cost-effectiveness analysis (CEA) that can be conducted for a program:

- *Cost-benefit analysis:* A method of economic evaluation where all benefits and costs of a program are measured in dollars. Programs have value when their benefits are equal to or exceed their costs, or the ratio of \$benefits/\$costs is equal to or greater than 1.0, or when the benefit/cost ratio of Program A is equal to or greater than 1.0 and exceeds the benefit/cost ratio of Program B.
- *Cost-minimization analysis:* A type of CEA where Program A and Program B have identical benefit outcomes, and the goal of the analysis is to determine which program has the lower cost.
- *Cost-utility analysis:* A type of CEA in which the outcomes of Program A and Program B are weighted by their value, or quality, and measured with a common metric, such as "quality-adjusted life years." The goal of the analysis is to determine which program produces the most quality-adjusted life years at the lowest cost.

The 10 basic steps to conducting a CEA are:

1. Define the problem and objectives.
2. Identify alternatives.
3. Describe production relationships, or the CEA's conceptual model.
4. Define the perspective of the CEA.
5. Identify, measure, and value costs.
6. Identify and measure effectiveness.
7. Discount future costs and effectiveness.
8. Perform a sensitivity analysis.
9. Address equity issues.
10. Use CEA in decision making.

A CEA can be an intense and complicated evaluation endeavor. If a planning team has minimal experience with this concept, they may find it

Strategy Tip

Evaluation is an essential element in the planning process. When developing plans, groups need to consider what types of evaluation they wish to conduct. Most evaluation plans will include several elements and will deal with analysis of both the outcome and the effectiveness of programs. Several models and references are available for teams when they are developing plans for evaluation components of programs.

necessary to partner with individuals with skill and experience in conducting CEA evaluation processes.

Sustaining Your Program Planning Efforts

Once the hard work of planning, implementing, and evaluation a public health program, it is important for the planning team to consider sustaining the program that has been created. Sustainability refers to the ability to maintain programming and its benefits over time. Without planning for sustaining a program, all of the hard work developing the initiative may dissolve. There are several factors that can impact sustainability such as funding stability, environmental support, partnerships, organizational capacity, program evaluation, program adaptation, and communication.

Washington University of St Louis has created a program sustainability tool (PSAT) that can assist a project team in completing a sustainability assessment, which can then lead to the creation of a sustainability plan.[22] The PSAT program provides work groups with sustainability assessment so they can develop a sustainability plan for their project. The site also provides the work group with links to numerous other sustainability resources.

Program Planning During COVID-19

COVID-19, a disease caused by a novel coronavirus, became a major global human threat that turned into a pandemic. The COVID-19 pandemic caused national and international public health programs to have to develop program planning with speed and efficiency. Knowledge of program planning tools were essential resources in helping public health organizations to coordinate a variety of key elements of support to communities such as COVID-19 testing, COVID 19 vaccinations, and supporting communities in accessing vital resources such as food.

The World Health Organization (WHO) recommended the use of the ecological model of health behavior in order to provide structured programming plans to support mental and physical health.[23] The CDC suggested the use of a logic model to help with program planning regarding community mitigation strategies to reduce or prevent COVID-19 transmission in the United States.[24]

Food insecurity increased during the COVID-19 pandemic. Community and public health dietitians/nutritionists were called upon to assist in program planning for food access initiatives such as increased need at emergency food and school nutrition settings. The CDC provided several tools that schools and food pantries could use to provide and plan for the provision of food to their community members.[25,26]

Summary

Proper planning, implementation, evaluation, and sustainability of programs are important managerial functions for the community and public health dietitian/nutritionist. A great deal of information is available for reference and support when taking on this critical community health program function. Several models are available for both planning and evaluation. The decision of which prototype to use will depend on the nature of the planning task and the team assembled to complete the work. Spending time planning before approaching an endeavor will be rewarded by a resulting product or program that positively impacts the community's health, thus contributing to professional success for the public health nutritionist and the planning team.

Pandemic Learning Opportunity

Describe the opening of food pantries across the United States during the Covid-19 pandemic. Do you believe a planning process was utilized to make this possible? Was the implementation successful? Evaluate their efforts.

Learning Portfolio

© olies/Shutterstock.

Issues for Discussion

1. Planning an important skill for a public health nutritionist to possess and justify spending time doing it. Justify your answer.
2. A public health nutritionist can potentially be involved in three types of planning. What types of work situations may cause a public health nutritionist to apply skills in strategic planning? Long-term planning? Operational planning?
3. Discuss how a project manager could make decisions regarding which team members and stakeholders to include in a public health project.

Practical Applications

1. You are working in a public health department and are assigned to implement a weight management program for the community.
   a. Choose a planning model presented in this chapter and draw how to apply the model to the assigned project.
   b. Create an implementation plan for your weight-management program using either a task development timeline, Gantt chart, or PERT diagram.
2. You are continuing work on your community weight-management program. Discuss and draw what types of data and evaluation methods you would use in order to evaluate the program.

Key Terms

	page
Socio-ecological model	159
Needs assessment	160
Ecological model	161
Consumer-based model	161
Logic model	161
Program implementation	169
Formative evaluation	175
Summative evaluation	175
Process evaluation	175
Impact evaluation	175
Cost-effectiveness evaluation	175

Case Study 1: COVID-19 Pandemic Food Pantry Using the Gantt Chart

You are a community dietitian/nutritionist and want to set up a food pantry for your township. Use the Gantt Chart model to accomplish this task.

Case Study 2: COVID-19 Pandemic Food Pantry Set Up Using the PERT Chart

You are a community dietitian/nutritionist and want to set up a food pantry for your township. Use the PERT Chart to accomplish this task.

Resources

Online Resources

1. Logic Model
   a. https://www.wkkf.org/resource-directory/resources/2004/01/logic-model-development-guide
   b. http://www.uwex.edu/ces/pdande/progdev/index.html

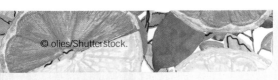

© olies/Shutterstock.

Learning Portfolio

2. APEXPH
   a. https://wonder.cdc.gov/wonder/prevguid/p0000089/p0000089.asp
3. PATCH
   a. http://www.lgreen.net/patch.pdf
4. Precede-Proceed
   a. http://www.lgreen.net/precede.htm
5. MATCH
   a. https://prezi.com/kvsjj8dyvkyo/multilevel-approach-to-community-health-match/
6. CDCynergy
   a. http://www.orau.gov/cdcynergy/soc2web/content/activeinformation/about.htm
7. The P Process Model
   a. http://www.thehealthcompass.org/sites/default/files/strengthening_tools/P%20Process%20Eng%20%26%20Fr.pdf
8. The Health Communication Process
   a. http://www.cancer.gov/publications/health-communication/pink-book.pdf
9. MAPP
   a. https://www.naccho.org/programs/public-health-infrastructure/performance-improvement/community-health-assessment/mapp

10. MAP-IT
    a. http://www.healthypeople.gov/2020/tools-and-resources/Program-Planning
11. Guide for Effective Nutrition Interventions and Education (GENIE)
    a. http://genie.webauthor.com/public/partner.cfm?partner_name=GENIE
12. Intervention Mapping
    a. http://www.interventionmapping.com/
13. COMMUNITY HEALTH ASSESSMENT AND GROUP EVALUATION (CHANGE)
    a. http://www.cdc.gov/nccdphp/dch/programs/healthy communitiesprogram/tools/change/downloads.htm
    b. http://www.cdc.gov/nccdphp/dch/programs/healthy communitiesprogram/tools/change/pdf/changeaction guide.pdf
14. Protocol for Assessing Community Excellence in Environmental Health (PACE-EH)
    a. http://archived.naccho.org/topics/environmental/PACE-EH/index.cfm

References

1. McKenzie JF, Neiger BL, Thackeray R. *Planning, Implementing, & Evaluating Health Promotion Programs: a Primer*. Pearson Education; 2017.
2. Centers for Disease Control and Prevention. *FastStats - Deaths and Mortality*. Centers for Disease Control and Prevention. 2021. https://www.cdc.gov/nchs/fastats/deaths.htm
3. García MC, Bastian B, Rossen LM, et al. Potentially preventable deaths among the five leading causes of death—United States, 2010 and 2014. *MMWR Morb Mortal Wkly Rep*. 2016;65:1245-1255. https://www.cdc.gov/mmwr/volumes/65/wr/mm6545a1.htm
4. Healthy People 2030. nd. https://health.gov/healthypeople.
5. McLeroy KR, Bibeau D, Steckler A, Glanz K. An ecological perspective on health promotion programs. *Health Educ Behav*. 1988;15(4):351-77. doi: 10.1177/109019818801500401. PMID: 3068205.
6. Koletzko B, Fishbein M et al. Prevention of childhood obesity: a position paper of the global Federation of International Societies of Paediatric Gastroenterology, Hepatology and Nutrition (FISPGHAN). *J Ped Gastro Nutr*. 2020;70(5):702-710. doi: 10.1097/MPG.0000000000002708
7. Plan 4 Health. nd *Policy, systems, and environmental change strategies*. nd. http://plan4health.us/policy-systems-and-environmental-change-strategies/
8. Schwartz P, Rauzon S, Cheadle A. *Dose matters: an approach to strengthening community health strategies to achieve greater impact. Nat Acad Med*. https://nam.edu/wp-content/uploads/2015/08/Perspective_DoseMatters.pdf

9. Gold RS, Green LW, Kreuter MW. *EMPOWER: Enabling Methods of Planning and Organizing Within Everyone's Reach*. Sudbury, MA: Jones and Bartlett; 1998.
10. Simons-Morton DG, Simons-Morton BG, Parcel GS, Bunker JF. Influencing personal and environmental conditions for community health: a multilevel intervention model. *Fam Commun Health*. 1988;11(2):25-35.
11. Centers for Disease Control and Prevention. *CDCynergy "Lite"*. 2010. Centers for Disease Control and Prevention. https://www.cdc.gov/healthcommunication/cdcynergylite.html
12. Johns Hopkins University Center for Communication Programs. *The P Process. Steps in strategic communication*. Accessed April 25, 2021. http://www.thehealthcompass.org/sbcc-tools/p-process
13. National Cancer Institute. *Pink Book—Making Health Communication Programs Work*. Accessed April 25, 2021. https://www.cancer.gov/publications/health-communication/pink-book.pdf
14. Mobilizing for Action through Planning and Partnerships (MAPP). National Association of County and City Health Officials. 2009. Accessed April 25, 2021. http://www.naccho.org/topics/infrastructure/mapp/
15. *Program Planning*. Program Planning | Healthy People 2030. n.d. https://www.healthypeople.gov/2020/tools-and-resources/Program-Planning
16. Academy of Nutrition and Dietetics; Academy of Nutrition and Dietetics Foundation; Con Agra Foundation. *Guide for Effective Nutrition Interventions and Education (GENIE)*. Available

at: http://genie.webauthor.com/public/partner.cfm?partner_name=GENIE

17. Bartholomew LK, Markham CM, Ruiter RAC, Fernàndez ME, Kok G, Parcel GS. Planning health promotion programs: an intervention mapping approach (4th ed.). Hoboken, NJ: Wiley; 2016.

18. Bartholomew LK, Parcel GS Kok G. Intervention mapping: a process for designing theory and evidence-based health education programs. *Health Edu Behav.* 1998;25:545-563.

19. Centers for Disease Control and Prevention *Community Health Assessment and Group Evaluation (CHANGE): Building a foundation of knowledge to prioritize community health needs: an action guide.* Available at: http://www.cdc.gov/nccdphp/dch/programs/healthycommunitiesprogram/tools/change/pdf/changeactionguide.pdf

20. National Association of County and City Health Officials. *PACE EH: Protocol for assessing community excellence in environmental health.* Accessed January 24, 2021. Available for order at: http://archived.naccho.org/topics/environmental/PACE-EH/

21. Grembowski D. *The practice of health program evaluation.* SAGE; 2016.

22. University of Washington at St Louis. *Program Sustainability Assessment Tool (PSAT).* n.d. PSAT/CSAT. https://www.sustaintool.org/psat/

23. Naja F, Hamadeh R. Nutrition amid the COVID-19 pandemic: a multi-level framework for action. *Eur J Clin Nutr.* 2020;74: 1117-1121. https://doi.org/10.1038/s41430-020-0634-3

24. Centers for Disease Control and Prevention. *Monitoring and Evaluating Community Mitigation Strategies.* nd. Centers for Disease Control and Prevention. https://www.cdc.gov/coronavirus/2019-ncov/php/monitoring-evaluating-community-mitigation-strategies.html

25. Centers for Disease Control and Prevention. (n.d.). *Guidance for Covid-19 Prevention; K-12 Schools.* Centers for Disease Control and Prevention. https://www.cdc.gov/coronavirus/2019-ncov/community/schools-childcare/k-12-guidance.html

26. Centers for Disease Control and Prevention. *Food Pantries & Food Distribution Sites.* n.d. https://www.cdc.gov/coronavirus/2019-ncov/community/organizations/food-pantries.html

CHAPTER 7

Serving Those at Highest Nutrition Risk

Julie M. Moreschi MS, RDN, LDN

(We would like to acknowledge the work of Rachel Colchamiro, MPH, RDN, LDN, and Jan Kallio, MS, RDN, LDN, in past editions of Nutrition and Public Health.)

Learning Outcomes

AFTER STUDYING THIS CHAPTER AND REFLECTING ON THE CONTENTS, YOU SHOULD BE ABLE TO:

1. List social and environmental factors that contribute to nutrition risk in communities, families, and individuals.
2. Describe the extent to which these factors affect various populations in the United States and how these factors impact nutrition status in families and individuals.
3. Communicate information needed by nutritionists to assess and effectively respond to factors in communities, families, and individuals that increase nutrition risk.
4. Identify the community services available to provide food, nutrition education, financial assistance, and health insurance to at-risk populations in the United States.
5. Describe the impact that the Coronavirus (COVID-19) pandemic has had on the nutrition risk of communities, families, and individuals.

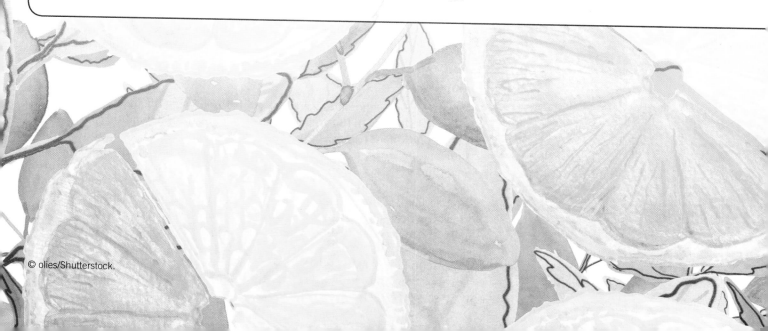

© olies/Shutterstock.

Introduction

Nutrition and health professionals have an essential role in collaborating with communities to effectively provide integrated, comprehensive, coordinated services to at-risk individuals and families to improve their nutrition status, health, and well-being. This chapter will explore factors that impact nutrition risk in communities, families and individuals, provide information to consider in assessing and identifying risks, and present information on Federal programs that are available for assistance.

Defining High-Risk Factors

Risk/High risk A greater-than-usual likelihood of a negative outcome may be caused or will happen.

A high-risk factor is a biological, economic, environmental, or social insult that increases risk—the likelihood of developing a disease or poor health condition. Factors that place individuals, families, and communities at risk must be investigated and described in the community needs assessment. Social, economic, and environmental factors that contribute to nutrition risk include but are not limited to:

- Poverty
- Unemployment and underemployment
- Inadequate education and literacy
- Immigration and cultural background
- Substandard housing and homelessness
- Hunger and food insecurity
- Geographic or social isolation
- Limited or inadequate health care
- Safe and accessible transportation
- Neighborhood and built environment

Health disparities The differences or inequalities in the incidence, prevalence, burden, or outcome of health conditions among populations, communities, families, and individuals.

These complex societal issues require the concerted attention of all those who are concerned about the nutrition health and well-being of community members. The impact of these issues often results in a range of **health disparities** (the differences in the incidence, prevalence, burden, or outcome of health conditions) among populations, communities, families, and individuals. The immediate needs of families and individuals are a shared responsibility of the interdisciplinary teams and networks that provide health and human services to reduce or eliminate population or community health disparities, as well as to prevent or diminish negative health outcomes on individuals. Many clients and their families are known to multiple programs and agencies. Assessment and eligibility information should be shared among service providers, and services should be coordinated to ensure comprehensive, unduplicated efforts.

Poverty

Poverty income guidelines were first set in 1964, using the index developed by Mollie Orshansky of the Social Security Administration. Findings of the 1955 U.S. Department of Agriculture (USDA) National Food Consumption Study indicated that at that time, the average American family spent approximately one-third of its net income on food. In the early 1960s, the USDA developed cost-specific, nutritionally balanced food plans and designated the Economy Food Plan as the least expensive food-purchasing plan to meet a family's nutrition needs. Therefore, the poverty line was established at three times the cost of the Economy Food Plan for a family of three or more persons.

In 1975, the USDA replaced the Economy Food Plan with the similarly cost-defined Thrifty Food Plan, which became the national standard for a low-cost, nutritious diet. Poverty thresholds continue to be based on the

1963–1964 calculation of the Economy Food Plan for a specific household size multiplied by three, with adjustments for price changes using only the Consumer Price Index. Poverty guidelines—a simplification of poverty thresholds created for administrative use—are used by federal agencies as criteria for eligibility for various federal assistance programs and as a basis for compiling data on poverty. **Table 7–1** shows the 2021 poverty income guidelines used by federal government agencies.[1]

TABLE 7–1
2021 Poverty Guidelines for the 48 Contiguous States and the District of Columbia[a]

Size of Family Unit	Poverty Guideline
1	$12,880
2	$17,420
3	$21,960
4	$26,500
5	$31,040
6	$35,580
7	$40,120
8[b]	$44,660

[a]There are separate poverty guideline figures for Alaska and Hawaii that reflect the Office of Economic Opportunity administrative practice, which began in the 1966–1970 period.

[b]For family units with more than eight members, $4,540 is added for each additional member.
Source: https://aspe.hhs.gov/poverty-guidelines

There are two slightly different versions of the federal poverty measure: poverty thresholds and poverty guidelines.

The **poverty thresholds** are the original version of the federal poverty measure. They are updated each year by the **Census Bureau**. The thresholds are used mainly for **statistical** purposes—for instance, preparing estimates of the number of Americans in poverty each year. (In other words, all official poverty population figures are calculated using the poverty thresholds, not the guidelines). Poverty thresholds since 1973 (and for selected earlier years) and weighted average poverty thresholds since 1959 are available on the Census Bureau's website. For an example of how the Census Bureau applies the thresholds to a family's income to determine its poverty status, see "How the Census Bureau Measures Poverty" on the Census Bureau's website.

The **poverty guidelines** are the other version of the federal poverty measure. They are issued each year in the Federal Register by the **Department of Health and Human Services (HHS)**. The guidelines are a simplification of the poverty thresholds for use for **administrative** purposes—for instance, determining financial eligibility for certain federal programs.

The poverty guidelines are sometimes loosely referred to as the "federal poverty level" (FPL), but that phrase is ambiguous and should be avoided, especially in situations (e.g., legislative or administrative) where precision is important.

Key differences between poverty thresholds and poverty guidelines are outlined in a table under Frequently Asked Questions (FAQs). See also the discussion of this topic on the Institute for Research on Poverty's website.

The January 2021 poverty guidelines are calculated by taking the 2019 Census Bureau's poverty thresholds and adjusting them for price changes between 2019 and 2020 using the Consumer Price Index (CPI-U). The poverty thresholds used by the Census Bureau for statistical purposes are complex and are not composed of standardized increments between family sizes. Since many program officials prefer to use guidelines with uniform increments across family sizes, the poverty guidelines include rounding and standardizing adjustments.

U.S. Department of Health and Human Services. Poverty Guidelines for the 48 Contiguous States and the District of Columbia. Retrieved from https://aspe.hhs.gov/topics/poverty-economic-mobility/poverty-guidelines

Strategy Tip

Unfortunately, the current poverty guidelines may no longer accurately measure poverty. Since the creation of the original poverty thresholds in the 1960s, the relative prices of the basic necessities of life for a family have changed considerably. Housing, transportation, childcare, and health care now comprise a larger proportion of a family's budget, while the relative cost of food has declined.

Poverty guidelines are set annually by the U.S. government. Check http://aspe.hhs.gov for current guidelines.

Discussion Prompt

Describe how poverty affects the population as a whole. Brainstorm on some solutions.

Pandemic Learning Opportunity

Data have also shown that poverty rates do improve when government stimulus has been provided to citizens.[4]

Discussion Prompt

Select an income from Table 7–1 and family size. Calculate how that family would be able to live fiscally in today's world. As a result of your findings, discuss some solutions to the problems.

Many food insecure families receive benefits from the Supplemental Nutrition Assistance Program (SNAP); however, many of these families still do not have enough money to cover their monthly food expenses. In addition, the Thrifty Meal Plans have been criticized due to the economics of the plan covering only food costs and not the costs of labor associated with food procurement and preparation.[2]

In 2019, an estimated 10.5% of the U.S. population lived in poverty (34.0 million individuals). This is the fifth consecutive, annual decline in poverty. Poverty rates differed by race and origin, as 18.8% of African Americans, 15.7% of Hispanic Americans, and 7.3% of Asian Americans were living at or below the poverty line, compared with 7.3% of non-Hispanic White Americans.[3]

A large number of children live in poverty. Children represent 22.3% of the total population account for 14.4% of the population living in poverty. In 2019, 6.2% of all children lived in extreme poverty or below 50% of the federal poverty level. Child poverty rates are highest for African American children (25.6%), and Hispanic American children (20.9%). The most at-risk children are those living in female single-parent–headed households. In 2019, 22.2% of children living in female single-parent-headed households lived in poverty, compared with 11.5% in male single-parent–headed households, and 4.0 in married-couple households.[3]

Data from the United States Census Bureau have a lag time due to the data collection and analysis aspects of the system. During the 2019 Coronavirus Disease pandemic (COVID-19), researchers at Columbia University have attempted to gather poverty data on a monthly basis in order to monitor the financial impact of the pandemic on the citizens of the United States. Findings show that the monthly poverty rate increased from 15 to 16.7% from February to September of 2020.

Poverty is a clear predictor of health status. Babies in households near or below the poverty line are at greater risk for infant mortality than babies born to more affluent families. Infant mortality rates have become more equal across the poorest and least poor counties in the United States between 1960 and 2000, with our estimate of mortality inequality declining by 76%. However, mortality inequality has remained roughly constant between 2000 and 2016 without improvement.[5] This has led to adverse health outcomes, which can affect child physical health, socioemotional development, and educational achievement.[6] One study reported that children at or below 100% of poverty were nearly nine times more likely to be reported to have a fair or poor health status compared with children at or above 400% of the poverty line.[7]

The health disparities associated with poverty grow more apparent with age and persist through adulthood. Thirty-three percent of adults ages 45 to 64 living under the poverty line report having two or more chronic health conditions (heart disease, high blood pressure, stroke, emphysema, cancer, diabetes, current asthma, chronic bronchitis, or kidney disease).[8]

Assessing an individual's or family's income with the poverty guidelines can give initial critical information regarding the ability to meet immediate basic needs. Even if a family does not meet the definition of poverty, their housing and utility costs may use up the major portion of their income. Therefore, they are left with little or no money for food and other basic household essentials. To determine an individual's or family's ability to buy food, dietitians/nutritionists must compare total net income with fixed costs for housing, utilities (heat, gas, electricity, water, telephone), medical care and insurance, transportation to and from work, and childcare. This calculation will assist in identifying their needs for financial and food assistance, health care, and social service programs.

Unemployment and Underemployment

The Great Recession, which began in December of 2007, hit the labor market particularly hard with increases in unemployment during 2008 representing the largest increase since 1982.[9] However, unemployment rates continued to improve through 2019. By the fourth quarter of 2019, the number of unemployed people, at 5.8 million, was down by 341,000 from a year earlier. The number of people experiencing long-term unemployment (those who had been looking for work for 27 weeks or longer) edged down by 91,000 in 2019. In the fourth quarter of 2019, 1.2 million people were long-term unemployed, representing 20.9% of the total unemployed. The proportion of long-term unemployed remained higher than it was before the 2007–2009 recession (17.8% in the third quarter of 2007), but it was much lower in 2019 than it had been during the recession.[10]

In early 2020, the unemployment rates were again on the rise due to the COVID-19 pandemic. The pandemic had a significant effect on unemployment in every state, industry, and major demographic group in the United States. The unemployment rate peaked at an unprecedented level, not seen since data collection started in 1948, in April 2020 (14.8%) before declining to a still-elevated level in December (6.7%). Job loss for those involved with in-person services were particularly hard hit. For example, the leisure and hospitality industry experienced an unemployment rate of 39.3% in April, before declining to 16.7% in December. Racial and ethnic minorities had relatively high unemployment rates beginning in April and were persistent through December of 2019 (16.7% for African American workers compared with 14.2% for Non-Hispanic White American workers, and 18.9% for Hispanic American workers).[11]

Although most policy and service planners focus on issues related to unemployment, **underemployment** is a hidden issue and is rarely recognized. Individuals employed in low-paying jobs, particularly at minimum wage, do not earn a "living wage," which means sufficient earnings to provide for basic household needs. An individual earning the federal minimum wage (set in 2009 and still in place in 2021) of $7.25 per hour, working 40 hours a week, 52 weeks a year, will earn only $15,080 annually, about 56.9% of the 2021 poverty level for a family of four. It should be noted that some cities and states have minimum wage laws that exceed the federal minimum wage.

Underemployment also applies to individuals that are employed, but do not have full-time or year-round work. This group is sometimes referred to as the working poor. The working poor are people who spend at least 27 weeks in the labor force (that is, working or looking for work) but whose incomes still fall below the official poverty level. In 2018, the working-poor rate of people in the labor force for 27 weeks or more was 4.5%. Additionally, full-time workers continued to be much less likely to be among the working poor than part-time workers. Among people in the labor force for 27 weeks or more, 2.8% of those usually employed full time were classified as working poor, compared with 11.1% of part-time workers.[12]

With the rapid advances in technology, there are fewer blue-collar jobs (industrial or factory jobs with unskilled or skilled manual labor) than ever before. Service jobs (maids, housecleaning, janitorial, maintenance, food

Pandemic Learning Opportunity

How did the type of jobs Americans held during the pandemic change? Is this a temporary change or a permanent one? What do you think will remain changed?

Discussion Prompt

What is the reason companies want minimum wage to remain low? (Hint: In some cases, employees are eligible for social programs if they live below the poverty line. Thus, the government subsidizes U.S. company employees.

Underemployment Employment that is insufficient in some important way for the individual, including individuals who are highly skilled but working in low paying jobs, individuals who are highly skilled but work in low skill jobs, and part-time workers who would prefer to work full time.

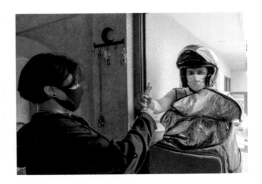

The working poor in America do so below the poverty line. Has minimum wage caught up with current living expenses?

© Arturo Garcia Martinez/Shutterstock.

Read more about food insecurity in Chapter 13.

See National Center for Education Statistics at: https://nces.ed.gov/programs/digest/d19/tables/dt19_104.10.asp

---

Literacy Ability to read and write; have competence or knowledge in a specific area.

Discussion Prompt

What are some of the factors that affect literacy, numeracy, and problem-solving skills? What can be done to improve this? Are these improvements being carried out now? What is the result for the population as a whole if people fall behind in these skill sets?

---

service) continue to be low paying and very often inadequate to meet family household needs.

Recent years have experienced instability of high-tech jobs, resulting in workers who once thought they had secure jobs being laid off. Assessment of the food intake of the unemployed and underemployed may show consistent inadequacy or an episode when the individual or family had little, or no food and nutrient intake was poor. One of the initial consequences of unemployment is to cut back on the spending for food as well as to postpone medical or dental treatment.[13]

It must be realized that the needs of the newly unemployed differ from the needs of those who have been unemployed for extended periods of time. For the newly unemployed, it is important to know if their income prior to unemployment was moderate, low, or below the poverty level; if their previous work had been continuous or sporadic; and if there is another wage earner in the household. First-time unemployed individuals and families working in low-paying jobs are less likely to know about available food and financial assistance programs and services and may not be familiar with their eligibility and the application processes.

Inadequate Education and Literacy

According to 2019 data from the National Center for Education Statistics, 9.9% of adults aged 25 years and older in the United States have an 11th-grade education or less. This varies widely by race and ethnicity with 8.7% of Asians/Pacific Islander Americans, 5.4% of Non-Hispanic White Americans, 11.2% of African Americans, and 28.2% of Hispanic Americans having not graduated from high school.[14] Low-income youth fail to graduate at five times the rate of middle-income students and at six times the rate of those who are high-income.[12]

The 2017 Program for the International Assessment of Adult Competencies found that 19% of adults in the United States had "below a Level 1" **literacy** level.[15] In a 2012 international survey of literacy, numeracy, and problem-solving skills, 18% of U.S. adults scored at the bottom two levels of proficiency on the literacy scale. The percentage of Non-Hispanic White American adults ages 16 to 65 years scored at the highest proficiency level (4/5) on the literacy scale and was higher than the percentages of their African American or Hispanic American peers.[16]

Education has been greatly impacted by the COVID-19 pandemic. The pandemic has exacerbated well-documented opportunity gaps that put low-income students at a disadvantage relative to their better-off peers. Access to the devices and Internet access critical to learning online is one of the most critical opportunity gaps. It is expected that the interruptions to education during the pandemic will further impact the limitations of standardized testing, which even prior to the pandemic have favored affluent students with access to specialized instruction.[17]

Most jobs require basic skills in reading, writing, mathematics, and computer skills. As the educational requirements of jobs increase, people with less education do not qualify. Among adults, poor reading skills are linked to poor economic potential and, therefore, to poverty and its associated likelihood of poor health outcomes. Among children whose parents have less than a high school degree, 82% live in low-income families and 50% live in poor families.[18] For families in the cycle of inadequate education, unemployment, and poverty, improving the education of one or more family members can be the key to breaking the cycle. Efforts focused on improving literacy of young children hold great potential; reading proficiency by the third grade is the most important predictor of high school graduation and career success. In 2019, the average reading score for 4th-grade students in high-poverty schools (score of 206) was lower than the scores for 4th-grade students in mid-high poverty schools (score of 217), mid-low poverty schools (score of 227), and low-poverty schools (score of 240).[19]

Refugees and immigrants may have limited literacy in their own language, making learning to communicate in a new language even more difficult. They may learn to understand some English to meet basic needs for daily living before they learn to speak, read, and write in this new language.

Low literacy affects the nutrition health of individuals and families by limiting access to the understanding of basic nutrition and health information, including food labels, medical or food preparation instructions (e.g., infant formula preparation), and dietary plans. Dietitians/Nutritionists should provide educational interventions and materials that consider the clients' ability to speak, read, write, and comprehend English.

Programs presented to non–English-speaking populations must build on their cultural food preferences and customs. Written materials should use pictorial graphics to communicate nutrition messages. Pictures and text should be field tested with the target audience to assure that the materials are acceptable and easy to understand. Data regarding educational attainment and language spoken is collected by many public health assistance programs. This information can be utilized to plan and respond more effectively to the needs of the populations served.

In most cases, dietitians/nutritionists will not be assessing an individual's literacy level. However, it should not be assumed that all clients are able to read either in English or in their native language. There are simple, informal methods to easily identify individuals with low literacy skills, without causing embarrassment to the client. Methods include asking open-ended questions about the materials received or handing written materials to clients upside down to observe if they turn it right side up to read. Dietitians/Nutritionists should also listen for comments commonly given to mask the inability to read, such as "I left my reading glasses at home" or "I'll read this later."

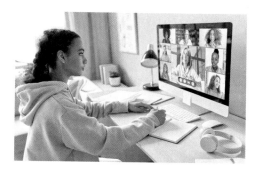

What were the advantages and disadvantages of learning by video during the pandemic?

© Insta_photos/Shutterstock.

> Many literacy tools are available, including the Simple Measure of Gobbledygook (SMOG) Readability Formula and the Fry Graph Reading Level Index, which can be used to evaluate written materials to determine the appropriateness of their reading level. See http://library.med.utah.edu/Patient_Ed /workshop/handouts/smog_formula.pdf for more information.

Cultural Barriers

In 2019, 1,031,765 persons were granted lawful permanent residence (i.e., immigrants who receive a "green card"), admitted as temporary nonimmigrants, granted asylum or refugee status, or are naturalized in the United States.[20] It is estimated that over 10.5 million individuals without documentation resided in the United States in 2017.[21] The U.S. foreign-born population reached a record 44.8 million in 2018, and immigrants today account for 13.7% of the U.S. population, which is nearly triple the share (4.8%) in 1970.[21] New immigrants need guidance and support as they resettle in an adopted land.

Citizenship status affects family members' employability, income, and eligibility for tax-supported services. Immigrants and refugees, who are not naturalized citizens or legal residents, may have difficulty finding jobs with adequate pay or even finding work at all. They may hesitate to follow through on referrals to government assistance programs, because they fear deportation or future problems in obtaining citizenship.

The COVID-19 pandemic did place some limitations of new persons moving into and out of the United States due to travel bans. However, immigrants already living in the United States may have a higher risk of contracting COVID-19 for a variety of reasons. These reasons could include higher incidence of poverty, overcrowded housing conditions, and high concentration in jobs where physical distancing is difficult.[22]

Within each cultural group, patterns and practices of families and individuals differ according to their socioeconomic status, religion, education, and age when they immigrated to the United States. Immigrants face an unfamiliar choice of foods in large and impersonal supermarkets, more "high-tech" kitchen and other equipment, and high prices for their traditional foods. They frequently give up their more nutrient-dense traditional foods in favor of U.S. snack foods and fast foods. Many choose to feed their babies formula instead of following traditions of breastfeeding.

Religion, tradition, beliefs, taboos, medical uses and philosophies, and the traditional roles of family members influence food habits. Dietitians/nutritionists should be knowledgeable about common cultural food patterns and should complete an individual assessment to determine the core foods that are a regular part of a client's daily diet, considering the nutrient contributions and typical preparation of these foods. This knowledge should serve as the beginning point for nutrition education, suggesting more emphasis on familiar or similar foods before introducing new foods.

When working with undocumented clients, their fears and concerns must be respected. Professionals must know about program eligibility, make referrals on a case-by-case basis, and maintain the family's confidentiality.

Substandard Housing and Homelessness

The past few decades have brought dramatic rises in rents and housing costs, a decreased availability of newly built government-subsidized housing, and condominium conversion of sizeable amounts of rental property. The homeownership and mortgage crisis of 2008 forced many families into foreclosure, further burdening a system in which secure housing is either unavailable or unaffordable to families who must live on a fixed income, limited budget, or public assistance allowance.

Housing is the largest single annual expenditure for households. In 2019, the lowest 20% of income consumer unit spent about 40.2% of their total expenditure on housing versus 15.3% on food.[23] African American renters had the highest share of housing cost burdens (53.7%), followed closely by American Hispanic renters (51.9%) and households identifying as multiracial or another race (46.6%). By comparison, 41.9% of Non-Hispanic White American renters were cost-burdened last year, along with 42.2% of American Asian renters.[24] From 2010–2019, the national average rent increased by 36%. The number of Americans who rent housing reached 108.5 million (M) in 2018, up from 99.4M in 2010. At the same time, the share of renters now makes up 34% of the general population and is the largest that it has been since 1960, when 36% of Americans were tenants.[25] On average, a renter earning the federal minimum wage must work 97 hours per week to afford a two-bedroom rental unit at the fair market rent.[26]

Households that reported being behind on rent payments were more likely to experience food and/or energy insecurity and made tradeoffs regularly between using available resources to pay for housing, food, utility, or medical expenses. Lack of affordable housing can have a lasting social–emotional impact on individuals, parents, and children.[27] Housing cost burdens, especially at high levels, are risk factors for negative outcomes for children, including eviction and homelessness, overcrowding, poor nutrition, frequent moving, lack of supervision while parents are at work, and low cognitive achievement.[28]

Strategy Tip

Community Health Departments should assign culturally competent dietitians/nutritionists to speak and guide their immigrant clients.

As housing costs rise beyond the means of low-income families and as affordable rental units are more difficult to obtain, many move in with friends and extended family. Families who are guests in someone else's household have little or no control over the kinds or quality of foods purchased or how foods are prepared.

Although they may have a roof over their heads, many low-income families live in substandard housing, lacking an adequate refrigerator, range, oven, or running water to prepare foods. Facilities to wash dishes, pots, and pans may be inadequate. There may be improper food storage or trash and garbage disposal, with rampant rodent and insect infestation. Older housing buildings may have lead-containing paint that is peeling, cracked, or chipped. Lead poisoning can result in impaired growth, learning disabilities, and even mental retardation for infants and children if the peeling paint is ingested.

For some families, the housing crisis has resulted in homelessness, which is a growing problem among women, children, and young families. In 2019, approximately 567,715 individuals in the United States were homeless on any given night; 171,670 of these individuals are part of a homeless family with children.[29] The number of identified, enrolled students reported as experiencing homelessness at some point during the last three school years increased by 15%, from 1,307,656 students in 2015–2016 to 1,508,265 students in 2017–2018.[29] Housing that is inadequate, crowded, or too expensive can pose serious problems to children's physical, psychological, and material well-being.[30]

Pandemic Learning Opportunity

The COVID-19 pandemic has resulted in increased rates of homelessness, which is largely associated with the rising rates of unemployment that have resulted from the crisis. There are estimates that the United States may experience a rise of homeless individuals by as many as 250,000 more people. Being homeless presents many complications to control the risk of contracting COVID-19. These complications include the inability to socially distance, limited access to proper handwashing and personal protective equipment, and difficulty in obtaining appointments for vaccinations.[31]

Many homeless families are housed temporarily in hotels, motels, or shelters, while some find themselves on the street. Often, mothers who live in shelters or on the streets feel guilty when they are not able to prepare adequate, nutritious meals for their children. Some shelters for the homeless serve meals or provide refrigerators and hot plates. However, many of the hotels and motels do not provide refrigerators, hot plates, group kitchens, or any place to store food, and they may even prohibit the use of small appliances to cook food in the rooms. These hotel and shelter residents may need to choose between spending their few dollars on high-priced restaurants or ready-to-eat foods and not eating.

Residential segregation, especially the separation of whites and blacks or Hispanics in the same community, continues to have lasting implications for the well-being of people of color and the health of a community. When neighborhoods are segregated, so too are schools, public services, jobs,

See University of Wisconsin Population
Health Institute School of Medicine and
Public Health as well as the Robert Wood
Johnson Foundation's County Health
Rankings and Roadmaps at: https://www
.countyhealthrankings.org/

Food insecurity The condition assessed
in the food security survey and represented in
USDA food security reports—is a household-
level economic and social condition of limited
or uncertain access to adequate food.

- **Low food security:** Reports of reduced
quality, variety, or desirability of diet. Little
or no indication of reduced food intake.
- **Very low food security:** Reports of multiple
indications of disrupted eating patterns
and reduced food intake.

Hunger An individual-level physiological
condition that may result from food insecurity.

Food security Physical, social, and
economic accessibility to sufficient, safe,
nutritious food at all times to meet dietary
needs and food preferences for a healthy
and active life.

- **High food security:** No reported indications
of food-access problems or limitations.
- **Marginal food security:** One or two reported
indications—typically of anxiety over food
sufficiency or shortage of food in the house.
Little or no indication of changes in diets or
food intake.

Discussion Prompt

What would happen to food insecure
persons without food assistance programs
in the United States? Would this affect the
population as a whole?

and other kinds of opportunities that affect health. African Americans and Hispanic Americans who live in highly segregated and isolated neighborhoods have lower housing quality, higher concentrations of poverty, and less access to good jobs and education. As a consequence, they experience greater stress and have a higher risk of illness and death. Conversely, for some population groups, living among others who share their cultural beliefs and practices can help build social connections that can lessen the health risks of hardship and neighborhood disadvantage. It is important for dietitians/nutritionists to help every community in paying attention to the ways that residential patterns may be a barrier to good health.[32] The Robert Wood Johnson Foundation's County Health Rankings and Roadmaps can provide an invaluable source of data to help in improving neighborhood equity.[33]

Dietitians/nutritionists should assess the housing issues in their community and identify potential problems experienced by families or individuals who relate to food access. These health professionals should be aware of the food storage and food preparation resources available to individuals and families living in hotels, motels, or shelters. Dietitians/nutritionists must identify individuals potentially at-risk for nutrition deficiencies in the homeless population. They must advocate and assist in improving the availability of nutritious food for homeless individuals and families and those living in substandard housing. Nutrition education and food assistance should be responsive to the needs and resources of the individual or family.

Hunger and Food Insecurity

Food insecurity and **hunger** are persistent problems in our society. **Food security** is defined as the assured access at all times to enough food for an active, healthy life, as well as access to enough food that is safe, nutritious, and acquired in socially acceptable ways. Hunger is an outcome of limited or uncertain access to food.[32]

A 2019 survey by the United States Department of Agriculture found that 10.5% of all participating households, and 6.5% of households with children, were food insecure at least some time during the year. Food insecurity rates were substantially higher than the national average in households with incomes at or below the Federal poverty line; in households with children and particularly households with children headed by single women or single men; women and men living alone; African and Hispanic American–headed households; and principal cities and nonmetropolitan areas.[34]

In 2019, 4.1% of food-insecure households had very low food security. This means that, at times during the year, the food intake of one or more adults in the household was reduced and their eating patterns were disrupted because of a lack of money and other resources for food. Food-secure households typically spent 24% more on food than food-insecure households of the same size and household composition. Approximately, 58% of all food-insecure households participated in one or more of the three largest federal food and nutrition-assistance programs during the month prior to the survey.[35]

Dietitians/nutritionists can help families to achieve food security by assuring that all eligible families utilize the federally funded Supplemental Nutrition Assistance Program (SNAP; formerly known as the Food Stamp Program), Child Nutrition programs including the Special Supplemental Nutrition Program for Women, Infants and Children (WIC), and elderly meal programs in combination with local food banks, soup kitchens, and food

Pandemic Learning Opportunity

The COVID-19 pandemic has significantly impacted food insecurity in the United States. Feeding America projects that 42 million people (one in eight), including 13 million children (one in six), may experience food insecurity in 2021. Citizens who were food insecure or at risk of becoming food insecure prior to the pandemic are facing greater hardship during the pandemic. Racial disparity that was present prior to the pandemic is expected to become even more pronounced.[36]

pantries. The federal food assistance programs are described in **Table 7–2**. The SNAP and Child Nutrition (National School Lunch Program (NSLP) School Breakfast Program, Summer Food Service Program for Children (SFSP) and Child and Adult Care Food Program (CACFP) programs are federally funded entitlement programs that are available in every community to serve all people who meet eligibility criteria. Some federally funded nutrition programs, such as WIC, are discretionary, meaning that programs will serve eligible individuals based on annually appropriated funding. Household income is a criterion for eligibility for federally funded food and nutrition assistance programs.

Participation in one or more food assistance programs extends the family's food purchasing power to meet the nutrition needs of family members

TABLE 7–2
Nutrition Assistance Programs

Program	Services/Benefits	Who Qualifies	Funding and Administration
Special Supplemental Nutrition Program for Women, Infants and Children (WIC) http://www.fns.usda.gov/wic /women-infants-and-children -wic	Provides supplemental food, nutrition education, referrals, and access to health care to low-income pregnant, postpartum, and breastfeeding women; infants; and children to 5 years of age at nutrition risk Monthly foods include infant cereal, baby foods, iron-fortified adult cereal, fruits and vegetables, vitamin C-rich fruit or vegetable juice, eggs, milk, cheese, yogurt, soy-based beverages, tofu, peanut butter, dried and canned beans/peas, canned fish, whole wheat bread, and other whole grain options. For infants of women who do not fully breastfeed, they should receive iron-fortified infant formula. Special infant formulas and medical foods may also be provided if medically indicated. Provides low-income households with coupons and electronic benefit transfer (EBT) cards to purchase eligible foods at authorized food stores	Pregnant women, postpartum women (6 months), breast-feeding women (up to 1 year), infants, and children (up to 5 years); must be certified to be at nutrition risk; household income determined to be at or below 185% of poverty level	Funded by USDA (some states offer supplemental funding) Administered by state health agencies Services provided by state or local agencies

(continues)

TABLE 7–2
Nutrition Assistance Programs   *(continued)*

Program	Services/Benefits	Who Qualifies	Funding and Administration
Supplemental Nutrition Assistance Programs (SNAP) http://www.fns.usda.gov/snap /supplemental-nutrition -assistance-program-snap	Provides low-income households with electronic benefit (EBT) cards to purchase eligible foods for a nutritionally adequate diet at authorized food stores	U.S. citizen: eligible, lawfully present noncitizen, based on immigration status and other SNAP eligibility requirements, limited benefits to able-bodied adults without dependents; eligibility and allotments are based on household size, income, resources, assets, and other factors	Funded by USDA Administered by state welfare, social services, or human service offices Services provided by local social service or human service offices
National School Lunch Program http://www.fns.usda.gov/nslp /national-school-lunch -program-nslp	Provides nutritious, low-cost lunch at full or reduced prices, or free to children enrolled in school	All children attending school may participate: free meals to children from families with incomes at or below 130% of poverty level; reduced-price meals to children from families with incomes between 131 and 185% of the poverty level; full price meals to children from families with incomes over 185% of poverty	Funded by USDA Administered by state department of education and local school districts Services provided by all public schools, voluntary in private schools
School Breakfast Program https://www.fns.usda.gov/sbp /school-breakfast-program	Provides nutritious, low-cost breakfast at full or reduced prices, or free to children in participating schools or institutions	Children under 18 years who come to an approved site; persons over 18 years who are enrolled in school program for persons with disabilities	Funded by USDA Administered by state department of education and local school districts Services provided by all public schools, voluntary in private schools
Summer Food Service Program (SFSP) https://www.fns.usda.gov/sfsp /summer-food-service-program	Provides free nutritious meals and/or snacks to children when school is out in the summer to fill the gap for the National School Lunch and School Breakfast programs	Children under 18 years who come to an approved site; persons over 18 years who are enrolled in school program for persons with disabilities	Funded by USDA Administered generally by state department of education, but state health or social service department or an FNS regional office may be designated Services provide by public and nonprofit private schools, public—local, municipal county, tribal or state—government, nonprofit private organizations; public or private nonprofit camps
Special Milk Program https://www.fns.usda.gov/smp /special-milk-program	Provides milk to children in schools, summer camps, and childcare institutions who have no federally supported meal program	Children attending schools or half-day pre-kindergarten programs and institutions with special milk program; milk is free to child from family eligible for free meals	Funded by USDA Administered by state department of education Services provided by public or nonprofit private schools of high school grade and under, eligible camps, and public or nonprofit private childcare institutions not participating in other federally supported meal programs

WIC Farmers Market Nutrition Program https://www.fns.usda.gov/fmnp /wic-farmers-market-nutrition -program	Provides coupons to WIC participants to purchase fresh, unprepared, locally grown fruits and vegetables at approved farms and farmers' markets	Women, infants (over 4 months), and children who have been certified to receive WIC program benefits or who are on a waiting list for WIC certification. States may serve some or all of these categories	Funded by USDA Administered by state agencies such as state agriculture departments, health departments, or Indian tribal organizations. Services provided by state or local agencies
Senior Farmers' Market Nutrition Program https://www.fns.usda.gov/sfmnp /senior-farmers-market-nutrition -program			Funded by USDA Administered by state agencies such as state agriculture departments, health departments, or Indian tribal organizations. Services provided by state or local agencies
Child and Adult Care Food Program https://www.fns.usda.gov/cacfp	Provides cash reimbursements and commodity foods for meals served in child and adult daycare centers, and family and group daycare homes, homeless shelters, and approved after-school care programs	Children 12 years and under and adults who attend eligible daycare programs; children of migrant workers 15 years and younger; physically/mentally handicapped individuals provided care in a center where the majority are age 18 years or younger; children residing in homeless shelters; snacks and suppers to youths participating in eligible after-school care program; income eligible for free or reduced-priced meals Adults who are functionally impaired and are enrolled in adult day care centers or who are 60 years of age or older	Funded by USDA Administered by state department of education or alternate state agency (state health or social service department) Services provided by public or nonprofit private licensed child and adult daycare centers and homes, outside after-school-hours care centers, Head Start, other licensed/approved daycare centers, homeless shelters
The Emergency Food Assistance Program (TEFAP) http://www.fns.usda.gov/tefap /emergency-food-assistance -program-tefap	Provides commodity foods to low-income persons, including elderly people, food banks, food pantries, and soup kitchens	Each state sets criteria for household eligibility; households may participate in another federal, state, or local food health or welfare program for which eligibility is based on income; homeless, including low-income seniors, can receive a meal in a congregate setting. There are no eligibility criteria for using a soup kitchen	Funded by USDA Administered by state agencies Services provided by food banks, food pantries, soup kitchens, and other public/ private nonprofit organizations that distribute food to the needy through the distribution of food for home use or meal preparation
Food Distribution Program on Indian Reservations https://www.fns.usda.gov/fdpir /food-distribution-program -indian-reservations	Provides commodity foods and nutrition education to low-income families who live on Indian reservations and to Native American families who live in approved areas near reservations. Serves as an alternate to the Supplemental Nutrition Assistance Program	Low-income households, including American Indian and non-Indian, living on a reservation or households who live in approved areas near reservations or in Oklahoma with at least one person who is a member of a federally recognized tribe. Must meet income and resource eligibility standards. Food package selected from over 70 food products. Cannot participate in the Supplemental Nutrition Assistance Program in the same month	Funded by USDA Administered by Indian Tribal councils or a state agency Services provided by the Indian Tribal council or a state agency

(continues)

TABLE 7–2
Nutrition Assistance Programs   *(continued)*

Program	Services/Benefits	Who Qualifies	Funding and Administration
Nutrition Assistance Program: Puerto Rico, American Samoa, and the Commonwealth of the Northern Marianas Islands https://www.fns.usda.gov/nap /nutrition-assistance-program -block-grants	Block grant program to provide cash and coupons to participants to buy nutritious foods in place of SNAP and commodities	The U.S. territories establish eligibility and benefit levels for their nutrition assistance programs	Funded by USDA
Nutrition Services Incentive Program (Nutrition Program for the Elderly) Each state's Agency on Aging provides information about nutrition programs in their state https://www.hhs.gov/aging/state -resources/index.html	Provides meals for senior citizens at senior citizen centers or delivered by meals-on-wheels programs through the receipt of cash and/or commodities from USDA; nutrition screening and assessment; nutrition education; links to other in-home and community-based services, transportation, and home-repair programs	People age 60 or older with greatest economic or social need, with special attention given to low-income minorities and rural older people; spouses of eligible people; disabled persons under age 60 who reside in housing facilities occupied primarily by the elderly where congregate meals are served, disabled persons who reside at home and accompany older persons to meals; nutrition service volunteers	Funded by DHHS, Administration on Aging (AoA); private donations Administered by state Units on Aging funded through Title III of the Older American Act (OAA); Indian tribal organizations Funded through Title VI of OAA. Services provided by senior centers, faith-based settings, schools, homes of homebound older adults
Head Start, Early Head Start https://www.acf.hhs.gov/ohs /about/head-start	Provides comprehensive medical, educational, nutrition, social, and dental services, referrals to social services, and other services to low-income children from birth to age 5, pregnant women and their families through assessment, early intervention, and prevention; provides nutritious meals and snacks	Children birth to 5 years, pregnant women and their families from low-income families receiving public assistance (TANF—Temporary Assistance for Needy Families or SSI—Supplemental Security Income) or total annual income not more than 100% of poverty level; children in foster care; at least 10% of total enrollment available for handicapped children	Funded by DHHS, Administration for Children and Families Administered by DHHS regional offices Services provided by local public agencies, private nonprofit and for-profit organizations, Indian Tribes, and school systems

Pandemic Learning Opportunity

How did pop-up food pantries help during the pandemic? Were community dietitians/ nutritionists involved in this effort?

better. In assessing family needs, each household member's participation in or eligibility for food assistance programs must be determined. When their household incomes are very low, families may not be able to meet their food needs even when they participate in one or more federal food assistance programs. In these cases, families may turn to emergency food assistance programs such as food pantries and soup kitchens. The community needs assessment should include the number of requests to food pantries and visits to soup kitchens, particularly by families with children. Although these emergency food assistance programs provide food to satisfy immediate needs, they are not designed to provide food for extended periods of time.

Over the long term, increased utilization of the federal food assistance programs could decrease the need for families to regularly use emergency food programs and reduce the growing burden on private food assistance programs. In addition, increased utilization could improve the stability of meeting basic food and nutrition needs of communities, families, and individuals. Many families still do not know about these programs or have inaccurate or insufficient information regarding their eligibility requirements. Complicated application forms and procedures, excessive eligibility documentation, and/ or inconsistent administrative operations deter many families from applying for food assistance. Dietitians/nutritionists must be familiar with eligibility requirements and be aware of administrative barriers so that they can assist potentially eligible clients in applying for benefits and navigating the food assistance system. Dietitians/nutritionists should also advocate, both locally and nationally, for measures that make it easier for individuals and families to use these services.

Some families believe that there is a stigma attached to the use of food assistance programs. The negative perceptions and attitudes associated with these programs may foster shame and embarrassment and prevent families in need from applying for food assistance. Dietitians/nutritionists should be sensitive to these feelings so that they can support clients and break down negative stereotypes attributed to people using food assistance programs.

Geographic and Social Isolation

Families who live in remote areas, distanced from settled communities, or blocked from social support systems are considered isolated. A family that does not have transportation, or the money to pay for it, may not be able to obtain adequate food at affordable prices or be able to access and/or utilize food assistance or healthcare programs. The geographically isolated include migrant and seasonal farm workers, rural families, Native Americans on reservations, and displaced and/or homeless families without access to transportation, even in urban areas.

Social isolation occurs when individuals or families are unable to establish supportive relationships with others. Social isolation is more subtle and difficult to recognize, as well as to overcome, than geographic isolation. Socially isolated individuals have difficulty establishing or maintaining supportive interpersonal relationships, either within their community or their family. This may occur when people move to new communities or when their cultural or ethnic background and/or their primary language differs from that of the community. Individuals and families experiencing homelessness, unemployment, marriage dissolution, mental illness, emotional breakdowns, or depression often distance themselves from their friends and family. Drug use, alcoholism, violence, and abuse dramatically change family dynamics and communication, often resulting in unstable families.

Social isolation may prevent an individual from seeking health care, food, financial or housing assistance, or other services they need. Social isolation has been identified as a contributor to inadequate food consumption for the elderly. Fewer calories are consumed at meals when eating alone than when eating with others.[37] In addition, an individual who lacks social support may find it difficult to continue ongoing health care or follow through on care plan recommendations. It may be difficult for individuals and families to access services when one family member or decision maker, often referred to as the "gatekeeper," controls the use of assistance programs.

Single and/or teen parents are often overwhelmed by parenting responsibilities; limited employment opportunities; low incomes; and lack of transportation, childcare, and family support. Parents caring for a handicapped or chronically ill child, or adults caring for a disabled or homebound spouse or parent, are also stressed emotionally, physically, and often financially. As such, these individuals may be socially isolated and less likely to seek services. In addition, they may experience difficulties with buying and preparing nutritious meals for themselves and their children due to meeting the demands of their children and family.

COVID-19 resulted in stay-at-home orders, quarantine, and social distancing recommendations, which further exacerbated the already serious problem of loneliness and social isolation. If a person was not an "essential worker,"

Strategy Tip

Brainstorm on how a dietitian/nutritionist can be sensitive to clients using food assistance programs.

the pandemic limited social contact to those whom a person might be living with. It is approximated that approximately 28% of Americans live alone, thus these people had little to no personal contact due to the pandemic. Some surveys have been conducted that estimate that rates of emotional stress have tripled and loneliness has increased by 20–30%. In addition, there have been some population that have been disproportionately impacted by COVID-19, such as those with low income, people of color, older adults, and those living in congregate settings such as nursing homes and prisons.[38]

Dietitians/Nutritionists should not expect to be able to single-handedly address or resolve the social issues of isolation that may affect their clients. They must identify the immediate needs of the individual or family and be sensitive and supportive in their response. The community needs assessment (see Chapter 5) must identify other health services and social services available in their community so that dietitians/nutritionists can make appropriate and timely referrals. Additionally, dietitians/nutritionists must recognize an individual's or family's ability to navigate service delivery systems to receive needed services and provide assistance as considered necessary. Most importantly, dietitians/nutritionists must work with other members of the health and human service agency teams to address the multiple and often long-standing problems faced by many families and advocate, both locally and nationally, for solutions.

Limited or Inadequate Health Care

The Affordable Care Act (ACA), the United States' health reform law, was enacted in March of 2010. The law intended to reform both private and public health insurance systems, in order to expand coverage to the 24 million uninsured Americans by 2023. Since the ACA was passed, healthcare coverage has expanded to over 20 million Americans.[39] The 2019 National Health Interview Survey found that adults aged 18–64 (14.7%) were the most likely to be uninsured, followed by children aged 0–17 years (5.1%), and adults aged 65 and over (0.9%).[40] Those who remain uninsured after ACA implementation may consider the cost of coverage to be too expensive, may not have access to insurance through a job, or may be lower-income individuals, earning above the basic Medicaid eligibility guidelines, living in states that declined to implement Medicaid expansion. Additionally, individuals without legal resident status are ineligible for Medicaid or insurance coverage through the ACA's insurance marketplace. Even among those with insurance, high-cost deductibles or copayments for certain types of health services may present a barrier to receiving care. Regular medical care helps individuals avoid health crises and ultimately protects their nutrition status.

Dietitians/nutritionists should know the availability of medical care services in the community and the barriers that low-income families face in accessing these services. They need to work with health providers and community members to support regular medical care, including nutrition services, and ensure that it is accessible and responsive to the needs of at-risk families. It is essential to advocate for nutrition intervention, referral, and follow-up to be integrated into medical services.

Transportation Environment

Health can be impacted by the availability of safe and accessible transportation systems within a community. Areas that can influence the transportation environment include safety, access to an active transportation alternative such as safe bike/walking paths, and the impact of transportation of air quality. The quality of a neighborhood's transportation system, such as connectivity and the variety of transportation modes available, can impact citizens' ability to

Medicaid: A U.S. government program that pays for medical assistance for certain individuals and families with low incomes. Learn more at: http://www.cms.gov

Medicare: A U.S. government medical benefit program for certain individuals when they reach age 65. Learn more at: http://www.medicare.gov

access food, healthcare services, access to green spaces, and the ability to get to jobs. Vulnerable members of the community, such as low-income residents, communities of color, children, and older adults, are often affected by the negative health of transportation.[41]

It is important for dietitians/nutritionists to better understand the links between transportation and health and to identify strategies to improve public health through transportation planning and policy. One tool that can assist in better understanding the transportation quality in the communities where a dietitian/nutritionist is working is to use the U.S. Department of Transportation's Transportation and Health Tool. This tool provides data on a set of transportation and public health indicators for each U.S. state and metropolitan area that describe how the transportation environment affects safety, active transportation, air quality, and connectivity to destinations.[42]

> See the U.S. Department of Transportation's Transportation and Health Tool at: transportation.gov

Neighborhood and Built Environment

The neighborhoods people live in have a major impact on their health and well-being[43] Neighborhood issues that can impact health include issues such as violence rates in the community, access to clean air and water, noise exposure, and exposure to smoking at places of work and where people live. Racial/ethnic minorities and people with low incomes are more likely to live in places with these risks.[44]

The social determinants of health are not equally distributed across all neighborhoods. Rather, residents of low-income and minority neighborhoods are much more likely to experience the harmful conditions that influence health. Dietitians/nutritionists can work to establish partnerships among community development, public health, and the medical field to document disparities, identify the most efficacious investments, design thoughtful interventions, and track their effectiveness. This work is critical in assisting communities in reducing disparities in health and economic opportunity, enabling everyone to reach their full potential, and making all neighborhoods healthy places to live and thrive.[44]

Improving Services to At-Risk Families

A thorough and comprehensive community's needs-assessment is key to providing targeted nutrition services that will support and respond to the needs of at-risk individuals and families. (See Chapter 5 for a refresher on Community Needs Assessment.) **Table 7–3** presents key factors to include in the assessment. This information documents needs and suggests priorities for developing community services. Additionally, this information identifies family and individual needs to assist in developing family and individual care plans. Identification of nutrition-related risk factors can be used to plan professional in-service training, mobilize resources, develop and implement health and nutrition programs, and ensure policies that respond to the nutrition needs of at-risk individuals and families and community nutrition efforts.

Ethics of Health

Throughout this chapter, it has been noted that some individuals, families, and communities are disproportionally at nutrition risk. Dietitians/nutritionists working in community health and public health must be aware of these disparities and engage in the ethical activities that can help to improve the issues related to all people not having access to equal tools, which aid them in living a long and healthy life.

TABLE 7–3
Assessing At-Risk Factors in the Community, Families, and Individuals

At-Risk Factor	Community Assessment	Family/Household Assessment	Individual Assessment
Income	Median family income; per capita income; % of population below 100% poverty level; % of population below 200% of poverty level; TANF benefit levels; availability of community-based assistance programs for food, childcare, fuel, etc., housing, and basic household costs (utilities, health care, etc.)	Family/household income; family size; Number of wage earners; participation in federal/state nutrition programs; income supplements such as TANF, unemployment benefits, fuel assistance; educational expenses; childcare costs; housing and basic household costs	Individual's monthly income; lives alone or with others; household expenses, child support; participates in federal/state food assistance; income supplement such as TANF, unemployment benefits, fuel assistance; educational expenses; childcare; single parent; homebound, disabled; elderly
Employment	State or local unemployment rate; median wage; predominance of minimum-wage, service-sector jobs; layoff, shutdowns, or strike in community; jobs available; seasonal jobs (e.g., agriculture, construction, tourism)	Household member laid off, work hours reduced, or on strike	Individual unable to find work at a wage that meets basic needs; laid off, work hours reduced, or on strike; barriers that prevent individual from finding adequate employment (lack of childcare, job opportunities, transportation/transportation costs)
Educational-level Literacy	% of adults over age 18 who did not graduate from high school; % of adults over age 18 who are low literacy proficiency; % of teen high school dropouts (by race)	Education level of head of household and mother; education obtained in country of origin	Education level; education obtained in country of origin; ability to read, speak, write English; computer/technology skills; if school age, grade level
Culture or language	Ethnic/cultural distribution in community; languages spoken, read, and/or written; availability of services representing the ethnic community; signs and information in appropriate languages; availability of traditional foods; prevailing community attitude	Cultural traditions, ability of head of household to speak, read, write English; ability to read/write native language; use of traditional foods; use of traditional medicine; family structure; degree of acculturation; citizenship status	Ability to speak, read, write English; ability to read/write native language; cultural traditions; use of traditional foods; use of traditional medicine; role in family and decision-making; immigration and citizenship status
Housing	Rental unit vacancy rate; % of substandard housing; % of rental units built before 1950 (risk of lead paint); availability of subsidized housing and length of waiting list; average and range of rents for 1-2-3 bedroom units; median purchase price for a house; condo conversion in community; estimated number of homeless individuals and families	Family lives in substandard housing; problems with rodents, roaches, chipping or peeling paint or plaster; family living in a hotel, motel, shelter, car, or on the street; recently moved in with friends or relatives due to the inability to obtain adequate housing; % of the family-household income spent on rent and utilities	Individual lives in substandard housing; living in hotel, motel, shelter, car or on the street; lives in room without cooking facilities, without working refrigerator or stove, or with limited food preparation tools and utensils; % income spent on rent/utilities; inability to pay rent; evicted for nonpayment of rent
Food availability, food costs, accessibility of grocery stores	Supermarkets/grocery stores in the neighborhood offer a variety of nutritious, good-quality foods at competitive prices; Number of "mom and pop" neighborhood markets; availability of culturally preferred foods at a reasonable price; accessible by public transportation or within walking distance; food delivery or shopping services available; availability of Farmers' Markets; average cost of full market basket of food	Family access to food resources and grocery stores; transportation to food resources; cultural foods available at reasonable price	Individual's food needs met by himself/herself or other household members; access to acceptable grocery stores and food resources with healthy, low-cost food choices; cost of available nutritious food; cost of culturally desired food; elderly or disabled individual able to arrange for assistance with shopping for food

Geographic or social isolation	Public transportation available; dispersed rural community; geographic barriers; condition of roads; cultural, ethnic, rural hostilities; immigrant, refugee, or migrant community; highly transient community; community violence	Supportive relationships; transportation or money for transportation; cultural or language barrier; victim of cultural, ethnic, racial, social prejudice; immigrant refugee, migrant family; mobile family; homeless family; family stress, unstable family, alcoholism, drug abuse, domestic abuse; community violence	Single parent; teen parent; homebound living alone; physical or mental disability; lack of supportive relationships; lack of transportation or money for transportation; victim of cultural, ethnic, racial, social prejudice; immigrant, refugee, migrant; mobile; alcoholic, drug abuser; victim of domestic violence, mental illness, depression, homeless, unemployed; provide individual care for handicap/disability, mentally ill, or elderly
Access to health services	Public health, health centers, and medical practices available (e.g., obstetrics, pediatrics, family practice); sliding fee scale; number of persons receiving and eligible for Medicare and Medicaid; medical practices accepting new patients; Medicaid payments accepted; services near public transportation; preventive programs offered at no cost or reasonable cost	Family access and use of health services; satisfaction with health services available; family members go without needed care	Use of health services; satisfaction of individual with health services available; perceived barriers to utilization of services; repeatedly misses scheduled appointments; missed appointments to referred services
Health insurance coverage	Health insurance coverage provided by employers includes maternity, dental, and optical care; Medicaid available to low-income married couples; coverage for prenatal care for low-income teens living with parents; % of jobs with no health insurance benefits; sliding fee scale or free health care available; Medicaid payment accepted by community physicians	Household members covered by health insurance, HMO, or Medicaid coverage; uninsured families have access to sliding fee scale or free health care; Medicaid unavailable because teen lives in parents' household; family's insurance covers preventive, well-child, dental and optical care	Individual has health insurance, HMO, Medicaid coverage; types of services covered (health, dental, optical); deductible for primary services; deductible for referred services; denial of health care due to lack of medical coverage or Medicaid; services not received due to cost or accessibility
Health status	Infant mortality rate; hospital discharge data; leading causes of death and disability; nutrition status and nutrition-related health measurements—% of population by age groups with anemia, high serum cholesterol levels, overweight/obesity, high lead levels, cardiovascular disease, cancer, diabetes, stroke, hypertension; smoking rates; breastfeeding rates	Nutrient content of diet; knowledge, attitude, and behavior related to healthy behaviors (i.e., breastfeeding, physical activity, fat/sugar/salt intake, fruit/vegetable intake); family history of nutrition-related health conditions (cardiovascular disease, cancer, diabetes, stroke, hypertension); smoking in household	Nutrient content of diet; intake of key nutrients (calcium, iron, vitamin C, folate, etc.) and intake of fat, sugar, and salt; intake of fruits, vegetables, and whole grains; knowledge, attitude and behavior related to healthy behaviors (i.e., breastfeeding, physical activity, fat/sugar/salt intake, fruit/vegetable intake); health parameters—weight, hemoglobin/hematocrit, cholesterol level, blood glucose, blood pressure, dental health; tobacco/alcohol/drug use
Transportation	Available public transportation; available private transportation; safe walking routes; safe biking routes; busy intersections; adequacy of shelter while waiting for public transportation	Family vehicle; purpose of travel for each family member (work, school, shopping, healthcare; religious activities, organizations that provide needed services, leisure); Public transportation within walking distance	Ability to read and comprehend public transportation maps or schedules; ability to pay for transportation; safety concerns; physical or emotional issues that impair ability to access/use public transportation.
Neighborhood and Built Environment	Crime statistics, access to open spaces; air quality; water quality	Household/family safety, safety of home (water, electricity, lead paint)	Access to services needed is impacted by crime; daily exposure levels to possible pollutants

See Generation Public Health at: https://www.apha.org/What-is-Public-Health/Generation-Public-Health

See Public Health Code of Ethics at: https://www.apha.org/-/media/files/pdf/membergroups/ethics/code_of_ethics.ashx

See Good Decision Making in Real Time at: https://www.cdc.gov/os/integrity/phethics/trainingmaterials.htm

The American Public Health Association (APHA) notes that a person's lifespan may be impacted as much as 15 years based on where a person lives, income, education, race, and access to healthcare. APHA and other professional organizations have ethics sections that work on these issues as well as help to assure that members of their organizations are working in an ethical manner. The APHA has created a specific program called Generation Public Health to help to work on the ethical issue of health. This movement is a group people, organizations, and communities dedicated to creating conditions in which everyone can be healthy. The work of this movement is focused on helping communities to build environments to support health and wellness, as well as working toward policies that support health.[45]

It is important for public health organizations to regularly assess the ethics of their work and systems. The APHA has created a Public Health Code of Ethics, which can be utilized for these purposes.[46] In addition, it is important for all personnel working in public health to learn more about how ethics can impact provision of services. The Centers for Disease Control and Prevention have developed a training program called Good Decision Making in Real Time: Public Health Ethics Training for Local Health Departments can be used by groups and individuals to aid them in becoming more aware of ethics in public health with the intent of minimizing any unethical practices and making personnel more aware of how to identify ethical concerns.[47]

Summary

This chapter explores factors that impact nutrition risk in communities and families and individuals, and includes current data describing the status of various health and social indicators in the United States. This chapter provides the reader with information to consider in assessing and identifying nutrition risk and presents descriptions including links to more in-depth resources of federal programs that are available for assistance.

As a nutrition and health professional, it is your responsibility to collaborate to effectively provide integrated, comprehensive, coordinated services to at-risk individuals and their families to improve their nutrition status, health, and well-being. There are a number of biological, economic, environmental, and social factors that impact nutrition risk in communities and with families and individuals. These factors must be investigated, the impact on nutrition and health should be assessed, and ways to resolve must be identified and implemented.

Action to improve services to at-risk families should be well integrated into the healthcare and nutrition service delivery system. Ideas to consider include:

- Recruit health or nutrition aides, lay health advisors, peer counselors, or volunteers who represent the populations and cultural groups in the community and train them to provide services to at-risk families.
- Coordinate one-stop service delivery by arranging with food and nutrition services, public assistance, and social services agencies to enroll eligible clients in health and social services.
- Address specific barriers that prevent eligible individuals/families from participating in assistance programs and design outreach strategies and methods to overcome these barriers.
- Streamline application processes of all programs targeting at-risk populations and utilize electronic data systems to eliminate duplication in data collection, including eligibility determination criteria.

- Schedule clinic hours so families do not need to take time off from work and lose pay to obtain services; offer locations that are accessible to clients with limited/no transportation.
- Enlist volunteer groups or clubs to adopt a service project to provide layettes, clothing, diapers, nutritious foods, or other essentials for at-risk families.
- Apply for grants to research and provide innovative services that help at-risk families work toward self-sufficiency.

Concerned health professionals, in conjunction with political leaders and concerned citizens, can collaborate with and mobilize community partners to provide integrated, comprehensive, and coordinated services to at-risk clients and families. They can participate in policy development and plans to increase awareness of problems; identify short- and long-term goals; allocate resources; and define, implement, and assess strategies to address the many complex economic and social issues that today's families face. Community coalitions can recommend and advocate for state and federal legislation that will address universal food access, housing, job training, health care, and employment.

Community needs-assessment data can be presented in public meetings, legislative hearings, or other forums. An ongoing surveillance system can be used to monitor hunger, nutrition risk, diet-related health problems, and utilization of food assistance programs. Grant funding can be sought to implement outreach and nutrition-education projects and to improve access to and use of various food assistance programs.

The dietitian/nutritionist has a vital and critical role in effectively serving those at highest risk, monitoring those at-risk, and must take a leadership and advocacy role to promote, implement, and evaluate effective services to meet the needs of at-risk populations.

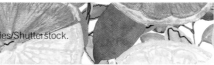
© olies/Shutterstock.

Learning Portfolio

Key Terms

	page
Risk/High risk	184
Health disparities	184
Underemployment	187
Literacy	188
Food insecurity	192
Hunger	192
Food security	192

Issues for Discussion

1. Discuss the impact of cuts to federal food and nutrition-assistance programs for those at highest risk. Place attendees in smaller groups and assign them to a specific food and nutrition assistance program. Regroup in full class and ask each subgroup to share the highlights of their discussion.

2. What food and nutrition assistance programs aid pregnant women? School-aged children? Families? The elderly?

3. Visit a website for a federal nutrition program. What features on the website were of good quality? What could be improved on the website?

4. Discuss how you would assess the nutrition risk of a community based on the at-risk factors reviewed in this chapter. What information would you gather? Are there specific data collection tools that might be useful when conducting your assessment?

Practical Activities

1. Individually or with a team of students, attempt a SNAP challenge. Plan a week of eating/menus on a SNAP allowance of $4.20 a day. Use resources such as https://frac.org/programs/supplemental-nutrition-assistance-program-snap/take-fracs-snap-challenge to help you get started.

2. Research the foods available to a WIC participant in your state. https://www.fns.usda.gov/contacts?f%5B1%5D=program%3A32 Visit a WIC-authorized grocery store and use your smartphone to take pictures of 20 items that are eligible for purchase. Using the foods that you took pictures of, plan a menu for the day for a family of three (two adults and one child).

3. Using a literacy assessment tool, determine the reading level of nutrition information available on the USDA or CDC website.

Case Study 1: Program Assistance

You are a dietitian/nutritionist in a community health center in a large urban area. You have received a referral from medical services to provide nutrition services for a young mother and her children who are new to the clinic. From the referral information and medical chart, you learn that the family is new to the community. The woman is 30 years old, with children 8 years old and 3 years old. The chart also notes the woman is non-English speaking, came to the United States 10 years ago, and both children were born in the United States. The mother came to the clinic seeking services for her current pregnancy; she is 4 months along. The family income is noted to be roughly $22,000 annually, with the father currently employed.

1. What are some of the social and environmental factors that could impact the health of this family and the different family members and how might these factors affect their health and nutrition status?

2. For the factors identified above, describe how you would gather data to assess each factor?

3. What federal nutrition and food assistance programs could this family be eligible for? How would the services of the nutrition and food assistance programs the family is eligible for potentially impact their nutrition status?

4. Consider your community. What programs and services are available that might be appropriate for this family?

5. After you have referred the family to the programs and services they are eligible for, what additional interventions might the family need or benefit from? What is your plan for follow-up with the family?

Case Study 2: Dietitians'/Nutritionists' Role in Community and Public Health Nutrition

What are the wide range of responsibilities the dietitian/nutritionist has in serving at-risk families in community nutrition as exemplified by this chapter?

Resources

1. United States Department of Agriculture, Food and Nutrition Service: www.fns.usda.gov
2. United States Census Bureau: www.census.gov
3. United States Census Bureau COVID 19 Site: https://covid19.census.gov/
4. CDC—National Center for Health Statistics: www.cdc.gov/nchs/
5. Children's Health Watch: www.childrenshealthwatch.org
6. Food Research and Action Center: www.frac.org
7. Kids Count Data Center: www.datacenter.kidscount.org

References

1. Office of the Assistant Secretary for Planning and Evaluation. Poverty guidelines. 2021. Retrieved March 12, 2021, from https://aspe.hhs.gov/poverty-guidelines
2. Carlson S, Llobrera J, Keith-Jennings B. . More adequate SNAP benefits would help millions of participants better afford food. 2019. Retrieved January 15, 2021, from https://www.cbpp.org/research/food-assistance/more-adequate-snap-benefits-would-help-millions-of-participants-better
3. Semega J, Kollar M, Shrider EA, Creamer J. Income and poverty in the United States: 2019. 2020. Retrieved January 15, 2021, from https://www.census.gov/library/publications/2020/demo/p60-270.html
4. Center on Poverty & Social Policy. Monthly poverty rates in the United States during COVID-19 policy. 2020. Retrieved January 15, 2021, from https://www.povertycenter.columbia.edu/news-internal/2020/covid-projecting-monthly-poverty
5. Turner N, Danesh K, Moran K. The evolution of infant mortality inequality in the United States, 1960–2016. *Sci Adv.* 2020;6(29):5908. doi: 10.1126/sciadv.aba5908
6. Council on Community Pediatrics. Poverty and child health in the United States. *Pediatrics.* 2016;137(4):e20160339. doi: 10.1542/peds.2016-0339
7. Schickedanz A, Dreyer BP, Halfon N. Childhood poverty: understanding and preventing the adverse impacts of a most-prevalent risk to pediatric health and well-being. *Pediatr Clin.* 2015;62(5):1111-1135.
8. National Center for Health Statistics. *Health, United States, 2011: with special feature on socioeconomic status and health.* Hyattsville, MD. 2012.
9. Borbely J. U.S. labor market in 2008: economy in recession. *Monthly Labor Rev.* Roxanna Edwards and Sean M. Smith, "Job market remains tight in 2019, as the unemployment rate falls to its lowest level since 1969," *Monthly Labor Review.* U.S. Bureau of Labor Statistics, April 2020. https://doi.org/10.21916/mlr.2020.8
10. Congressional Research Service. Unemployment rates during the COVID-19 pandemic: In brief. 2021. Retrieved January 30, 2021, from https://fas.org/sgp/crs/misc/R46554.pdf
11. U. S. Bureau of Labor Statistics. A profile of the working poor, 2018. 2020. Retrieved January 30, 2021, from https://www.bls.gov/opub/reports/working-poor/2018/home.htm

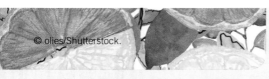
© olies/Shutterstock.

Learning Portfolio

12. Ganong P, Hsieh C, Blader S, Belot M. Consumer spending during unemployment: evidence from US bank account data. 2020. Retrieved January 14, 2021, from https://microeconomicinsights.org/consumer-spending-during-unemployment-evidence-from-us-bank-account-data/

13. National Center for Education Statistics (NCES). Digest of Education Statistics, 2019. 2019. Retrieved January 14, 2021, from https://nces.ed.gov/programs/digest/d19/tables/dt19_104.10.asp

14. The National Center for Education Statistics (NCES). Fast facts: Adult literacy. nd. Retrieved January 30, 2021, from https://nces.ed.gov/fastfacts/display.asp?id=69

15. Kena G, Aud S, Johnson F, et al. *The Condition of Education 2014* (NCES 2014-083). U.S. Department of Education, National Center for Education Statistics. Washington, DC. 2014. Retrieved January 8, 2016. http://nces.ed.gov/pubsearch

16. García E, Weiss E. COVID-19 and student performance, equity, and U.S. education policy: lessons from pre-pandemic research to inform relief, recovery, and rebuilding. 2020. Retrieved January 11, 2021, from https://www.epi.org/publication/the-consequences-of-the-covid-19-pandemic-for-education-performance-and-equity-in-the-united-states-what-can-we-learn-from-pre-pandemic-research-to-inform-relief-recovery-and-rebuilding/

17. Koball H, Jiang Y. Basic facts about low-income children: children under 18 years, 2016. 2018. Retrieved January 16, 2021, from https://www.nccp.org/publication/basic-facts-about-low-income-children-children-under-18-years-2016/

18. National Center for Education Statistics (NCES). The condition of education - Preprimary, elementary, and secondary 2020. Retrieved January 16, 2021, from https://nces.ed.gov/programs/coe/indicator_cnb.asp

19. Homeland Security. Table 1. Persons obtaining lawful permanent resident status: fiscal years 1820 to 2019. 2020. Retrieved January 16, 2021, from https://www.dhs.gov/immigration-statistics/yearbook/2019/table1

20. Budiman A. Key findings about U.S. immigrants. 2020. Retrieved January 16, 2021, from https://www.pewresearch.org/fact-tank/2020/08/20/key-findings-about-u-s-immigrants/

21. Organisation for Economic Co-operation and Development. What is the impact of the COVID-19 pandemic on immigrants and their children? 2020. Retrieved January 12, 2021, from https://www.oecd.org/coronavirus/policy-responses/what-is-the-impact-of-the-covid-19-pandemic-on-immigrants-and-their-children-e7cbb7de/

22. Statista Research Department. Percentage of average annual consumer expenditure on major components in the United States in 2019, by income Quintiles 2019. 2021. Retrieved January 16, 2021, from https://www.statista.com/statistics/247420/percentage-of-annual-us-consumer-spending-by-income-quintiles/

23. Joint Center for Housing Studies of Harvard University. The state of the Nation's housing 2020. 2020. Retrieved January 11, 2021, from https://www.jchs.harvard.edu/state-nations-housing-2020

24. Lupa I. The decade in housing trends: high-earning renters, high-end apartments and thriving construction. 2020. Retrieved January 11, 2021, from https://www.rentcafe.com/blog/rental-market/market-snapshots/renting-america-housing-changed-past-decade/

25. National Low Income Housing Coalition. Out of reach. n.d. Retrieved January 11, 2021, from https://reports.nlihc.org/oor

26. Habitat for Humanity. The impact of housing affordability on families. n.d. Retrieved February 01, 2021, from https://www.habitat.org/costofhome/housing-affordability-and-families

27. Childstats.gov. America's children in brief: key national indicators of well-being, 2020. 2020. Retrieved January 11, 2021, from https://www.childstats.gov/americaschildren/housing.asp

28. National Alliance to End Homelessness. State of homelessness: 2020 edition. 2021. Retrieved February 15, 2021, from https://endhomelessness.org/

29. National Center for Homeless Education. University of North Carolina Greensboro. Federal data summary school years 2014-15 to 2016-17 education for homeless children and youth. 2019. Retrieved January 11, 2021, from https://nche.ed.gov/wp-content/uploads/2019/02/Federal-Data-Summary-SY-14.15-to-16.17-Final-Published-2.12.19.pdf

30. Moses J. COVID-19 and the state of homelessness. May 19, 2020. Retrieved January 11, 2021, from https://endhomelessness.org/covid-19-and-the-state-of-homelessness

31. Schwarz D. What's the connection between residential segregation and health? 2020. Retrieved January 14, 2021, from https://www.rwjf.org/en/blog/2016/03/whats-the-connection-between-residential-segregation-and-health.html

32. Robert Wood Johnson Foundation. Explore health rankings. 2021. Retrieved January 14, 2021, from https://www.google.com/search?q=32.+Robert+Wood+Johnson+Foundation.+Explore+health+rankings&oq=32.%09Robert+Wood+Johnson+Foundation.++Explore+health+rankings&aqs=chrome..69i57.2761j0j4&sourceid=chrome&ie=UTF-8

33. US Department of Agriculture, Definitions of food security. 2019. Available online at: https://www.ers.usda.gov/topics/food-nutrition-assistance/food-security-in-the-us/definitions-of-food-security.aspx

34. Coleman-Jensen A, Rabbitt MP, Gregory C, Singh A. Household food security in the United States in 2019. 2020. Retrieved January 11, 2021, from https://www.ers.usda.gov/publications/pub-details/?pubid=99281

35. Feeding America. The impact of Coronavirus on food insecurity. 2021. Retrieved March 18, 2021, from https://www.feedingamerica.org/research/coronavirus-hunger-research

36. Boulos C, Salameh P, Barberger-Gateau P. Social isolation and risk for malnutrition among older people. *Geriatrics & Gerontology International.* 2017;17(2):286-294. doi: 10.1111/ggi.12711. Epub 2016 Jan 21. PMID: 26790629.

37. Holt-Lunstad J. Social Isolation and Health. 2020. *Health Affairs Health Policy Brief.* https://www.healthaffairs.org/do/10.1377/hpb20200622.253235/full/

38. Rapfogel N, Gee E, Calsyn M. 10 ways the ACA has improved health care in the past decade. 2020. Retrieved December 27, 2020, from https://www.americanprogress.org/issues/healthcare/news/2020/03/23/482012/10-ways-aca-improved-health-care-past-decade/

39. Centers for Disease Control and Prevention. Health insurance coverage. 2021. Retrieved March 6, 2021, from https://www.cdc.gov/nchs/fastats/health-insurance.htm

40. Centers for Disease Control and Prevention. National Center for Environmental Health. Healthy places. Transportation and health tool. 2015. Retrieved January 11, 2021, from https://www.cdc.gov/healthyplaces/healthtopics/transportation/tool.htm

41. US Department of Transportation. Transportation and Health tool. 2015. Retrieved January 12, 2021, from https://www.transportation.gov/transportation-health-tool

42. Centers for Disease Control and Prevention. Social determinants of health: Know what affects health. 2018. Retrieved from https://www.cdc.gov/socialdeterminants/index.htm

43. Robert Wood Johnson Foundation. How do neighborhood conditions shape health? An excerpt from *Making the Case for Linking Community Development and Health*. 2021. Retrieved February 1, 2021, from https://www.buildhealthyplaces.org/content/uploads/2015/09/How-Do-Neighborhood-Conditions-Shape-Health.pdf

44. American Public Health Association. Generation public health. n.d. Retrieved January 10, 2021, from https://www.apha.org/What-is-Public-Health/Generation-Public-Health

45. American Public Health Association. Public health code of ethics. 2019. Retrieved January 10, 2021, from https://www.apha.org/-/media/files/pdf/membergroups/ethics/code_of_ethics.ashx

46. Centers for Disease Control and Prevention. Public health ethics training materials. 2019. Retrieved January 10, 2021, from https://www.cdc.gov/os/integrity/phethics/trainingmaterials.htm

47. Office of the Assistant Secretary for Planning and Evaluation. Poverty guidelines. 2021. Retrieved March 12, 2021, from https://aspe.hhs.gov/poverty-guidelines

CHAPTER 8

Intervening to Change the Public's Eating Behavior

Jessica L. Garay, PhD, RDN, CSCS, FAND

April Pelkey, BS

(We would like to acknowledge the work of Brandy-Jo Milliron, PhD; Margaret-Claire Chenault, MS, AND; Dana Dychtwald, MS; and Yeemay Su Miller, MS, RDN on past editions of Nutrition in Public Health.)

Learning Outcomes

AFTER STUDYING THIS CHAPTER AND REFLECTING ON THE CONTENTS, YOU SHOULD BE ABLE TO:

1. Describe the social, economic, and environmental factors that influence eating behavior.
2. Identify characteristics of successful short- and long-term intervention strategies for improving dietary behavior.
3. Compare and contrast at least two commonly used theories or models that can be employed to develop health and nutrition interventions.
4. Explain how government policies and recommendations influence public health nutrition.
5. Understand how social marketing is used to affect individual health behavior.

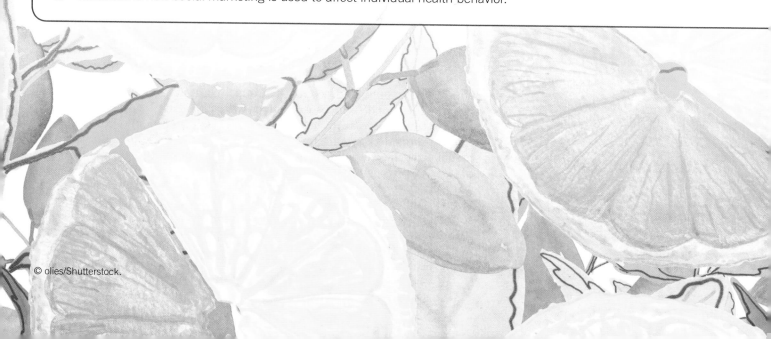

© olies/Shutterstock.

Obesity In adults aged 20 years and older, obesity is defined as a body mass index (BMI) ≥30 kg/m^2.

Overweight In adults aged 20 years and older, overweight is defined as a body mass index (BMI) ≥25 kg/m^2 but <30 kg/m^2.

Introduction

Consuming a diet rich in fruits, vegetables, and whole grains can reduce the risk of developing chronic diseases such as **obesity**, diabetes, heart disease, and certain cancers.[1] Unfortunately, rates of chronic disease continue to increase among both children and adults. Data from the National Health and Nutrition Examination Survey (NHANES) indicates that between 2003–2004 and 2013–2014, adult obesity (defined as BMI of 30 or greater) increased from 31.7% to 37.5%, respectively.[2] Furthermore, the prevalence of diabetes among U.S. adults has risen from 10.3% to 13.2% during this timeframe.[2] A similar trend emerges for U.S. children and adolescents. From 1999–2000 to 2015–2016, rates of **overweight** rose from 28.8% to 35.1% among 2–17 year olds, with obesity rates increasing from 19.5% to 26.5%, according to NHANES data.[3] These chronic diseases are not uniformly distributed across racial, ethnic, and socioeconomic groups—significant disparities exist. In the 2015–2016 NHANES dataset, 47% of Hispanic adults and 46.8% of non-Hispanic black adults were obese, compared with 37.9% of non-Hispanic white adults.[4] This pattern is also seen in youth—obesity rates are higher among Hispanic (32%), and non-Hispanic black (38%) than non-Hispanic white (19%) children and adolescents.[3]

Developing community and public health programs aimed at improving dietary intake is crucial to address the sobering statistics presented above. The good news is that research continues to confirm that a variety of approaches to changes in diet can lead to weight loss and overall reduction in risk of chronic disease.[5] However, interventions must address the specific and unique needs of the target audience. In addition to understanding personal and cultural preferences, an appreciation of the interrelated influence of biological, economic, and environmental factors on food choice is necessary.[6] Human beings have an innate preference for sweet and salty tastes, which is often easy to find in cheap, processed foods. For individuals who live in food deserts, lack of access to supermarkets, farmer's markets, or other sources of fresh, healthy foods, is a constant reality. Often, these same communities instead have a high density of convenience stores, fast-food restaurants, and other outlets (i.e., corner store markets or bodegas) that tend to sell calorie-dense foods that are nutritionally empty. Beyond food access, living in a neighborhood with a high crime rate may limit safe places for walking and bicycling and discourage an individual from participating in outdoor activities. Even when individuals are motivated to improve their health, and are given adequate education and support, barriers in their current environment may make it difficult to achieve success.

Although low socioeconomic status can make it more difficult to consistently obtain healthy food, resulting in the poverty-obesity paradox, it should be noted that high rates of preventable chronic disease exist across all racial, ethnic, geographic, and economic groups. Current community and public health efforts tend to focus on reducing the prevalence of specific diseases, such as cardiovascular disease or cancer, by reducing blood cholesterol levels or improving screening practices. However, these specific efforts should be balanced by simultaneously addressing behavioral and social influences on food choice that may cause or prevent disease. In particular, the ubiquitous nature of the obesity epidemic makes it clear that change must occur at many different levels—from personal to community to environmental to societal factors. Effective health promotion interventions need to address the reality that individuals deal with multiple layers of influence every day. Furthermore, while eating behavior is the focus of this chapter, community and public health programs striving to reduce chronic disease burden should also

Discussion Prompt

Plan a day's intake of food if fast-food and convenience stores were your only sources of food. What would be the result of eating like this for years?

address another important component related to achieving and maintaining a healthy weight, namely physical activity. Research has consistently shown that changes to dietary intake can lead to changes in body weight, but the best results are seen when improvement in eating habits is paired with an increase in physical activity.[7]

This chapter begins with an overview of several leading models and theories that community and public health and nutrition professionals need to consider during the development of interventions targeting eating behavior. Then we will consider current dietary recommendations and eating trends in the United States. Finally, we will highlight examples of recent nutrition-related interventions across various life cycle groups.

Strategy Tip

As you read, challenge yourself to think of ways in which interventions could be adapted to fulfill a broader or more specific scope to better facilitate change in new campaigns. Addressing all aspects of a problem is challenging and no one-size-fits-all solution exists. Keeping an open, inventive mind will better enable you to understand unique challenges that present in individuals and communities when it comes to dietary and lifestyle changes.

Models & Theories of Health Behavior

Interventions concerning eating behavior should be created while keeping a specific framework in mind to guide the development of the new program. Such frameworks can include the application of health-related models and theories in order to justify the structure and components of the intervention itself. These various paradigms typically consist of specific concepts that collectively help explain how or why a particular behavior occurs. Understanding the driving factors behind a behavior can be useful during the planning stages of an intervention to ensure that the main influences on the behavior will be targeted by the intervention. Several models and theories are commonly used in the public health and nutrition fields. A selection of these is summarized briefly below.

Diffusion of Innovation Theory

The Diffusion of Innovation Theory refers to how individual decision making is situated within a group or social context.[8] Individuals have varying levels of comfort regarding the adoption of a new behavior or "innovation." This theory has historically been applied to use of new technologies, but also helps to understand why or why not a person would begin a certain health behavior. The main concepts that support this theory include: how compatible the innovation is with the individual's values; the level of complexity of the innovation; how cost-effective the innovation is (cost vs. benefit); whether or not the innovation can be applied by the individual across different settings; the perceived advantages to adopting the innovation; the amount of risk and uncertainty associated with the innovation; and how easy or difficult it is to return to the prior behavior.[8] According to this theory, individuals fall into one of five categories: innovators, early adopters, early majority, late majority, and laggards.[8] Distribution across each category represents a bell curve, with most people classified as early or late majority. Use of a diet-tracking mobile

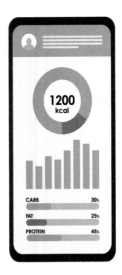

Phone apps help track food consumption and exercise.

© KW4NG/Shutterstock.

phone app among older adults is one nutrition-related intervention that may need to be developed while considering this theory, as older adults are more likely to fall in the late majority or laggard groups when it comes to using apps on their mobile phone. Interventions that focus on a newer diet trend, such as intermittent fasting, may need to specifically target individuals who self-identify as innovators or early adopters. A recent study applied the diffusion of innovations theory during the development of a nutrition education program for adult women.[9] Focus groups were used to identify which strategies and messages would best help participants to adopt the recommendations, which were based on the Dietary Guidelines for Americans.[9]

Health Belief Model

The Health Belief Model focuses on the idea that individuals undergo a cost-benefit analysis prior to deciding whether to engage in a health behavior.[10] The perceived threat(s) and benefit(s) are weighed against each other. The consequences related to avoiding the behavior, such as the individual's susceptibility to any illness that may result, and the severity of said illness, are balanced against the positive aspects of initiating the behavior and any anticipated barriers related to the behavior.[10] A healthy teenager may not be inclined to increase consumption of high-fiber foods in order to reduce heart disease risk because heart disease is not an urgent, perceived threat at that stage of life. The concept of self-efficacy also plays a role in the perceived threats and benefits. If an individual has low confidence in their ability to adopt the behavior, that will likely lead to decreased motivation. If the same teenager does not know which foods are considered high fiber, or where to access these foods, their self-efficacy regarding adding more fiber in their diet will be quite low. An additional component of the Health Belief Model, which has implications for interventions designed to improve diet quality, is the concept of "cues to action," such as having a bowl of fresh fruit on the kitchen counter instead of candy. A recent survey of college students determined their weight-related beliefs by asking questions related to the core concepts of the Health Belief Model.[11] Results showed that respondents who reported the higher perceived severity of being overweight had the lowest BMI while those who indicated a higher perceived susceptibility toward overweight had higher BMIs.[11]

Knowledge-Attitude-Behavior Model (KAB)

This straightforward model posits that obtaining new knowledge about a health issue will then cause a change in the individual's attitude and thus increase the likelihood that a new behavior is adopted. When seeking knowledge, it may fall into one of two categories: increasing awareness of an issue or health condition or providing specific direction regarding how to perform a new action. The type of knowledge provided will affect people differently, depending on their level of motivation prior to receiving the information. For someone who is completely unaware of the issue, they have low motivation and thus need the awareness knowledge to increase motivation. If someone is already motivated about that issue, the more concrete information is appropriate to better support the adoption of a new behavior. This model is similar to the Transtheoretical Stages of Change model discussed below. It should be noted that in today's day and age, individuals often seek health information online rather than traditional sources, such as medical professionals. Unfortunately, that means knowledge may not always be evidence-based but can still lead to changes in attitudes and, ultimately, behavior. Health professionals need to consider this when developing interventions to make sure that their content stands out as evidence-based compared with competing programs that may be more anecdotal in nature. Application of the KAB model in the nutrition field has been minimal; recently, a related model, the Value-Attitudes-Behavior model, has also been applied to eating behavior. This model implies that the value an individual assigns to a particular behavior will thus influence their attitude toward adopting the behavior or not, and this ultimately leads to actual behavior change (or behavior avoidance). Use of this model was seen in a study conducted to better understand the decision-making process behind choosing healthy food items at restaurants.[12] Individuals who value their health were more likely to select healthy foods. Therefore, interventions should encompass health-related values and concerns of the program's recipients.[12]

PRECEDE-PROCEED

The PRECEDE-PROCEED model was presented in Chapter 6 and is commonly used in community and public health programming. It is very comprehensive. It consists of nine distinct phases: 1–5 focus on assessing different levels of influence (i.e., social, environmental) while phase 6 is the actual implementation of the program and phases 7–9 deal with evaluation of the program, including impact and outcomes.[13]

The letters in the word PRECEDE represent Predisposing, Reinforcing, and Enabling Constructs in Education/Environmental Diagnosis and Evaluation.[13] This acronym corresponds to phases 1-5. The letters in the word PROCEED represent Policy, Regulatory, and Organizational Constructs in Education and Environmental Development.[13] This acronym corresponds to phases 6–9. Note that recent use of this model in the nutrition field includes the development of a website providing education to college students regarding healthy eating and the creation of an intuitive eating program to support weight management among military spouses.[14,15]

Social Cognitive Theory/Social Learning Theory

In the 1960s, psychologist Albert Bandura proposed the Social Learning Theory. This expanded in the 1980s to the Social Cognitive Theory. The main premise of this theory is that the process of learning is interactive among the individual, their environment, and their behavior, a concept known as reciprocal determinism.[16] In particular, the dynamic nature of social interaction is emphasized in this theory, with a strong focus on observational learning, both in past and current experiences.[16] Other core concepts of Social Cognitive Theory include the person's behavioral capacity to engage in the target behavior, the person's confidence (self-efficacy) in their ability to carry out the behavior, and the anticipated consequences, or outcome expectations, related to the behavior.[16] In some ways, this theory overlaps with the socioecological model as well as the Theory of Planned Behavior. The overall goal of the Social Cognitive Theory is to understand how an individual uses self-efficacy and positive or negative reinforcement to not only initiate a health behavior but also to maintain the behavior. A wide range of nutrition interventions have been developed using the social cognitive theory. For example, interventions that focus on increasing physical activity and improving diet among cancer survivors, for the purposes of weight management and reducing risk of future illness, have used a variety of delivery methods that are each rooted in this theory.[17] Assessing the impact of a nutrition education program for elementary school students not only focused on the change in knowledge and behavior but also on the self-efficacy of the students who received the intervention, as well as the interaction among all three outcomes.[18]

Strategy Tip

Brainstorm about where dietitians/nutritionists could be utilized to change food consumption behaviors. Is there an absence or a presence of nutrition professionals in strategic places for accessibility already?

Discussion Prompt

Because consumption behaviors include more than being guided on food selections, what other health professionals could be included on a team to change behavior?

Socioecological Model

The Socioecological Model is one of the most widely referred to frameworks in public health and nutrition. This model recognizes that there are multiple levels, or spheres, of influence on an individual, as seen in **Figure 8–1**. Many of the other models and theories focus primarily on the individual or interpersonal influences on behavior, which are the most tangible determinants of whether or not a person will engage in a particular behavior. The socioecological model also gives weight to the role of more abstract influences, such as the day-to-day environment of school or work, neighborhood and community factors, and even broader public policies that may impact an individual's level of choice related to certain health behaviors.

Using this model is prevalent in community-based participatory research, with the goal of addressing multiple spheres of influence using a multifaceted strategy. Such projects often target underserved communities and populations that are historically underrepresented in research. Recent examples include obesity prevention programs for African Americans[19] and improving beverage choices among young children.[20]

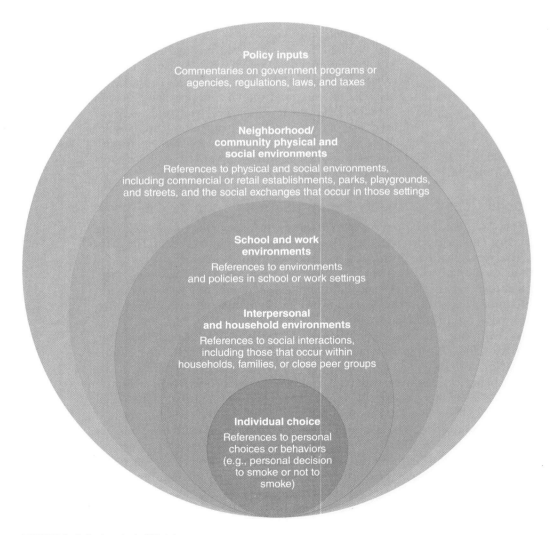

FIGURE 8–1 Socioecological Model.

FitzGerald, Elizabeth A. "Community-Generated Recommendations Regarding the Urban Nutrition and Tobacco Environments: A PHOTO-ELICITATION Study in Philadelphia." Preventing Chronic Disease, vol. 10, 2013, doi: 10.5888 /pcd10.120204. https://www.cdc.gov/pcd/issues/2013/12_0204.htm

Theory of Reasoned Action/Planned Behavior

The Theory of Reasoned Action suggests that an individual's intention to engage in a particular behavior is the biggest determinant of whether the behavior occurs.[21] Intention in this case is a reflection of both internal motivation and externally perceived social pressure. This theory was later expanded to the Theory of Planned Behavior, which proposes that in addition to intention, behavior is also influenced by perceived behavioral control.[21,22] Generally speaking, an individual will engage in a desired behavior with sufficient effort if they believe they have control over the decision to perform the behavior. On the other hand, if an individual feels as though they have little control over a behavior, they will be less likely to engage in it. When it comes to behavior change interventions, strategies such as modeling, goal setting, incentives, social support, and self-monitoring incorporate the Theory of Planned Behavior.[22] Indeed, a recent study developed a weight loss intervention for obese adolescents using this theory as a guiding framework.[23] A reduction in BMI was achieved following participating in multiple education sessions.[23] Furthermore, scores related to knowledge, intention, and perceived behavioral control all improved as a result of the intervention.[23]

(Transtheoretical) Stages of Change Model

The Transtheoretical model encompasses ideas from several theories related to interventions. The resulting model, which includes both stages of change and processes of change, reflects an integration of hundreds of theories that explain behavior change. The construct of stages of change is likely familiar to many readers. Individuals can be classified into one of six stages related to a particular behavior: precontemplation, contemplation, preparation, action, maintenance, and termination.[24] These stages indicate the individual's awareness of the behavior, their intention to start the new behavior, and the incorporation of the behavior into their daily life. The construct of processes of change is less commonly discussed but helps to understand how an individual progresses through the stages of change. The processes include consciousness raising, counterconditioning, dramatic relief, environmental and self-re-evaluation, helping relationships, reinforcement management, self and social liberation, and stimulus control.[24] These processes can be used to describe how and why individuals adopt or change behaviors.[24] This model has been applied to interventions related to eating behavior. Tailored text messages were developed for elementary school children based on their current dietary intake as well as their decision to make a future change and their self-confidence related to this change.[25] This type of program represents a cost-effective method to provide personalized nutrition education content to individuals of all ages.

Current Eating Trends

In the United States over the past 2 decades, consumers have witnessed a dramatic increase in the type and availability of fresh and processed foods, both healthy and unhealthy, at grocery stores, restaurants, and other outlets that sell food. According to the Economic Research Service (ERS) of the U.S. Department of Agriculture (USDA), in 2018, there were approximately 65 pounds of chicken available per person in the United States, an amount that surpassed beef.[26] Availability of corn products has also increased in recent years, although wheat flour is still the dominant grain in the U.S. food supply.[26] In 2019, the amount of caloric sweeteners (which includes both refined sugar, corn sweeteners, and honey) was 28 pounds lower per person compared with 1999 levels.[26] In addition to shifts in food availability, a 2016 regulatory update from the FDA brought changes to nutrition labels on packaged foods, including updated

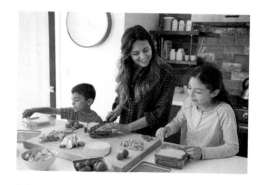

Being content to eat a healthy snack engages the action stage of the Stages of Change Model. Teachers assisted with the pre-action choices and child peers helped with the maintenance stage.

© Monkey Business Images/Shutterstock.

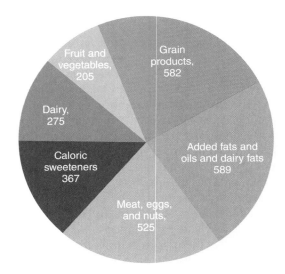

FIGURE 8–2 Daily Calories per Capita by Food Group.

USDA, Economic Research Service, Food Expenditure Series.

serving sizes and percent daily values, details regarding added sugars, and actual amounts of select micronutrients.[27] Despite these changes intended to improve the eating habits of Americans, many individuals still fail to meet the Dietary Guidelines recommendations for fruits, vegetables, and dairy products.[26,28] Furthermore, Americans do not consume enough seafood but overall consume too much from the protein and grains food groups.[26,28] In addition, most Americans consume excess foods containing added sugar and fat.[28] Part of the problem is the surplus food available in the U.S. food supply. Over a 50-year period, the total energy available per person per day increased by over 800 calories, from 2,880 in 1961 to 3,682 in 2013.[29] While this does not necessarily equal the number of calories consumed, it reflects an abundant supply of calories across all food groups, including high-calorie foods that contain unneeded sugar and fat. **Figure 8–2** displays total daily calories per person by food group in 2010. Specifically, increases in caloric intake were observed in all categories, with grains (mainly refined grains) accounting for 173 additional calories and added fats & oils providing 225 more calories. The remaining categories contributed less than 100 extra calories to the daily total. Only vegetable consumption declined during this time period. In 2017, meat, egg, and nut calories continued to increase, along with a small increase in vegetable calories.[26] The dairy and fruit food groups were stable in terms of calories available, while calories from the grain group and sugar/sweeteners decreased from 2010 levels.[26] Data from the 2011–2014 NHANES showed that roughly ⅔ of children and adolescents drank a sugar-sweetened beverage daily, providing approximately 120–165 calories per day.[30] During the same time period, roughly half of U.S. adults consumed a sugary beverage, with average calories ranging from 113 for women to 179 for men.[31]

Parallel to the rise in food availability is an unequal distribution of access to food, particularly healthy food. This disparity is seen in both rural and urban communities. Using data from the 2010 Census and other sources, researchers found that nearly 10% of Americans live more than one mile away from a grocery store.[32] About half of Americans have access to three grocery stores within 2 miles of their home.[32] More recent data from 2019 indicates that 10.5% of U.S. households are classified as food insecure, and over half of those households include children.[33]

Pandemic Learning Opportunity

Preliminary data assessing the impact of the COVID-19 pandemic on food insecurity in the United States suggests that levels of food insecurity among adults have increased significantly, especially among individuals who are low-income, Native American, Black, and Hispanic.[34]

Food Away from Home Is Impacting the Food Environment

Foods and beverages that are consumed outside of the home are an increasing source of calories and have been linked to weight gain and other health problems overall, but especially for women and low-income adults.[35] Since 2000, the number of quick-service restaurants across the United States has increased dramatically, including fast casual restaurants. According to the Economic Research Service of the U.S. Department of Agriculture (USDA), spending on foods consumed away from home now exceeds spending on foods eaten at home.[36] In 2011–2012, 34% of total daily calorie intake was attributed to foods and beverages consumed away from home.[36] Given this, it should come as no surprise that these food items tend to be higher in saturated fat and sodium while providing less fiber, calcium and iron compared with foods consumed at home.[36] The only exception is for school meals, which typically have a nutritional composition similar to foods eaten at home.[36] Recent findings from NHANES indicate that between 2015–2018, 36% of children and adolescents reported daily intake of fast food, which provided nearly 14% of total daily calories on average.[37] Children eat almost twice as many calories when they eat a meal at a restaurant compared with a meal at home.[38] One problem associated with foods provided at restaurants and snack foods found in convenience stores is the increased portion size, which has occurred concurrently with increases in the prevalence of obesity. Between 1986 and 2016, portion sizes of main dishes, side items, and desserts at 10 fast-food restaurant chains increased by 226%, leading to significant increases in calorie and sodium content.[39] The impact of the COVID-19 pandemic on foods consumed away from home is unclear, but given the extensive stay-at-home recommendations across much of the United States, it is expected that during 2020, there was an increase in foods consumed at home and a decrease in foods purchased and/or eaten at restaurants. Despite this short-term trend, reliance on foods and beverages from outlets like restaurants and convenience stores must be addressed in future public health interventions.

Hectic schedules and less time for food shopping, preparation, and cooking at home has moved convenience to the top of the list that dictates food choice. To combat the reliance on unhealthy foods offered at convenience stores and restaurants, change is needed across several layers of the socio-ecological model. At the policy level, imposing nutritional criteria for children's meals, along with regulations about advertising to children, may help. Requiring restaurants to display nutrition facts on menus is fairly widespread in the United States for chain restaurants; however, data are mixed regarding the impact that this has on purchase decisions. At the environmental level, restaurants and other establishments selling food need to provide additional options that are lower in calories, fat, sodium, and added sugar. Finally, at the individual level, there needs to be increased motivation to eat better, which may require more education on nutrition. This last factor is an opportunity for interventions focused on improving eating behavior.

Food away from home Meals and snacks eaten outside of the home, which comprise between 40 and 50% of weekly meals and snacks for the average American. These foods tend to be higher in calories and fat, lower in fiber, and larger in portion sizes, and consumption of food away from home has been associated with obesity.

Strategy Tip

Imagine that you are a dietitian/nutritionist employed at the main office of a fast-food chain. What dietary changes would you make to the menu, knowing that many adults and children eat there regularly?

Food Fads and Emerging Dietary Practices

Every year, nearly half of U.S. adults attempt to lose weight.[40] Of these, 88% report using two or more strategies.[40] The strategies most often used are shown in **Figure 8–3** and include eating less, exercising, and/or eating more fruits and vegetables. Recently, various trends have emerged regarding how best to eat for weight loss. Strategies such as counting macronutrients have replaced traditional calorie counting methods. Shifts in eating patterns, such as intermittent fasting, have also grown in popularity. Specific dietary practices are also widely used, ranging from long-standing recommendations such as the

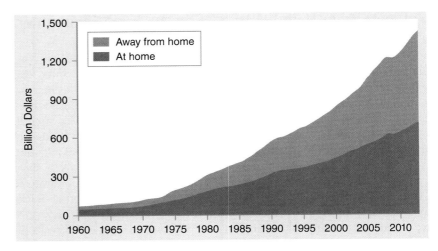

FIGURE 8–3 Food-at-home and Away-from-Home Expenditures in the United States, 1960–2013.
USDA, Economic Research Series, Food Expenditure Series.

Mediterranean and DASH (Dietary Approaches to Stop Hypertension) diets to the newer ketogenic, Paleo, and low-FODMAP diets.[41] Interest in, and adherence to, a plant-based diet is also on the rise among U.S. adults.[41] Consuming a gluten-free diet has developed into a diet trend. Typically reserved only for individuals with Celiac disease, now people are choosing to avoid gluten for a range of purported health benefits.[41] "Clean eating" and "real food" are also becoming popular buzzwords in the food industry and in the online nutrition community.[42] However, there is little to no consensus regarding the definition of these terms. Furthermore, consistent evidence to support any of the above approaches leading to an improvement in weight or overall health is lacking in general, although success has been seen in certain populations. The Mediterranean diet and the DASH eating plan are the two methods of eating that are routinely regarded as effective and realistic for chronic disease risk reduction.[43,44]

Many individuals who desperately want to lose weight are quick to start a diet that provides instant results, even at the expense of health, nutrition, and overall quality of life. Too often, misinformation about fad diets is spread through online sources, without sufficient factual support. Indeed, a recent survey of online nutrition content found that the most liked Facebook pages that discussed nutrition were hosted by celebrities, and only two of nine pages contained information aligned with healthy eating guidelines.[42] This is a major challenge for dietetic/nutrition professionals, whose attempt to educate the public on the harm of fad diets may be ignored by the determined dieter.

> Look up these diet trends for a better understanding: Mediterranean and DASH (Dietary Approaches to Stop Hypertension) ketogenic, Paleo, and low-FODMAP diets.

Changing Eating Behavior

According to the National Academy of Medicine (formerly the Institute of Medicine (IOM)), "Interventions must recognize that people live in social, political, and economic systems that shape behaviors and access to the resources they need to maintain good health."[43] The implication of this statement is that individual behavior changes are not likely to result in improved health and quality of life without an environment that supports the maintenance of those changed behaviors. Making dietary changes to better meet nutritional recommendations can cost more money and may require more knowledge, skill, time, or effort to prepare food. Therefore, understanding psychosocial and environmental influences on food choice and consumption is essential to creating nutrition programs, designing educational messages, and disseminating dietary recommendations that realistically help consumers make healthier dietary changes. In a previous IOM report, *Promoting Health: Intervention Strategies from Social and Behavioral Research,* they state that "The key to helping people enjoy longer, healthier lives are to understand how to promote behavioral change and create healthier environments."[44] However, some of the most meaningful changes that will have the greatest impact on the public's eating behavior are likely to be the most difficult to achieve. At the individual level, characteristics of successful nutrition education interventions include a person-centered approach that uses goal setting and self-monitoring.[45] Ideally, interventions should have a duration of at least 5 months, develop clear objectives (no more than three), and create theory-driven strategies to facilitate behavior change.[46] Changing eating behavior starts by helping an individual understand what it means to eat healthy. In the two sections that follow, we review current federal nutrition recommendations and nutrition education programs, namely Healthy People and the Dietary Guidelines.

Healthy People 2030

A multilevel approach will have the greatest, most sustaining effect on improving the population's eating behavior. Using a **socioecological model** as the theoretical framework from which one plans, creates, researches, applies, and evaluates nutrition interventions would be most effective. The socioecological perspective, as it has evolved in behavioral sciences and public health, focuses on the nature of people's transactions with their physical and sociocultural surroundings. **Healthy People 2030** is the premier socioecological program in the United States. Healthy People provides science-based, measurable objectives for improving the health of the nation and are updated every decade.[47] **Figure 8–4** depicts the social determinants of health that need to be considered with regard to food intake.

Healthy People 2030 tracks approximately 355 objectives organized into five health topics: Health Conditions, Health Behaviors, Populations, Systems and Settings, and Social Determinants of Health, each representing an important public health area. Currently, the overarching goals include attaining high-quality, long-lasting life that is free of preventable disease,

Socioecological model An approach in which interventions not only address individual intentions and skills but also the social and physical environmental context of a desired behavior, considering all social networks and organizations as well that share that environment and have the most potential for population-wide impact.

Healthy People 2030 Provides evidence-based objectives for improving the health of all Americans. Updated every 10 years, Healthy People tracks approximately 355 objectives organized into five health topics: Health Conditions, Health Behaviors, Populations, Systems and Settings, and Social Determinants of Health.

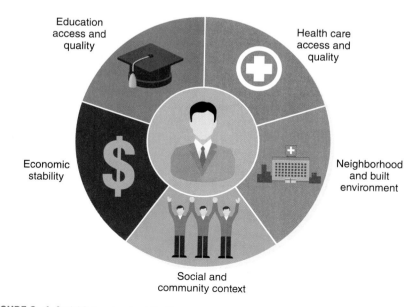

FIGURE 8–4 Social Determinants of Health.

U.S. Department of Health and Human Services. Social Determinants of Health. Retrieved from https://health.gov/healthypeople/objectives-and-data/social-determinants-health

To read more about Healthy People 2030, visit their website (http://www.healthypeople.gov) where you can find information about the wide variety of programs Healthy People supports and the progress that has been made since the program's inception.[47]

Dietary Guidelines for Americans A report jointly published every 5 years by the United States Departments of Health and Human Services (HHS) and Agriculture (USDA), which provides four overarching guidelines that encourage healthy eating patterns, including their food and nutrient characteristics.

To read more about the *Dietary Guidelines*, visit their website (DietaryGuidelines.gov) where you can find information about specific recommendations.

disability, injury, and premature death, the achievement of health equity and health improvement in all groups, the creation of social and physical environments that promote healthfulness, and quality-of-life promotion, healthy development, and behaviors across all life stages. These goals are based on multilevel approaches for successful achievement and the program provides benchmarks to measure outcomes from identification of health improvement priorities to their implementation and measurement. Furthermore, Healthy People 2030 addresses objectives that can help the United States become more resilient to community and public health threats like COVID-19.

Dietary Guidelines for Americans

Healthy eating patterns and regular physical activity can help people achieve and maintain good health and reduce the risk of chronic disease throughout all stages of the lifespan. This is reflected through the recommendations of the *2020 – 2025 Dietary Guidelines for Americans*, a report published every 5 years that contains nutritional and dietary information for the general public.[48] Jointly published by the United States Departments of Health and Human Services (HHS) and of Agriculture (USDA), the *Dietary Guidelines* is required under the 1990 National Nutrition Monitoring and Related Research Act. The statute requires that the *Dietary Guidelines* be based on the preponderance of current scientific and medical knowledge.

A growing body of research has examined the relationship between overall eating patterns, health, and risk of chronic disease, and findings on these relationships are sufficiently well established. As a result of this evidence, the 2020–2025 *Dietary Guidelines* recommendations focus on eating patterns as a whole and their food and nutrient characteristics at every life stage.[48] It is important to note that this is the first time since 1985 that the *Dietary Guidelines* include recommendations of healthy eating patterns for infants and toddlers. Additionally, previous editions of the *Dietary Guidelines* focused primarily on individual dietary components such as food groups and nutrients. However, people do not eat food groups and nutrients in isolation but rather in combination, and the totality of the diet forms an overall eating pattern. Furthermore, components of the eating pattern can have interactive and cumulative effects on health. These patterns can also be tailored to an individual's personal preferences. As shown in **Figure 8–5**, the 2020–2025 Dietary Guidelines provide four overarching guidelines that encourage healthy eating patterns.

The *Dietary Guidelines* is designed for professionals to help individuals at all life stages; infancy, toddlerhood, childhood, adolescence, adulthood, pregnancy, lactation, and older adulthood consume a healthy, nutritionally adequate diet.[48] The information in the *Dietary Guidelines* is used in developing federal food, nutrition, and health policies and programs; and provides the basis for Federal nutrition education materials designed for the community and public and for the nutrition education components of HHS and USDA food programs. It is developed for use by policymakers and nutrition and health professionals. Additional audiences who may use *Dietary Guidelines* information to develop programs, policies, and communication for the general public include businesses, schools, community groups, state and local governments, media, and the food industry.[48]

Currently, eating patterns in the United States are not meeting dietary guidelines. As shown in Figure 8–5, Americans consume more than the recommended share of added sugars, saturated fat, and sodium in their diets but less than the recommended share of fruit, dairy, and vegetables. Among the vegetable subgroups, red and orange vegetables are the least consumed. Additionally, Figure 8–5 shows that although total grains and protein foods meet or exceed recommendations, more than half of the U.S. population fails

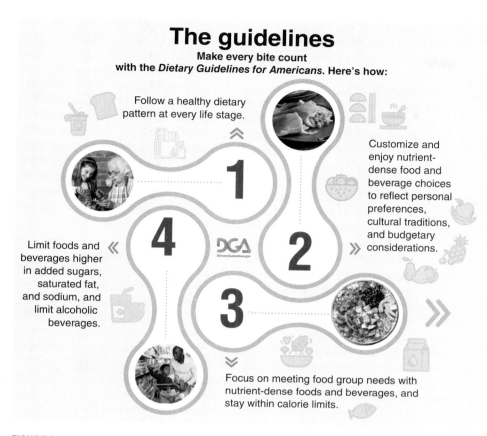

FIGURE 8–5 The 2020–2025 Dietary Guidelines Provide Four Overarching Guidelines that Encourage Healthy Eating Patterns.

Dietary Guidelines for Americans. Retrieved from https://www.dietaryguidelines.gov/sites/default/files /2020-12/DGA_2020-2025_The4Guidelines.png

to meet subgroup recommendations of whole grains and protein subgroups of nut/seeds and seafood.

The Influence of Media on Eating Behavior

Mass media has always exerted a powerful ability to persuade by altering norms, thinking, and behavior. The rise of social media has created another avenue just as influential on personal behaviors. Together, these external forces can lead individuals to change their behavior, even if they were not previously planning to do so. When food, eating, and dieting are portrayed in the media, many unhealthy, processed food products, fad diets, or unhealthy eating practices tend to be promoted. However, the media can also be a source of positive encouragement for a significant proportion of people to alter their dietary habits. This was exhibited by a simple "It Starts Here" campaign in Multnomah County, Oregon, which targeted women (specifically young mothers).[49] Messages were placed online (including social media), on billboards, television, community facilities such as libraries and parks, among other locations.[49] A toolkit was also developed for use by community organizations.[49] The campaign materials were adapted from the New York City Department of Health and Mental Hygiene materials regarding sugar and soda consumption. Results of a survey found that almost 70% of participants knew about at least one component of "It Starts Here."[49] A majority of respondents reported that they intended to reduce their sugar beverage consumption in the future.[49] Knowledge about the health implications of excess sugar was significantly greater among those who saw the campaign compared with those who did not.[49]

Similar interventions have been developed in both rural and urban sectors across the United States. The Los Angeles County Department of Public Health created a "Sugar Pack" campaign to decrease consumption of sugary beverages.[50] Graphics were placed on public transportation, billboards, and on social media. The reach of this campaign was impression—an estimated total of 515 million impressions.[50] Survey results indicate that over half of respondents saw the campaign materials, and of these, over 60% stated their intention to reduce intake of sugary beverages.[50] More recently, another intervention ("Live Sugarfreed") aimed at sugar-sweetened beverages was implemented in several rural counties across Virginia, Tennessee, and Kentucky.[51] The target audience was young adults, who tend to have the highest rates of sugary beverage intake.[51] The messages were developed to specifically focus on the risk associated with high sugar intake.[51] Messages ran on television as well as online platforms such as YouTube and Hulu; radio advertisements were played locally and on Internet radio.[51] The campaign resulted in over 26 million impressions.[51] Post-campaign survey results indicated that over half of the respondents saw an advertisement from the campaign, and 28% of them mentioned the contents to someone else.[51] The majority of individuals who saw the campaign agreed that sugary beverages were a contributing factor to weight gain and diabetes.[51] Sixty-four percent of respondents indicated they would decrease consumption of sugar-sweetened beverages in the future.[51]

Such positive results have not gone unnoticed. Attention has increasingly been given to the effect of advertising on eating behavior, healthy or otherwise. On the community level, there have been interventions that use subtle print advertisements and signage to promote healthier choices by identifying healthier foods and/or ways these foods can be incorporated into recipes. In one study, researchers not only posted shelf signs identifying healthy foods but provided sample shopping lists, tips, and other signage as well as conducted brief shopping education by a trained nutritionist.[52] Researchers noted that this one-shot intervention resulted in a significantly greater incidence of fruit and green and yellow vegetable purchases among those who received the intervention.[52] While this is an example of how to implement a point-of-purchase intervention using media, these scientists are not alone in their positive results. A systematic review conducted in 2014 evaluated 32 nutrition interventions made at the point-of-purchase.[53] These scientists found a range of interventions, including nutrition education plus increased availability of healthy food, nutrition education and promotion alone, monetary incentive plus nutrition education, monetary incentive alone, nutrition intervention through vending machines, and nutrition intervention through shopping online.[53] They found that monetary incentives for healthy foods were the most effective in promoting an increased purchase of healthier foods and recommended that more studies be completed to elucidate mediating factors and further examine effective ways to implement point-of-purchase interventions).[53] Future interventions must incorporate some of these best practices to increase rates of success. It is apparent that clever advertising, enticing promotions, and meaningful incentives work. Unfortunately, simply providing nutrition education is not enough to cause long-lasting behavior change.

The Food Industry

In 1988, the World Health Organization (WHO) recommended that free sugars should account for no more than 10% of daily energy intake.[54] This recommendation continues to be strong and as of 2015, WHO suggests a conditional recommendation to further reduce the intake of free sugars to below 5% of the

Strategy Tip

Are any dietitians/nutritionists social media influencers? Is this important? Why or why not?

Discussion Prompt

Analyze the statement, "Simply providing nutrition education is not enough to cause long-lasting behavior change." Is this true? Why or why not?

See more about the influence of social marketing in Chapter 19.

total energy intake under certain circumstances.[55] These recommendations were made from a large body of evidence supporting the relationship between free sugar intake and body weight and dental caries. These recommendations have not received universal acceptance, especially from the food industry. This is no surprise that the industry's most lucrative products are processed foods, laden with sugar and/or salt that are calorically dense. This explains why new products like these enter the marketplace almost daily. Given the plethora of choices, selecting a granola bar or snack cracker makes food shopping a much lengthier, more complicated process. A large array of choices can also contribute to overeating. When presented with more variety, individuals eat more. When food options are more monotonous, individuals tend to eat less.

The food industry is colossal and can exert powerful influence on government policy via lobbying techniques.[56] Although the food industry may be an important factor contributing to the poor nutritional habits of consumers, industry must be enlisted now as part of the solution. In the past, industry has been a key player in curing and preventing nutritional deficiencies by vitamin and mineral fortification of foods.[56] Remember also that the food industry is quite responsive to consumer and market demands; therefore, as more grassroots and consumer groups call for healthier food choices as a top priority, the industry can and will respond. More than ever, businesses have been realizing the economic value behind marketing their foods as healthier choices. More than ever, customers are willing to pay a premium for foods they consider to be good for them. Perhaps framing healthy foods through the lens that they can be just as profitable as "junk" food is one strategy when reconciling business interests with those of community and public health.

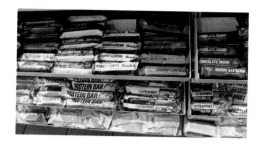

Consumers have an excessive number of choices leading to confusion about what is best.

© SophieOst/Shutterstock.

Schools

The school environment is an ideal place to reach large groups of children in one setting to deliver nutrition education. Scientific expert panels have consistently recommended that children and adolescents eat at least five servings of fruit and vegetables daily and participate in daily physical activity to reduce the risk of chronic disease and premature death; however, youth are not meeting policy standards for these health behaviors.[3,30,37] Children should be a major focus of intervention efforts because many of the risk factors observed in adults can be detected in childhood, such as high blood pressure and cholesterol as well as being overweight. There is considerable evidence that middle school years and adolescence are critical periods for influencing eating behavior, as more food choices are being made independently from parents as children grow older. A 2018 literature review examining key determinants for adolescent eating behaviors concluded that individual factors such as food beliefs, time constraints, and taste preferences were most influential on dietary behaviors, while social support, environmental factors, and policy factors were less likely.[57] Therefore, school-based interventions that encourage consumption of a variety of healthy foods while incorporating cooking and nutrition education should be developed, such as the Cookshop™ program. Evidence from this hands-on program suggests that 5th graders are more willing to try unfamiliar foods.[58]

The National Heart, Lung, and Blood Institute (NHLBI) sponsored one of the largest school-based health promotion trials, the Child and Adolescent Trial for Cardiovascular Health (CATCH), which was implemented in 96 public elementary schools from 1991 to 1995.[59] This study was designed to decrease cardiovascular risk factors in children through interventions implemented in the classroom, during physical education class, and in the cafeteria via the school food service. The most significant results were decreases in total fat and saturated fat consumption, as well as increases in physical activity in the children who received the interventions compared with the control

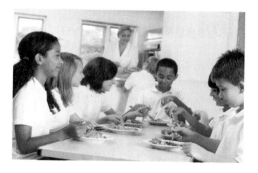

School-based interventions help introduce children to new foods.

© Monkey Business Images/Shutterstock.

schools. Five years after the intervention, follow-up studies were conducted and showed that it is possible to maintain and sustain environmental changes to promote healthy behaviors.[60,61] This is encouraging news because many positive health behavior changes seen immediately postintervention have not always been sustained long term (2+ years). Two of the most important factors in the viability and sustainability of the CATCH intervention in the schools were staff training and a more open and supportive school climate for the health promotion program.[62] In 2010, Michelle Obama announced a further initiative of CATCH, now known as Coordinated Approach to Child Health (CATCH), called *Let's Move!*. *Let's Move!* was a task force established as a national action plan to combat childhood obesity.[63,64] The various *Let's Move!* programs include *Let's Move!* Active Schools; *Let's Move!* Salad Bars to Schools; *Let's Move!* Cities, Towns and Countries; *Let's Move!* Child Care; *Let's Move!* Museums and Gardens; *Chefs Move to Schools; Let's Move!* Outside; *Let's Move!* in Indian Country; Let's Read, Let's Move! and *Let's Move!* Faith and Communities.[63,64] *Let's Move!* Active School implemented curriculum, training and equipment to support evidence-based physical activity and health programs among school age children.[64]

Schools are an efficient, practical place to influence children's eating habits, because one or two meals per weekday and many snacks per week are consumed there. The **Healthy, Hunger-Free Kids Act of 2010** included several requirements that had immediate impacts on the school food environment. First, it required the U.S. Department of Agriculture to update school meal nutrition standards (based on the Dietary Guidelines) for the first time since 1995.[65] This act also required all school districts to adopt wellness policies and created a requirement that water be made available (for free) during breakfast and lunch.[65,66] In addition, the U.S. Department of Agriculture had to develop standards for snack items that may be available during the school day.[65] This included items sold in vending machines and a la carte food items.[65] As a result of the new standards, which were officially published in 2012, immediate improvements were seen in school foods. From 2013–2015, a sample of 401 schools from across the United States found that 74% were currently meeting the reimbursable meal standards but only 54% were fully compliant with the nutrition standards for "competitive foods" (i.e., those sold in vending machines).[67] Importantly, no differences in adherence to the new standards were discovered when comparing schools by poverty level.[67] A 2017 review found that in 14 of 19 studies, the availability of healthy foods translated into improved sales and intake of these foods, along with decreased plate waste.[68] However, only two studies demonstrated that nutrition standards were being met as a result of the improved food consumption behavior.[68]

An additional component of the Healthy, Hunger-Free Kids Act of 2010 was the creation of a national Farm to School Program.[69] The goal of the program is to increase use of local foods in school meal programs. As of 2015, over 42,000 schools participate.[69] Recent research has shown that state laws regarding farm to school efforts have a significant impact on the availability of fruits and vegetables in school cafeterias.[70] Other initiatives related to this program include the creation of school gardens, use of local foods in the Summer Food Service Program, and salad bars containing local foods at school lunch.[69]

The **Fresh Fruit and Vegetable Program** is another initiative bringing healthy food to school meals. This program was established in 2002 through the Farm Bill and was initially intended to be a pilot project in only 25 states.[70] Currently, the operation and funding of this program are under both the Farm Bill and the Child Nutrition Reauthorization Act, each of which gets renewed every 5 years.[71] The Fresh Fruit and Vegetable Program provides a fresh fruit or vegetable for free to elementary school children at

Healthy, Hunger-Free Kids Act of 2010 Now part of the Child Nutrition and WIC Reauthorization Act, this legislation requires all school districts to adopt wellness policies and increases funding available for fresh, healthy school food.

Discussion Prompt

What is in the vending machines in your school or workplace? Discuss the changes that have occurred over the years.

Fresh Fruit and Vegetable Program Originally created in 2002 through the Farm Bill, this program provides a fresh fruit or vegetable snack to all students in participating schools. Program goals include increasing the variety of fruits and vegetables those children consume, creating healthier school food environments, and positively impacting the nutrition of students and their families.

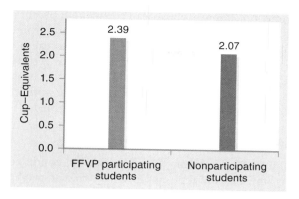

FIGURE 8–6 Impact of FFVP on Daily Fruit and Vegetable Intake.

Evaluation of the Fresh Fruit and Vegetable Program, 2013. Available at: https://fns-prod.azureedge
.net/sites/default/files/FFVP_Summary.pdf

eligible schools. The goals of this program are: increase the variety of fruits and vegetables that children consume, create healthier school food environments, and positively impact the nutrition of students and their families.[72] Elementary schools participating in the National School Lunch Program, who have at least 50% of students receiving free or reduced-price meals are eligible for this program.[72] In 2018–2019, 7,600 schools participated in this program with a reach of nearly 4 million students.[71] **Figure 8–6** shows how many days per week the fruits and vegetables purchased from this program are offered.[70] The majority of participating schools provides these healthy options at least 3 days per week.[70] A 2013 analysis of the program found that students from participating schools had a 0.32 cup higher intake of fruits and vegetables compared with students at nonprogram schools.[70] In addition, students from participating schools were more likely to report that they liked to try new fruits and vegetables.[70] **Figure 8–7** shows the difference in nutrition education provided by schools in the Fresh Fruits and Vegetables Program compared with nonparticipating schools.[70]

In summary, because school-aged children and adolescents spend much of their day in schools and eat numerous meals, snacks, and beverages there, offering healthy food choices is the socially responsible thing to do. The most effective interventions in schools are those that have comprehensive and multiple components. Specifically, the intervention components most critical to affecting change in fruit and vegetable consumption among young children

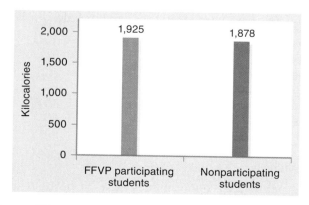

FIGURE 8–7 Impact of FFVP on Daily Energy Intake.

Evaluation of the Fresh Fruit and Vegetable Program, 2013. Available at: https://fns-prod.azureedge
.net/sites/default/files/FFVP_Summary.pdf

include environmental changes, classroom curriculum, parental involvement, and partnerships with local produce companies. In addition to providing a healthier food environment, students will be enabled to eat more nutritiously if: 1) access to junk food is limited; 2) healthy behavior is the group norm in the school environment; 3) peer leaders and others model nutritious choices; 4) the cafeteria offers appealing vegetables and fruits; and 5) cafeteria staff provide verbal encouragement to eat fruits and vegetables.

Organizational and Worksite Interventions

According to the 2019 American Time Use Survey, conducted by the U.S. Bureau of Labor Statistics, full-time employees worked an average of 8.5 hours per day on weekdays.[73] With so much time spent at work, it is no surprise that worksites have become a focus of eating interventions. The 2017 Workplace Health in America survey of 2,843 worksites found that 46% offered some type of wellness or other health promotion program.[74] The likelihood of a wellness program dramatically increases with company size—nearly 92% of companies with 500 or more employees offer a health promotion program.[74] Programs are most likely to exist in hospitals, and least likely in arts, recreation, food service, or entertainment businesses.[74] Use of incentives within the health promotion program was implemented by 53% of the worksites, and the majority of these companies relied on participation as the determining factor for awarding the incentive.[74] Incentives were most likely to be a gift or prize, cash reward, or discount on health insurance.[74]

Employees at their worksites are a captive audience and are ideal for intervention delivery. In particular, high traffic areas, such as the cafeteria and break rooms, are strategic places to deliver brief education. If the average worker eats lunch at work 5 days a week, that's around 24% of meals consumed away from home and at the workplace. And this says nothing of other snacks and beverages that may be consumed on work premises. A recent survey confirmed that 23% of adults acquire food at work, either by purchasing it onsite or receiving it for free.[75] The foods obtained at work tended to be low in diet quality.[75] **Worksite inventions** may include health education, cafeteria modifications, dietary consultations performed by registered dietitians/nutritionists, and physical activity education. Indeed, 23% of worksites include nutrition and healthy eating in their wellness programs, second only to physical activity (included in 28.5% of worksites).[74] Of these, 27% simply provide information, while 64% provide both education and skill-building activities.[74] This is a positive trend, because imparting knowledge and skills for new health behaviors is not enough; targeting and intercepting workplace norms and eating environments is necessary to support change. Furthermore, best practices for worksite health promotion programs have been identified,[76] and include:

- Leadership
- Relevance
- Partnership
- Comprehensiveness
- Implementation
- Engagement
- Communication
- Data driven
- Compliance

Regarding partnership, opportunities exist for health-related organizations, community organizations, and local or state public health agencies to provide some or all of the education and screening included in the healthy promotion program. Comprehensive health promotion programs typically include five components: allocation of adequate resources to support the

Worksite interventions Healthy lifestyle programs delivered at the workplace, including health education, cafeteria modifications, and dietary consultations performed by registered dietitian nutritionists and physical education.

program, health education, health screening, referrals to related programs, and a supportive environment (socially and physically).[74] Unfortunately, only one-quarter to one-third of companies include the first three components, while just under half of companies include the latter two components.[74]

Conducting formative, or background, research on perceptions and beliefs forms a basis from which researchers and health professions can identify barriers to change more effectively. This knowledge can be used to create interventions that are specifically tailored and relevant to a community or group. In addition, involving relevant stakeholders and key figures in planning and conducting the health-promoting activities will facilitate and allow maintenance of such interventions within an organization. Management plays an important role in creating a work culture that can make or break an otherwise perfectly suitable health intervention. For example, management can provide full hour or half hour breaks in which employees can take a reasonable amount of time to eat a healthy, relaxed lunch and take a mental break from the stresses of the day. Or management can contribute to a work environment where individuals are expected to just "work through lunch" or eat at their desk. Some examples of physical and environmental modifications include policies restricting or banning smoking on the premises, onsite exercise and kitchen facilities, and offering healthier fare in the cafeteria and vending machines. Also, having an understanding of the organizational climate and culture (e.g., attitudes, beliefs, needs, and resources of the members), including the organization's receptiveness to health interventions, is important to create effective behavioral change interventions. Incorporating a personally tailored behavioral component (e.g., personalized education and/or a follow-up phone call) can be an effective way to promote continued employee participation in follow-up health screening compliance.[76] Upper management should increase their efforts in building capacity for sustaining health-enhancing activities in the organization that will facilitate increased commitment and follow through by employees.[76] The Centers for Disease Control and Prevention (CDC) has developed a Worksite Health ScoreCard that can be used by employers to determine if their intervention strategies are effective and evidence based.[77] The ScoreCard was first developed in 2012 but updated in 2019.[77] The CDC also offers a Work@Health program to provide training to employers regarding how best to decrease chronic disease risk and increase productivity among employees. See **Figure 8–8** for a sample of the Worksite Health Scorecard.

Family and Friends

The important influence of supportive family relationships and other social ties for good health is widely accepted in the scientific community.[78,79] Family members and family dynamics are interconnected and mutually influential. Whether we realize or are conscious of this, family and friends influence our consumption of certain foods by modeling healthy or unhealthy choices by peer pressure (e.g., "You have to have some apple pie, I made it especially for you."). Parents or caregivers initially play the most influential role in a young child's development of eating preferences, habits, or patterns. Parenting and feeding styles will either foster or limit a child's ability to regulate their caloric intake by altering their responsiveness to internal or external cues of hunger and satiety.[80] Overprotective and authoritative parents are more likely to engage in positive practices such as modeling healthy eating and providing healthy foods, but overprotective parents are also inclined to pressure their children to eat while authoritative parents tend to use food as a reward.[81] Parents play a key role in preventing or treating overweight/obesity in their children.[82] More specifically, parents who are overweight and struggling to adopt healthier eating habits for themselves, or who are concerned about their

2019 Summary Benchmark Report - Any Town Office Park

Interventions in Place

ⓘ Resources for Action ▲ Score increased from prior year ▼ Score decreased from prior year

🖼 Export to Excel 📄 Export to PDF

TOPIC	2019 ScoreCard Total Points Possible	2019 Score	2019 Sample Scores Medium Worksites (250-749 employees)c	All Worksitesd
Organizational Supports ⓘ	44	25	32	32
Tobacco Use ⓘ	18	12	15	13
High Blood Pressure ⓘ	16	12	11	11
High Cholesterol ⓘ	13	9	9	9
Physical Activity ⓘ	22	18	15	15
Weight Management ⓘ	8	4	6	8
Nutrition ⓘ	24	16	12	11
Heart Attack and Stroke ⓘ	19	12	14	13
Prediabetes and Diabetes ⓘ	15	9	11	10
Depression ⓘ	16	10	11	10
Stress Management ⓘ	14	6	10	9
Alcohol and Other Substance Use ⓘ	9	8	7	6
Sleep and Fatigue ⓘ	9	0	4	3
Musculoskeletal Disorders ⓘ	9	6	6	5
Occupational Health and Safety ⓘ	18	18	15	14
Vaccine Preventable Diseases ⓘ	14	10	13	11
Maternal Health and Lactation Support ⓘ	15	7	11	10
Cancer ⓘ	11	6	7	6
TOTAL	294	188	209	196

Footnotes

cTotal number of worksites included in Medium Worksites 2019 average: 19

dTotal number of worksites included in All Worksites 2019 average: 93

Source

CDC Worksite Health ScoreCard Online

FIGURE 8–8 Worksite Health Scorecard Example.

https://www.cdc.gov/workplacehealthpromotion/initiatives/healthscorecard/pdf/CDC-ScoreCard-Sample-Benchmark-Reports-Final-Jan-2019-508.pdf

Discussion Prompt

How can parents foster the development of self-regulation in children?

children's risk for overweight, may adopt controlling or restrictive child-feeding practices in an attempt to prevent obesity in their children.[80-82] This type of eating environment, which is inadvertently created by caring parents who only want the best for their children, may create or exacerbate an unhealthy eating pattern or genetic predisposition already present in their children.

The development of self-regulation is grounded in a child's feelings of competence, autonomy, and connectedness.[80-82] When parents provide structure and guidelines for meals as well as the reasons behind the guidelines, this motivates compliance and internalization for children. In addition, when parents support autonomy in their children and provide a warm, positive connection with them, this motivates compliance and affirms competence.[80-82]

Families are embedded in a greater ecology, and, therefore, are subject to outside influences. Environments provide increased opportunities and resources, thus placing constraints on parental choices. An important public health goal is to identify families that are at greater risk for poorer eating habits, such as those with limited income, high levels of stress, obese parents, or a single working parent, and provide a family-focused intervention relevant to their circumstances. This would be an opportunity to provide social support and/or education, enabling the provision of healthy meals in the home. The advice parents receive from professionals must be practical, meaning that parents not only need to know what to do but also how to do it within the constraints of their present circumstances. The modality of the education provided must also match the parents' learning style. Printed materials can be helpful to some, but a video (available in different languages) can be a better method if there is a language barrier or literacy issues.

Interventions should take advantage of, and build upon, the momentum created by family transitions and changes, such as a couple expecting their first baby. Pediatric healthcare providers could begin disseminating advice to new parents during their baby's infancy on how to create a child who is a "healthy eater." This would give parents the opportunity and time it takes to begin the challenging process of altering suboptimal eating habits and replacing them with more healthful patterns. The result would be a home environment more conducive to healthy eating being the norm, because parental modeling of good habits is most influential in forming a child's eating pattern. How and where does a child initially learn about healthy foods and patterns of eating? Primarily, via exposure to foods from parents or caregivers. Parents also need to understand the detriments of coercive feeding practices and be given alternatives to restricting food and pressuring children to eat. Helpful practical advice for parents could include:

- How to promote acceptance of new foods by children, which entails offering the food repeatedly
- Providing parents with easy-to-use, healthy recipes and tips on simple, quick, and inexpensive meals
- Recommendations on proper portion sizes from each food group
- How to avoid food struggles with picky eaters

Feeding children healthily and handling picky eaters can be two of the more stressful or frustrating aspects of child rearing. Picky eaters (those resistant to eating many familiar foods) and children with **neophobia** (reluctance to try new foods) are two different and distinct consumption behaviors. It is no surprise that vegetables are the one food group children are less likely to consume in adequate amounts, compared with children with neither pickiness nor neophobia. Given that vegetable intake among children is well below recommended levels in the United States, finding effective means to increase vegetable intake among children is important and needed.

One encouraging research study involving 192 7-year-old girls and their parents revealed predictors of pickiness in girls, which are primarily environmental or experiential factors subject to change,[83] and not a genetically linked or normal trait of children as some may believe. Picky girls had mothers who:

- Perceived their family to have little time to eat healthful foods
- Had less variety in their vegetable intake
- Breastfed for fewer than 6 months

One explanation for this last finding is that breastfed children are exposed early in life to a diversity of flavors via breast milk (if the mother consumed a variety of foods in her diet).[83] These findings reveal important ways for dietitians, nutritionists, and other healthcare practitioners to intervene and prevent pickiness in children's eating habits. Education should include encouraging:

- Longer duration of breastfeeding
- Parental modeling of eating a greater variety of vegetables
- The use of simple methods and time-saving preparation techniques for vegetables

Neophobia Reluctance to try new foods.

Strategy Tip

Research creative ways to increase vegetable intake among children. What did you find?

For adolescents, the strongest correlations for vegetable and fruit intake are home availability of these foods and taste preferences for them.[84] However, this study found that even if taste preferences for fruits and vegetables was low among these adolescents, if fruits and vegetables were available, intake increased, nevertheless. Parents, therefore, need to be encouraged to purchase produce regularly and have fruits and vegetables available in the home and offered at all meals as much as possible.

An example of a family nutrition intervention program includes "The High 5 Low Fat" nutrition intervention as part of the Parents as Teachers Program, which targets African American parents.[85] Trained African American parents act as role models and disseminate the information via personal visits, group sessions, and newsletters to other parents. This intervention has been shown to improve the intake of fruits and vegetables, as well as lower overall dietary fat for parents receiving the intervention.

Another example of the importance of family support in promoting better health was shown in a study conducted with individuals with diabetes in a Diné (Navajo) Native American population. Individuals with active family nutritional support showed greater control in HgA(1c) (an indicator of longer-term blood glucose control) and total cholesterol and triglyceride levels, compared with individuals with less family involvement.[86] The type of support these individuals received and reported included a family member helping with shopping and cooking healthy meals, or family members who would eat low-fat, low-sugar foods with them. These persons with diabetes and this type of family support demonstrated and improved self-care behavior.

The family environment, particularly parents, plays an important role in child and adolescent eating habits. From role modeling healthy eating behavior, to ensuring that healthy foods are available, to adopting family mealtime routines, opportunities exist for interventions to provide concrete strategies for families to implement to increase the quality of their diet.

Community Interventions

Community Any grouping of individuals who have a shared sense of identity or a common thread that draws all members together.

A **community** is any grouping of individuals who have a shared sense of identity or a common thread that draws all of them together. Most commonly, a community is thought of as a geographic area of persons but is not necessarily limited to this factor.[43] Communities can be a certain ethnic group; a professional group, such as small business owners; or a group of individuals who are all cancer survivors. The collective strength of a community to promote its own health is beyond the ability of any single person to control or change. It is important to note that although community interventions may be implemented by any group or organization, their success relies on that acceptability of the intervention in the view of the target population. For example, WHO or National Institutes of Health may implement a campaign encouraging a certain community to eat more vegetables, but for the campaign to be successful, the desires and needs of the target community must be considered. There are good reasons why institutions and other groups invest in community interventions. When compared with individual nutrition therapy, community interventions have the ability to reach more people, are cost-effective, and have the potential to facilitate sustained health behavior change through permanent environmental (and other) modifications. Community-based interventions include several different channels: health departments, worksites, schools, supermarkets, physicians' offices, community organizations, restaurants, and the media. Key community nutrition intervention strategies involve using these channels to promote national health objectives and develop interventions based on theories of behavior change. Additionally, it is recognized that to have a community-wide effect, multiple channels must be utilized.[87]

Valuable lessons have been learned from prior community-focused behavior change interventions.[88] They include the following:

- Engaging the community, rather than an outside organizer or researcher, to define needs and priorities
- Identifying and building upon the strengths, assets, and resources of the community's members
- Being flexible and tailoring the change strategies to each particular community's context and environment
- Building long-term sustainability of programs and identifying diversified sources of funding

Places of Worship

Despite continued efforts to reduce health disparities among diverse populations in the United States, certain ethnic groups are faced with higher disease risk and death rates. African Americans continue to be disproportionately affected by all causes of disease compared with other groups. Greater effort is needed to reach this segment of the population with prevention strategies. Unfortunately, African Americans are more likely to be distrustful of investigators given negative historic events (e.g., the Tuskegee experiment) and subpar medical access and care they tend to receive. The church, therefore, has become an ideal channel and setting for reaching members of this community with health education, given the high regard and level of trust members have for their pastors. For many African American families, life centers on the church and its activities, and; therefore, the church exerts a high degree of influence.[89,90]

Several interventions conducted in churches have shown clinically meaningful decreases in disease risk outcomes, such as body weight, blood pressure, and waist circumference.[89,90] Some of the specific successful behavioral and dietary outcomes these programs have achieved include decreased fat and sodium intake; increased fruit, vegetable, and fiber intake; and increased physical activity. One example of this type of intervention is the PRAISE! (Partnership to Reach African Americans to Increase Smart Eating!) project, conducted in 60 churches in eight North Carolina counties, which used a community-based participatory research (CBPR) approach.[91] The CBPR approach views community participants as partners in the research process, rather than just subjects of the research conducted. At least one randomized clinical trial so far has found that research designed with a CBPR approach is associated with high levels of trust and a perceived benefit of satisfaction with the research process.[92]

Meals, coffee, and refreshments are common accompaniments to fellowship in church social gatherings and meetings. These gatherings afford an opportune setting for dietary intervention, such as offering lower-fat dishes and recipes and incorporating more vegetables and fruits. This is one reason the National Institute of Health (NIH) has created a program titled, "Body & Soul: A Celebration of Healthy Eating and Living."[93] This program helps empower church members to be more physically active and to eat five to nine servings of fruits and vegetables every day for better health. The combined elements of this program include pastoral leadership, health education, an environment in church that supports healthy eating, and peer counseling.

Reaching Older Adults

Innovative and effective health promotion interventions targeted at older adults, within a public health framework, are becoming increasingly important as the U.S. population ages. The benefits of healthier lifestyles for older adults include increased functional ability, delaying the onset of disease, and an improved quality of life, which are important goals in program planning for this population.[94]

Specific nutritional goals for elders should include increasing the intake of vegetables, fruits, and calcium-rich foods, just like most segments of the population.[94] Some may think that interventions targeting adults over age 55 years seem to have a limited effect, given the difficulty of changing nearly a lifetime of eating habits and behaviors. However, a review of nutrition interventions targeting older adults discovered that active participation and opportunities for collaboration were consistent qualities of successful interventions.[95] Additional features to consider when designing an intervention for older adults include the application of an appropriate behavior change theory; limiting the education to one or two key messages; providing hands-on activities, incentives, and access to health professionals; reinforcing and personalizing the health messages; and a social environment that supports healthy behavior.[95,96]

An example of a community intervention targeting older adults was a creative partnership established among Tri-Parish Nursing Ministries, The Arthritis Foundation, Missouri Extension Services, and the Saint Louis County Department of Health.[97] The goal was to promote the quality of life for older adults through physical activity and health education messages. Twenty-nine participants met twice a week in a local church to exercise for 1 hour with a trainer from PACE (People with Arthritis Can Exercise).[97] The participants received 30 minutes of nutrition education from a Saint Louis County registered dietitian using the Missouri Extension's Health for Everybody program.[97] The participation rate for the program was 62% at the end of 6 weeks.[97] The mean age of participants was 74 years. All participants reported favorably, indicating that they enjoyed sessions and "learned something new."[97] Feedback also revealed that participants even asked for more ways to exercise outside of class.[97] Providing older adults with encouragement, a place to exercise, and an opportunity to learn healthy eating tips could potentially make a significant difference in improving quality of life for this segment of the population.

Individual and Group Counseling

Until greater social change occurs and the long-term solution to improve our nation's nutrition and health is realized, dietitians/nutritionists and other health educators play an important role in helping individuals manage better within our current "toxic food environment," as some have termed it.[56] Educating individuals and equipping people with tools and strategies is critical to resist or combat the powerful "eat more" marketing messages that is constantly bombarding us by the food and restaurant industries.[56]

Brief counseling that incorporates principles of **motivational interviewing (MI)** and patient-centered behavioral change strategies have shown promise in medical settings. A recent intervention among obese adults who relapsed in their treatment found that using MI techniques in a group setting was successful.[98] The groups met once per week for seven weeks, and were then followed up for six months.[98] Using the stages of change model, the number of patients who were in precontemplation or contemplation regarding behavior changes to target their obesity was significantly decreased, while the number in action or maintenance increased for both dietary intake and physical activity.[98] The specific behaviors that patients were engaging in included reducing calorie intake, increasing physical activity, and decreasing sedentary time.[98] As a result, patients lost an average of 3% of their body weight at the end of the 6 months.[98] Group MI sessions were also used in a pilot study targeting African American women who were obese and had Type 2 Diabetes.[99] The women met five times for sessions that included nutrition education as well as motivation-based activities.[99] As a result of this intervention, the participants experienced a

---

See more about community and public health nutrition for older adults in Chapter 11.

Motivational interviewing A directive, client-centered counseling style for eliciting behavior change by helping clients to explore and resolve ambivalence. Compared with traditional counseling, it is more focused and goal directed. Motivation to change is elicited from the client and not imposed by the counselor.

significant improvement in hemoglobin A1C scores, a marker of long-term blood glucose levels.[99] Perhaps more importantly, all of the participants indicated they would recommend the intervention to a peer.[99]

Unfortunately, MI techniques do not appear to be universally effective. A meta-analysis of studies involving obese adolescents found that the use of MI alone is not an effective strategy for improvement in BMI or other metabolic syndrome criteria.[100] However, the use of MI in combination with other strategies likely improves health behaviors.[100] Indeed, best practices for MI include the following:

- Intervention delivered by a health professional trained in MI[101]
- Multi-component intervention combining education and goal-setting strategies[101]
- Blended approach (in-person and telephone/text/e-mail)[101]
- Appropriate session length (ideally 30–40 minutes each)[102]

Recently, the U.S. Preventive Services Task Force (USPSTF) performed a systematic review of research involving behavioral counseling related to diet and physical activity among adults who have risk factors for cardiovascular disease.[103] The goal of the review was to determine effectiveness of the behavioral counseling and establish a consensus on best practices for this target population. The results of the review showed a benefit of behavioral counseling interventions on risk of a cardiovascular event as well as measures of blood pressure, blood lipids, blood glucose, and body fat.[104] As a result, the USPSTF recommends use of behavioral counseling for adults who are predisposed to cardiovascular disease. They identified the following best practices[103]:

- Approximately 6 hours of contact in 1 year, including a combination of individual and group sessions
- Use of nonphysician health professionals to deliver the intervention
- Use of MI and other behavior change techniques including self-monitoring
- Dietary advice focused on:
  - Decreasing consumption of saturated fat, sugar, and sodium
  - Increasing consumption of whole grains, fruits, and vegetables
- Recommending 90–180 minutes per week of exercise that is moderate or vigorous in intensity
- Inclusion of family members in the intervention

> Read more about motivational interviewing for nutrition counseling at: https://eatrightpa.org/members/blog/become-proficient-motivational-interviewing/

Role of Government

Individual counseling in a healthcare setting and public health interventions in a variety of settings play significant roles in bringing preventative nutrition to the forefront. However, those methods, as presently implemented, are still limited in their effectiveness. In contrast, laws and regulations have proven to play a decisive and more effective role in advancing the public's health, especially with the passage of the Affordable Care Act. Public health's contribution is particularly evident in the prevention and control of communicable diseases and in the realm of injury prevention, which were the leading causes of death at the beginning of the 20th century.[105] Today, tobacco use and chronic diseases are the leading causes of death and disability, especially as more countries undergo the demographic transition.[105] Our strength in protecting the public has still primarily been in our means of responding to acute threats such as the recent COVID-19 pandemic or, perhaps, terrorism since the attack on September 11, 2001. It is imperative for all countries to move from a palliative medical model to one that is prevention-based if we are to make noticeable improvements in the worldwide quality of life and control rising healthcare costs. In the United States, the role of law has been

Pandemic Learning Opportunity

What did America learn as a nation with regard to prevention and the spread of Covid-19?

fully applied to the prevention and control of chronic diseases and their risk factors (e.g., tobacco control and smoking prevention). There has been a noteworthy impact on community and public health, such as a major decrease in smoking rates across the country for most segments of the population.

We have reached a point in healthcare history where we need to fully explore and create comprehensive legal frameworks for preventing and controlling the growing epidemics of obesity, heart disease, stroke, diabetes, and other chronic diseases and their related major risk factors.[105] Laws and regulations that implement widespread change will be a crucial addition to the tools available to the public health workforce, especially state and local health departments, as well as state and national policymakers. Legal steps or laws may take the form of constitutional provisions, statutory enactments, regulations, ordinances, government-initiated litigation, court rulings, or policies adopted by public-sector bodies, such as schools and zoning boards. For example, we have seen bans on trans fats, limits on portion sizes of sodas, and heightened nutrition standards for schools. However, as of 2021, laws such as the Treat and Reduce Obesity Act (last reintroduced in 2019 as H.R.1530/S.595) and Preventing Diabetes in Medicare Act (last reintroduced in 2017 as H.R.3124/S.1299) continue to languish in the U.S. Congress, serving as prime examples of the legal challenges in enacting new policy, as well as making changes to existing ones.

Law can also include policies or treaties adopted by international bodies, such as the International Code of Marketing of Breast-Milk Substitutes ("The Code") passed in 1981 by the WHO. It states that governments should provide information about the superiority of breastfeeding.[106] The Code also outlines measures that would control use of inappropriate marketing practices that can undermine a woman's ability to successfully initiate and continue breastfeeding.[106] The enactment of The Code was an effort to mitigate the aggressive marketing of infant formula by companies in developing countries, where infant mortality rates increased when mothers were disingenuously persuaded to formula-feed instead of breastfeed.

In 2004, WHO published the Global Strategy on Diet, Physical Activity, and Health.[107] One of the main objectives of their Global Strategy was to encourage the creation of policies at any level that can lead to improvements in both eating behavior and physical activity.[107] In this report, WHO makes it clear that governments around the world are in a position to cultivate health-promoting environments: "The role of government is crucial in achieving lasting change in public health".[107] WHO also points out that governments will need to engage with key stakeholders such as the media.[107] One particular area that was mentioned in the Global Strategy was the need for governments to work with the private sector regarding the marketing of food to children, both in terms of advertising and promotion. Six years later, in 2010, WHO tackled the issue of food marketing to children head on. It recommended that countries create or enforce policies that would limit marketing unhealthy foods to children.[108] This statement was preceded by a position from the American Heart Association in 2008, which recommended that in the United States, the Federal Trade Commission and the Federal Communications Commission be given the authority to regulate food companies who market their products to children.[109] In addition, it stated that only healthy foods should be marketed to children, and that toys or promotions should only accompany healthy food items.[109] Furthermore, the recommendations were made to reduce product placement of unhealthy foods in movies, television shows, etc., that target children, and that sponsorships by food companies should be eliminated in school settings.[109] Most recently, in 2020 the American Academy of Pediatrics (AAP) released a policy statement regarding digital advertising aimed at children for foods, alcohol, and tobacco products, among others.[110] The statement provided recommendations for parents, healthcare providers, and policymakers. The latter set of recommendations emphasized the need for education and research regarding digital literacy, concerns over privacy, and banning in-app sales or advertisements, including product placements.[110] Specific to nutrition, AAP recommended reducing what they called "targeted advertising" to children and adolescents that "exacerbates disparities when combined with structural sources of inequality."[110]

In response to these strong statements, Chile, Canada, Taiwan, South Africa, and the European Union have developed policies that specifically target promotion of unhealthy foods and marketing directly to children.[111] The impact of these policies on individual eating behavior, and ultimately, body weight status and chronic disease risk, remains to be seen. However, it has been demonstrated that food marketing has the potential to influence eating behavior.[111] The interaction of food marketing with the socioecological model is complex but has effects on the food environment (macro level), which then trickles down to direct effects on individual choice and behavior.[111]

Beyond marketing, other aspects of eating behavior have been targeted by regulations. A 2015 final ruling from the U.S. Food and Drug Administration (FDA) requires calories on chain restaurant menus and menu boards. In conjunction with the nutrition labeling provision of the Affordable Care Act, besides requiring calories on menus, menu boards and drive-through displays, the legislation requires chains with 20 or more outlets to provide additional nutrition information upon request.[112] At the time, these new requirements were met with much fanfare and optimism that having the nutrition information available at the point of purchase would dramatically influence personal choice. However, available evidence suggests mixed results. On one hand, menu labeling at Starbucks did lead to a small but significant decrease in the number of calories from food and/or beverages that were "purchased" at each transaction.[113] However, many studies have shown that there has been no significant change in eating behavior as a result of menu labeling.[113,114] This lack of an effect is seen in both children and adults.[113]

The challenge in developing public health effective legislation is the balance between human rights and public health legislation. According to Thomas Friedman, former director of the CDC, governments have three core responsibilities[105]:

- To promote truth in advertising
- To protect citizens from harm (i.e., unhealthy or unsafe food)
- To intervene (for the purposes of improving public health) when citizens are unable to carry out the intended action on their own

Similarly, Jonathan Mann, a pioneer advocating for the combination of public health, ethics, and human rights, developed a Four-Step Impact Assessment with his colleagues at the Francois-Xavier Center for Health and Human Rights at the Harvard School of Public Health.[115] The assessment measures the respective overlap or infringement of human rights and public health and asks the following questions:

1. To what extent does the proposed policy or program represent "good public health"?
2. Is the proposed policy or program respectful and protective of human rights?
3. How can we achieve the best possible combination of public health and human rights quality?
4. Does the proposed policy or program (as revised) still appear to be the optimal approach to the public health problem?

Mann's paradigm can effectively assist public health personnel in drafting policy that promotes the public health agenda that is cognizant and respectful of human rights. However, even the best intentions of public health may not be without controversy, especially as it relates to individual rights.

Discussion Prompt

Recent examples of arguments of personal freedoms include the debate over compulsory vaccination policies for children, mask-wearing during the pandemic, and legal attempts at restricting the portion sizes of sugary drinks available for sale and consumption. Discuss individual rights versus mandating action for the greater good.

Price Adjustments, Taxation, and Subsidies

Many factors influence our food choices; however, the top four considerations of why we eat what we do are taste, convenience, cost, and nutritional value.[116] In fact, simple strategies such as lowering the price of healthier foods, including fruits, vegetables, and salad bars in cafeterias, offering healthy snacks in vending machines at schools and worksites, can each lead to an increase in the sales of those items.[117,118] At minimum, this change in cost can positively change the proportion of sales of healthier choices versus less nutritious ones.[117,118] Price reductions of healthier foods in cafeterias or vending machines in 12 worksites and 12 secondary schools led to increased sales volume, which provided a constant level of profit, indicating a win-win situation for both consumers and food companies. This type of pricing strategy was pilot tested in a Midwestern suburban high school cafeteria during an entire school year.[119] Seven foods were targeted during the intervention: three popular higher-fat foods (French fries, cookies, and cheese sauce) and four lower-fat foods (fresh fruit, low-fat cookies, low-fat chips, and cereal bars).[119] Prices ranged from 35¢ to $1.00. Prices on the higher-fat foods were raised by approximately 10% and prices on the lower-fat foods were reduced by approximately 25% for the school year.[119] Sales data collected from school food services showed that the revenue from the seven foods were within 5% of revenues estimated for usual price conditions.[119] Therefore, students purchased based on price, which included a larger quantity of lower-fat foods at lower prices, as revenue remained relatively unchanged.[119] In addition, the impact of a 50% price reduction on fresh fruit and baby carrot consumption in two secondary school cafeterias was examined.[120] Compared with usual price conditions, price reductions resulted in a fourfold increase in fresh fruit sales and a twofold increase in baby carrot sales.[120] These studies demonstrate the efficacy of price reductions in increasing purchases of more healthful foods in community-based settings, such as worksites and schools.

A strategy taken from the public health approach to tobacco is to impose taxation on nonnutritious food and soda. The expectation is that the higher pricing on these food items would decrease consumption since cost is an important factor in food choice. This approach was originally suggested in the WHO's *1988 Healthy Public Policy Report*, which stated, "Taxation and subsidies should discriminate in favor of easy access for all to healthy food and improved diet."[121] In other words, taxations on unhealthy food could and should be used to subsidize fruits, vegetables, and whole grains. Several countries in Europe have enacted a fat, soda, or "junk food" tax, along with 40 states in the United States. Typically, these taxes are minimal (i.e., one or two cents). As of January 1, 2014, 34 states and the District of Columbia

Discussion Prompt

Is there a moral dilemma in distributing subsidies to the producers of such sweeteners while simultaneously taxing the consumers?

(D.C.) apply sales to sugar-sweetened sodas sold through grocers, while 39 states and D.C. apply that same sales tax to vending machine sales.[122] Revenue generated from these nominal taxes varies—over a 4-month span in Cook County, IL (home to Chicago), the sugar-sweetened beverage tax raised over $60 million but was ultimately repealed.[123] In the city of Berkeley, CA, revenue has exceeded $9 million since implementation in 2015.[124] This money could be used for health promotion programs as well as subsidies for produce companies. There are dissenters, however, who believe that these types of economic or governmental measures are infringing on personal choice and amount to "food policing." The question becomes, "How do we determine what foods are clearly 'unhealthy,' and therefore should be subject to taxation?" The United States faces the arduous task of creating and passing legislation for food and health policies that protect the health of Americans. Another complication in these taxes exists. The corn industry is the recipient of numerous subsidies, but a byproduct of this industry is corn syrup, which inevitably makes its way to candy bars and soda to be used as a sweetener.

Social Marketing

Social marketing is a powerful tool for reaching an enormous number of people via a well-designed campaign. To improve personal and social welfare, social marketing campaigns apply commercial marketing strategies to influence the voluntary behavior of target audiences. The three main attributes of a successful social marketing campaign are the following:

1. Its primary goal is to influence the voluntary behavior of target market members.
2. It offers benefits for changing behavior and reduced barriers to perform the behavior.
3. It primarily benefits members of the target audience, or society at large, rather than the organization that initiated it.[125]

This is what makes social marketing distinctly different from commercial marketing.

> See more about social marketing in Chapter 19.

The VERB Campaign

VERB was a multiethnic media campaign sponsored by the CDC, the goal of which was to increase and maintain physical activity among "tweens," that is, children aged 9 to 13 years.[126] The campaign ran from 2002–2006 and encouraged young people to get off of the sofa, choose their "cool verb," and be active in sports and other hobbies (dance, swing, swim, play, etc.). It was an excellent example of successful social marketing that successfully reached youth and changed their behavior. Parents and other influential community members (i.e., teachers, youth program leaders, and coaches) were the secondary audiences of the VERB initiative. VERB is not an acronym but a word that indicates action: "It's what you do."[126]

VERB successfully applied sophisticated commercial marketing techniques to address the public health problem of the sedentary lifestyles of American children. The social marketing principles addressed product, price, place, and promotion. Additionally, this initiative was successful because it was focused and consumer-centric and was designed specifically for and by kids of a specific age range.[126] A sufficient budget to carry this message into all media that children used was essential to "break through the clutter" of competing media messages. VERB spent a total of $125 million in 1 year, which predominantly went to paid advertising on television programs most watched by tweens.[126] VERB's financial resources were a major factor contributing to the campaign's success; unfortunately, many other well-designed campaigns do not have this amount of funding. Additionally, more than 450 partners were involved in the initiative to promote more physical activity in children.

The VERB campaign strived for high brand awareness and affinity among tweens. The theory was that when tweens bonded positively with VERB, they were more receptive to messages about physical activity. Many, if not most, would hopefully take the next step and be active. VERB was successfully "sold" to tweens as "their brand for having fun" because the campaign associated itself with popular kids' brands, athletes, celebrities, and activities and products that were appealing, fun, and motivating. When asked about VERB, the majority of children familiar with it responded with, "It's cool."[126]

Best Bones Forever!

In 2001, the U.S. Department of Health and Human Services' Office on Women's Health, in collaboration with the National Osteoporosis Foundation and the CDC, launched the National Bone Health Campaign aimed at girls 9–14 years old.[127] The goal of this social marketing campaign is to educate and encourage girls to establish lifelong healthy habits, especially increased calcium consumption and weight-bearing physical activity to build and maintain strong bones.[127] The initial tagline was "Powerful Bones, Powerful Girls" but in 2009, it was updated to "Best Bones Forever!"[128] As of 2014, oversight of the program was transferred from the Office of Women's Health to the nonprofit American Bone Health.[127]

This social marketing campaign includes the following features that have contributed to its success in reaching its target audience[128]:

- Paid print and radio advertising for girls and parents
- An award-winning website for girls—this girl-friendly website helps girls understand how weight-bearing physical activity and calcium can be a fun and important part of everyday life. The site's key features include interactive games and quizzes, recipes for tasty foods with calcium, and ideas to help girls get plenty of weight-bearing physical activity.
- A downloadable calendar—this free calendar for girls and parents allows girls to track their calcium intake and physical activity, with their parents' input
- Collaboration with Radio Disney, the Girl Scouts of the USA, Girls Inc., the National Association of School Nurses, and the President's Council on Fitness, Sports, and Nutrition

Several community organizations have implemented materials and messages from the Best Bones Forever! campaign, in particular through the Body-Works program.[129] As a result, knowledge of bone health, attitudes toward the importance of bone health, and confidence in making changes to enhance bone health, all improved.[129] However, whether these improvements lead to long-lasting behavior change has not been evaluated.

Fuel Up/Lift Off! LA/Sabor y Energia!

A Los Angeles County Department of Health Services social marketing campaign, Fuel Up/Lift Off! LA/Sabor y Energia! is targeted at obesity control in predominantly African American and Latino American communities.[130,131] Primary interventions include demonstrations and training in strategies to integrate physical activity and healthy food choices into routine business activities.[130,131] Examples include incorporating activity breaks with music into lengthy meetings, offering healthy food choices when refreshments are served, and hosting walking meetings.[130,131] A randomized, controlled trial tested the feasibility of including physical activity breaks as a part of lengthy meetings. The trial demonstrated success in the feasibility of engaging more than 90% of a sample of predominantly middle-aged and older women in 10 minutes of moderate physical activity, regardless of their fitness level or overweight status.[131]

Health Communication Technology

Printed educational materials and face-to-face communication are two basic and simple methods to increase knowledge and understanding of health risks and how to make healthful behavior changes. However, these two traditional methods for health education are now supplemented by or even being replaced by cell phones, e-mail, social media, and other online platforms. Newer technologies have opened up an unprecedented range of options for communicating and facilitating health behavior change strategies. A variety of software and apps now make it quick and easy to produce personalized health information tailored to an individual's needs or stage of change. The question of whether tailored or general materials are more effective has not been definitively established yet. Among obese adults in the SMART trial, the use of tailored feedback delivered remotely had significant reductions in calorie and saturated fat intake compared with the traditional intervention group.[132] There is also a role for tailored materials in the long-term maintenance of weight loss and health behaviors, as evidenced by the use of text messages (approximately eight delivered every 2 weeks for 6 months) in a group of individuals who recently finished a weight-loss program.[133] Participants who received the text messages were better able to prevent weight regain, and maintained physical activity post-intervention, compared with similar interventions with no long-term follow-up.[133] Framing and tailoring the messages delivered in a behavior change intervention is a key predictor of success, according to a recent evaluation of the literature.[134] The Comprehensive Messaging Strategy for Sustained Behavior Change was designed with the stages of change model in mind.[134] There are four phases: detection, decision, implementation, and maintenance.[134] Each phase will require a specific focus to the messages in order to resonate with the individual. Successful messaging campaigns need to tailor the messages to the participant's current phase.

For those seeking a program for weight loss, individuals are able to enroll and participate in one without leaving home or even engaging in face-to-face contact. A number of online programs can provide sound nutrition and exercise advice from qualified fitness professionals and registered dietitians. The top-rated websites may include the following:

- Personal nutrition, exercise, and behavioral assessments
- Customized meal planning tools, healthy recipes, online food journal, and exercise logs
- Scientifically sound, up-to-date nutrition information and weight loss tips
- Personalized exercise plan appropriately matched to ability, interest, and fitness level
- Information addressing emotional and behavioral issues (e.g., stress) related to food, along with coping strategies and support
- An online "community" and chat rooms to motivate and provide support on a regular basis

Studies examining the effectiveness of online support groups for weight loss have shown mixed results. Results from Weight Watchers members who participate in their Facebook group revealed three different types of individuals: Passive Recipients, Active Supporters, and Casual Browsers.[135] These terms describe the overall level of interaction a group member has in the online setting, with varying types and amounts of support provided and received. The first two groups receive the most support (information-based and emotion-based) from other group members.[135]

However, as Internet access continues to grow ubiquitous in everyday life and many are finding that online group therapy is convenient and may have a bigger impact than originally thought. Recently, scientists examined the effects of a therapist-guided, Internet-based behavior therapy on patients suffering from generalized anxiety disorder.[136] Researchers found moderate to large effects on symptoms of patients' anxiety and moderate effects on depressive symptoms.[136] Certainly, mental health counseling is different from medical nutrition therapy, but there are still lessons to be learned. While in-person therapy may have more benefits to the patients, online therapies may be well suited to serve as a complement to traditional therapies. In other scenarios, online therapy may provide to be a more accessible and cheaper alternative to in-patient sessions. It is easy to imagine cases where patients cannot afford or are unable to make time for numerous in-patient sessions. Researchers continue to evaluate and invent novel approaches for online therapies and healthcare professionals should expect this particular administration of therapy to grow.

Thousands of electronic, health-related, peer-to-peer support groups in the form of mailing lists, chat rooms, and discussion forums are available on the Internet. Internet access has created opportunities to access health information on any topic and has led some people to self-diagnose. This can either be a favorable or an unfortunate phenomenon, depending on whether the individual is then prompted to seek qualified medical advice in person. Numerous online support groups exist that serve as important social networks, especially for people with stigmatizing diseases such as AIDS, alcoholism, and certain cancers. For individuals suffering from chronic pain, rare diseases, or conditions for which modern medicine has no effective remedy, and/or for those who are socially isolated with no family, these virtual friends and support groups can be life-giving.

The rise in use of social media can be capitalized on by developing interventions that include messages delivered through an online social media platform.[137] It is too early to tell if incorporating social media into behavior change interventions will be meaningful on success rates, or if it will simply contribute more to the feelings of anxiety that are associated with excess social media use.[137] Being mindful of the target audience for the intervention is important when deciding whether or not to include new technologies or methods of communication.

Pandemic Learning Opportunity

Online doctor visits were made available due to the Covid-19 pandemic. Discuss the potential expanded use of social media that can be utilized from this example.

Summary

A variety of strategies has been used to target improvements in eating behavior. At present, the most effective interventions are likely based on the socioecological model. This theoretical model utilizes a multilevel approach and acknowledges the role of individual choice as well as environmental influence when it comes to supporting healthy eating. While recognizing the continued importance of intervening at all levels of society (from individual to population-wide), future efforts should recognize the power and influence of media along with governmental policy on individual behaviors. Better health and quality of life can be achieved for every individual when all sectors of society work together in minimizing barriers to health and capitalizing on each other's strengths.

Learning Portfolio

© olies/Shutterstock.

Issues for Discussion

1. The socioecological model was used throughout the chapter to illustrate the various levels of influence on an individual's behavior. Which level do you think is the most influential on day-to-day decisions regarding healthy eating? Which level do you think is the easiest to modify to improve eating habits?

2. Accountability, incentives, and self-monitoring are often included in behavior change intervention programs. How practical do you feel these strategies are if you were going to implement an intervention in your own school, organization, or work setting? How would you modify the interventions and campaigns discussed in this chapter to best fit your own community?

3. Taxation of sugary drinks has been promoted as one strategy for reducing consumption of sugar-sweetened beverages. This so-called "soda tax" has been applied to soft drinks sold through both supermarkets and vending machines. In small groups, discuss the pros and cons of state and local governments implementing a "soda tax." What are two alternative strategies that could lead to a reduced consumption of sugar-sweetened beverages?

Practical Activities

1. Approximately 2 billion of the world's population lives on less than $3/day. The goal of this activity is to see if you can meet your food and nutrient needs on $3/day for 5 days.
   a. How did it might feel—physically, emotionally, and cognitively—to be food insecure?
   b. What foods did you buy with your $15? Where did you shop?
   c. What strategies did you use to maximize your budget?
   d. Do you think meeting the Dietary Guidelines 2020–2025 will be challenging? Why or why not?

2. Conduct a search on social media (i.e., Instagram, Pinterest, Facebook) for weight loss ideas. How are these effective or noneffective for healthy eating while losing weight? How do these impede the efforts of the government to help the population to eat right?

Key Terms

	page
Obesity	210
Overweight	210
Food away from home	217
Socioecological model	219
Healthy People 2030	219
Dietary Guidelines for Americans	220
Healthy, Hunger-Free Kids Act of 2010	224
Fresh Fruit and Vegetable Program	224
Worksite interventions	226
Neophobia	229
Community	230
Motivational interviewing	232

Case Study: Improving Health Behaviors Among Pregnant Women

You work for a county health department that includes a mid-sized city with a high population of non-Hispanic Black women. This demographic group has a significantly higher risk of both obesity and maternal mortality compared with non-Hispanic white women in your community. In addition, the city recently lost a locally owned grocery store chain. Now there are only three full-scale grocery stores in the entire city, which spans 25 square miles. Your county is situated in an area of the United States that experiences cold, snowy winters and public transportation is limited to city buses. A large farmer's market is centrally located in the city and remains open year-round. Several small parks are located within the city, and a larger park with an extensive walk/bike trail exists on the northern side of the city.

The local hospitals (who each have an ob/gyn clinic in the city) contact you with a request to help develop an intervention that will address dietary intake and physical activity during pregnancy. The target population is non-Hispanic Black women who are obese and currently pregnant.

Consider the following questions:

1. What do you want to know about the target population as you develop the intervention? How do you intend to obtain this information?

2. Which behavior change theory seems most appropriate to guide you in the development of the intervention? Why?

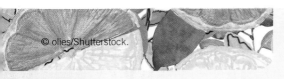
© olies/Shutterstock.

Learning Portfolio

Case Study: Improving Health Behaviors Among Pregnant Women

3. How will you structure the intervention? Specifically:

   a. How will you recruit women to participate?

   b. Who will deliver the intervention?

   c. How long will it last?

   d. What (if any) incentive will be provided?

4. How will you determine if the intervention is successful?

Case Study: Poor Healthy Food Access

Consider a community suffering from poor food access, especially when it comes to healthful food choices. You've been tasked with developing a community-driven program that aims to increase the community's access to healthy foods, especially fruits and vegetables. After careful consideration, the city government has decided to dedicate funding to your project that specifically targets local stores with the objective of improving stocking practices of healthful foods. The hope is that if these foods are available to purchase, people will start to make healthier choices. You decide to host a townhall-style meeting where storeowners and interested citizens can learn more about this new program. In attendance are several local storeowners who are excited about the idea of helping improve their community—but have some concerns about the feasibility of stocking these items, especially perishable produce. Specifically, some of the smaller storeowners tell you that it is already difficult to compete with larger stores because of their lower buying power and they are worried about their thin profit margins. Consult the textbook and conduct a brief literature search as you consider the following questions. Please answer thoroughly—questions have multiple answers to select from—and cite at least one source for each answer. These sources can come from peer-reviewed literature or the textbook.

1. What would make local merchants consider changing their stock to meet the city's goals of increased fruits and vegetables available to purchase?

2. Would more availability of fruits, vegetables, and other healthy foods be enough to sway citizens into purchasing these items? If not, what other ideas would you suggest the city consider investing in? Are these ideas cost-effective?

3. What fruits and vegetables would you suggest the storeowner stock at first to minimize loss?

4. What tips and strategies could the storeowner implement to increase sales of these perishable items within the store? Think in terms of product placement, marketing, and price point.

Resources

1. Dietary Guidelines for Americans 2020–2025: https://www.dietaryguidelines.gov/
2. Healthy People 2030: https://health.gov/healthypeople
3. Academy of Nutrition and Dietetics: https://www.eatright.org/
4. World Health Organization: https://www.who.int/health-topics/nutrition
5. School Nutrition Association: https://schoolnutrition.org/
6. Society for Nutrition Education and Behavior: https://www.sneb.org/

7. National Farm to School Network: http://www.farmtoschool.org/

8. Centers for Disease Control and Prevention: https://www.cdc.gov/nutrition/index.html

9. Feeding America (Hunger Relief): https://www.feedingamerica.org/

10. Motivational Interviewing: https://motivationalinterviewing.org/

11. Healthy Children (from the American Academy of Pediatrics): https://www.healthychildren.org/English/healthy-living/nutrition/Pages/default.aspx

12. U.S. Department of Health and Human Services' Office on Women's Health: https://www.womenshealth.gov/

References

1. Rychter AM, Ratajczak AE, Zawada A, Dobrowolska A, Krela-Kaźmierczak I. Non-systematic review of diet and nutritional risk factors of cardiovascular disease in obesity. *Nutrients.* 2020;12(3):814. https://doi.org/10.3390/nu12030814

2. Palmer MK, Toth PP. Trends in lipids, obesity, metabolic syndrome, and diabetes mellitus in the United States: An NHANES analysis (2003-2004 to 2013-2014). *Obesity.* 2019;27(2):309-314.

3. Skinner AC, Ravanbakht SN, Skelton JA, et al. Prevalence of obesity and severe obesity in U.S. Children, 1999–2016. *Pediatrics.* 2018;141(3):e20173459.

4. Hales CM, Carroll MD, Fryar CD, Ogden CL. Prevalence of obesity among adults and youth: United States, 2015–2016. NCHS data brief, no 288. Hyattsville, MD: National Center for Health Statistics. 2017.

5. Koliaki C, Spinos T, Spinou M, Brinia M-E, Mitsopoulou D, Katsilambros N. Defining the optimal dietary approach for safe, effective and sustainable weight loss in overweight and obese adults. *Healthcare.* 2018;6(3):73. https://doi.org/10.3390/healthcare6030073

6. de Villiers A, Faber M. Changing young people's food-related behaviour: a socio-ecological perspective. *Public Health Nutrition.* 2019;22(11):1917-1919. doi: 10.1017/S136898001900123X

7. Johns DJ, Hartmann-Boye J, Jebb SA, Aveyard P. Diet or exercise interventions vs combined behavioral weight management programs: a systematic review and meta-analysis of direct comparisons. *J Acad Diet Nutr.* 2014;114(10):1557-1568. https://doi.org/10.1016/j.jand.2014.07.005

8. Rogers, EM. *Diffusion of innovations.* 4th ed. Simon and Schuster; 2010.

9. Huye HF, Molaison EF, Downey LH, Landry AS, Crook LB, Connell CL. Development of a nutrition education program for the Mississippi Communities for Healthy Living Nutrition Intervention using the Diffusion of Innovations. *JHSE.* 2017;5(3).

10. Green EC, Murphy EM. Gryboski K. The Health Belief Model. In: Cohen LM, ed. *The Wiley Encyclopedia of Health Psychology.* Wiley; 2020:211-214.

11. McArthur LH, Riggs A, Uribe F, Spaulding TJ. Health belief model offers opportunities for designing weight management interventions for college students. *J Nutr Educ Behav.* 2018;50(5):485-493.

12. Kang J, Jun J, Arendt SW. Understanding customers' healthy food choices at casual dining restaurants: Using the Value–Attitude–Behavior model. *Int J Hosp Manag.* 2015;48:2-21.

13. Crosby R, Noar SM. What is a planning model? An introduction to PRECEDE-PROCEED. *J Public Health Dent.* 2011;71:S7-S15.

14. Whatnall M, Patterson A, Hutchesson M. A brief web-based nutrition intervention for young adult university students: development and evaluation protocol using the PRECEDE-PROCEED model. *JMIR Res Protoc.* 2019;8(3):e11992. doi: 10.2196/11992

15. Cole RE, Horacek T. Applying PRECEDE-PROCEED to develop an intuitive eating nondieting approach to weight management pilot program. *J Nut Educ Behav.* 2009;41(2):120-126.

16. Schunk DH. Theories, constructs, and critical issues: social cognitive theory. In: Harris KR, Graham S, Urdan T, McCormick CB, Sinatra GM, Sweller J, eds. *APA handbooks in psychology®. APA educational psychology handbook.* Vol. 1. American Psychological Association; 2012:101-123. https://doi.org/10.1037/13273-005

17. Stacey FG, James EL, Chapman K, Courneya KS, Lubans DR. A systematic review and meta-analysis of social cognitive theory-based physical activity and/or nutrition behavior change interventions for cancer survivors. *J Cancer Surviv.* 2015;9(2):305-338. doi: 10.1007/s11764-014-0413-z

18. Hall E, Chai W, Koszewski W, Albrecht J. Development and validation of a social cognitive theory-based survey for elementary nutrition education program. *Int J Behav Nutr Phys Act.* 2015;12:47. https://doi.org/10.1186/s12966-015-0206-4

19. Coughlin SS, Smith SA. Community-based participatory research to promote healthy diet and nutrition and prevent and control obesity among African-Americans: a literature review. *J Racial Ethn Health Disparities.* 2017;4(2):259-268. doi: 10.1007/s40615-016-0225-0

20. Grummon AH, Cabana MD, Hecht AA, et al. Effects of a multipronged beverage intervention on young children's beverage intake and weight: a cluster-randomized pilot study. *Public Health Nutr.* 2019;22(15):2856-2867. doi: 10.1017/S1368980019001629

21. Conner M, Sparks P. Theory of planned behaviour and health behaviour. In: Conner M, Norman P, eds. *Predicting Health Behaviour* 2nd Ed. Open University Press; 2005:170-222.

22. Steinmetz H, Knappstein M, Ajzen I, Schmidt P, Kabst R. How effective are behavior change interventions based on the theory of planned behavior? A three-level meta-analysis. *Zeitschrift für Psychologie.* 2016;224(3):216-233. https://doi.org/10.1027/2151-2604/a000255

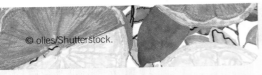

Learning Portfolio

© olies/Shutterstock.

23. Mazloomy-Mahmoodabad SS, Navabi ZS, Ahmadi A, Askarishahi M. The effect of educational intervention on weight loss in adolescents with overweight and obesity: Application of the theory of planned behavior. *ARYA Atheroscler.* 2017;13(4): 176-183.

24. Prochaska JO, Redding CA. Evers KE. The transtheoretical model and stages of change. In: Glanz K, Timer BK, Viswanath K. eds. *Health behavior: Theory, research, and practice* 2nd Ed. Jossey-Bass; 2015:125-148.

25. Lee JE, Lee DE, Kim K, et al. Development of tailored nutrition information messages based on the transtheoretical model for smartphone application of an obesity prevention and management program for elementary-school students. *Nutr Res Pract.* 2017;11(3):247-256. doi: 10.4162/nrp.2017.11.3.247

26. United States Department of Agriculture. Food availability and consumption. Available at: https://www.ers.usda.gov /data-products/ag-and-food-statistics-charting-the-essentials /food-availability-and-consumption/

27. US Food and Drug Administration. Food Labeling: Revision of the Nutrition and Supplement Facts Labels. 2016;FDA-2012-N-1210.

28. Bentley J. U.S. trends in food availability and a dietary assessment of loss-adjusted food availability, 1970-2014. Err-166, U.S. Department of Agriculture, Economic Research Service, January 2017.

29. Roser M, Ritchie H. "Food Supply". Published online at OurWorldInData.org. 2013. Retrieved from: 'https://ourworldindata .org/food-supply' [Online Resource]

30. Rosinger A, Herrick K, Gahche J, Park S. Sugar-sweetened beverage consumption among U.S. youth, 2011–2014. NCHS data brief, no 271. Hyattsville, MD: National Center for Health Statistics. 2017.

31. Rosinger A, Herrick K, Gahche J, Park S. Sugar-sweetened beverage consumption among U.S. adults, 2011–2014. NCHS data brief, no 270. Hyattsville, MD: National Center for Health Statistics. 2017.

32. Ver Ploeg M, Breneman V, Dutko P, et al. Access to affordable and nutritious food: updated estimates of distance to supermarkets using 2010 data. ERR-143, U.S. Department of Agriculture, Economic Research Service, November 2012.

33. Coleman-Jensen A, Rabbitt MP, Gregory CA, Singh A. Household food security in the United States in 2019. ERR-275, U.S. Department of Agriculture, Economic Research Service; 2020.

34. Fitzpatrick KM, Harris C, Drawve G, Willis DE. Assessing food insecurity among U.S. adults during the COVID-19 pandemic. *J Hunger Environ Nutr.* 2021;16(1):1-18. doi: 10.1080/19320248.2020.1830221

35. Strupat C, Farfán G, Moritz L, Negre M, Vakis R. Obesity and food away from home: What drives the socioeconomic gradient in excess body weight? *Econ Hum Biol.* 2021. [In press]

36. Saksena MJ, Okrent AM, Anekwe TD, et al. American's eating habits: food away from home. EIB-196, U.S. Department of Agriculture, Economic Research Service; 2018.

37. Fryar CD, Carroll MD, Ahluwalia N, Ogden CL. Fast food intake among children and adolescents in the United States, 2015–2018. NCHS Data Brief, no 375. Hyattsville, MD: National Center for Health Statistics. 2020.

38. Powell LM, Nguyen BT. Fast-food and full service restaurant consumption among children and adolescents: Effect on energy, beverage, and nutrient intake. *JAMA Pediatrics.* 2013;167(1): 14-20.

39. McCrory M, Harbaugh AG, Appeadu S, Roberts SB. Fast-food offerings in the United STates in 1986, 1991, and 2016 show large increases in food variety, portion size, dietary energy, and selected micronutrients. *J Acad Nutr Diet.* 2019;119(6): 923-933.

40. Martin CB, Herrick KA, Sarafrazi N, Ogden CL. Attempts to lose weight among adults in the United States, 2013–2016. NCHS Data Brief, no 313. Hyattsville, MD: National Center for Health Statistics. 2018.

41. Hills Jr. RD, Erpenbeck E. Guide to popular diets, food choices, and their health outcome. *Health Care Curr Rev.* 2018;6(2): 223-228.

42. Ramachandran D, Kite J, Vassallo AJ, et al. Food trends and popular nutrition advice online - implications for public health. *Online J Public Health Inform.* 2018;10(2):e213-e227.

43. Institute of Medicine. *Health and Behavior.* Washington, DC: National Academy Press; 2001.

44. Institute of Medicine, Smedley BD, Syme SL, eds. *Promoting Health: Intervention Strategies from Social and Behavioral Research report.* Washington, DC: National Academy Press; 2000.

45. Samdal GB, Eide GE, Barth T, et al. Effective behaviour change techniques for physical activity and healthy eating in overweight and obese adults; systematic review and meta-regression analyses. *Int J Behav Nutr Phys Act.* 2017;14:42. https://doi .org/10.1186/s12966-017-0494-y

46. Murimi MW, Kanyi M, Mupfudze T, et al. Factors influencing efficacy of nutrition education interventions: a systematic review. *J Nut Ed Behav.* 2017;49(2):142-165.

47. U.S. Department of Health and Human Services. *Healthy People 2030.* Washington, DC: Department of Health and Human Services. Accessed January 8, 2021. www.healthypeople .gov

48. U.S. Department of Health and Human Services and U.S. Department of Agriculture. 2020 - 2025 Dietary Guidelines for Americans. 9th Edition. December 2020. Available at: https://www.dietaryguidelines.gov/

49. Bole M, Adams A, Gredler A, Manhas S. Ability of a mass media campaign to influence knowledge, attitudes, and behaviors about sugary drinks and obesity. *Prev Med.* 2014;67(S1): S40-S45.

50. Barragan NC, Noller AJ, Robles B, et al. The "Sugar Pack" health marketing campaign in Los Angeles County, 2011-2012. *Health Promot Pract.* 2014;15(2):208-216.

51. Farley TA, Halper HS, Carlin AM, et al. Mass media campaign to reduce consumption of sugar-sweetened beverages in a rural area of the United States. *AJPH.* 2017;107:989-995.

52. Milliron BJ, Woolf K, Appelhans BM. A point-of-purchase intervention featuring in-person supermarket education affects healthful food purchases. *J Nutr Educ Behav.* 2012;44(30):225-232.

53. Liberato SC, Baillie R, Brimblecombe J. Nutrition interventions at point-of-sale to encourage healthier food purchases: a systematic review. *BMC Public Health.* 2014;14:919.

54. World Health Organization Regional Office for Europe. *The Adelaide Recommendations: Healthy Public Policy*. Geneva, Switzerland; WHO; 1988.

55. Guideline: Sugars intake for adults and children. Geneva: World Health Organization; 2015.

56. Nestle M. *Food Politics: How the Food Industry Influences Nutrition and Health*. Berkeley: University of California Press; 2002.

57. Stok FM, Renner B, Clarys P, et al. Understanding eating behavior during the transition from adolescence to young adulthood: A literature review and perspective on future research directions. *Nutrients*. 2018;10(6):1-16. https://doi.org/10.3390/nu10060667

58. Quinn LJ, Horacek TM, Castle J. The impact of Cookshop™ on the dietary habits and attitudes of fifth graders. *Top Clin Nutr*. 2003;18(1):42-48.

59. Perry CL, Stone EJ, Parcel GS, et al. School-based cardiovascular health promotion: the Child And Adolescent Trial For Cardiovascular Health (CATCH). *J Sch Health*. 1990;60:406-413.

60. Hoelscher DM, Feldman HA, Johnson CC, et al. School-based health education programs can be maintained over time: results from the CATCH institutionalization study. *Prev Med*. 2004;38:594-606.

61. Osganian SK, Hoelscher DM, Zive M, Mitchell PD, Snyder P, Webber LS. Maintenance of effects of the Eat Smart School Food Service program: results from the Catch-On study. *Health Educ Behav*. 2003;30:418-433.

62. Parcel GS, Perry CL, Kelder SH, et al. School climate and the institutionalization of the Catch program. *Health Educ Behav*. 2003;30:489-502.

63. "Let's Move!" *National Archives and Records Administration*, National Archives and Records Administration. Accessed on February 2, 2021. https://letsmove.obamawhitehouse.archives.gov/achievements

64. Miller GF, Sliwa S, Michael S, et al. Evaluation of Let's Move! active schools activation grants. *Prev Med*. 2018;108:36-40. https://doi.org/10.1016/j.ypmed.2017.12.024

65. Hayes D, Contento IR, Weekly C. Position of the Academy of Nutrition and Dietetics, Society for Nutrition Education and Behavior, and School Nutrition Association: comprehensive nutrition programs and services in schools. *J Acad Nutr Diet*. 2018;118(5):913-919.

66. Council on School Health, Committee on Nutrition. Snacks, sweetened beverages, added sugars, and schools. *Pediatrics*. 2015;135(3):575-583.

67. Au LE, Ritchie LD, Gurzo K, et al. Post-Healthy, Hunger-Free Kids Act adherence to select school nutrition standards by region and poverty level: The Healthy Communities Study. *J Nutr Ed Behav*. 2020;52(3):249-258.

68. Mansfield JL, Savaiano DA. Effect of school wellness policies and the Healthy, Hunger-Free Kids Act on food-consumption behaviors of students, 2006–2016: a systematic review. *Nutr Rev*. 2017;75(7):533-552. https://doi.org/10.1093/nutrit/nux020

69. U.S. Department of Agriculture. The Farm-to-School Census. 2015. Accessed February 7, 2021. https://farmtoschoolcensus.fns.usda.gov/

70. Bartlett S, Olsho L, Klerman J, et al. Evaluation of the Fresh Fruit and Vegetable Program (FFVP): Final evaluation report. Contract No. AG-3198-D-09-0053. 2013. Alexandria, VA: U.S. Department of Agriculture, Food and Nutrition Service.

71. United Fresh Produce Association. Fresh fruit and vegetable program. 2020. Accessed February 7, 2021. https://www.unitedfresh.org/nutrition/fresh-fruit-vegetable-program/

72. U.S. Department of Agriculture, Food and Nutrition Service. The Fresh Fruit and Vegetable Program Fact Sheet. December 2017. Accessed February 7, 2021. https://fns-prod.azureedge.net/sites/default/files/resource-files/FFVPFactSheet.pdf

73. U.S. Bureau of Labor Statistics. American time use survey - 2019 Results. USDL-20-1275. 2020. Accessed February 7, 2021. https://www.bls.gov/news.release/pdf/atus.pdf

74. Centers for Disease Control and Prevention. Workplace Health in America 2017. Atlanta, GA: Centers for Disease Control and Prevention, U.S. Department of Health and Human Services, 2018.

75. Onufrak SJ, Zaganjor H, Pan L, Lee-Kwan SH, Park S, Harris DM. Foods and beverages obtained at worksites in the United States. *J Acad Nutr Diet*. 2019;119(6):999-1008.

76. Pronk N. Best practice design principles of worksite health and wellness programs. *ACSMs Health Fit J*. 2014;18(1):42-46. doi: 10.1249/FIT.0000000000000012

77. Centers for Disease Control and Prevention. CDC Worksite Health ScoreCard. January 2019. Accessed February 7, 2021. https://www.cdc.gov/workplacehealthpromotion/initiatives/healthscorecard/introduction.html

78. House JS, Landis KR, Umberson D. Social relationships and health. *Science*. 1988;241:540-545.

79. Hill PL, Weston SJ, Jackson JJ. Connecting social environment variables to the onset of major specific health outcomes. *Psych Health*. 2014;29(7):753-767.

80. Balantekin KN, Anzman-Frasca S, Francis LA, Ventura AK, Fisher JO, Johnson SL. Positive parenting approaches and their association with child eating and weight: A narrative review from infancy to adolescence. *Ped Obes*. 2020;15(10):e12722.

81. van der Horst K, Sleddens EF. Parenting styles, feeding styles and food-related parenting practices in relation to toddlers' eating styles: A cluster-analytic approach. *PloS ONE*. 2017;12(5):e0178149.

82. Golan M, Crow S. Parents are key players in the prevention and treatment of weight-related problems. *Nutr Rev*. 2004;62:39-50.

83. Galloway AT, Lee Y, Birch LL. Predictors and consequences of food neophobia and pickiness in young girls. *J Am Diet Assoc*. 2003;103:692-698.

84. Neumark-Sztainer D, Wall M, Perry C, Story M. Correlates of fruit and vegetable intake among adolescents. Findings from Project EAT. *Prev Med*. 2003;37:198-208.

85. Haire-Joshu D, Brownson RC, Nanney MS, et al. Improving dietary behavior in African Americans: the Parents As Teachers High 5, Low Fat Program. *Prev Med*. 2003;36:684-691.

86. Epple C, Wright AL, Joish VN, Bauer M. The role of active family nutritional support in Navajos' type 2 diabetes metabolic control. *Diabetes Care*. 2003;26:2829-2834.

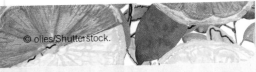

Learning Portfolio

87. Wallerstein N, Minkler M, Carter-Edwards L, Avila M, Sánchez V. Improving health through community engagement, community organization, and community building. In: Glanz K, Timer BK, Viswanath K. eds. *Health behavior: Theory, research, and practice* 2nd Ed. Jossey-Bass; 2015:125-148.

88. Viadro CI, Farris RP, Will JC. The WISEWOMAN projects: lessons learned from three states. *J Womens Health (Larchmt)*. 2004;13:529-538.

89. Berkley-Patton J, Thompson CB, Bradley-Ewing A, et al. Identifying health conditions, priorities, and relevant multilevel health promotion intervention strategies in African American churches: A faith community health needs assessment. *Eval Program Plann*. 2018;67:19-28. doi: 10.1016/j.evalprogplan.2017.10.012

90. Yanek LR, Becker DM, Moy TF, Gittelsohn J, Koffman DM. Project Joy: Faith based cardiovascular health promotion for African American women. *Public Health Rep*. 2001;116 (suppl 1):68-81. doi: 10.1093/phr/116.S1.68

91. Ammerman A, Corbie-Smith G, St. George DMM, Washington C, Weathers B, Jackson-Christian B. Research expectations among African American church leaders in the PRAISE! Project: a randomized trial guided by community-based participatory research. *Am J Public Health*. 2003;93:1720-1727.

92. Corbie-Smith G, Ammerman AS, Katz ML, et al. Trust, benefit, satisfaction, and burden: a randomized controlled trial to reduce cancer risk through African-American churches. *J Gen Intern Med*. 2003;18:531-541.

93. Body & Soul: A Celebration of Healthy Eating & Living. Accessed February 7, 2021. http://www.floridahealth.gov/programs-and-services/minority-health/body-and-soul-toolkit/index.html

94. Shlisky J, Bloom DE, Beaudreault AR, et al. Nutritional considerations for healthy aging and reduction in age-related chronic disease. *Adv Nutr*. 2017;8(1):17-26. doi: 10.3945/an.116.013474

95. Bandayrel K, Wong S. Systematic literature review of randomized control trials assessing the effectiveness of nutrition interventions in community-dwelling older adults. *J Nutr Ed Behav*. 2011;43(4):251-262.

96. Zhou X, Perez-Cueto FJA, Santos QD, et al. A systematic review of behavioural interventions promoting healthy eating among older people. *Nutrients*. 2018;10(2):128. https://doi.org/10.3390/nu10020128

97. Chapel DL, McCulla MM, Reinsch B, Warren C. Moving right along: a creative partnership to engage older adults in physical activity and nutrition programs. Abstract. Preventing Chronic Disease. 2004. Accessed April 6, 2010. http://www.cdc.gov/pcd/issues/2004/apr/03_0034d.htm

98. Centis E, Petroni ML, Ghirelli V, et al Motivational interviewing adapted to group setting for the treatment of relapse in the behavioral therapy of obesity. A clinical audit. *Nutrients*. 2020;12(12):3881.

99. Miller ST, Oates VJ, Brooks MA, Shintani A, Gebretsadik T, Jenkins DM. Preliminary efficacy of group medical nutrition therapy and motivational interviewing among obese African American women with type 2 diabetes: a pilot study. *J Obes*. 2014. https://doi.org/10.1155/2014/345941

100. Vallabhan MK, Jimenez EY, Nash JL, et al. Motivational interviewing to treat adolescents with obesity: a meta-analysis. *Pediatrics*. 2018;142(5):e20180733.

101. Mifsud JL, Galea J, Garside J, Stephenson J, Astin F. Motivational interviewing to support modifiable risk factor change in individuals at increased risk of cardiovascular disease: A systematic review and meta-analysis. *PloS ONE*. 2020;15(11): e0241193.

102. Schneider JK, Wong-Anuchit C, Stallings D, Krieger MM. Motivational interviewing and fruit/vegetable consumption in older adults. *Clin Nurs Res*. 2017;26(6):731-746. https://doi: 10.1177/1054773816673634

103. U.S. Preventive Services Task Force. Behavioral counseling interventions to promote a healthy diet and physical activity for cardiovascular disease prevention in adults with cardiovascular risk factors: U.S. Preventive Services Task Force Recommendation Statement. *JAMA*. 2020;324(20):2069-2075. https://doi: 10.1001/jama.2020.21749

104. O'Connor EA, Evans CV, Rushkin MC, Redmond N, Lin JS. Behavioral counseling to promote a healthy diet and physical activity for cardiovascular disease prevention in adults with cardiovascular risk factors: updated evidence report and systematic review for the US Preventive Services Task Force. *JAMA*. 2020;324(20):2076-2094. https://doi: 10.1001/jama.2020.17108

105. Frieden TR. The future of public health. *N Engl J Med*. 2015;373(18):1748-54.

106. World Health Organization. *International Code of Marketing of Breast-milk Substitutes*. Geneva, Switzerland. WHO;1981.

107. World Health Organization. *Global Strategy on Diet, Physical Activity and Health*. Geneva, Switzerland. WHO; 2004.

108. World Health Organization. *Marketing of food and non-alcoholic beverages to children*. WHA63.14. Geneva, Switzerland. WHO; 2010.

109. American Heart Association Advocacy Department. *Policy Position Statement on Food Advertising and Marketing Practices to Children*. Washington, DC. AHA; 2008.

110. Radesky R, Chassiakos YR, Ameenuddin N, Navsaria D, Council on Communication and Media. Digital advertising to children. *Pediatrics*. 2020;146(1):e20201681. https://doi.10.1542/peds.2020-1681

111. Cairns G. A critical review of evidence on the sociocultural impacts of food marketing and policy implications. *Appetite*. 2019;136(1):193-207.

112. United States Food and Drug Administration. Menu and vending machines labeling requirements. May 2020. Accessed February 7, 2021. https://www.fda.gov/food/food-labeling-nutrition/menu-and-vending-machine-labeling

113. VanEpps EM, Roberto CA, Park S, Economos CD, Bleich SN. Restaurant menu labeling policy: review of evidence and controversies. *Curr Obes Rep*. 2016;5(1):72-80.

114. Cantu-Jungles TM, McCormack LA, Slaven JE, Slebodnik M, Eicher-Miller HA. A meta-analysis to determine the impact of restaurant menu labeling on calories and nutrients (ordered or consumed) in U.S. adults. *Nutrients*. 2017;9(10):1088.

115. MacNaughton G. Human rights impact assessment: a method for healthy policymaking. *Harvard Health*

Reports. 2015. Accessed February 7, 2021. https://sites.sph.harvard.edu/hhrjournal/2015/04/human-rights-impact-assessment-a-method-for-healthy-policymaking/

116. Glanz K, Basil M, Maibach E, Goldberg J, Snyder D. Why Americans eat what they do: taste, nutrition, cost, convenience, and weight control concerns as influences on food consumption. *J Am Diet Assoc.* 1998;98:1118-1126.

117. Steenhuis IHM, Waterlander WE, de Mul A. Consumer food choices: the role of price and pricing strategies. *Pub H Nutr.* 2011;14(12):2220-2226. https://doi: 10.1017/S1368980011001637

118. Kushida O, Murayama N. Effects of environmental intervention in workplace cafeterias on vegetable consumption by male workers. *J Nutr Educ Behav.* 2014;46(5):350-358.

119. Hannan P, French SA, Story M, Fulkerson JA. A pricing strategy to promote purchase of lower fat foods in a high school cafeteria: acceptability and sensitivity analysis. *Am J Health Promot.* 2002;17:1-6.

120. French SA. Pricing effects on food choices. *J Nutr.* 2003;133:841S-843S.

121. World Health Organization. Technical Report Series. *Diet, Nutrition and the Prevention of Chronic Diseases.* Geneva, Switzerland: WHO; 2003:916.

122. Bridging the Gap. State sales taxes on regular soda. Accessed February 7, 2021. http://bridgingthegapresearch.org/research/sodasnack_taxes/index.html

123. Chriqui JF, Sansone CN, Powell LM. The sweetened beverage tax in Cook County, Illinois: lessons from a failed effort. *Amer J Pub H.* 2020;110:1009-1016. https://doi.org/10.2105/AJPH.2020.305640

124. Falbe J, Grummon AH, Rojas N, Ryan-Ibarra S, Silver LD, Madsen KA. Implementation of the first U.S. sugar-sweetened beverage tax in Berkeley, CA, 2015–2019. *Amer J Pub H.* 2020;110:1429-1437. https://doi.org/10.2105/AJPH.2020.305795

125. Lee NR, Kotler P. *Social marketing: Changing behaviors for good.* Los Angeles: Sage Publications; 2015.

126. Wong FL, Greenwell M, Gates S, Berkowitz JM. It's What You Do!: Reflections on the VERB™ Campaign. *Amer J Prev Med.* 2008;34(6):S175-S182.

127. Office of Women's Health. *Best Bones Forever!.* U.S. Department of Health and Human Services. 2015. Accessed February 7, 2021. https://www.girlshealth.gov/about/best-bones/best-bones.html

128. Abercrombie A, Sawatzki D, Lotenberg LD. Building partnerships to build the Best Bones Forever!: Applying the 4Ps to partnership development. *Soc Mark Q.* 2012;18(1):55-66. https://doi: 10.1177/1524500411435484

129. Sadler MD, Saperstein SL, Golan E, et al. Integrating bone health information into existing health education efforts. *ICAN.* 2013;5(3):177-183. https://doi: 10.1177/1941406413487769

130. Yancey AK, Miles OL, McCarthy WJ, et al. Differential response to targeted recruitment strategies to fitness promotion research by African-American women of varying body mass index. *Ethn Dis.* 2001;11:115-123.

131. Yancey AK, McCarthy WJ, Taylor WC, et al. The Los Angeles Lift Off: a sociocultural environmental change intervention to integrate physical activity into the workplace. *Prev Med.* 2004;38(6):848-856.

132. Ambeba EJ, Ye L, Sereika SM, et al. The use of mHealth to deliver tailored messages reduces reported energy and fat intake. *J Cardiovasc Nurs.* 2015;30(1):35-43.

133. Spark LC, Fjeldsoe BS, Eakin EG, Reeves MM. Efficacy of a text message-delivered extended contact intervention on maintenance of weight loss, physical activity, and dietary behavior change. *JMIR Mhealth Uhealth.* 2015;3(3):e88.

134. Pope JP, Pelletier L, Guertin C. Starting off on the best foot: a review of message framing and message tailoring, and recommendations for the comprehensive messaging strategy for sustained behavior change. *Health Comm.* 2018;33(9):1068-1077.

135. Ballantine PW, Stephenson RJ. Help me, I'm fat! Social support in online weight loss networks. *J Cons Behav.* 2011;10(6):332-337.

136. Dahlin M, Andersson G, Magnusson K, et al. Internet-delivered acceptance-based behavior therapy for generalized anxiety disorder: A randomized controlled trial. *Behav Res Ther.* 2016;77:86-95.

137. Dahl AA, Hales SB, Turner-McGrievy GM. Integrating social media into weight loss interventions. *Curr Opin Psych.* 2016;9:11-15.

PART IV

Promoting the Public's Nutritional Health

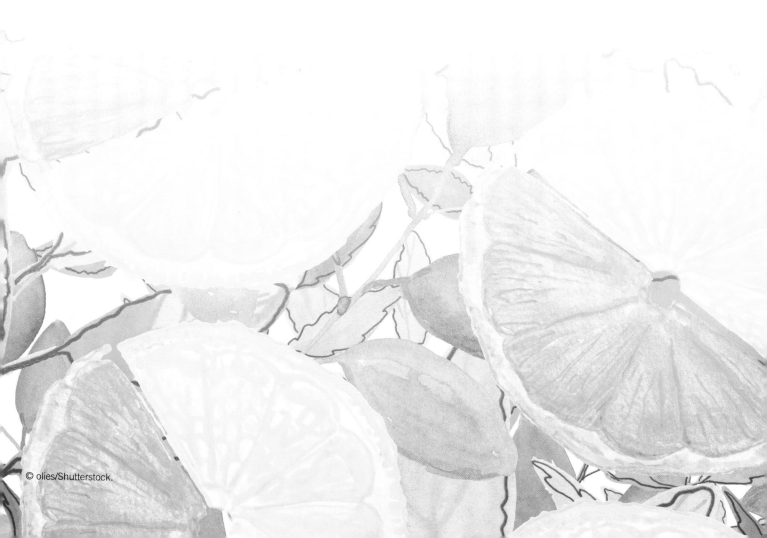

CHAPTER 9

Growing a Healthier Nation: Maternal, Infant, Child, and Adolescent Nutrition with an Emphasis on Childhood Overweight and Health Equity

Meg Bruening, PhD, MPH, RDN

Gabriela Martinez, BS

Molly Jepson, BS

(We would like to acknowledge the work of Shortie McKinney, PhD, RDN, LDN, FADA; Beth Leonberg, MS, RDN, CSP, FADA, LDN; Bonnie Spear, PhD, RDN; Edna Davis, MS, MPH, RDN, LDN; and Inger Stallman, MS, RDN, LDN for their work on past editions of Nutrition in Public Health.)

Learning Outcomes

AFTER STUDYING THIS CHAPTER AND REFLECTING ON THE CONTENTS, YOU SHOULD BE ABLE TO:

1. Discuss the need for community and public health nutrition services for women, infants, children, and adolescents.
2. Identify the health maladies that can occur without community and public health nutrition services in maternal, infant, and child health.
3. Forecast how adolescent mothers may fare in society without community and public health programs.
4. List the growing challenges related to overweight in children.
5. Describe the societal and environmental changes that have contributed to increased nutrition-related health disparities in children and opportunities for community and public health dietitians/nutritionists to address these conditions in children.

Introduction

Ensuring adequate food and nutrition throughout the various stages of growth from prenatal development to adolescence is crucial to lifelong health and optimal functioning. Numerous studies have documented the physiological and mental deficits that can occur when pregnant women, infants, and children are not provided with the nutritional resources and advice they need for optimal health. With medical interventions becoming more sophisticated than ever, society must determine ways to support the provision of nutrition and health care to these vulnerable groups to minimize the strain on our already-overburdened healthcare system. Numerous negative outcomes, such as preterm births, small-for-gestational-age infants, **fetal alcohol syndrome**, gestational diabetes, anemia, obesity, stunting, nutrient deficiencies, and eating disorders, can result when adequate food and nutrition are not provided during pregnancy and the early stages of life.

Pregnancy, infancy, childhood, and adolescence are all life stages in which nutrients are needed for the development of important body systems. For the first time ever, the 2020 Dietary Guidelines for Americans (DGAs) considered the nutritional needs for pregnancy, lactation, and birth to 24 months (all previous versions of the DGAs limited to Americans aged 2 years and older),[1] highlighting the critical dietary needs and the state of the science for these important populations. The behavioral and epigenetic programming that especially occurs during pregnancy, infancy, and early childhood are critical for lifelong health. At the same time, systemic health disparities persist (e.g., increased rates of maternal mortality for black women, increased prevalence of food insecurity for households of color, and those with children), which are especially harmful during these critical life stages. A lens for health equity is needed more than ever in addressing health disparities. Nutrition education and system-level promotion activities are essential for women of childbearing age a time when nutrition education can help promote an optimal environment for a healthy pregnancy, and for children and adolescents to develop positive lifelong eating and exercise habits.

Along with the essential need for optimal nutrition during developmental stages, the nation needs to sharpen its focus on energy balance at all stages of life. The balance between caloric intake and expenditure is out of alignment for many children and adults, leading to overweight and obesity. Despite significant research and an increase in public health focus, the obesity epidemic continues to be a public health issue. The early stages of life from infancy through adolescence are important times to establish positive food and exercise patterns to support a healthy pattern.

Healthy People 2030 Objectives

The *Healthy People (HP) 2030* objectives were established to promote improved health across the nation. Maternal and child health programs provide key interventions to help achieve these objectives.[2] **Table 9–1** lists the HP 2030 objectives that relate to maternal child health: pregnancy, lactation, infancy, childhood, and adolescence, as well as nutrition and weight. The table summarizes selected HP 2030 objectives that relate to Maternal Infant and Child Health (MICH) and Nutrition and Weight Status (NWS) that public health professionals should consider. The HP 2030 Maternal Infant and Child Health objectives listed in Table 9–1 focus on a variety of issues related to healthy pregnancies, infant birth rates, child growth and development, and preventable health consequences during development. The HP 2030 Nutrition and Weight Status (NWS) objectives listed focus on food, nutrition, and weight goals. Most of the nutrition goals listed apply to mothers and children and

Fetal Alcohol Syndrome Mental and physical deficits caused by alcohol intake, primarily during the first trimester.

TABLE 9–1
Healthy People 2030: Selected Maternal, Infant, and Child Health (MICH) and Nutrition and Weight Status (NWS) Goals

Maternal Infant and Child Health	
Women—Baseline only	
MICH-01.	Reduce the rate of fetal deaths at 20 or more weeks of gestation.
MICH-04.	Reduce maternal deaths.
MICH-05.	Reduce severe maternal complications identified during delivery hospitalizations.
MICH-06.	Reduce Cesarean births among low-risk women with no prior births.
MICH-07.	Reduce preterm births.
MICH-08.	Increase the proportion of pregnant women who receive early and adequate prenatal care.
MICH-09.	Increase abstinence from alcohol among pregnant women.
MICH-10.	Increase abstinence from cigarette smoking among pregnant women.
MICH-11.	Increase abstinence from illicit drugs among pregnant women.
MICH-12.	Increase the proportion of women of childbearing age who get enough folic acid.
MICH-13.	Increase the proportion of women who had a healthy weight before pregnancy.
Women—Developmental only	
MICH-D01.	Increase the proportion of women who get screened for postpartum depression.
MICH-D02.	Reduce the proportion of women who use illicit opioids during pregnancy.
Infants—Baseline only	
MICH-02.	Reduce the rate of infant deaths.
MICH-14.	Increase the proportion of infants who are put to sleep on their backs.
MICH-15.	Increase the proportion of infants who are breastfed exclusively through age 6 months.
MICH-16.	Increase the proportion of infants who are breastfed at 1 year.
Infants—Developmental only	
MICH-24.	Increase the proportion of live births that occur in facilities that provide recommended care for lactating mothers and their babies.
Children—Baseline only	
MICH-03.	Reduce the rate of deaths in children and adolescents aged 1 to 19 years.
MICH-17.	Increase the proportion of children who receive a developmental screening.
MICH-18.	Increase the proportion of children with autism spectrum disorder who receive special services by age 4 years.
MICH-19.	Increase the proportion of children and adolescents who receive care in a medical home.
MICH-20.	Increase the proportion of children and adolescents with special healthcare needs who have a system of care.
Nutrition and Weight Status	
Nutrition and Healthy Eating—General—Baseline only	
NWS-01.	Reduce household food insecurity and hunger.
NWS-02.	Eliminate very low food security in children.
NWS-06.	Increase fruit consumption by people aged 2 years and over.

(continues)

TABLE 9–1
Healthy People 2030: Selected Maternal, Infant, and Child Health (MICH) and Nutrition and Weight Status (NWS) Goals   *(continued)*

Nutrition and Weight Status

Nutrition and Healthy Eating—General—Baseline only

NWS-07.	Increase vegetable consumption by people aged 2 years and older.
NWS-08.	Increase consumption of dark green vegetables, red and orange vegetables, and beans and peas by people aged 2 years and over.
NWS-09.	Increase whole grain consumption by people aged 2 years and over.
NWS-10.	Reduce consumption of added sugars by people aged 2 years and over.
NWS-11.	Reduce consumption of saturated fat by people 2 years and over.
NWS-12.	Reduce the consumption of sodium by people aged 2 years and over.
NWS-13.	Increase calcium consumption by people aged 2 years and over.
NWS-14.	Increase potassium consumption by people aged 2 years and over.
NWS-15.	Increased vitamin D consumption by people aged 2 years and over.
NWS-16.	Reduce iron deficiency in children aged 1 to 2 years.

Nutrition and Healthy Eating- Women—Baseline only

NWS-17.	Reduce iron deficiency in females aged 12 to 49 years.

Physical Activity—Overweight and Obesity—Baseline only

NWS-03.	Reduce the proportion of obese adults.
NWS-04.	Reduce the proportion of obese children and adolescents.
NWS-05.	Increase the proportion of healthcare visits by adults with obesity that include counseling on weight loss, nutrition, or physical activity.

U.S. Department of Health and Human Services, *Healthy People 2030*. Available at http://www.healthypeople.gov

Pandemic Learning Opportunity

Imagine the effects of the pandemic on persons already nutrition challenged. What could have been done to prevent more vulnerability in these populations?

their diets, and some objectives specifically address children's issues. Detailed information about the 2030 goals and progress to the goals are available on the Healthy People 2030 website. Many of the goals are quite ambitious and will require organized public health efforts along with the ongoing support of maternal infant and child programs to be successful.

As a result of persistent health disparities, many of the HP goals of the past were not reached, and some categories moved even further away from the target goals; new goals were added to some of these pressing issues. For example, in the HP 2030, goals for food insecurity were introduced. While some of these indicators were showing trajectories of improvement prior to the COVID-19 global pandemic, it is expected that issues like food insecurity and even overweight and obesity among vulnerable populations is likely to drastically increase. These goals provide a unique opportunity to community and public health dietitians/nutritionists to prioritize activities to address social determinants of health and promote health equity, particularly among low-income and underrepresented minority populations.

Maternal Health

The health of the mother is especially important to the health of the child. The nutritional status of the mother before she conceives establishes the quality of the environment in which the fetus will develop and is a key determinant in the life of the newborn. The mother's nutritional health also affects her ability to breastfeed the infant and provide postnatal nurturing. The interconceptional period before the woman becomes pregnant again is vital to the health of both the mother and the next baby she will conceive. If she becomes pregnant too soon after her previous pregnancy or does not have sufficient food intake before she becomes pregnant, she will not be able to replenish her depleted body stores that will put both the mother and the fetus at risk. Beyond pregnancy and infancy, the mother's health impacts her interactions with her family and her ongoing ability to feed her children and provide them with an optimal maternal–child experience as they move to adulthood. Health professionals who work with women of childbearing age have the potential to make significant impacts on the entire society by focusing on ways to improve the health of the mother. This is a global challenge and women in many parts of the world lack access to prenatal care and education.

Preconceptional Period

The preconceptional period is the time before a woman becomes pregnant. Women who are trying to become pregnant are more likely to be aware of their food intake and the importance of nutrition in relation to the success of their eventual pregnancy. But most women are pregnant for 6 to 8 weeks before they know it. This early pregnancy period is especially important in fetal development, and women who have health problems, nutritional deficiencies, or who consume alcohol or illicit drugs have a much higher risk of poor pregnancy outcomes. For this reason, health messages directed at women in the preconceptional period need to focus on information about the importance of a healthy diet before becoming pregnant so any future baby will be healthy. Women are most likely to receive this advice during visits to their gynecologist, family physician, or family planning clinic.

The primary nutrition messages for women in their childbearing years relate to weight management and nutritional and alcohol intake. Women who are at extremes of either underweight or obesity are at a higher risk of delivering preterm or experiencing health problems during pregnancy. For this, as well as other reasons, these women should be advised to maintain their weight in the normal range or at the very least, not to gain additional weight. With increasing numbers of women in the overweight and obese categories, this issue takes on more importance in relation to pregnancy and childbirth. Adequate nutritional intake in the preconceptional period is important to ensure that the woman enters pregnancy with fully replete body stores; this is especially important for women who are in the interconceptional period. Nutrient intake should be kept in the recommended range to avoid both deficiencies and excesses. Women should be evaluated for dietary practices that may put them at increased risk for either. Alcohol intake during the first trimester is associated with higher rates of fetal alcohol syndrome. Because no level of alcohol has been identified as being safe, women should be advised to keep their alcohol intake levels low if they decide to drink alcohol during this time period.

Nutritional Assessment and Intervention During the Preconceptional Period

The following are guidelines for nutritional assessment and intervention for women in their childbearing years that should be conducted by the health professional:

1. Screen and assess women for preconceptional nutritional status. A self-administered questionnaire can be used to collect pertinent

Strategy Tip

How should health professionals counsel women of childbearing ages? What should be included in these counseling classes/sessions?

data, which is then reviewed by a healthcare professional. Criteria for referral to the dietitian can be established.

2. Nutrition information should be provided to all women. Women categorized as healthy and with no nutritional problems can be given a standard pamphlet to review. Women with low-risk problems can be counseled by the healthcare provider who is monitoring her care. Women identified as high risk should be referred to the community or public health dietitian/nutritionist for more intensive nutrition counseling.

3. Specific nutritional guidance should include:
   - Maintaining a healthy weight in the normal Body Mass Index (BMI) range
   - Consuming a healthy diet that meets the Dietary Guidelines
   - Maintaining adequate intake of all nutrients, with special attention to iron, folic acid, calcium, vitamin C, vitamin D, and protein
   - Stopping smoking due to its impact on infant—development
   - Avoiding alcohol
   - Monitoring medical conditions, such as diabetes and hypertension

Prenatal Care

Once a woman learns she is pregnant, she needs to be evaluated and provided with appropriate guidance to assist her in staying healthy and delivering a healthy full-term baby. Nutritional assessment and advice, though similar to the preconceptional period, becomes more precise to the woman's particular status and needs.

Weight Gain

Prepregnancy weight, in conjunction with height, provides the baseline for determining weight gain ranges for the pregnant woman. Recommendations of the Institute of Medicine (IOM), now the National Academy of Science, are based on the BMI of the woman when she became pregnant. Women are placed in one of four categories (underweight, normal weight, overweight, or obese) based on the BMI table. Women in the normal weight category (BMI 18.5–24.9) should gain between 25- and 35-pounds during pregnancy. Underweight women (BMI <18.5) should gain between 28 and 40 pounds. Overweight women (BMI 25–29.9) should gain between 15 and 25 pounds; obese women (BMI ≥30) should gain 11 to 20 pounds. If a woman is carrying twins, she should gain 37 to 54 pounds depending on her prepregnancy weight status.

Once the woman has been placed in a weight category, her weight should be measured and plotted at each prenatal visit. Weight gain should be low during the first trimester (range 2–5 pounds). Weight gains higher than this indicate that too many calories are being consumed. During the second and third trimesters, most women should gain one pound per week, on average. Underweight women should gain slightly more (1—1.3 lb.), and overweight women should gain only two-thirds of a pound weekly. Maternal weight gain is an important factor in reducing the incidence of preterm delivery.[3]

Weight gain components include the fetus, fat stores, extracellular fluid, blood volume, uterus, amniotic fluid, placenta, and breast tissue (listed in order from highest to lowest weight for a term pregnancy). After delivery of a full-term infant weighing 7.5 to 8.5 pounds on average, most mothers will retain 10 to 20 pounds. By 6 weeks postpartum, most women continue to retain 5 to 10 pounds above preconception levels.[4-6]

Although excessive weight gain can be harmful, weight loss and dietary restrictions are not recommended during pregnancy. A woman may be advised to slow her rate of weight gain, but women should never be told to lose weight while pregnant.

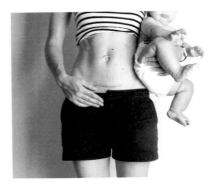

By 6 weeks postpartum, most women continue to retain 5 to 10 pounds above preconception levels.[4-6]

© Troyan/Shutterstock.

Nutrient Intake

In order to support the recommended level of pregnancy weight gain, the pregnant woman needs to eat and drink wisely. Although health professionals know that pregnant women should not "eat for two," many women tend to eat more than advised, leading to extra weight gain. Review of food intake during pregnancy can help the pregnant woman eat the food she needs to maintain a healthy pregnancy and deliver a healthy baby, while ensuring that she does not consume more calories than she needs.

Calories

The Dietary Reference Intakes (DRIs) for pregnant women vary by trimester. The Estimated Energy Requirements (EER) for a woman in the first trimester is the same as a nonpregnant woman due to the low level of additional energy needed to sustain the pregnancy. A pregnant woman needs an additional 340 kcal/day in the second trimester and 452 kcal/day in the third trimester. These calorie goals may need to be adjusted for women who are in the underweight or overweight/obese weight categories.

These additional calories need to be used wisely to ensure that they are nutrient-rich foods that contribute to the other nutrients that need to be consumed in levels higher than for a nonpregnant woman. Recommended intake for nearly all nutrients is higher in pregnancy. Vitamin/mineral supplementation should be evaluated on an individual basis. Supplements cannot replace the combination of nutrients found in food. Some women tend to rely on supplements and are less careful about their food intake. Nutrients that may require supplementation include iron, calcium, and folic acid. Additional nutrients may be indicated in some cases, such as an adolescent or a woman who is carrying multiple fetuses.

Protein

Protein intake is especially important in pregnancy. Growth and development of the fetus, as well as the tissues to support the pregnancy, rely on adequate protein for tissue development. The 2020 DGAs for protein in pregnancy is a total of 71g/protein per day (an additional ~25 g/day) for all three trimesters.[1,5] This level of additional protein is relatively easy for most women to consume. This is a key example of wise food selection. If one cup of nonfat milk is consumed, protein, calcium, vitamin D, and numerous other nutrients are significantly increased with only 100 kcal added to the diet. Dairy products are not appropriate for all women; for example, women with lactose intolerance will need alternate solutions.

Smoking

Smoking cessation should be advocated as part of the nutrition education session. Smoking is totally contraindicated during pregnancy due to the profound impact it has on development of the fetus. Less oxygen is available to the fetus of a mother who smokes, so the baby is likely to be small for gestational age (SGA). SGA babies are at higher risk of complications of birth and have higher rates of problems during the first year of life. Pregnant women who smoke need to be referred to an appropriate smoking cessation program if they are willing to try to stop smoking.

Alcohol

Alcohol abstinence is an essential element of pregnancy. Alcohol is known to cause birth defects and is linked to fetal alcohol syndrome (FAS). Infants born with FAS exhibit numerous permanent developmental problems,

Discussion Prompt

Describe the nutritional stress of a pregnant adolescent. What effects could the fetus experience?

Foetal alcohol syndrome

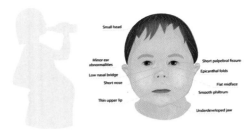

Small head

Minor ear abnormalities

Low nasal bridge

Short nose

Thin upper lip

Short palpebral fissure

Epicanthal folds

Flat midface

Smooth philtrum

Underdeveloped jaw

Fetal alcohol syndrome can also affect facial changes.

© Maniki_rus/Shutterstock.

Strategy Tip

Can a case be made that all pregnant women would benefit from a session with a dietitian/nutritionist? What is the cost? Is the cost worth the potential outcome difference?

including mental retardation. Infants who have been exposed to alcohol in utero may have fetal alcohol effects even if they are not diagnosed with FAS. Most pregnant women willingly abstain from alcohol to eliminate any risk of FAS.

Nutritional Assessment and Intervention in Pregnancy

Professional guidelines for nutritional assessment and intervention in pregnancy include[5]:

1. Screen and assess the nutritional status of pregnant women. A self-administered questionnaire can be used to collect pertinent data, which is then reviewed by a healthcare professional. Criteria for referral to the community and public health dietitian/nutritionist can be established.
2. Nutrition counseling should be provided to all pregnant women. Counseling strategies can be based on:
   - Women categorized as healthy and with no nutritional problems can be provided routine prenatal nutrition advice as part of their routine care.
   - Women with low-risk problems can be counseled by a healthcare provider who is monitoring their care using materials provided by the community and public health dietitian/nutritionist.
   - Women identified as high risk should be referred to the dietitian/nutritionist for more intensive nutrition counseling. High-risk women may include those who are not gaining sufficient weight; those who are gaining excessive amounts of weight; women with preexisting health conditions, such as diabetes, who require dietary intervention; and women who develop diseases requiring nutrition advice.
3. Specific nutritional guidance for women during pregnancy can include:
   - Maintaining a healthy weight gain as appropriate for her BMI category. Weight should be plotted at every prenatal visit to monitor growth.
   - Increasing calorie and protein intake during the second and third trimesters.
   - Consuming a healthy diet that meets the Dietary Guidelines. Emphasis should be placed on fruits and vegetables, whole grains, dairy products, and protein foods.
   - Maintaining adequate intake of all nutrients, with special attention to iron, folic acid, calcium, vitamin C, vitamin D, and protein. Supplements should be recommended if needed.
   - Maintaining physical activity as advised.
   - Consuming adequate amounts of fluid.
   - Stopping smoking due to its impact on infant development.
   - Abstaining from alcohol.
   - Learning about infant feeding methods; strong consideration should be given to breastfeeding with an emphasis on the benefits for both the mother and the baby.
   - Monitoring medical conditions, such as diabetes and hypertension.
   - Providing nutrition intervention as needed.

Special Conditions

Adolescent Pregnancy

Recommended weight gains during pregnancy may be slightly higher for the teenager than for the adult.[6] The current recommendation is that pregnant adolescents should gain weight within the upper range of that currently recommended for adults (i.e., 30–35 lb.).[7] For adolescents with a below-normal, prepregnancy weight, a 35- to 40-lb weight gain may be desirable.[5,7]

Pregnant adolescents who are of young gynecologic age (the number of years between the onset of menses and the date of conception) or who are undernourished at the time of conception have the greatest nutritional needs. A young woman who conceives soon after her first menstrual period is at greatest physiologic risk. It was once thought that adolescents with advanced physiologic maturity had no more physical complications during pregnancy than adult women, but the Camden Study[8] showed that both adolescents and their infants are at increased risk. This **longitudinal study** sought to explain why, with increasing maternal weight gains in adolescent mothers, the infant birth weights remained low. This increased risk of fetal growth restriction may be attributed to disruption in fetal-placental blood flow and in the transmission of nutrients to the fetus as a result of the physiology associated with maternal growth.

Longitudinal studies The researcher follows a cohort of subjects over time, performing repeated measurements at prescribed intervals.

Aside from the consequences to the outcome of pregnancy, adolescents who begin their childbearing early (while still growing themselves) may be at particular risk for overweight and obesity. The Camden Study[9] has documented that the excessive accrual of subcutaneous fat stores at central body sites often leads to the development of cardiovascular disease, non–insulin-dependent diabetes mellitus, and hypertension later in life.

A clinically practical method of ensuring nutritional adequacy is to encourage the pregnant adolescent to gain the recommended amount of weight by consuming nutrient-rich foods. Most important, contact with health professionals during prenatal care provides the opportunity to teach adolescents about feeding themselves and their families.[7] Because of the frequency of economic instability of the pregnant adolescent, it is impossible to assume that she will have an adequate food supply. Health professionals can help provide access to and information about resources, such as the Supplemental Nutrition Assistance Program (SNAP), food banks, and the Special Supplemental Nutrition Program for Women, Infants and Children (WIC Program).

Gestational Diabetes

Gestational diabetes is a form of diabetes that develops in some women when they become pregnant but resolves once the pregnancy ends. Many of these women will go on to have type 2 diabetes later in life, particularly if they become obese. Gestational diabetes can have harmful effects on both the mother and the infant. The mother has an increased risk of **preeclampsia** and delivering by Cesarean section. Infants born to women with all types of diabetes have a higher risk of becoming too large in utero (macrosomia: weighing more than 10 pounds). The infant is also at higher risk to be stillborn, to have hypoglycemia at birth, and to develop hypertension, diabetes, and obesity as an adult.

Preeclampsia A hypertensive disorder of pregnancy that is characterized by the presence of protein in the urine and swelling, putting both mother and infant in danger.

Women in moderate- to high-risk categories need to be screened for gestational diabetes using a glucose tolerance test. This is usually done by weeks 24 to 27 of the pregnancy. Once diagnosed, an intervention plan is developed to bring the diabetes under control. Interventions generally start with diet and exercise and move to include medications as necessary to control blood glucose levels. Women with gestational diabetes need to be counseled and monitored by a community dietitian/nutritionist.[5]

Opioids

Opioids are a class of prescription drugs that are typically prescribed initially for pain relief. Commonly known prescription medications within this class include OxyContin, Percocet, Vicodin, and morphine. These substances are highly addictive and have contributed to an increase in dependence on the drug after the recommended treatment period has ended. Drugs such as heroin and fentanyl have been described to have similar effects as prescription drugs. It has been estimated by the Centers for Disease Control and Prevention (CDC) that 14–22% of pregnant women filled a prescription for an opioid.[10] The current standard treatment for pregnant women who are taking opioids is methadone maintenance treatment. Methadone is an opioid replacement prescription medication that serves to reduce withdrawal symptoms and reduces cravings. Pregnant women who take methadone while pregnant will reduce risk of birth defects and maternal mortality during childbirth.[11]

Opioids impact the gastrointestinal system directly, impacting nutrient absorption, especially the essential vitamins and minerals needed to maintain proper nutritional status for pregnancy. There is a lack of literature regarding the nutritional needs of pregnant women who are receiving methadone treatment. A pilot study conducted found lower total levels of plasma folate, serum β-tocopherol, and lycopene, docosahexaenoic acid (DHA) and eicosapentaenoic acid (EPA), and higher levels of plasma homocysteine compared with non–methadone-using pregnant women.[12]

Infancy

The infant's first 12 months of life are a critical period for establishing health and health-related habits. Key issues include the parent's decision to breastfeed or formula feed; monitoring growth and development; introducing appropriate complementary foods when the infant is developmentally ready; and providing adequate amounts of key nutrients such as vitamin D, iron, and fluoride. This section provides an overview of these key issues and describes several initiatives aimed at helping infants to get a good start.

Breastfeeding

Breast milk is the undisputed optimal food for both term and pre-term newborn infants.[13] The unique characteristics of breast milk and breastfeeding confer many advantages, including health, nutritional, immunological, developmental, psychological, social, economic, and environmental benefits. The American Academy of Pediatrics (AAP) Breastfeeding Working Group,[14] Academy of Nutrition and Dietetics (AND),[15] and World Health Organization[16] (WHO) support exclusive breastfeeding of infants for the first 6 months. The AAP further recommends that breastfeeding be continued for the first 12 months and beyond for as long as it is mutually desired by the mother and the toddler.

Breastfeeding rates continue an upward trajectory in the United States. In 2010, 76.7% of mothers initiated breastfeeding and 47.5% continued to breastfeed at six months.[17,18] The HP 2020 goals targeted 81.9% initiation of breastfeeding and the 2017 level was 84.1%, with 58.3% continuing to breastfeed at 6 months and 35.3% continuing to breastfeed at 12 months.[19]

Achievement of the ambitious goals of 2020 is an indication of the positive efforts to promote breastfeeding. Rates of breastfeeding are different across demographic groups within the United States. Mothers who are less educated, single, adolescents, have other children, work, or are African American may be less likely to breastfeed. The latest Breastfeeding Report Card revealed that African American infants are less likely to ever be breastfed (73.7%) compared with White (86.7%) and Hispanic infants (84.1%). The report also found that infants who were eligible and participating in WIC's (Women, Infant and Children) Special Supplemental Nutrition Program were less likely to ever be breastfed (77%) compared with infants who were ineligible to participate in WIC (92.1%).[20] Check the Breastfeeding Report Card website for current national and state differences. The report card is updated every 2 years.

Research has demonstrated that exclusive breastfeeding can meet the nutrient needs of infants through the first 6 months. There are very few instances in which breast milk and/or breastfeeding are not recommended.[21] These include infants with **galactosemia** or certain other metabolic disorders, infants whose mothers abuse illegal drugs, or those mothers with certain other medical conditions, as recommended by the infant's pediatrician. In the United States, breastfeeding is not recommended for infants of mothers with human immunodeficiency virus (HIV).

New mothers returning to work may decide against breastfeeding or may nurse their infants for only a very limited time because of the real and/or perceived obstacles involved with breastfeeding their infants while holding a job. This is unfortunate, as breast milk is the ideal food for infants. However, all mothers should be encouraged to breastfeed for any length of time that they are willing to do so.

Some reports indicate that women who breastfeed are able to lose fat tissue more readily than women who formula-feed their infants,[22] but a systematic review was not able to confirm this hypothesis.[23] Appropriate strategies should be used to help mothers to lose the weight gain of pregnancy. Postpartum weight retention contributes to the high nationwide obesity rates for women.

Nutritional Needs to Support Breastfeeding

Lactation requires excess energy (~500 kcal/day for the first 6 months) to produce breast milk.[24] Like pregnancy, there are additional nutrient needs for lactation such as protein, vitamin C, most B vitamins, vitamin E, zinc, iodine, and selenium.[25] Some have promoted breastfeeding as a mechanism for women to quickly return to prepregnancy weight, especially when paired with a healthy diet. However, the 2020 Dietary Guidelines Advisory Committee concluded that there was not sufficient evidence to link dietary patterns during lactation and postpartum weight loss.[26]

Potential Benefits of Breastfeeding to Child Weight Status

Evidence is emerging that breastfeeding may offer some protection against obesity.[27-29] Proposed mechanisms for this effect include more normal growth patterns (lower early weight gain) possibly associated with lower basal insulin levels in the breastfed infant compared with an infant-fed formula, and the inherent control of food intake maintained by the breastfed infant.[30] Breastfeeding on demand as opposed to on schedule is thought to teach infants to regulate their intakes appropriately, based on internal cues for hunger and satiety and in response to their individual growth needs.[31] Formula-fed infants may have fewer opportunities to develop this important skill, perhaps because parents or caregivers want to follow a set feeding schedule or encourage the

Galactosemia Digestive problem resulting from absence of the enzyme that breaks down galactose.

Discussion Prompt

Describe the many benefits of breastfeeding. Why is there an outlash against it in some public places?

baby to consume a certain amount of formula. Both of these feeding behaviors override the infant's internal cues and may result in overfeeding and lessening of the infant's ability to self-regulate energy intake.[30]

A literature review by the WHO concluded that breastfeeding conferred a small protection against overweight later in life.[28] A 2020 multinational, cross-sectional study conducted by Ma et al., found that breastfeeding is significantly associated with decreasing obesity risk in children aged 9–11 years in 12 countries (including the United States).[32] Differences in the nutritional content of infant formula compared with breast milk may contribute to breastfeeding being protective against overweight. Breast milk nutritional content changes over time so that it contains less protein after the first few months when the infant's need for protein is less. It is thought that the more rapid gains in weight and length from about 2 months of age to the end of the first year of life of formula-fed infants may be due to the higher protein content of formula that exceeds the infant's needs after about 1–2 months of age. Differences in adiposity appear only at about 12 months when evidence suggests that breastfed infants are leaner than formula-fed infants.[33]

Strategies to Promote Breastfeeding

Because breastfeeding may be an early intervention to prevent childhood obesity, breastfeeding promotion should occur in various settings. Community and public health dietitians/nutritionists could consider the following listed projects. These initiatives support the HP 2030 objectives related to increasing the proportion of women who breastfeed their babies.[2,34]

Coalition An alliance, sometimes temporary, of people, factions, or parties.

- Develop a breastfeeding **coalition** that focuses on developing breastfeeding policies at worksites, hospitals, or public areas. In addition, coalition members may monitor and evaluate the interventions implemented.
- Collaborate with partners or participate in coalitions to increase breastfeeding awareness and promotion through World Breastfeeding Week, health fairs, or other community events.
- Train other dietitians/nutritionists, nurses, doctors, or other medical professionals on breastfeeding management and support ways to increase breastfeeding initiation and duration rates.
- In a clinical setting, a public health dietitian/nutritionist may provide one-on-one breastfeeding education, counseling, and support of pregnant and lactating women to increase the breastfeeding initiation and duration rates.

Formula Feeding

Infant formula is the appropriate food for infants who are not breastfed and for infants who are weaned from the breast before 12 months. Infant formulas sold in the United States must meet safety and nutritional guidelines that are established and updated periodically by the U.S. Food and Drug Administration.[34] The WHO International Code of Marketing of Breast-milk Substitutes recommends that infant formulas should not be advertised or promoted to the general public and that manufacturers should not provide samples of products to pregnant women, mothers, or members of their family.[35] In agreement, the AAP has stated their disapproval of direct advertising because it may negatively impact breastfeeding initiation or continuation.[36] Some hospitals continue the practice of providing a starter package of formula to new mothers when they leave the hospital. Community and public health dietitians/nutritionists should consider this an opportunity to educate professionals and leadership in the facility about the disadvantages of promoting formula feeding.

Infant formulas are available as ready-to-feed liquid, or as concentrated liquid or powder to which water must be added. These products tend to be a costly item for mothers on limited resources. The majority of infant formulas are made from modified cow milk; however, soy-based and specialty formulas designed for medical conditions are also available. Cow milk-based infant formulas are available either as iron-fortified or low iron. Both the AAP and the CDC recommend that infants less than 12 months old be fed only iron-fortified infant formula.[36,37]

Soy-based formulas are appropriate for infants with galactosemia, hereditary lactase deficiency, documented lactose intolerance following acute gastroenteritis, and for vegetarian infants. However, the routine use of soy-based formulas has not been demonstrated to be effective in preventing or managing colic or in preventing the development of food allergies and is not appropriate for preterm infants.[38] Infants who develop symptoms of food allergies may benefit from using a soy-based formula or a hypoallergenic formula in which the protein is partially or totally hydrolyzed.[38,39]

Infant Growth and Development

Infancy is a period of rapid growth and development. Most infants double their birth weight by the 6th month and triple it by the 12th month.[40] However, there are normal differences in growth between healthy breastfed and formula-fed infants during the first 6 months of life. Breastfed infants tend to gain weight more rapidly than formula-fed infants in the first 3 months, but less rapidly from 3 to 12 months; these differences in weight gain and growth tend to disappear in the second year.[41]

Growth can best be assessed by plotting weight and length for age, and weight for length on an appropriate National Center for Health Statistics Growth Chart. These charts have been constructed using data from large population groups over time and are a way to assess an individual's growth against group norms. However, each infant will establish and follow his or her own growth curve.[42]

Rapid development during the first year is responsible for the infant changing from a newborn who needs head support to feed and is capable of a simple suck-swallow-breathe pattern during feeding, to an older infant who can easily feed herself with her fingers and can drink from a cup. The Start Healthy Feeding Plan reflects an evaluation of many years of research and graphically represents the advancement of developmental and feeding skills throughout infancy.[43]

Healthcare providers can monitor growth and development by comparing an infant's progress using these tools. Periodic visits allow the provider to establish a relationship with the infant and his caregivers, through which a dialogue can be held. At the appropriate times, questions about the child's development and feeding will provide the basis for anticipatory guidance or counseling to help provide a smooth transition between developmental stages as the child grows.[44]

Complementary Foods

Most infants are developmentally ready for the introduction of complementary foods and beverages by 4 to 6 months. Parents need to make wise decisions about which foods and beverages to give to their children.

See The Start Healthy Eating Plan at: https://www.cdc.gov/healthyweight /healthy_eating/index.html

See what beverages to offer toddlers at: https://www.cdc.gov/nutrition /infantandtoddlernutrition/foods-and -drinks/foods-and-drinks-to-encourage .html

Solid Food

In the United States, an infant's first solid food is typically an iron-fortified, single-ingredient (rice) infant cereal. The 2020–2025 Dietary Guidelines affirm that iron is an important source for breastfed infants by 6 months in meeting daily requirements.[1] This can be provided by iron-fortified infant cereal and later by meats. Following cereal, single-ingredient pureed fruits and vegetables are offered to the infant, with at least 2 to 4 days between introductions of each new food. Whether fruits or vegetables should be offered first has long been a subject of debate, but a review of the literature indicates the order in which they are introduced isn't critical.[45] It is well-established that it can take 10 to 15 exposures to a new food for it to be accepted by an infant or toddler, and parents should be encouraged to present the food repeatedly to encourage acceptance.[45,46]

Juice

Juice manufacturers have successfully marketed 100% fruit juice as a healthy beverage. However, some fruit juices, such as prune, apple, and pear, contain a significant amount of sorbitol (a sugar alcohol) and proportionally more fructose than glucose. Infants can only absorb a portion of the sorbitol (as little as 10%) and fructose in these juices.[47] The unabsorbed carbohydrate is fermented in the lower intestine, causing diarrhea, abdominal pain, or bloating. These symptoms are commonly reported in infants and toddlers who drink excessive amounts of juice.

The AAP has concluded that fruit juice offers no nutritional benefit for infants younger than 6 months and no benefit over whole fruits for infants older than 6 months. They recommend that juice not be introduced to infants before 1 year old, should not be given in a bottle or easily transported covered cup, should not be given at nap- or bedtime, and should be limited to 4 to 6 ounces daily for infants and children up to 6 years old.[48] Unfortunately, many infants and children receive more juice than recommended. The caloric load of juice may have an impact on development of lifelong preference for sweet beverages.

Important Nutrients in Infancy

Infants need a full complement of nutrients starting from calories and protein and moving through all of the essential vitamins and minerals. Additional background on all nutrient requirements for infants can be obtained from the AAP. Described below are three elements that are of special concern.

Vitamin D

Rickets is a disease of vitamin D and/or calcium deficiency, characterized in infants by poor bone growth leading to bowing of the legs. Although the incidence of rickets in developed countries is very low, cases have continued to be reported regularly over the last 20 years. Most cases have occurred in breastfed infants of dark-skinned mothers who had minimal exposure to sunlight[49-51] and in toddlers on vegetarian diets.[52] Although rickets can be prevented by regular exposure to sunlight, increasing concern over the long-term effects of early sun exposure on the development of skin cancer have led to new recommendations for vitamin D supplementation of all infants. The AAP now recommends that all breast-fed infants receive 400 IU of vitamin D daily.[52] They further recommend that formula-fed infants who consume less than 1 L of formula daily receive 400 IU vitamin D daily in an alternative way.

Iron

Iron deficiency anemia in infancy has been associated with significant developmental deficits, including language difficulties, poor motor skills and balance, and poor attention, responsiveness, and mood, which may be only partially reversible with subsequent supplementation.[53] Fetal iron stores are exhausted by 4 to 6 months of age, making it necessary that iron be supplied by the diet.[21] This need corresponds well with the introduction of high-iron complementary foods, such as iron-fortified infant formula, iron-fortified infant cereals, and/or meats. The AAP recommends that full-term breastfed infants need a supplemental source of iron beginning at 4 to 6 months and that only iron-fortified formula should be used for weaning or supplementing breast milk for infants up to 12 months. The immature gastrointestinal (GI) tract of infants is unable to digest and absorb cow's milk during the first year, and its ingestion is responsible for GI blood loss leading to anemia.[54,55] The AAP recommends the avoidance of regular cow, goat, or soy milk for the milk-based part of the diet before 12 months of age.[21]

Fluoride

Exposure to appropriate levels of fluoride is effective in reducing the prevalence of dental caries. Most public water supplies are fluoridated to provide 0.7–1.2 ppm of fluoride. The need for fluoride supplementation depends on the total amount of fluoride available to the infant from all sources, including infant formula, water, and commercial and home-prepared baby foods. Breast milk contains little fluoride, even in areas with fluoridated water.[56] The amount of fluoride in commercial concentrated or powdered infant formula depends on the amount of fluoride in the formula and in the water used for mixing. Infants fed formula made with fluoridated water may receive up to 1.0 mg/day of fluoride.[57] Ready-to-feed infant formulas are manufactured with nonfluoridated water. The AAP, the American Academy of Pediatric Dentistry, and the CDC recommend no fluoride supplementation for infants less than 6 months old.[57-59] For infants older than 6 months whose community drinking water contains 0.3 ppm fluoride, they recommend supplementation of 0.25 mg sodium fluoride/day.

Nutritional Assessment and Intervention in Infancy

Guidelines for nutritional assessment and intervention in infancy are recommended in the following steps.

Birth to 6 months:

1. Breastfeed for the first 4–6 months. Supplement with iron and vitamin D.
2. If breastfeeding is not selected, provide a fortified infant formula that approximates breast milk. Ensure that the formula is prepared under sanitary conditions and according to directions.
3. Begin complementary foods when the infant is developmentally ready.
4. Measure length and weight growth status and plot on NCHS growth charts.

Six months to 1 year:

1. Continue breast milk or formula.
2. Continue to introduce foods as directed by pediatrician or dietitian/nutritionist.
3. Include infant in family meals.
4. Provide finger foods and child-sized utensils to encourage self-feeding.

Discussion Prompt

How is your dental health? Can you assess whether you grew up in a fluoridated area or had fluoride supplementation as an infant from your dental history?

5. Measure length and weight growth status and plot on NCHS growth charts.
6. Provide opportunities to develop physical abilities.
7. Refer to WIC when indicated.
8. Provide appropriate care for disease or other health conditions.

Access the growth charts at: https://www.cdc.gov/growthcharts/index.htm

Childhood and Adolescence

Beyond infancy, children move through various stages of growth and development on their journey to becoming young adults. Each age level has different nutrient needs. Toddlers have a slower growth rate that continues through childhood until the growth spurt of adolescence starts. Children also move from being dependent on parents to provide healthy food choices to making all of their own food choices when they are in late adolescence. An important role for parents and other caregivers is to provide a wide variety of healthy foods and let the children decide which foods and the amount to eat. Mealtime struggles can create an unpleasant environment for everyone and do little to encourage children to a variety of foods. This period from early childhood through adolescence is very important for establishing a balance between food intake and physical activity that promotes a healthy weight throughout childhood and into young adulthood.

Nutrient Requirements for Children and Adolescents

Children and adolescents require a full complement of macro- and micronutrients as they move through their developmental years. In this chapter, the focus will be on the major nutrients that may put children at risk. Focus will be on those nutrients and food and beverage components that can be impacted by community and public health nutrition programs and professionals. Additional background on all nutrient requirements can be obtained from governmental sources such as the USDA and the CDC.

Energy

Energy requirements are designed to maintain health, promote optimal growth and maturation, and support a desirable level of physical activity. Children who limit energy intake or have food security issues that limit energy intake may limit ultimate adult growth. In 2002, the National Academy of Sciences released new guidelines for energy requirements (access at www.nap.org). Estimated Energy Requirements (EER) are based on energy expenditure, requirements for growth, and level of physical activity. Variability in the EER exists for both males and females because of variations in growth rate and physical activity.

Protein

Protein needs, like those for energy, correlate more closely with the growth pattern than with chronological age. The Dietary Reference Intakes for protein are based on the amount of protein needed for growth and positive nitrogen balance.[24] The DRIs provide for both the Estimated Average Requirements (EAR) and the Recommended Dietary Allowances (RDA). The DRIs recommend using the EAR when assessing nutrient intakes of groups. The EAR provides for adequate intake of 50% of the population. The RDA is recommended for assessing the intake of an individual. Average intakes of protein for adolescents are well above the RDA for all age groups. There is little evidence to show that insufficient protein intake is common in the adolescent population.

If energy intake is inadequate for any reason (i.e., food security issues, chronic illness, or attempts to lose weight), dietary protein may be used to meet energy needs and will, therefore, be unavailable for synthesis of new tissue or for tissue repair. This may result in a state of insufficient protein, which will lead to a reduction in growth rate and a decrease in lean body mass. When children or adolescents voluntarily restrict calories in an effort to control weight, the impact can be harmful, especially when protein sources are used to meet energy needs. Conversely, a high protein intake can interfere with calcium metabolism as well as increase fluid needs.

Minerals and Vitamins

Micronutrients (vitamins and minerals) play an important role in the growth and health of all children and adolescents. Fruits and vegetables are the major contributors to vitamin and mineral intake. Because of the many health benefits associated with fruits and vegetables, national recommendations support increased consumption of these foods. The U.S. 2020 Dietary Guidelines for Americans recommended 2 cups of fruit and 2½ cups of vegetables per day and focuses on increasing variety (i.e., dark green, red and orange, legumes, whole fruit) in addition to quantity.[1] Unfortunately, many children and adolescents do not consume that level of fruits and vegetables (CDC).

Despite the low levels of fruits and vegetables, most children get sufficient amounts of vitamins and minerals until they reach adolescence, when requirements increase dramatically due to growth demands. Because of increased energy demands during this period, increased quantities of thiamine, riboflavin, and niacin are required for the release of energy from carbohydrates. With tissue synthesis, there is an increased demand for vitamin B_6, folic acid, and vitamin B_{12}. There is also an increased requirement for vitamin D (for rapid skeletal growth), and vitamins A, C, and E are needed for new cell growth.

Calcium

Because of accelerated muscular, skeletal, and endocrine development, calcium needs are greater during puberty and adolescence than in childhood or during the adult years. At the peak of the growth spurt, the daily deposition of calcium can be twice that of the average during the rest of the adolescent period. In fact, 45% of the skeletal mass is added during adolescence.[60]

Some evidence suggests a role for calcium in modulating body fat.[61] National Health and Nutrition Examination Survey (NHANES) III data showed an inverse relationship between calcium and BMI, indicating that individuals with higher calcium intake had lower BMIs.[62] The results from several studies are not definitive.[63] With no disadvantages to increasing calcium intake, even the slightest decrease in body fat could help in preventing comorbidities associated with overweight/obesity.[64]

Iron

Iron is a key indicator nutrient throughout childhood and adolescence. Iron deficiency anemia is fairly common, with 4–7% of children exhibiting low hemoglobin and hematocrit. During adolescence, iron requirements are increased. Dallmon (1989) noted that in boys, there is a sharp increase in the requirements for iron from approximately 10 to 15 mg/day.[65] After the growth spurt and sexual maturation, growth increases rapidly and so does the need for iron. In girls with marginal intakes, iron deficiency anemia may result from growth demands. Conversely, iron deficiency may be a limiting factor for growth during adolescence. Additionally, anemia in adolescence may impair the immune response. Adolescent girls, who typically have lower caloric intakes than boys, may have more difficulty in obtaining adequate levels of iron from their diets. Iron deficiency is prevalent in adolescents of both genders and in teens of all ethnicities and socioeconomic levels. In its recommendations to prevent and control iron deficiency in the United States, the CDC includes guidelines for prevention, screening, and treatment of iron-deficiency anemia.[37]

Assessment of Growth and Weight Status

Growth assessment is the best way to determine if children are well nourished. When children are getting enough to eat and do not have health problems, they should be growing normally. Plotting height (or length for very young children) and weight on the NCHS standardized growth charts can help determine if a child's growth is appropriate.

Weight and height can be plotted on growth grids to determine whether individuals are maintaining their growth pattern or growth channel. The relationship between weight and height can be evaluated by using the CDC/NCHS BMI tables. Appropriate weights for height, according to age and sex, lie between the 10th and 85th percentiles, a range that allows for individual differences in body build.[44]

Use of BMI, which is highly correlated with body fatness, can also indicate weight status. BMI is calculated by dividing body weight (expressed in kilograms) by the square of height (in meters), that is, BMI 5 kg/m^2. Children with BMIs below the fifth percentile should be assessed for organic diseases or eating disorders. Children with BMIs between the 85th and 95th percentiles are at risk for overweight, and a nutritional screening/assessment should be performed to determine health risk. Children with BMIs at the 95th percentile for age and gender are overweight and should have an in-depth medical assessment[64] that includes data on family history, blood pressure, total cholesterol level, any major change in BMI, and concern about weight.[44,66]

A skinfold evaluation yields a further degree of precision. For example, a low skinfold measurement in an individual who is above the 85th percentile BMI indicates a state of being overweight, but not overfat. An assessment of muscle and arm circumference can confirm the muscular composition. However, a skinfold in the 90th percentile or greater with a BMI greater than the 95th percentile suggests overfat or truly overweight.[66]

Excessive or less-than-normal growth can be detected by plotting height changes on the CDC growth charts.[42] The major cause of short stature during adolescence is genetically late initiation of puberty, although other conditions, such as chronic disease or skeletal and chromosomal abnormalities, can also account for certain children being shorter than normal. Hormonal imbalances leading to abnormal growth are rare.

In the pediatric population, the body mass index (BMI) is used as a screening tool and is not a diagnosis for overweight in children. The CDC has revised and published growth charts for children 2 to 20 years of age in 2000: BMI-for-Age, Weight-for-Age, and Stature-for-Age. The BMI-for-Age nutrition status indicators for children classified as Overweight are ≥85th percentile to <95th percentile and for Obese in the ≥95th percentile.[67] Study results have found that many children with overweight will become obese adults.[68,69] However, the BMI-for-Age assessment should be applied carefully so as not to label children as with overweight or obese in error. It is important to determine whether a child indeed has extra fat mass and not extra muscle mass, particularly across genders and ethnicity.[70,71]

Access the growth charts at: https://www.cdc.gov/growthcharts/index.htm

Access Body Mass Index charts at: https://www.nhlbi.nih.gov/health/educational/lose_wt/BMI/bmicalc.htm

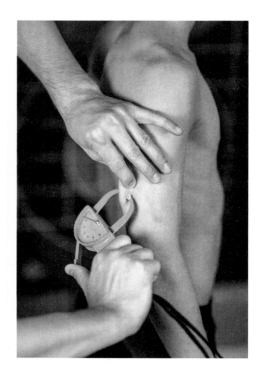

Skinfold evaluation, when performed correctly, can indicate degree of body fat.

© Microgen/Shutterstock.

The terms *at-risk for overweight* and *overweight* were the classification terms previously used by the CDC; *at-risk for obesity* and *obese* are terms used in the childhood overweight literature. The use of different terms may have contributed to some difficulty in interpreting and comparing data from different studies and countries. The term *at-risk for overweight* was sometimes erroneously understood to mean that the child was at risk for becoming overweight/obese in the future, when it actually referred to a child who might be obese with regard to having excess body fat, but who should undergo a second-level screen for a more in-depth assessment.[67] However, four terms—at-risk for overweight, overweight, obese, and obesity—are used throughout publications on the issue of overweight in children, and sometimes the two sets of terms are synonymous and at other times they have different meanings. Both sets of terms will be used throughout the chapter and when citing other literature to reflect the meaning intended by the original author.

Weight status is a single indicator, and it is critical not to focus on weight alone. Research has consistently shown that conversations about weight with children are related to unhealthy weight control behaviors and potentially disordered eating.[72,73] Public health nutrition professionals should focus on the creation of healthy eating environments and promote healthy eating and physical activity behaviors to promote better lifelong health for children.

School-based Weight Screening

In response to the increasing epidemic of childhood obesity across the nation, many state and local governments have implemented programs to measure children's growth and educate and inform parents about their child's weight status. These screening programs are designed to provide a process by which parents of high-risk children are:

- Informed about their child's risk of overweight
- Educated on the risks of childhood overweight on health
- Referred for available community and school-based interventions

While screening programs were initially thought of as a way to identify youth who needed more support to maintain a healthy weight, research has demonstrated that a screening program alone has no effect on children's weight status.[74] Screening programs provide a way for parents and children to more easily access the needed resources to address childhood overweight in an effective manner and facilitate collaboration between school, family, primary-care providers, and interested community partners.

BMI measurement screening programs can be controversial.[75] Although many states have developed policies to require screening of children's weight status, many others do not have policies. In response to a request from the IOM, the CDC developed a report to guide states and schools in developing BMI screening programs. The key guidance provided was concerned about the potential risk of harming students and included the following points: "introduce the program to school staff and community members and obtain parental consent, train staff in administering the program (ideally, implementation will be led by a highly qualified staff member, such as the school nurse or dietitian), establish safeguards to protect student privacy, obtain and use accurate equipment, accurately calculate and interpret the data, develop efficient data collection procedures, avoid using BMI results to evaluate student or teacher performance, and regularly evaluate the program and its intended outcomes and unintended consequences."

Discussion Prompt

Describe the lifelong effects of both undernutrition and obesity in childhood.

Strategy Tip

Discuss the benefits of having a dietitian in the school system for nutrition referrals.

Early Childhood Specifics

After the rapid growth of infancy, the toddler and preschool child's growth slows. Toddlers (age 1–3) gain about half a pound and grow ¼ inch to ½ inch per month. Preschool children gain about 4 to 5 pounds and grow 2 inches per year. Children generally lose some of the body fat that they accumulate as an infant, their bodies elongate, and they begin to look more like children. All baby teeth should be in place by age 2. Brain development continues to be important, with brain growth 75% complete by age 2, and attaining adult size during the elementary school years.

Total energy needs continue to increase to support body maintenance and a slow rate of growth, but calories per kilogram declines until the growth spurt of adolescence. Along with the gradual increase in total calories, the need for protein, vitamins, and minerals also increases.

Eating Patterns

Young children develop lifelong eating patterns in response to the food environment in which they live. This is easily demonstrated by the diverse foods eaten by children of different cultures. Children learn to prefer the foods that they are exposed to at mealtimes. Parents and other adults have an important role to play as food and nutrition gatekeepers by ensuring that a wide variety of nutritious foods are served. Foods rejected by children should continue to be offered on other occasions. Children are naturally neophobic about new foods, and frequency of exposure to food promotes increased preference. Food choices of other children in the home or in childcare settings also influence what children like to eat. Children often go on food jags where they want to eat the same foods; fortunately, these periods generally don't last long enough to impact their nutritional intake. Families need to take care in encouraging children to try new foods and to help ensure that children enjoy a wide diversity of foods. All children should be encouraged to eat the same foods as the rest of the family.

Young children respond well to small frequent meals; snacks contribute as much as 20% of daily calories. Portion sizes need to be kept in balance with the child's appetite. Children like foods with interesting shapes, colors, and contrasting temperatures. Foods that might cause choking if swallowed whole, such as grapes, popcorn, hard candy, and hot dogs, should be avoided. Added sugars should be avoided among young children. Parents and caregivers can help promote a healthy variety of food choices by maintaining a positive attitude toward food and minimizing mealtime conflicts.[76]

Nutritional Assessment and Intervention in Early Childhood

Guidelines for nutritional assessment and intervention in early childhood, ages 1 to 5, may include the following:

1. Screen and assess growth status and plot on NCHS growth charts.
2. Provide a wide variety of healthy foods with emphasis on nutritious choices such as whole grains, fruits, vegetables, dairy foods, and lean meats and protein alternatives.
3. Continue to serve new foods even if not initially preferred.
4. Avoid using food as a reward or punishment.
5. Provide opportunities for physical activity through active play.
6. Avoid low nutrient-dense foods as snack choices.
7. Evaluate nutrition services in childcare facilities to ensure that standards are met.

8. Provide appropriate care for disease or other health conditions.
9. Teach children to wash their hands before eating.

Childcare Programs

The majority of parents in the United States have jobs outside of the home, which means that many children are in childcare programs during the pre-school years. Generally, these programs provide some level of food service to the children they serve. AND's position paper on childcare programs recommends that childcare menus provide one-third of a child's nutritional requirements in the meals and snacks provided.[76] This report indicated benchmarks to promote the development of healthy eating behaviors in this early life stage. Specifically, it was recommended that early childcare centers should:

1. Serve a variety of healthy foods in appropriate portion sizes.
2. Limit less-healthy foods (e.g., those foods high in sugar, fat, and salt).
3. Consider food safety, foodborne illness, and food allergies.
4. Create environments that promote healthy physical and social eating.
5. Respect children's hunger and satiety cues.
6. Encourage childcare provider role modeling.
7. Work with parents to encourage parents to send healthy foods from home to childcare.
8. Respect culture and encourage cultural foods.
9. Be mindful of food security and family resources.
10. Consider barriers to serving healthy foods and beverages from the provider perspective
11. Provide training and technical assistance to childcare providers

Childcare centers are advised to use the services of a community or public health dietitian/nutritionist in planning the menus and to include nutrition education in the classroom. Cleanliness in food production and service are important to minimize foodborne illness. The Child and Adult Care Food Program administered by the USDA provides assistance to childcare programs in setting food standards and gives financial support to provide nutritious foods for low-income children.[77]

Lead Exposure

Lead absorption is highest during stages of rapid growth such as early childhood. Lead intake is harmful to children because it contributes to iron deficiency and anemia. Low levels of lead toxicity can be difficult to diagnose because the symptoms, such as diarrhea, irritability, and fatigue, are nonspecific. Early identification is important due to the permanent damage that can occur, leading to nerve damage and mental retardation.[78] Concerns about lead in the environment have resulted in numerous bans on the use of lead in such items as gasoline and paint. Although these efforts have had a positive impact, the lingering lead in the environment continues to contribute to lead poisoning in young children. Many young children are exposed to lead in their homes. Lead is present in old paint and water pipes.

The lead in water pipes resulted in a public health disaster in Flint Michigan in 2015–2016. The City of Flint changed its source of water from the well-established Detroit water system to implementing their own water purification system of sanitizing water from the Flint River in an effort to save money. Unfortunately, the Flint water department failed to add the chemicals necessary to provide the correct pH of the water to prevent the corrosive

Strategy Tip

What benefit would a dietitian consultant associated with a childcare program bring?

Flint River water from stripping lead from the water pipes in the city and in homes. As a result, the majority Black population of Flint was exposed to high levels of lead while city and state leaders insisted that nothing was wrong with the water despite evidence to the contrary and the citizens' complaints. Initially, it was reported that at least 100 children were determined to have high levels of lead in their system; it has been now determined that over 100,000 residents were exposed to high levels of lead. Research has found seven times elevated cord blood lead levels among infants born in Flint.[79] Long-term damage to the children and residents may be the result of this failure to protect the public health. This situation is an example of health disparities and **environmental justice**.

Food Allergies

Food allergies are caused when the body's immune system reacts to a whole food protein. Allergic responses can range from inflammation of the nasal passages to skin rashes to anaphylactic shock. Food allergies can be difficult to identify, particularly if the response is delayed. Nonallergenic adverse reactions to foods can be misidentified as food allergies. Many children outgrow food allergies as their gastrointestinal system matures. Foods likely to cause allergies include eggs, milk, fish, peanuts, and soybeans. Children with severe allergic reactions need to be evaluated by a physician and will require careful monitoring of their food intake. Some children may need access to an epinephrine (epi) pen in case of accidental exposure to an allergenic food. To reduce this problem, many school systems strive to reduce food elements that are common allergens; an example is peanuts. Due to the high allergenic response to peanuts and the relative ease of eliminating them, schools often eliminate them from the menu and ask families not to provide foods containing peanuts in lunches and snacks brought from home.

School-Aged Child Specifics

By the time a child enters school, they should weigh twice as much as they did at age 1. During the elementary school years, children continue to grow at a steady rate, gaining approximately 2.5 inches and 5 to 7 pounds per year. Children's appetites will ebb and wane as their growth patterns change, with increased food intake during a growth spurt. Families continue to play an important role in food choices, but peer pressure and media influences begin to play a strong role in food decisions.

Children mature physically and mentally during this time span. They become progressively stronger, and their motor coordination increases. Body image becomes important in relation to peers, as children don't want to be seen as different. Their independence grows and they learn how to make decisions for themselves. This can lead to conflicts over food choices and emotional struggles with parents.

Changes in the Food Environment

One of the most noticeable changes affecting our food environment during the past three decades is the rapid growth in the number of restaurants, especially the $208 billion fast-food industry.[80] Fast-food restaurants are found throughout our communities, even inside public schools and hospitals. The effective marketing and advertising of these restaurants to adults and children have fueled the growth of this industry.

Fast Foods

Fast-food items are convenient and relatively low cost.[81] The amount of food dollars spent purchasing meals at dine-in and take-out restaurants has increased significantly to comprise about 46% of total household food budgets. Thirty-seven percent of the family food dollar is spent on fast-food meals. Meals eaten outside of the home tend to have large portion sizes, have higher energy content, and include fewer fruits and vegetables than meals eaten in the home. Unfortunately, fast-food restaurant fare is usually high in calories, fat, salt, and sugars, while low in fiber content.[81] As a result, the increase in out-of-home meal consumption may have a negative impact on diet quality health risk of children and their families.[82,83] Fast-food intake among adolescents negatively impacts their intake of fruits, milk, and vegetables and their likelihood of meeting MyPlate recommendations.

The use of fast foods for meals or snacks is especially popular with adolescents. Fast foods include foods from vending machines, self-service restaurants, convenience grocery stores, and franchised food restaurants. Fast foods tend to be low in iron, calcium, riboflavin, and vitamin A, and there are few sources of folic acid. The vitamin C content of fast foods is also low unless fruit or fruit juice is consumed. Although most fast-food restaurants offer a selection of healthy foods, many of the general menu items provide more than 50% of their calories from fat. Fast-food restaurants have recently received increasing pressure to make improvements in the quality of food components. Adolescents should be counseled on how to make wise and healthy choices when eating out in a restaurant.

> See MyPlate recommendations at: myplate.gov

Food Modifications

Product innovations launched during the past two decades have included many products designed to lower the fat content of popular foods to address consumers' concerns about dietary fat and unwanted weight gain. Despite an explosive growth in low-fat food products in many food categories, these food supply changes have seemingly not had the desired effect on our obesity rates. Many food manufacturers offset the lower fat content of the reformulated foods by increasing sugar and carbohydrate contents to maintain product acceptance by consumers. In the end, the caloric content of the lower fat product is often similar to the original version. There is also concern that so-called low-fat foods may encourage the consumer to actually eat more calories overall because the low-fat food provides a "license to eat more."[84] The consumption of unprocessed/limited processed foods should be promoted whenever possible.

Beverages

The American Heart Association recommends no more than 6 teaspoons—or less than 25 grams—of added sugar daily for children aged 2 to 18 years.[85] Most children consume added sugars through sugar-sweetened beverages. High-sugar beverage intake is linked to fast-food consumption because soft drinks are typically marketed and bundled with meal packages in fast-food restaurants. Twice as many children and adolescents drank carbonated soft drinks if they had consumed fast foods on one of two survey days than if they had not consumed fast foods.[86] High consumption of soft drinks among children and adolescents has been shown to be associated with higher energy intakes.[87,88] An association between school children's sugar-sweetened drink consumption and their BMI has consistently demonstrated a link to overweight and obesity in children.[89]

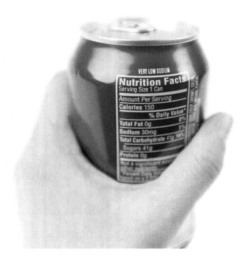

Sugar-sweetened sodas add many grams of sugar to the diet. Water would be a welcome replacement.

© Jorik/Shutterstock.

The typical 12-fluid-ounce can of soda is rapidly being replaced by the 20–24 fluid-ounce bottles at convenience stores and in vending machines, encouraging increased consumption of these drinks. Many brands offer a 32-fluid-ounce version that is packaged in a bottle shape that is easy to tote around, thereby encouraging increased consumption. Average portion sizes of soft drinks have increased by 12–18% for persons aged 2 and older.[88] Soft drink consumption (per capita) has increased by approximately 500% over the past 50 years, with adolescents consuming between 36 grams and 58 grams of sugar daily from this source.[87] It is important to note that some research indicates that there is increased sugar-sweetened beverage marketing to communities and youth of color,[90,91] which likely contributes to some of the nutrition-related health disparities and health inequities for these populations.

Nutritional Assessment and Intervention in School-Aged Children

Guidelines for nutritional assessment and intervention in school-aged children, ages 6 to 10, should include:

1. Screen and assess growth status and plot on NCHS growth charts.
2. Children identified as at risk for overweight or who are overweight should be referred for further evaluation and possible treatment.
3. Provide a wide variety of healthy foods with emphasis on nutritious choices, such as whole grains, fruits, vegetables, dairy foods, and lean meats and protein alternatives.
4. Ensure that children eat breakfast before going to school or receive breakfast at school.
5. Promote regular physical activity at school and at home.
6. Reduce sedentary activity with an emphasis on reduction of screen time.
7. Provide nutrition education in school.
8. Ensure regular meals and snacks.
9. Encourage reduced levels of low nutrient-dense beverages.
10. Support school lunch and breakfast programs.
11. Provide appropriate care for disease or other health conditions.

School Meals

The USDA National School Lunch and Breakfast Programs started in 1946 to provide financial support to schools to provide nutritious lunches to low-income children. The National School Lunch program is in over 100,000 schools nationwide and cost $11.6 billion in 2012. Since it started, over 224 billion lunches have been served. In addition, these programs mandate food and nutrition criteria for schools to use in planning school meals. The USDA's Team Nutrition was established to provide resources and technical support to help schools improve healthy eating and physical activity patterns.[92]

After many years with no changes in the nutrient requirements for school menus, the USDA significantly revamped nutrient requirements in July of 2014. The new program is called the Healthy Hunger Free Kids Act (see USDA Lunch and Breakfast website for more details). All schools that want to participate in the free and reduced meal programs must comply with the new stricter requirements for participation. Prior to the new guidelines, schools did not need to meet restrictions related to competitive foods; these are foods sold a la carte, from vending machines, school stores, or any other location on the school campus. Essentially, the National School Lunch and Breakfast Programs have brought competitive foods from their frequent role of nonhealthy options within schools that provide free and reduced lunches into being a component of a healthy food environment on the school campus and thus, improved the nutrient composition of competitive foods. As part of the new program, over 22,000 schools nationwide that serve primarily low-income students will be eligible to serve free lunch and breakfast to all students. This new option will be a benefit to schools by eliminating the extensive process of individual qualification of students.

Requirements in these new nutrient standards include types and sizes of beverages that can be sold and definitions for allowable nutrient levels including calories, sodium, fat, and sugar. Lower calorie beverages must be no larger than 20 ounces and cannot contain more than 10 calories per 20 fluid ounces. Milk and juice may be sold as 8-oz portions in elementary schools and 12 oz in middle and high schools. Calories, fat, and sodium will be carefully monitored with snacks containing no more than 200 calories, 35% fat, and 230 mg of sodium. Entrees cannot have more than 350 calories, less than 10% fat, and 480 mg of sodium.

Many states and large school districts already had policies in effect for beverages and competitive foods, but not all. Beverage policies and vending machines in schools have been a particular focus point. A review of policies across the nation found that 38 states had laws or policies for snack foods and beverages in schools. Although no state met all of the new requirements, 16 states fully met one provision, 10 states partially met at least one, and seven states met none of the provisions.[93] The fact that so many states already have policies means that they realize the need for change in foods and beverages provided in schools. Although the new law will require substantial changes in most school districts, schools and states are well positioned to make the adjustments necessary in order to maintain the free lunch and breakfast program.

In fact, elementary schools have been making steady progress in terms of providing healthier options with more fruits and vegetables and fewer fried potatoes and pizza, for example.[94] During that time period, the availability of whole grains increased from 76–97%, an impressive change. Since the new standards went into effect, students are selecting and eating more fruits and vegetable and overall plate waste has gone down.[95]

The impact of the new nutrition standards has shown positive results. A study of over 1.7 million meals in three middle and three high schools in Washington State before and after implementation of the Healthy Hunger-Free Kids Act (HHFKA) found improvements in nutritional quality of meals selected. Energy density was reduced and meal participation remained steady.[96] A review on the effects of Healthy, Hunger-Free Kids Act found that most studies in the post-HHFKA period indicate a positive influence on students' eating behaviors.[97] Research analyzing the National Survey of Children's Health, shows that there is not yet an association between HHFKA and childhood obesity trends.[98] Recent study on HHFKA exposure from 2007–2016 found that the dietary quality of lunch improved in low, low middle, and middle high income NSLP participants.[99]

The School Breakfast Program extends free nutritious food to the breakfast period. More schools in low-income neighborhoods should be encouraged to participate in this program. Many low-income children go to school hungry or eat low-nutrient foods before starting school. A healthy breakfast has been shown to improve school performance.

Discussion Prompt

Describe the difference in identifying students who can qualify for a free school meal and just providing a free meal for all. What will this mean to students on the border of qualifying for meals?

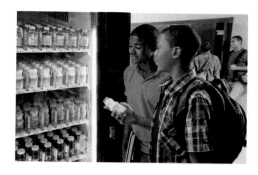

Vending machines are slowly changing over to more healthy choices.

Courtesy of USDA.

School Wellness Policy

School Wellness policies are required for all schools that participate in either the School Lunch or Breakfast programs. The purpose of school wellness policies is to provide local guidance on the implementation and support of school nutrition and physical activity environments. Although the majority of school districts have implemented a school wellness policy, most lack the details that would support effectiveness.[100]

School wellness councils or committees that involve stakeholders was mandated by the Healthy, Hunger-Free Kids Act of 2010. Although schools are mandated to have a school wellness policy, the data indicates that many schools have not embraced the benefit of the policy. From 2009–2011, the percentage of children who were in a school district that had a school wellness policy decreased from 54–46%.[101,91] Resources were not funded for support of Wellness policies, but technical support is approved. During the 2012–2013 school year, only 49% of districts required a health advisory of wellness committee. The required improvements in school wellness policies is another step to ensure that schools provide a positive environment for nutrition and physical activity, and has been shown in multiple studies to be effective at increased selection, intake, and sales of healthy foods, and decreased plate waste in schools.[97] This is an opportunity for involvement of community and public health dietitians/nutritionists.

In 2014, First Lady Michelle Obama joined USDA Secretary Tom Vilsack to announce new guidelines for school wellness policies. The new guidelines ensure that unhealthy foods are not marketed within schools. A website was established by the USDA to support implementation of the school wellness policies, School Nutrition Environment, and Wellness Resources.

CDC School Health Index

The School Health Index (SHI) is a self-assessment and planning guide developed for grades K–12 by the CDC. It consists of eight modules based on the coordinated school health program model and aligns with the Whole School, Whole Community, Whole Child (WSCC) model, in an effort to promote health equity. The modules have assessment questions in health education, physical education, health services, nutrition services, counseling, psychological and social services, healthy school environment, health promotion for staff, and family/community involvement. The current version focuses on physical activity; nutrition; tobacco use; asthma; unintended injury/violence; and sexual health in elementary, middle, and high schools. This tool identifies the strengths and weaknesses of a school's health promotion policies and programs. The SHI assists teachers, parents, students, and community members to develop an action plan for improving the health of the student population.[102]

The SHI is easy to administer and complete. The role of the community public health dietitian/nutritionist is to present current trends of poor eating habits and physical inactivity nationally, statewide, and locally. In addition, an existing partnership with local tobacco-use prevention educators is important because they may discuss trends of tobacco use in children. Once the evidence of health problems is described, the dietitian/nutritionist should review resources, such as the SHI, and examples of policy and environmental interventions for targeted schools. Some examples of policy interventions are to: serve breakfast to all students; serve low-fat milk, fresh fruits and vegetables, and whole grain products; limit access to vending machines during school hours and/or provide healthy options in the vending machines; provide opportunities for vigorous physical activity for all students; and offer healthy food options in school stores. Some examples of environmental interventions include building a walking track for student, staff, and community members to use; purchasing playground equipment for students; and planning an annual community health event for community members, parents, teachers, and children.

The community and public health dietitian/nutritionist acts as a consultant to the SHI site coordinator, who assembles and supports the SHI team members. Team members complete the assessment questions and planning guide. They develop an action plan with interventions tailored for their school. The role of the public health dietitians/nutritionists is to ensure the development of an appropriate action plan that results in interventions of healthy eating practices and physical activity, especially among the student population.

Community and public health dietitians/nutritionists should attend the planning meeting to assist SHI members in developing an action plan. Although the site coordinator should facilitate the meeting and solicit ideas and opinions, the dietitian/nutritionist serves as a consultant by helping the team members to focus on healthy eating and physical activity. In addition, the public health dietitians/nutritionists can assist with funding efforts to provide an incentive to improve the school's health policies and programs. The SHI is an excellent tool in developing partnerships with local school staff and community, obtaining and dispersing grant funding to promote health, and monitoring and evaluating interventions that benefit children's health.

> Access the School Health Index at: https://www.cdc.gov/healthyschools/shi/index.htm

Nutrition Education in Schools

School settings are ideal for nutrition education. The majority of U.S. children between the ages of 5 and 17 years are enrolled in school, and this provides a unique learning community through which children are able to participate in nutrition-based education. A familiar environment and the support of teachers and peers strengthens the impact of nutrition education. Programs are likely to be more widely accepted by the participants when they are culturally and socially sensitive. Multidimensional strategies including health/physical education, parental involvement, and food-service involvement along with nutrition education helps to promote learning and behavior change. Children seem most interested in teaching methods that use discovery learning, student learning stations, cooperative groups, situation analysis, and cross-age and peer teaching. Extensive research on school-based methods to improve nutritional intake supports their continued use but confirms that behavioral change is slow. Nutrition education needs to be part of the comprehensive school health education program to strengthen and advance positive food and nutrition messages consistently and over the course of childhood.

Screen Time

Television viewing and other media outlets such as video games and computer usage have displaced a more natural environment of family interactions for growing children, such as learning and playing. Children who spend more time in sedentary activities tend to weigh more and be at greater risk of being overweight. Several studies conclude that children who watch four or more hours of TV are more likely to be overweight than those who watch less TV.[103-105] In addition, African American (30%) and Hispanic American (22%) children are both more likely than Caucasian (12%) children to spend more than 5 hours a day watching TV/screens.

There may be some question about leisure activities in the United States, indicating that U.S. children overall are less active than children in other countries and cultures. The trend toward increasingly sedentary lifestyles is obvious to many older adults, as they compare the children's activity level in this current generation to that of children two or three generations earlier. Learning, playing, and being physically active were an integral part of family life, and television viewing was a special occasion. Today, television viewing, which is a sedentary behavior, is a prominent part of family life in many families.[106]

Food Advertising

Television, magazines, and other social media probably have a greater influence on children's eating habits than any other source. Children are exposed to 4.4K to 7K food advertisements per year depending on their age and the number of hours of screen-time they view.[107,108] Food advertisements use a variety of techniques to appeal to children such as cartoon characters, catchy songs, colorful images, appealing colors and tastes, and celebrity endorsers. Many advertisers use prizes and other incentive items as well as special pricing to encourage food purchases. Advertisements for low nutrient-dense foods, such as soda, candy, and snacks, have a dominant presence in the time slots in which children's programming is aired. Young consumers predictably request the products or even purc-hase these themselves during trips to the grocery store, as they recognize their favorite cartoon characters on the colorful packages that are strategically placed at their eye level when riding in the grocery cart. Excessive television viewing by children creates a cycle of physical inactivity and high-calorie consumption due to the influence of TV food advertising, which might be a perfect formula for fueling the growth in numbers of overweight children.

Food manufacturers have been under tremendous pressure to modify their advertising to children. Some fast-food outlets and food manufacturers have started to respond with plans to eliminate some advertising directed at children. Efforts such as these will help to improve the unhealthy food environment in children's television.

Adolescence Specifics

Adolescence is one of the most challenging periods in human development. Because of the extent of the physical and psychological changes taking place, a number of important issues arise that influence the nutritional well-being of the teenager. Knowledge of the developmental processes is a prerequisite to understanding the nutritional aspects of this period of life. Understanding the nutritional and physical activity needs of adolescents will help nutrition professionals provide counseling and programs that can impact the future health of these individuals.

Adolescence is a time of dramatic change in the life of every human being. The relatively uniform growth of childhood is suddenly altered by an increase in the velocity of growth. This sudden spurt is also associated with hormonal, cognitive, and emotional changes. All of these changes create special nutritional needs. Adolescence is considered an especially nutritionally vulnerable period of life for several reasons. First is the greater demand for nutrients due to the dramatic increase in physical growth and development. Second is the change of lifestyle and food habits of adolescents that affect both nutrient intake and needs. Third are those adolescents with special nutrient needs, such as those who participate in sports, have a chronic illness, diet excessively, or use alcohol or drugs.[109,110]

Physiologic Changes

Puberty, the process of physically developing from a child to an adult, is stimulated by physiological factors and includes maturation of the entire body. Adolescence is the only time following birth when the velocity of growth actually increases. The adolescent gains about 20% of adult height and 50% of adult weight during this period.

This growth continues throughout the approximately 5–7 years of pubertal development. A great percentage of this height will be gained during the 18- to 24-month period of the growth spurt. The growth spurt or peak height gain velocity occurs at different ages for different individuals, as does the initiation of puberty. In general, girls began the pubertal process approximately 2 years earlier than boys. Although growth slows following the achievement of sexual maturity, linear growth and weight acquisition continue into the late teens for young women and early twenties for men. Most girls gain no more than 1–2 inches following menarche, although girls who have early menarche tend to grow more after its onset than those having later menarche.

In the process of total body maturation, the composition of the body changes. Prepubertal boys and girls tend to be similar, with body fatness averaging approximately 15 and 19%, respectively. Girls gain more fat than boys during puberty, and in adulthood, they have about 22–26% body fat, compared with approximately 15–18% in men. During puberty, boys gain twice as much lean tissue as girls. This is an especially important time for nutrition education efforts to support positive energy balance. Children who enter the growth spurt with excess body fat have a great opportunity to use those fat stores to fuel growth as long as adequate protein is provided.

Psychological Changes

Adolescence is a period of maturation for both mind and body. Along with the physical growth of puberty, emotional and intellectual development is rapid. Adolescents' capacity for abstract thinking, as opposed to the concrete thought patterns of childhood, enables them to grow cognitively during adolescence. Many of these tasks have implications for their nutritional well-being.

Cognitive and emotional development can be divided into early, middle, and late adolescence. Determining the adolescent's stage can be very helpful in providing nutritional counseling as well as in designing educational programs.[111] The younger adolescent:

- Is preoccupied with body and body image
- Trusts and respects adults
- Is anxious about peer relationships
- Is ambivalent about autonomy

The nutritional implications are that adolescents in this stage are willing to do or try anything that will make them look better or improve their body image. However, adolescents at this stage want immediate results, so nutrition counseling should be geared to short-term goals and to addressing nutritional concerns that impact the teen's appearance, performance (e.g., dance, sports), or both.

A teen in middle adolescence:

- Is greatly influenced by their peer group
- Is mistrustful of adults
- Considers independence to be very important
- Experiences significant cognitive development

During this stage, the teen will listen to peers more than to parents or other adults. Teens are becoming more in charge of the foods they eat. The drive toward independence often results in temporary rejection of the family dietary patterns. At this age, adolescents often experiment with vegetarianism. Nutritional counseling should include making wise decisions when eating away from home.

The teen in late adolescence:

- Has established a body image
- Is oriented toward the future and is making plans
- Is increasingly independent
- Is more consistent in their values and beliefs
- Is developing intimacy and permanent relationships

By late adolescence, teens are thinking about the future and are interested in improving their overall health. Nutritional counseling during this stage can address long-term goals. Adolescents in this stage still want to make their own decisions but are open to information provided by healthcare professionals. Nutritional counselors should not only present current recommendations but also explain the rationale behind them.

As adolescents strive for independence, they often take risks. Many of these risks are important to becoming independent (e.g., trying out for a sports team, applying to college, dating), but many risk behaviors can be dangerous. Resnick et al.,[112] found that serious behaviors, termed *acting out behaviors*, can be grouped together and include the following: drug use, school absenteeism, and unintended injury risk, such as drinking and driving, not wearing seatbelts, and not using a bicycle helmet. The second group of serious behaviors, termed *quietly disturbed behaviors*, are of concern to dietitians/nutritionists because these behaviors include the following: poor body image; disordered eating, including binging, bulimia, and chronic dieting; fear of loss of control overeating; emotional stress; and suicidal ideation.

Food Habits

Recommendations for fulfilling the nutritional needs of adolescents arise from a small research base. Part of the difficulty lies in the fact that studies of requirements must consider not only age but also stage of physical maturity.

Adolescents search for identity, strive for independence and acceptance, and are concerned about appearance. Irregular meals, snacking, eating away from home, and following alternative dietary patterns characterize the food habits of adolescents. These habits are further influenced by family, peers, and the media.

Irregular Meals and Snacking

Meal patterns of adolescents are often chaotic. Teenagers miss an increasing number of meals at home as they get older. Breakfast and lunch are often the meals most frequently missed, but social and school activities may cause a teen to miss an evening meal as well. Adolescent girls tend to miss more meals than their boy counterparts.[44]

Although concern has been expressed about the habit of snacking, teenagers may obtain substantial nourishment from foods eaten outside of traditional meals. Thus, the choice of foods is more important than the time or place of eating.

As a result of health and science education at school, most adolescents know what they should and should not eat.[44,108,113] However, overcoming barriers to act on that knowledge is the concern. Teens identify the biggest barrier as time. Teens perceive themselves as too busy to worry about food, nutrition, meal planning, or eating right. Additionally, adolescents form mainly

Strategy Tip

The second group of serious behaviors, termed *quietly disturbed behaviors*, are of concern to dietitians/nutritionists because these behaviors include the following: poor body image; disordered eating, including binging, bulimia, and chronic dieting; and fear of loss of control overeating.

negative associations with healthy foods, but positive associations with junk foods.[107] In order for adolescents to change their eating habits to better behaviors, counseling must center on fitting proper nutrition into allowable time, making the selection of healthy foods easier, and making healthy foods appealing to teens and their peers.

During the time of peak growth velocity, adolescents usually need to eat large amounts of food often. They are able to use foods with a high concentration of energy; however, they need to be increasingly careful about the amounts and frequency of eating when growth has slowed. This transition can lead to weight gain if intake changes are not made. Habits of overeating adopted during adolescence may ultimately contribute to adult obesity and a number of related diseases.

Adolescents as Food Purchasers

For marketers, being a teenager is a matter of lifestyle and spending habits, not age. Marketing to teens has become a multi-billion-dollar business. It is estimated that the nation's approximately 23 million teens spend nearly $100 billion annually.[114,115] Teenagers spend $15 billion annually on fast food and other food and snacks. Teens not only spend money themselves, but also wield a tremendous influence over purchases made by their parents.[114]

Teens are frequent visitors to different stores. In a 30-day period, the top two types of stores teens visited were food stores, with more than 200 million visits to convenience stores and supermarkets. Teens eat in fast food restaurants often, with most visits occurring either immediately after school or at a weekday dinnertime.

Nutritional Assessment and Intervention in Adolescence

Guidelines for nutritional assessment and intervention in adolescence may include:

1. Screen and assess growth status and plot on NCHS growth charts.
2. Refer adolescents identified as at risk for overweight or who are overweight for further evaluation and possible treatment.
3. Provide a wide variety of healthy foods with emphasis on nutritious choices such as whole grains, fruits, vegetables, dairy foods, and lean meats and protein alternatives.
4. Promote daily physical activity that fits with the adolescent's interests.
5. Reduce sedentary activity with an emphasis on reduction of screen time.
6. Provide nutrition education in school.
7. Ensure regular meals and snacks.
8. Encourage reduced levels of low nutrient-dense beverages and promote intake of milk and dairy foods.
9. Provide appropriate care for disease or other health conditions.

Situations with Special Needs

Vegetarian Eating Practices: Adolescents tend to be attracted to vegetarian and/or vegan eating practices, especially during middle or late adolescence, because of their concerns about animal welfare, ecology, the environment, or personal health. Additionally, concerns about body weight motivate some adolescents to adopt a vegetarian diet, because this is a socially acceptable way to reduce dietary fat. Vegetarian eating is often seen in adolescents with anorexia nervosa, who adopt the diet in an attempt to hide their restriction of food intake.[116,117]

Vegetarian and vegan diets are consistent with the Dietary Guidelines for Americans and can meet the DRIs/RDAs for nutrients. With planning, vegetarian and vegan diets can provide a variety of nutrient-dense foods that promote health, growth, and development. Diets need to be planned to provide adequate energy, protein, calcium, iron, zinc, and vitamins B_{12} and D. The bioavailability of calcium, iron, and zinc should also be ensured. When adolescents become vegetarians or vegans, parents are often concerned about the diet's nutritional adequacy, especially about meeting protein requirements. Parents need reassurance that a vegetarian diet can meet their adolescent's nutrition needs, and they should receive information on the principles of healthy vegetarian eating for adolescents. But both parents and adolescents should be informed that overly restricted or inappropriately selected vegetarian/vegan diets can result in significant malnutrition. Some vegetarian adolescents have suffered from a delayed growth spurt, iron-deficiency anemia, and vitamin B_{12} deficiency.[117,118]

Eating Disorders: Eating disorders rank as the third most common chronic illness in adolescent females, with an incidence of up to 5%. The prevalence has increased dramatically over the past three decades.[117,119] Just as adolescents are at increased risk for developing eating disorders, they are also more vulnerable to the complications of these disorders. The impact of malnutrition on linear growth, brain development, and bone acquisition can be longstanding and irreversible. Yet, with early and aggressive treatment, there is also the potential for a better outcome than in adults who have more longstanding disease.[117,119]

Early identification of adolescents with disordered eating habits has been linked to improved long-term outcome, but this is difficult to accomplish. Often, parents will bring an affected teen in for another reason, such as gastrointestinal complaints, amenorrhea, or unexplained weight loss. A screening for disordered eating should include questions about fear of becoming fat, amount of dieting, use of laxatives, fasting or frequent meal skipping to lose weight, fear of certain foods (e.g., foods containing fat or sugar), vomiting, binging, and excessive exercise.

Because adolescence is the greatest period of risk for development of an eating disorder, efforts must be made to reduce the incidence of malnutrition, or at least provide early intervention to prevent its serious complications.[119] Work should be done to promote body positivity and a healthy relationship with food and physical activity.

Physical Activity

Physical Activity and Health: A Report of the Surgeon General is a comprehensive overview of research related to physical activity and health.[120] The report: 1) summarizes the benefits of physical activity; 2) reinforces the importance of promoting physical activity; 3) states that many children and adolescents are at risk for health problems because of inactive lifestyles; and 4) states that everyone should participate in a moderate amount of physical activity (e.g., 15 minutes of running, 30 minutes of brisk walking, 45 minutes of playing volleyball) on most, if not all, days of the week. Results from the Youth Risk Behavior Surveillance (YRBS) indicate that a large number of children and adolescents don't achieve the levels recommended. Consult the YRBS maintained by the CDC for the latest information.

These findings are disturbing in view of the numerous health benefits that children and adolescents derive by being physically active on a regular basis. Physical activity can lead to improved body composition (e.g., increased lean muscle mass, reduced total body fat) and can help reduce other coronary

See Youth Risk Behavior Surveillance (YRBS) at: https://www.cdc.gov/healthy youth/data/yrbs/index.htm

heart disease (CHD) risk factors among adolescents. For example, increased physical activity levels can favorably alter blood lipid profiles in adolescents at high risk for CHD (e.g., children and adolescents who are obese or who have type 1 or 2 diabetes mellitus) and can reduce blood pressure, especially in adolescents whose blood pressure is elevated. Physical activity plays a substantial role in the development of bone mass during adolescence and can help maintain the structure and functional strength of bone throughout life.[121,122]

Efforts to increase physical activity levels among children and adolescents have been most successful in school settings. However, less attention has been focused on promoting physical activity among children and adolescents in settings other than schools, including healthcare settings (i.e., health professionals counseling children and adolescents about physical activity during health supervision visits).[122]

Health professionals, families, peers, and communities can influence children's and adolescents' physical activity levels. Parents who participate in physical activity themselves and who support and encourage physical activity in their adolescents have a positive influence on adolescents' physical activity levels. In addition, older children and adolescents whose friends are physically active tend to be more physically active themselves.

Little is known about which factors motivate children and adolescents to become physically active, remain physically active, and increase their physical activity levels as they become older. In addition, it is not clear why these factors differ for girls and boys or for different racial and ethnic groups. However, it is clear that girls are less likely than boys to participate in vigorous physical activity, participate in strengthening or toning activities, or participate on sports teams. Strategies different from those used to promote physical activity in young and adolescents boys may be needed to promote physical activity in young and adolescent girls.[115] Strategies that take into account children's and adolescents' race or cultural background could also be beneficial. The Physical Activity Guidelines for Americans (2018) recommends the following intervention strategies to promote physical activity in children and adolescents[122]:

- Preschool-aged children (ages 3 through 5 years) should be physically active throughout the day to enhance growth and development. Adult caregivers of preschool-aged children should encourage active play that includes a variety of activity types.
- Provide young with people opportunities and encouragement to participate in physical activities that are appropriate for their age, that are enjoyable, and that offer variety.

Other recommendations include the following:

- Help adolescents succeed and increase their confidence in their ability to be physically active.
- Support adolescents' efforts to be physically active.
- Help adolescents learn about the benefits of physical activity and help them develop positive attitudes toward it.
- Help adolescents overcome barriers that keep them from being physically active.

Physical Inactivity Affecting Overweight Status in Children

Physical inactivity among children is one of the major public health concerns regarding overweight children. Children learn to be physically inactive by emulating adults who are inactive and having limited access to community recreation activities, unsafe neighborhoods, and perhaps, unlimited access to television viewing and other media outlets, including computers. In addition, many newly developed communities are poorly planned and don't include "built-in" access to physical activity. Often, children are bused to school or driven by parents because walking to school is not an option due to safety issues and distance. Although further research is needed for a better understanding of the influence of the human-built environment on physical activity, it appears clear that urban sprawl has caused some relationship between land use, transportation, and health, particularly children's health.[123]

School Physical Education

At school, children may not find many opportunities to be physically active on a daily basis. Often, school academic curriculums and programs take priority over physical education and recess time. Decreased school budgets are a contributing factor. Physical education (PE) curriculums and recess have slowly diminished over the last few years.

The percentage of schools that require physical education in each grade declines from around 50% in grades one through five, to 25% in grade eight, to only 5% in grade 12. Although the National Association for Sport and Physical Education (NASPE) and National Association of State Boards of Education (NASBE) discourage student exemption from physical education based on participation in other school and community activities, some states, districts, and schools allow such exemption from required physical education.[124]

Data from the Youth Risk Behavior Surveillance System (YRBSS) show that 55.7% of students nationwide were enrolled in PE classes 1 or more days in an average week, while only 28.4% of students nationwide attended PE classes 5 days in an average week. Of the 55.7% of students enrolled in PE classes nationwide, 80.3% of students actually exercised or played sports for more than 20 minutes. Improvements in PE are also needed to decrease inappropriate teaching practices, such as prohibiting physical activity as a form of punishment or physical activity games that may cause embarrassment or aggressive behavior (e.g., dodge ball).[124] Although some PE improvements are needed, a nationwide effort to establish laws or policies to increase student enrollment and participation in daily PE is desirable, especially in the older student population. The goal is for children to establish healthy lifestyle habits that may carry over into adulthood as well as to support caloric balance during growth periods.

While the majority of children spend much of their waking hours in school, it is a threat to children's health and fitness when the school infrastructure does not mandate daily physical activity. Advocacy for increasing student participation in daily recess and physical activity should be a top priority of schools and health and community leaders to help prevent overweight in children. This is an area where community and public health dietitians/nutritionists can play a role.

Family Mealtime

Increasing emphasis is being placed on family mealtime because of its positive impact on child development and food intake. Project EAT surveyed middle school and high school students from ethnically and socioeconomically diverse communities.[125] Results show that almost one-third of participants reported eating only one to two meals with their family each week, or never eating meals together as a family. Children eating more than three family meals per week were significantly less likely to skip breakfast or report poor consumption of fruits, vegetables, and dairy foods, compared with children eating less than three family meals per week. African Americans and Hispanic Americans were less likely to skip breakfast and to report poor fruit consumption compared with Caucasian children. A higher frequency of family meals is associated with significantly lower odds of the following variables: use of cigarettes, alcohol, or marijuana use; low grade-point average; high depressive symptoms; and suicidal ideation. Family meal frequency had a strong positive association with intake of energy; percentage of calories from protein; calcium; iron; vitamins A, C, E, B_6; folate; and fiber.[44]

A family meal study from the ongoing Nurses' Health Study II found that children who ate family dinner every day consumed an average of 0.8 more servings of fruits and vegetables than those who never ate family meals or did so only on some days. Additionally, consumption of fried food and soda was inversely associated with frequency of family meals. Participants who ate family meals more often reported slightly higher energy intakes and also higher intakes of several nutrients including fiber; calcium; folate; vitamins B_6, B_{12}, C, and E; and iron. In addition, they consumed less *trans*-fat and saturated fat as a percentage of energy intake.[126] Family mealtime may be a potentially protective factor in the lives of children for nearly all of these variables.

See more about Project EAT at: https://snaped.fns.usda.gov/library/materials/project-eat

Impact of Families on Childhood Weight Status

Genetic differences are estimated to account for approximately 30–50% of the variance of BMI within a population, but these estimates do not describe the complex interactions taking place between genetics and the environment.[127] Parents who are struggling with personal weight issues may hamper their children's ability to self-regulate energy intake. Aiming to avoid overweight in their children, parents may impose greater restrictions on their children's intake. If these same parents exhibit uninhibited eating styles themselves, they will serve as poor role models. These behaviors in combination can cause the transfer of eating styles that pose an increased risk for the development of overweight in the child. As a result, well-intentioned parents may actually produce the very outcome they sought to avoid.[128]

A common strategy employed by families is to control children's intake by restricting their access to high-calorie foods or using favorite foods as a reward to shape behavior. At first, these behaviors may seem reasonable enough; however, restricting certain foods has been shown to increase the child's desire to consume these foods. When available, these desirable foods will likely be consumed in greater amounts. Again, such family dynamics around food may set up patterns of poor self-control of energy intake in the child.[129]

Families often have a mistaken perception of their children's food and beverage intake versus their actual intake. Children are eating fewer fruits and vegetables and drinking more high-sugar beverages than recommended.[130,131] The researchers also assessed parents adherence to the Academy of Pediatrics 5-2-1-0 recommendations, which recommends five servings of fruits and vegetables per day, 2 hours of screen time per day, 1 hour of physical activity per day, and 0 servings of sugary beverages. For infants, 97% of parents reported a "very healthy" intake whereas for preschool children, the rate dropped to 38% of parents. Eighty percent of parents thought their children were getting enough fruits and vegetables when only 38% were. About half of the families limited the intake of sugary beverages and only 2% of toddlers met the recommendation of zero screen time.

An optimal environment for children to develop self-control of energy intake is when parents provide nutritious food and allow children to determine when and how much to eat. These principles of division of responsibility are discussed extensively in other resources.[132-134]

Household Food Insecurity

Food insecurity relates to lack of sufficient food and is often found in low-income households. Although seemingly paradoxical, lower-income households compared with higher-income households appear to experience increased rates of overweight for some individuals. A proposed mechanism for low socioeconomic status (SES) being related to overweight and obesity is that higher intakes of cheaper, more calorie-dense foods may lead to excessive energy intakes.[135] Persons from low-income, food insecure households may overeat during periods of relative abundance and gain weight as a result. Food insecurity in low-income households appears to play a role in the increased overweight rates among older Caucasian girls (8–16 years of age) compared with children from low-income households who do not experience food insecurity.[136] However, family participation in programs such as the National School Breakfast and Lunch Programs and Supplemental Nutrition Assistance Programs (SNAP, formerly known as Food Stamps) may be protective for these girls. Girls who participated in all three programs were 68% less likely to become overweight compared with nonparticipants from families experiencing food insecurity.[136] On the other hand, another study found a 42.8% increase for young girls and a 28.8% decrease for young boys in the predicted probability of obesity with participation in SNAP for the previous 5 years. This study did not control for food insecurity within households, which may help to explain the differing results.[137] However, a more recent study (2021) found that increased benefit in SNAP was beneficial to the weight status of both sexes of youth, but the effect varied by age: younger children who had household SNAP benefits were less likely to have overweight compared with older children.[138] Personal characteristics such as age, race, and sex may influence the relationship between overweight and obesity in individuals within households and SES. Among boys aged 2 to 9 years, those of high SES had the lowest prevalence of BMI above the 95th percentile compared with their peers, while young girls showed only small differences according to SES. See more about food insecurity in Chapter 13.

In contrast, there was a strong inverse association between low SES and high BMI (greater than the 95th percentile) for white adolescent girls, but not for boys. High-SES Black girls, in contrast to their white counterparts, were at increased risk for high BMI.[134] Additional studies that are **retrospective**, longitudinal, and include assessment of food security and hunger status of each household member are needed to help explain why some children are affected more than others. This is important because not all members of a household may be experiencing food insecurity to the same extent. Understanding these dynamics better will help to focus attention on those within a household who may be at a greater risk of being overweight.

Retrospective studies These studies examine events that have occurred in the past or they represent attribute variables that cannot be manipulated; therefore, the researcher does not have direct control of the variables under study.

Supplemental Nutrition Assistance Program Education (SNAP-Ed)

The Supplemental Nutrition Assistance Program (SNAP) was formerly known as Food Stamps. The food stamp program has been part of the food safety net since the Food Stamp act of 1964. The processes have changed over time and many elements have been expanded. The name SNAP went into effect in 2008. A key component of SNAP is the provision of nutrition education, titled SNAP-Ed.

SNAP-Ed is provided across the country to groups of individuals who meet low-income requirements. SNAP-Ed is provided in a wide variety of settings ranging from schools to daycare to senior care settings and many venues in between. Individuals who live in high intensity areas for SNAP-Ed have been found to have improved intake of fruits and vegetables and less use of fast foods. These changes may have a positive impact on obesity rates over time.[135]

SNAP-Ed interventions focused on children have been found to have a positive impact on improvements on the use of low-fat milk rather than whole milk. Children in these interventions were more willing to try new fruits and vegetables. Unfortunately, the parents did not show a similar willingness to purchase and serve fruits and vegetables for snacks and dinner. More efforts are needed in these communities to support parental change.[139]

Overweight in Children from a Public Health Perspective

Obesity and obesity-related diseases are some of the biggest public health challenges of the 21st century. The rate of overweight in children is especially alarming. Ultimately, the cry for partnerships and resources to prevent overweight and obesity will be heard because of the unparalleled rise in U.S. medical and healthcare costs for treatment of obesity and related conditions. To maximize effectiveness, overweight and obesity prevention efforts must focus on policy and environmental interventions.

The topic of children with overweight is a very complex issue. Changes in the food and nutrition environment have made a dramatic impact of food and calorie intake. Individual interventions alone have not proven to be highly effective and will not stop this epidemic. Population-based interventions will be needed to achieve the greatest effect. In addition, children with overweight will be improved using a prevention-based approach by applying the public health model (assessment, policy development, and assurance) and **evidence-based** efforts (increase physical activity and healthy eating and decrease television viewing). Advocacy and education will be crucial to motivate community stakeholders and gain their support. Innovative prevention-based approaches for overweight in children are definitely needed.

Evidence-based A concept whereby analysis is based on scientific proof.

Overweight Rates in the United States

There was a rapid increase in our nation's rates of adults with obesity over the past 3 to 4 decades. The United States is not alone in facing this serious public health problem. Obesity has been declared one of the top 10 risk conditions in the world and one of the top five in the developed world by WHO. In recognition of the challenges of obesity, the nation has developed many strategies to slow the growth of overweight and obesity. Fortunately, the latest NHANES study found that obesity rates, for both adults and children, have remained stable with one-third of adults and 17% of children categorized with obesity.

For children and adolescents aged 2–19 years, the prevalence of obesity has remained fairly stable at about 17% and affects about 12.7 million children and adolescents. For some subgroups such as low-income, preschool children who participate in government food assistance programs and participants in a multisite pediatric practice, the obesity level has declined slightly in the United States and some other countries. Although these are positive signs, the obesity epidemic remains a real problem and strong consistent efforts are needed to promote healthy eating and physical activity in children and adults.[140]

Health Effects of Overweight

The incidence of overweight in children is especially concerning because of the predicted health consequences later in life when overweight status begins in childhood. In the Bogalusa Heart Study, Freedman et al.,[141] evaluated the longitudinal relationship between children's BMI and their adult levels of lipids, insulin, and blood pressure. The mean time interval between first and follow-up measurements was 17 years. Over this time period, 77% of overweight children remained overweight as adults. This study was done at a time when the rates of childhood obesity were lower than today; thus, the implications for long-term health and economic consequences of childhood overweight are significant. The persistence of being overweight, once it occurs, is of great concern because being overweight is more strongly linked to chronic disease than living in poverty, smoking, or drinking.[142] The impact of obesity on overall health has been likened to aging by 20 years[143]: "Childhood obesity precedes insulin resistance/hyperinsulinemia and strongly predicts the risk of developing a constellation of metabolic, hemodynamic, thrombotic, and inflammatory disorders of syndrome X."

Although there is well-justified concern for overweight in children tracking into adulthood and increasing the risk of adult health problems, health professionals must not ignore the acute physical and psychological health issues that may affect the child with overweight. Many body functions are often affected by being overweight, including the nervous, pulmonary, cardiovascular, skeletal, gastrointestinal, endocrine, and reproductive systems. In addition, children with overweight may suffer from mental health problems such as depression, anxiety, lowered self-esteem, and sometimes eating disorders.[144,145]

Pediatricians are diagnosing the most children and adolescents with obesity with hypertension, dyslipidemia, and non–insulin-dependent diabetes mellitus (NIDDM). Even if the overweight status does not track into adulthood, there may be long-lasting medical and psychosocial effects for children with overweight.[146]

Health Disparities

Ethnic, cultural, gender, genetic, socioeconomic, and regional differences exist that influence which children are at greater risk for being overweight. For example, Hispanic American boys, African Americans, and those residing in the South are especially likely to experience higher rates of being overweight.[140,147] The ethnic differences in the degree to which certain population groups are affected by overweight prevalence may exacerbate long-term health outcomes and economic disparities that already exist in the United States.[148]

Economic Effects of Overweight

The burden of being overweight stresses individuals, families, and society. For the individual, quality of life issues such as family income, rates of marriage, and educational attainment were all lower, while poverty rates were higher for women who had been obese in late adolescence and young adulthood.[145,148] Financially, child hospitalizations for conditions related to obesity cause parents or caregivers to be absent from work, stressing family budgets and causing loss of productivity for the parents' employer(s).

The full economic consequences of overweight children cannot yet be known with certainty. For example, type 2 diabetes historically has been

Strategy Tip

Dietitians/nutritionists need to promote their services to pediatricians to allow more referrals of children for good nutrition.

considered an adult-onset condition, with negative effects on a person's health generally limited to the adult years. In adults, type 2 diabetes may show a certain pattern of development of health complications, such as peripheral neuropathy and impaired vision. The onset of such diabetic complications appears to depend to some extent on the length and severity of exposure to the diabetes condition. Thus, weight-related type 2 diabetes, which could begin in youth, has the potential to cause excess morbidity, mortality, and diminished quality of life and productivity for many. It is reasonable to expect that the longer the duration of complications of being overweight, the greater the healthcare costs incurred with their treatment.[149]

On a societal level, healthcare costs related to childhood obesity could have serious implications. The new generation of young adults that is expected to "carry" the nation's productivity and pay into social security, Medicare, Medicaid, and support federal and state social programs with their tax dollars may find themselves disabled or with limited earnings potential due to overweight-related impairments in health. National and state budgets will be doubly strained as healthcare payouts to program recipients soar while the funds supplying the tax coffers are diminishing by a less-productive workforce. In the private sector, health insurance premiums can be expected to increase to keep pace with the increased costs of health care associated with treatment for overweight and its complications. Also important are the lost "opportunity costs" of society not being able to fund other important social, educational, and public programs due to the drain on budgets from the healthcare costs of treating individuals with overweight.

Environmental Influences on Children Who Are with Overweight
Societal Factors

Many people with overweight have experienced discrimination because of the negative attitudes and judgmental behaviors of others who may see them as lazy and lacking willpower. Viewing children with overweight within a construct of "personal responsibility" has allowed past treatment interventions to focus on the child and, perhaps, the family unit. Experience has shown that this treatment model used by itself often has failed as many overweight children have grown up to be overweight adults.

Today, it is widely recognized that the microenvironment (home and family setting) and the macroenvironment (the setting in which the family is embedded) are the major contributors to child weight status, ranging from underweight to overweight.[123,150] The mission of public health is to fulfill society's interest in assuring conditions in which people can be healthy. Altering both the micro- and macroenvironments to promote healthy behaviors in children is vital to the mission of public health.

Overweight and Energy Balance

The environmental factors underlying the recent increase in obesity rates in the United States are multiple; however, diet and physical activity play a crucial role. Basic to this concept is the fact that to maintain a stable weight, energy intake and output must be balanced. When physical activity level is low, weight status can be maintained with a diet appropriately lower in calories. However, if an adjustment is not made by either increasing physical activity or decreasing energy intake, energy intake will exceed expenditure and will result in weight gain.

Programs and Resources That Support Evidence-Based Practices in Preventing Overweight in Children

A great many programs are available to support efforts to improve food intake and increase physical activity. Although research is limited on successful practices in various settings, the following are a few programs and resources that may be used by a public health dietitian/nutritionist when addressing overweight in children. Note that these programs will benefit all children to establish healthy eating and physical activity behaviors.

Walking Promotions

Many communities across the country are making efforts to increase the number of children who walk to school when they have a reasonable walking distance. These programs have taken many forms over the years; they mobilize community members such as school staff, the Parent Teacher Association, police departments, businesses, civic associations, and so on to work together to increase safe routes to and from school for children to walk or use their bicycles. Overall, the community becomes aware of the importance of children participating in daily physical activity, thereby changing an unwalkable community into a walkable community, which is an environmental intervention. This program supports the HP 2030 objectives related to children's trips to school by walking or bicycling.[1]

Reducing Screen Time

Various programs have been used to make the public and families aware of the amount of time spent with computers, cell phones, and other digital devices. Sometimes, the focus is on reducing screen time spent in front of the TV and other screens. The goal of these efforts is to encourage children and adults to turn off the television and replace that time with quality activities that promote healthier living and communities. In the past, the last week of April of every year was used to focus attention on reducing screen time. Programs promoting reduced screen time encouraged physical activities, such as running, skating, dancing, walking, bicycling, or playing a sport, along with other nonphysical activities. Since a link has been established between excessive TV viewing and increased BMI in children, decreasing TV viewing may encourage children to be more physically active.[151] Programs promoting screen-free activities support the HP 2020 objectives related to increasing the number of adolescents watching 2 hours or fewer of television on school days.

Nutrition

Have a Plant: The Produce for Better Health Foundation is a consumer education organization that sponsors national campaigns to encourage greater intake of fruits and vegetables. Have a Plant is observed monthly and encourages people to consume seven to 13 servings a day of colorful fruits and vegetables. Researchers have studied the relationship between fruit and vegetable intake and weight maintenance and loss in the pediatric population. Similarly, Team Fruits and Vegetables (FNV) is a campaign targeted to adolescents to promote more consumption of fruits and vegetables, using memes and celebrity endorsements. A message to increase fruits and vegetable intake has the benefit of being positive and guiding people to eat healthy foods, rather than using a negative approach such as recommending that people do not eat high fat and sugary foods.[152] Fruit and vegetable campaigns are useful because they have adaptable toolkits and other promotional items that fit various settings. In particular, the concepts of a rainbow on your plate and eating a rainbow are used in various nutrition education campaigns to educate children on the importance of healthy eating by consuming a variety of colorful fruits and vegetables. This initiative supports the HP 2030 objective related to persons 2 years and older consuming several servings of fruits and vegetables daily.[1]

Other Programs: Beyond breastfeeding, healthy eating habits among toddlers, and children are vitally important, as these lay the foundation for lifelong eating habits. There are many good sources of information on healthy eating practices among toddlers. Public health dietitians/nutritionists should identify successful programs that support the HP 2030 objective (developmental) related to increasing the proportion of children and adolescents who consume meals and snacks that are of good overall dietary quality.

The programs and resources discussed above are only a few avenues to explore and suggest to partners. To accomplish the ultimate goal of healthy children in healthy communities, the public health dietitian/nutritionist should be resourceful when suggesting programs, initiatives, and campaigns related to overweight in children. They must have a toolbox of information ready when entering various settings: coalition, community, school, worksite, healthcare facility, or other organizations. This toolbox of information and resources will vary depending on the target population. New resources become available regularly as the government and nongovernmental agencies fund efforts to develop evidence-based solutions. Community and public health dietitians/nutritionists must be creative and timely in sharing their vision and potential solutions to address childhood obesity.

Public Health Initiatives

Special Supplemental Nutrition Program for Women, Infants and Children

For more than 40 years, the WIC Program (Special Supplemental Nutrition Program for Women, Infants and Children) has provided supplemental foods and nutrition education for low-income women, infants, and children up to 5 years of age. The ultimate goal of WIC is to improve the nutritional status of low-income pregnant or lactating women, infants, and young children who have been identified as being at nutritional risk. The primary method of achieving that goal is through the provision of specific nutrient-dense foods paid for through program checks, vouchers or electronic debit cards by eligible pregnant or lactating women and mothers/caregivers of infants and children.[153]

WIC is funded at the federal level by the U.S. Department of Agriculture and is administered by states through public and private organizations, such as county and regional health departments. Breastfeeding promotion and support are central to the WIC program, and it has been credited with improving breastfeeding rates among vulnerable populations.[18,154] WIC program participation includes regular nutrition risk screening, growth assessment, and counseling by healthcare providers. During the infant's first year, WIC supplemental food packages for breastfeeding mothers provide milk, iron-fortified breakfast cereals, 100% juice containing vitamin C, eggs, and either dried beans/peas or peanut butter. Mothers of exclusively breastfed infants also receive cheese, tuna, and carrots. Breastfed infants do not receive food packages until they are weaned. Food packages for infants who are weaned provide iron-fortified infant formula for the first 6 months with the addition of iron-fortified infant cereal and infant juices at 4 to 6 months.

Access Team Fruits and Vegetables at: FNV.com

WIC provides nutritional services to a very large proportion of the population, with 24% of children aged 1 to 4 years receiving benefits, 35% of all pregnant and postpartum women, and 50% of all infants in the United States.[153] Food availability and food insecurity are problems for many WIC recipients, and approximately one-third of all WIC recipients also receive SNAP. WIC has been shown to be effective against food insecurity.[155] Any barriers that decrease food resources for these individuals make them more vulnerable to food insecurity as well as nutritional risk.[153,156-158]

Numerous studies have been conducted to evaluate WIC. Many have focused on specific outcomes such as the incidence of low–birth-weight infants,[154] nutritional assessment of pregnant women,[159] and the nutrient intakes of infants and young children.[160] Studies have investigated barriers to WIC usage. Woelfel et al.,[157] identified several key barriers to the use of WIC services. Their survey of over 3,000 WIC recipients rated 68 potential barriers to WIC use as measured by likelihood of not picking up WIC checks. Some changes have already taken place in many settings and the food package has been improved since this study. These barriers can be broken down into three broad categories: office procedures, the WIC food package, and nutrition education.

Office Procedures

The office setting is a key area where improvements are possible. The most frequently reported barrier relates to the long waiting times to receive WIC services.[157,161] When combined with three related items from the top 11 (more than an hour to recertify, overcrowded waiting rooms, and no activities for children), office procedures become a logical target for improvement. The image of unhappy, crying children waiting with their mothers in a cramped waiting room does not create a positive response. Less wait time results in fewer clients and children in the waiting room. In addition, all WIC sites should provide enjoyable activities for infants and children. Creatively developed activities could become nutrition education opportunities for children and caregivers. By 2020, Congress required that all states disburse WIC benefits through an Electronic Benefits Transfer (eWIC) system, which improves stigma and wait time for WIC.[158] This strategy alone has been found to be effective in states that implemented eWIC before 2020: spending on non-WIC eligible foods did not change but redemptions of WIC benefits increased,[162] thereby increasing the reach of the WIC program to eligible families.

WIC Food Package

The WIC Food Package was revised by USDA in 2014 in response to feedback from consumers, nutrition professionals, and state and local agencies. Dissatisfaction with the WIC food package had been recognized by many practitioners primarily for the lack of flexibility. A significant improvement was the 30% increase in dollars that can be used to purchase fruits and vegetables for children. This increase in funds for fruits and vegetables is accompanied by the option to purchase fresh fruits and vegetables instead of jarred infant food for older infants. Taken together, these changes will likely have an important benefit to the nutritional intake of children. Additional changes include allowance to use yogurt as a partial milk substitute, expanding whole-grain options and allowing states and local WIC agencies flexibility to meet the nutritional and cultural needs of WIC participants. If clients have problems identifying appropriate foods and package sizes or are uncertain about store policies, dietitians and public health dietitians/

nutritionists can design a learning activity that simulates the options available in the store.

WIC Nutrition Education

To be effective, nutrition education must engage the client in the learning process in a meaningful way. Less than optimal nutrition education could result from a variety of reasons, ranging from staff training and available nutrition education materials to inappropriate techniques, as well as insufficient nutrition staff and requirements for time efficiency. Very often, the WIC dietitian/nutritionist is an entry-level position for a dietitian/nutritionist, dietitian, or other health professional or paraprofessional, and this position often suffers from frequent turnover. These frontline nutrition educators need to be provided with the skills and resources to be most effective in making meaningful connections with their clients and to be a stimulating and vibrant part of the WIC experience. WIC dietitians/nutritionists need to evaluate objectively the effectiveness of their customary nutrition education programs and involve clients in determining pros and cons of current practices and ways to improve eating habits. In addition, more work is doing to better serve WIC clientele and improve nutrition education research through telehealth efforts and other technology-based nutrition education to support the needs of eligible families with young children.

Improvements in WIC office procedures, the WIC food package, and WIC nutrition education can have a significant impact on the nutritional status of WIC clients. The more barriers encountered by WIC recipients, the less likely they are to obtain the nutritious food needed to improve nutrition status. WIC nutrition practitioners can make the greatest impact by identifying and eliminating barriers in their locale.

Bright Futures

Launched in 1990 by the Health Resources and Services Administration's Maternal and Child Health Bureau, Bright Futures is an initiative aimed at improving health promotion and preventive services for infants, children, and adolescents. Bright Futures has produced a series of guidelines and supportive materials for health supervision focused on the areas of oral health, nutrition, physical activity, and mental health. The nutrition guidelines include recommendations for nutrition supervision from infancy through adolescence, common nutrition issues and concerns, and nutrition tools.[44] In 2002, collaboration with the AAP led to the establishment of the Bright Futures Education Center and Pediatric Implementation Project, whose objective is to support the implementation of the guidelines. For more information, see the Bright Futures website.

Opportunities for Community and Public Health Dietitians/Nutritionists to Intervene and Prevent Overweight in Children

Public health dietitians/nutritionists are challenged to think of new ways to address the problem of childhood obesity within existing venues and frameworks. To be most successful, the emphasis must be on population-based approaches and prevention, as traditional and clinical-based practices clearly have failed to adequately address the obesity epidemic. The public health dietitians/nutritionists thus may examine existing nutrition, social, and other programs and seize opportunities to advance goals. Some suggestions for opportunities are listed in the following sections.

WIC

- Develop policies and provide outreach activities to recruit pregnant women into prenatal care during the first trimester. This may improve nutrition delivery to the unborn child to avoid pregnancy under- or overnutrition, and thereby lower the risk of future obesity.[123,149]
- Grocery store tours are conducted in some clinics to teach shopping skills for healthy eating to program participants.
- Assess monitoring systems and develop policies or protocols to target high-risk children older than 2 years who exhibit rapid weight gain and ensure that they receive intensive guidance through culturally appropriate interventions.
- Train the healthcare team in anticipatory guidance and counseling, with regard to infant and child feeding and physical activity consistent with obesity prevention, to enable the team to serve as positive role models.
- Assess the clinic environment for inconsistencies (deliberate as well as unintended) in the healthy eating and physical activity messages and develop policies that promote a healthy environment for staff and program participants.
- Develop policies and environmental interventions that promote, support, and protect breastfeeding.

Head Start/Preschool/Daycare

- Develop policies that ensure healthy menu items and eating environments for children.
- Develop policies that ensure that children participate in recommended physical activity daily.
- Train childcare providers and the food service team in obesity prevention strategies through provision of nutritious food choices and daily physical activity appropriate for age and development.
- Assist with efforts to provide environmental intervention (e.g., playground, equipment for physical activity).
- Support training in healthy eating practices for children for staff and parents.
- Sponsor community events that involve families and staff to adopt healthy living practices, such as reducing sedentary behavior and increasing physical activity.

School Systems

- Advocate for daily recess and active physical education for all children through school boards, parent and teacher organizations, and school administrators.
- Develop policies that limit competitive foods and beverages.
- Serve fresh fruits and vegetables daily on the breakfast and lunch menus.
- Develop nutrition standards for vending machines and school stores.
- Advocate for a unified message for healthy eating and physical activity throughout the school (no candy fundraisers, no food and/or candy rewards for good behavior in the classroom, healthy snacks at parties and school events, and a campus that is friendly to physical activity, such as walkways, bicycle racks, and safe outdoor play equipment).
- Advocate for universal school breakfast and lunch program participation.
- Advocate for strengthening nutrition education throughout the entire school curricula (K–12) and make an impact on student behavior (50 hours/year minimum).

- Develop monitoring systems to assess children's health and behaviors (e.g., height and weight, BMI, blood pressure, fruit and vegetable consumption, TV viewing, transportation modes to school, and actual physical activity during recess and PE classes).

After-School Care

- Train staff to support obesity prevention efforts (healthy snacks, physical activity for all children).
- Survey the environment for consistency of health messages, minimizing the availability of competitive foods of poor nutritional quality.
- Make the environment friendly to physical activity.
- Assist with obtaining grants to provide facilities and equipment to enable and encourage physical activity (e.g., walking track, basketball court, playground equipment, etc.).

Other Possible Venues

- Advocate for child participation in federal summer feeding programs for needy children.
- Advocate for a healthful environment at various settings for children, such as Boys and Girls Clubs, YMCA/YWCA, summer camps, and other programs through provision of training opportunities and materials in obesity prevention to directors and their staff.

Opportunities for Community and Public Health Dietitians/Nutritionists to Promote Health Equity

As social determinants of health have been increasingly documented to be key factors in supporting health outcomes, it is critical for community and public health dietitians/nutritionists to consider how to more effectively develop interventions and prevention programs for underrepresented populations. Successful activities will likely include the following:

- An asset-based approach that values the lived experience of the target population.
- Co-created activities and nutrition education with the target population.
- Understanding of the historical and systemic issues that resulted in the disparities.
- Partnerships with key stakeholders that have an impact on social determinants of health.
- Systems-level solutions to address the root cause of the issue. While nutrition education is important, it cannot be the only approach as it tends to focus on individual-level change and not more upstream issues.

Envisioning the Future of Public Health Nutrition for Maternal, Infant, Child, and Adolescent Health

Growing a healthier nation will require input from everyone interested in the health of our children. This dream requires action from many individuals and in many locations. Based on the information in this chapter, this vision of a healthier nation described below is possible.

What a Healthier Nation Will Look Like

- Prenatal care is provided for all pregnant women in the first trimester.
- Health professionals provide anticipatory counseling for families to encourage breastfeeding and prevent feeding problems.
- Working mothers are given adequate breastfeeding support before and after returning to work.
- Food programs provide access to fresh produce at low cost for low-income families.
- Children learn early to love foods that will sustain their health.
- Children feel secure that they will have enough to eat.
- Schools serve nutritious lunches that children enjoy.
- Recess time allows for daily physical activity for all children.
- Vending machines at school are stocked with healthful choices that supply nutrients important to children's health.
- After-school programs offer ample opportunities to play.
- After-school programs provide nutritious snacks.
- Neighborhoods are planned with adequate green space for play and recreation.
- New parks are added during urban renewal projects.
- Children can walk or ride their bikes safely to and from school on walking trails and bike paths.
- Neighborhoods are planned for mixed use so that it is possible to walk to the store or other local businesses.
- Government agricultural support is increased for growing fruits and vegetables.
- Healthy foods are affordable.
- High-fat and high-sugar foods are expensive.
- Food companies don't advertise high-fat and sweetened foods to children during and between children's TV programming.
- Children participate in daily physical activities.
- Children's weight is appropriate for their growth and development.

Summary

Community and public health nutrition programs that provide services to women in the childbearing years, pregnant and lactating women, infants, children, and adolescents are vital to the health of the nation. Dietitians/nutritionists and other health professionals have important roles to play in improving the health of the nation by ensuring that these vulnerable groups get the services they need to grow and develop to their full potential. Attaining the Healthy People 2030 goals that relate to maternal, child, and adolescent issues can be used as an indicator of how successful public health programs are in providing the necessary services. Refer to the list of websites at the end of this chapter for extensive information, regular updates and announcements of new programs. Many public health nutrition programs undergo change on a regular basis. Recommendations in this chapter are based on information at the time of writing and are subject to change as the government and nongovernmental organizations adjust to newer information.

The stages of growth and development covered in this chapter are the most nutritionally challenging periods in human development. Knowledge of the developmental processes is a prerequisite to understanding the nutritional aspects of these life stages. Understanding these groups' nutritional and physical activity needs will help nutrition professionals provide individual counseling, group and community programs, and environmental solutions that can impact the future health of these individuals and of the nation.

Community and public health dietitians/nutritionists may use existing nutrition and social programs as opportunities to promote evidence-based strategies for health promotion and disease prevention. However, many programs are designed for specific groups (such as WIC and SNAP) and do not serve or reach all segments of the population that are involved in the care of children. Because many nutrition and social programs have a narrow focus, population-based services are essential to helping communities, schools, worksites, other organizations, and especially families to adopt healthy behaviors. Healthy eating among children cannot be addressed without including the family as a whole and the environment.

Children with overweight continue to be a public health concern; preventive efforts must target the parents and caregivers as well as the children. Improving family interactions through healthy eating practices and physical activity is essential to preventing childhood obesity. Healthy lifestyle behaviors can be taught in parenting classes and discussed during doctor's office visits, at worksites, at health fairs, in parent–teacher organizations, and at other sites. Understanding the social determinants of health and how they impact the nutritional intake and overall health disparities in these populations is critical. In particular, food insecurity and overall access to affordable health foods is a challenge for many communities and families, especially those with children, impacting the ability for certain populations to maintain health. In addition, population-based services and partners can develop and implement policy and environmental interventions that make it convenient for families to include healthy eating practices and daily physical activity.

Healthy eating practices and physical activity are interrelated when addressing normal growth. Although some traditional public health nutrition roles, as nutrition educator or a consultant to medical professionals, are valuable, the role of public health nutrition practitioners has expanded to include stepping outside of the office and into the community. Working with partners and stakeholders is essential, as is obtaining financial resources to implement programs in the community or schools. The media offers endless opportunities to reach target populations with various health messages and social marketing campaigns. Policy and advocacy will be crucial in developing standard nutrition and physical activity policies within various settings.

Public health dietitians/nutritionists have abundant opportunities for innovation, creativity, and personal development as this challenge demands the use of each person's unique skills: up-to-date knowledge of evidence-based care, communication and media skills, grant writing and budget know-how, research and presentation skills, advocacy and policy development, cultural competency, and relationship and coalition building. Population-based approaches should be comprehensive so that environmental changes will support healthy eating and regular physical activity and encourage optimal health for people of all ages.

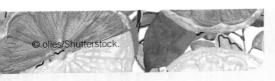
© olies/Shutterstock.

Learning Portfolio

Key Terms

	page
Fetal Alcohol Syndrome	252
Longitudinal studies	259
Preeclampsia	259
Galactosemia	261
Coalition	262
Environmental Justice	272
Retrospective studies	286
Evidence-based	287

Issues for Discussion

1. Which social determinants of health impact nutrition-related health equity for pregnant and lactating women, infants, children, and adolescents?
2. Which changes have occurred in lifestyles over the past 25 years that could have contributed to the rapid rise in the prevalence of overweight in children?
3. What types of challenges might you expect in a school district as you strive to improve food, beverage, and physical activity options?
4. Physical activity and exercise are as important as healthy eating in the pediatric population. Which partnership strategies could you use to promote physical activity as an intervention for children from early childhood to adolescence?
5. Evaluate the effectiveness of a current public and/or private effort to reduce childhood obesity. Discuss what improvements are needed to increase effectiveness.
6. List ways a public health dietitian/nutritionist can measure the success of an intervention related to preventing overweight in children.

Case Study: Community Nutrition

The dietitian/nutritionist and director of nursing for the public health department in a small southern rural community were concerned that a large number of children were food insecure in the school-aged student population. They contacted the local university and learned about a surveillance study that had recently been conducted with 4th, 8th, and 11th graders.

They reviewed the data and conducted an assessment of the limited amounts of healthy food outlets, low level of nutrition education, and physical activity in the school district as well as nutrition-related public programs available in the county. Based on their findings, the community dietitian/nutritionist and the county nurse decided to work together to seek funds to develop an intervention.

They identified key partners in the county (chief medical officer in the public health department, school superintendent, mayor, and community leaders) to gain support for a grant. The grant application was submitted, describing the county demographics, assessment of the problem, goals, objectives, strategies, time frame, stakeholders, and budget along with letters of support. The community dietitian/nutritionist and the director of nursing were awarded $25,000 to work with the school district to address food insecurity.

The goals of the project were to conduct the School Health Index (SHI) and develop policy and environmental interventions related to physical activity and nutrition within the school district. The project provided an opportunity for the dietitian/nutritionist and the director of nursing for the public health department to mobilize the school district and the community to participate in healthy lifestyle choices to improve the health of local children and the entire community.

1. List five possible problem areas that were identified in the SHI.
2. Identify some possible activities, policies, and environmental solutions to each of the problem areas developed by the team.
3. Describe three possible strategies to evaluate the outcome of the grant.
4. Identify three benefits that could be expected from this project.

Case Study: Screening for Overweight and Obese Children in the Schools

ABC Elementary School had their school nurse screen the children for overweight and obesity in the 5th grade as a part of a community health outreach program. After the screening was done using the NCHS growth charts and skinfold arm thickness, notes were sent home with the overweight and obese children informing the parents of their findings.

1. Why was sending home notes with the children a potential mistake?

2. What other methods could have been used to notify parents of their child's health?

3. What support should the school offer the parents for their children?

Resources

1. **Breastfeeding Report Card:** www.cdc.gov/breastfeeding/data/reportcard.htm
2. **Bridging the Gap:** www.bridgingthegapresearch.org
3. **Bright Futures:** brightfutures.aap.org
4. **CATCH:** www.childtrends.org/Lifecourse/programs/ChildandAdolesentTrialforCardiovascularHealth.htm
5. **CDC/NCHS BMI tables:** www.cdc.gov/growthcharts
6. **Child and Adult Care Program:** www.fns.usda.gov/cacfp
7. **Center for Health and Health Care in Schools:** www.healthinschools.org
8. **DHHS HRSA Maternal and Child Health Bureau:** www.mchb.hrsa.gov
9. **Dietary Guidelines:** www.health.gov/dietaryguidelines
10. **DRI:** ods.od.nih.gov/HealthInformation/Dietary_Reference_Intakes.aspx
11. **Food Allergy & Anaphylaxis Network:** www.foodallergy.org
12. **Food and Nutrition Information Center:** www.nal.usda.gov/fnic
13. **Food portions:** www.niddk.nih.gov/health-information/weight-management/just-enough-food-portions
14. **Food Research and Action Center:** www.frac.org
15. **Healthy People 2030:** www.healthypeople.gov
16. **International Lactation Consultants Association:** www.ilca.org
17. **Kids Count:** www.kidscount.org
18. **La Leche League:** www.lalecheleague.org
19. **Let's Move: First Lady Michelle Obama anti-obesity campaign:** letsmove.obamawhitehouse.archives.gov/
20. **National Assoc. of State Boards of Education State School Policy Database:** www.nasbe.org/healthy_schools
21. **National Center for Education in Maternal and Child Health:** www.ncemch.org
22. **Nurses' Health Study II:** www.channing.harvard.edu/nhs
23. **CDC Growth Charts:** www.cdc.gov/growthcharts
24. **National Early Childhood Technical Assistance Center:** http://www.nectac.org
25. **Physical Activity and Health: A Report of the Surgeon General:** www.cdc.gov/nccdphp/sgr/sgr.htm
26. **Planet Health:** www.hsph.harvard.edu/prc/projects/planet/
27. **Project EAT:** www.sphresearch.umn.edu/epi/project-eat/
28. **School Health Index (SHI):** www.cdc.gov/healthyschools/shi/index.htm
29. **School Meals Programs:** www.fns.usda.gov/cnd/
30. **School Nutrition Environment and Wellness Resources:** healthymeals.nal.usda.gov/school-wellness-resources-2
31. **Spark:** www.sparkpe.org
32. **Start Healthy, Stay Healthy:** www.starthealthystayhealthy.in
33. **Team FNV:** https://fnv.com/team/
34. **Team Nutrition:** www.fns.usda.gov/tn/
35. **U.S. Breastfeeding Committee:** www.usbreastfeeding.org
36. **U.S. government's food and nutrition site:** www.nutrition.gov
37. **USDA Center for Nutrition Policy and Promotion:** www.usda.gov/cnpp
38. **USDA Food and Nutrition Information Center:** fnic.nal.usda.gov/
39. **USDA Women, Infants and Children (WIC) Program:** www.fns.usda.gov/wic/

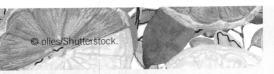
© olies/Shutterstock.

Learning Portfolio

References

1. U.S. Department of Agriculture and U.S. Department of Health and Human Services. Dietary Guidelines for Americans, 2020-2025. 9th ed. 2020.

2. U.S. Department of Health and Human Services. Healthy People 2030. Accessed September 1, 2021. https://health.gov/healthypeople

3. Schieve LA, Cogswell ME, Scanlon KS. Maternal weight gain and preterm delivery: differential effects by body mass index. *Epidemiology*. 1999;10:141-147.

4. Gunderson E, Abrams B, Selvin S. Does the pattern of post-partum weight change differ according to pregravid body size? *Int J Obes*, 2001;25(6):853-862.

5. Procter SB, Campbell CG. Position of the Academy of Nutrition and Dietetics: nutrition and lifestyle for a healthy pregnancy outcome. *J Acad Nutr Diet*. 2014;114(7):1099-1103.

6. Zhao R, Xu L, Wu M, Huang S, Cao XJ. Maternal pre-pregnancy body mass index, gestational weight gain influence birth weight. *Women and Birth*. 2018;31(1):e20-e25.

7. Stang J, Story M, Feldman S. Nutrition in adolescent pregnancy. *Int J Childbirth Educ*. 2005;20(2):4-11.

8. Scholl TO, Hediger ML, Schall JI. Maternal growth and fetal growth: pregnancy course and outcome in the Camden Study. *Ann N Y Acad Sci*. 1997;817(1):292-301.

9. Hediger ML, Scholl TO, Schall JI. Implications of the Camden Study of adolescent pregnancy: interactions among maternal growth, nutritional status, and body composition. *Ann N Y Acad Sci*. 1997;817(1):281-291.

10. Centers for Disease Control and Prevention. Data and statistics about opioid use during pregnancy. Accessed September 1, 2021. www.cdc.gov/pregnancy/opioids/data.html

11. Zedler BK, Mann AL, Kim MM, et al. Buprenorphine compared with methadone to treat pregnant women with opioid use disorder: a systematic review and meta-analysis of safety in the mother, fetus and child. *Addiction*. 2016;111(12):2115-2128.

12. Tomedi LE, Bogen DL, Hanusa BH, Wisner KL, Bodnar LM. A pilot study of the nutritional status of opiate-using pregnant women on methadone maintenance therapy. *Subst Use Misuse*. 2012;47(3):286-295.

13. Wambach K, Spencer B. *Breastfeeding and human lactation*. Jones & Bartlett Learning; 2019.

14. Eidelman AI. Breastfeeding and the use of human milk: an analysis of the American Academy of Pediatrics 2012 Breastfeeding Policy Statement. *Breastfeed Med*. 2012;7(5):323-324.

15. Lessen R, Kavanagh K. Position of the academy of nutrition and dietetics: promoting and supporting breastfeeding. *J Acad Nutr Diet*. 2015;115(3):444-449.

16. The World Health Organization. The optimal duration of exclusive breastfeeding. In. *A systematic review*. Geneva, Switzerland 2001.

17. Ryan AS, Wenjun Z, Acosta A. Breastfeeding continues to increase into the new millennium. *Pediatrics*. 2002;110(6):1103-1109.

18. Crowther SM, Reynolds LA, Tansey E. *The resurgence of breastfeeding, 1975–2000*. Vol 35: Wellcome Trust Centre for the History of Medicine at UCL; 2009.

19. U.S. Department of Health and Human Services. Healthy People 2020. In: Washington, DC.

20. Kuehn B. Breastfeeding report card. *JAMA*. 2018;320(14):1426-1426.

21. Kleinman RE. Pediatric nutrition handbook. *Actividad Dietética*. 2009;13(1):46.

22. Kramer FM, Stunkard AJ, Marshall KA, McKinney S, Liebschutz J. Breast-feeding reduces maternal lower-body fat. *J Am Diet Assoc*. 1993;93(4):429-433.

23. Neville C, McKinley M, Holmes V, Spence D, Woodside JV. The relationship between breastfeeding and postpartum weight change—a systematic review and critical evaluation. *Int J Obes*. 2014;38(4):577-590.

24. Table M. *Dietary reference intakes for energy, carbohydrate, fiber, fat, fatty acids, cholesterol, protein, and amino acids*. Vol 5: National Academy Press: Washington, DC, USA; 2005.

25. Picciano MF. Pregnancy and lactation: physiological adjustments, nutritional requirements and the role of dietary supplements. *J Nutr*. 2003;133(6):1997S-2002S.

26. Dietary Guidelines Advisory Committee. Scientific Report of the 2020 Dietary Guidelines Advisory Committee: Advisory Report to the Secretary of Agriculture and the Secretary of Health and Human Services. In: U.S. Department of Agriculture ARS, ed. Washington, DC. 2020.

27. Armstrong J, Reilly JJ., The Child Health Information Team. Breastfeeding and lowering the risk of childhood obesity. *Lancet*. 2002;359(9322):2003-2004.

28. Uwaezuoke SN, Eneh CI, Ndu IK. Relationship between exclusive breastfeeding and lower risk of childhood obesity: a narrative review of published evidence. *Clin Med Insights: Pediatr*. 2017;11:1179556517690196.

29. Baidal JAW, Locks LM, Cheng ER, Blake-Lamb TL, Perkins ME, Taveras EM. Risk factors for childhood obesity in the first 1,000 days: a systematic review. *Am J Prev Med*. 2016;50(6):761-779.

30. Dietz WH. Breastfeeding may help prevent childhood overweight. *JAMA*. 2001;285(19):2506-2507.

31. Shloim N, Vereijken C, Blundell P, Hetherington M. Looking for cues–infant communication of hunger and satiation during milk feeding. *Appetite*. 2017;108:74-82.

32. Ma J, Qiao Y, Zhao P, et al. Breastfeeding and childhood obesity: A 12-country study. *Matern Child Nutr*. 2020;16(3):e12984.

33. Ziegler EE. Growth of breast-fed and formula-fed infants. *Protein and Energy Requirements in Infancy and Childhood*, 2006;58:51-63.

34. Raiten DJ, Talbot JM, Waters JH. Assessment of nutrient requirements for infant formulas. *Journal Nutr*. 1998;128(11).

35. Forsyth J. International code of marketing of breast-milk substitutes—three decades later time for hostilities to be replaced by effective national and international governance. *Arc Dis Child*. 2010;95(10):769-770.

36. Hernell O, Fewtrell MS, Georgieff MK, Krebs NF, Lönnerdal B. Summary of current recommendations on iron provision and monitoring of iron status for breastfed and formula-fed infants in resource-rich and resource-constrained countries. *J Pediatr.* 2015;167(4):S40-S47.

37. Centers for Disease Control and Prevention. Iron - Infant and Toddler Nutrition. Accessed September 1, 2021. www.cdc.gov /nutrition/infantandtoddlernutrition/index.html

38. Bhatia J, Greer F. Use of soy protein-based formulas in infant feeding. *Pediatrics.* 2008;121(5):1062-1068.

39. Committee on Nutrition. Soy protein-based formulas: Recommendations for use in infant feeding. *Pediatrics.* 1998;101(1):148-153.

40. Butte NF, Hopkinson JM, Wong WW, Smith EOB, Ellis KJ. Body composition during the first 2 years of life: an updated reference. *Pediatr Res.* 2000;47(5):578-585.

41. Gale C, Logan KM, Santhakumaran S, Parkinson JR, Hyde MJ, Modi N. Effect of breastfeeding compared with formula feeding on infant body composition: a systematic review and meta-analysis. *Am J Clin Nutr.* 2012;95(3):656-669.

42. Centers for Disease Control and Prevention. Use and Interpretation of the CDC Growth Charts. Accessed September 1, 2021. www.cdc.gov/growthcharts/index.htm

43. Butte N, Cobb K, Dwyer J, Graney L, Heird W, Rickard K. The start healthy feeding guidelines for infants and toddlers1. *J Am Diet Assoc.* 2004;104(3):442-454.

44. Story M. *Bright futures in practice.* National Center for Education in Maternal and Child Health; 2002.

45. Nicklaus S. Complementary feeding strategies to facilitate acceptance of fruits and vegetables: A narrative review of the literature. *Int J Envir Res Public Health.* 2016;13(11):1160.

46. Mura Paroche M, Caton SJ, Vereijken CM, Weenen H, Houston-Price C. How infants and young children learn about food: a systematic review. *Front Psychol.* 2017;8:1046.

47. Lifschitz CH. Carbohydrate absorption from fruit juices in infants. *Pediatrics.* 2000;105(1):e4.

48. Heyman MB, Abrams SA. Fruit juice in infants, children, and adolescents: current recommendations. *Pediatrics.* 2017;139(6).

49. Kreiter SR, Schwartz RP, Kirkman Jr HN, Charlton PA, Calikoglu AS, Davenport ML. Nutritional rickets in African American breast-fed infants. *J Pediatr.* 2000;137(2):153-157.

50. Pugliese MT, Blumberg DL, Hludzinski J, Kay S. Nutritional rickets in suburbia. *J Am Coll Nutr.* 1998;17(6):637-641.

51. Welch TR, Bergstrom WH, Tsang RC. Vitamin D–deficient rickets: the reemergence of a once-conquered disease. *J Pediatr.* 2000;137(2):143-145.

52. Wagner CL, Greer FR., & the Section on Breastfeeding and Committee on Nutrition. Prevention of rickets and vitamin D deficiency in infants, children, and adolescents. *Pediatrics.* 2008;122(5):1142-1152.

53. Nokes C, van den Bosch C, Bundy DA. The effects of iron deficiency and anemia on mental and motor performance, educational achievement, and behavior in children. *A report of the INACG Washington, DC: Int Life Sci Inst.* 1998.

54. Ziegler EE, Jiang T, Romero E, Vinco A, Frantz JA, Nelson SE. Cow's milk and intestinal blood loss in late infancy. *J Ped.* 1999;135(6):720-726.

55. Fernandes SMR, de Morais MB, Amancio OMS. Intestinal blood loss as an aggravating factor of iron deficiency in infants aged 9 to 12 months fed whole cow's milk. *J Clin Gastro.* 2008;42(2):152-156.

56. Hale TW, Rowe HE. *Medications and mothers' milk 2017.* Springer Publishing Company; 2016.

57. Palmer CA, Gilbert JA. Position of the Academy of Nutrition and Dietetics: the impact of fluoride on health. *J Acad Nutr Diet.* 2012;112(9):1443-1453.

58. American Academy of Pediatric Dentistry. Guideline on fluoride therapy. *Ped Dent,* 2013;35(5):E165-E168.

59. Kohn WG, Maas WR, Malvitz DM, Presson SM, Shaddix KK. Recommendations for using fluoride to prevent and control dental caries in the United States. 2001.

60. Greer FR, Krebs NF. Optimizing bone health and calcium intakes of infants, children, and adolescents. *Pediatrics.* 2006;117(2):578-585.

61. Zemel MB. Role of dietary calcium and dairy products in modulating adiposity. *Lipids.* 2003;38(2):139-146.

62. Alaimo K, McDowell MA, Briefel RR, et al. Dietary intake of vitamins, minerals, and fiber of persons ages 2 months and over in the United States: Third National Health and Nutrition Examination Survey, Phase 1, 1988-91. 1994.

63. Skinner JD, Bounds W, Carruth BR, Ziegler P. Longitudinal calcium intake is negatively related to children's body fat indexes. *J Am Diet Assoc.* 2003;103(12):1626-1631.

64. Song Q, Sergeev IN. Calcium and vitamin D in obesity. *Nutrion Res Rev.* 2012;25(1):130-141.

65. Dallman PR. Iron deficiency: does it matter? *J Int Med,* 1989;226(5):367-372.

66. Barlow SE, Dietz WH. Obesity evaluation and treatment: Expert committee recommendations. *Pediatrics.* 1998;102(3):e29.

67. Flegal KM, Tabak CJ, Ogden CL. Overweight in children: Definitions and interpretation. *Health Educ Res,* 2006;21(6):755-760.

68. Serdula MK, Ivery D, Coates RJ, Freedman DS, Williamson DF, Byers T. Do obese children become obese adults? A review of the literature. *Prev Med.* 1993;22(2):167-177.

69. Krassas GE, Tzotzas T. Do obese children become obese adults: childhood predictors of adult disease. *Pediatric Endocr Rev.* 2004;1:455-459.

70. Ellis KJ, Abrams SA, Wong WW. Monitoring childhood obesity: Assessment of the weight/height^2 index. *Am J Epidemiol.* 1999;150(9):939-946.

71. Taylor RW, Jones IE, Williams SM, Goulding A. Body fat percentages measured by dual-energy X-ray absorptiometry corresponding to recently recommended body mass index cutoffs for overweight and obesity in children and adolescents aged 3–18 y. *The Am J Clin Nutr* 2002;76(6):1416-1421.

72. Puhl RM. What words should we use to talk about weight? A systematic review of quantitative and qualitative studies examining preferences for weight-related terminology. *Obes Rev.* 2020;21(6):e13008.

73. Yourell JL, Doty JL, Beauplan Y, Cardel MI. Weight-talk between parents and adolescents: a systematic review of relationships with health-related and psychosocial outcomes. *Adolesc Res Rev.* 2021:1-16.

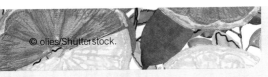
© olies/Shutterstock.

Learning Portfolio

74. Madsen KA, Thompson HR, Linchey J, et al. Effect of school-based body mass index reporting in California public schools: a randomized clinical trial. *JAMA Pediatr,* 2020;175(3):251-259. doi: 10.1001/jamapediatrics.2020.4768

75. Patel AI, Sanchez-Vaznaugh EV, Woodward-Lopez G. The importance of body mass index assessment and surveillance in schools. *JAMA Pediatr,* 2021;175(6):645. doi: 10.1001/jamapediatrics.2021.0016

76. Benjamin-Neelon SE. Position of the Academy of Nutrition and Dietetics: Benchmarks for nutrition in child care. *J Acad Nutr Diet.* 2018;118(7):1291-1300.

77. Stang J. Position of the American Dietetic Association: Child and adolescent nutrition assistance programs. *J Am Diet Assoc.* 2010;110(5):791-799.

78. Farley D, Alert F. Dangers of lead still linger. *FDA Consumer.* 1998;32(1):16-21.

79. Hanna-Attisha M, Gonuguntla A, Peart N, LaChance J, Taylor DK, Chawla S. Umbilical cord blood lead level disparities between Flint and Detroit. *Am J Perinatol.* 2020.

80. Schlosser E. *Fast food nation: The dark side of the all-American meal.* Houghton Mifflin Harcourt; 2012.

81. Bowman SA, Gortmaker SL, Ebbeling CB, Pereira MA, Ludwig DS. Effects of fast-food consumption on energy intake and diet quality among children in a national household survey. *Pediatrics.* 2004;113(1):112-118. https://doi.org/10.1542/peds.113.1.112

82. Slawson DL, Fitzgerald N, Morgan KT. Position of the Academy of Nutrition and Dietetics: the role of nutrition in health promotion and chronic disease prevention. *J Acad Nutr Diet.* 2013;113(7):972-979.

83. Nicklas TA, Baranowski T, Cullen KW, Berenson G. Eating patterns, dietary quality and obesity. *J Am Coll Nutr.* 2001;20(6):599-608.

84. Kurtzweil P. *Taking the fat out of food.* Department of Health and Human Services, Public Health Service, Food and Drug Administration; 1996.

85. Vos MB, Kaar JL, Welsh JA, et al. Added sugars and cardiovascular disease risk in children: a scientific statement from the American Heart Association. *Circulation.* 2017;135(19):e1017-e1034.

86. Paeratakul S, Ferdinand DP, Champagne CM, Ryan DH, Bray GA. Fast-food consumption among US adults and children: dietary and nutrient intake profile. *J Am Diet Assoc.* 2003;103(10):1332-1338.

87. Ludwig DS, Peterson KE, Gortmaker SL. Relation between consumption of sugar-sweetened drinks and childhood obesity: a prospective, observational analysis. *Lancet.* 2001;357(9255):505-508.

88. Rosinger A, Herrick KA, Gahche JJ, Park S. Sugar-sweetened beverage consumption among US youth, 2011-2014. *NCHS Data Brief, 271,* 1-2.

89. Luger M, Lafontan M, Bes-Rastrollo M, Winzer E, Yumuk V, Farpour-Lambert N. Sugar-sweetened beverages and weight gain in children and adults: a systematic review from 2013 to 2015 and a comparison with previous studies. *Obes Facts.* 2017;10(6):674-693.

90. Backholer K, Gupta A, Zorbas C, et al. Differential exposure to, and potential impact of, unhealthy advertising to children by socio-economic and ethnic groups: A systematic review of the evidence. *Obes Rev.* 2020;22(3);e13144.

91. Nguyen KH, Glantz SA, Palmer CN, Schmidt LA. Transferring racial/ethnic marketing strategies from tobacco to food corporations: Philip Morris and Kraft General Foods. *Am J Pub Health.* 2020;110(3):329-336.

92. Bergman E. Position of the American Dietetic Association: Local support for nutrition integrity in schools. *J Am Diet Assoc.* 2010;110(8):1244-1254.

93. Chriqui JF, Piekarz E, Chaloupka FJ. USDA snack food and beverage standards: how big of a stretch for the states? *Child Obes.* 2014;10(3):234-240.

94. Turner L, Chaloupka FJ. Improvements in school lunches result in healthier options for millions of US children: Results from public elementary schools between 2006-07 and 2013-14 (A BTG Research Brief). *Chicago: University of Illinois at Chicago.* 2015.

95. Cohen J, Schwartz MB. Documented success and future potential of the healthy, hunger-free kids act. *J Acad Nutr Diet.*2020;120(3):359-362.

96. Johnson DB, Podrabsky M, Rocha A, Otten JJ. Effect of the Healthy Hunger-Free Kids Act on the nutritional quality of meals selected by students and school lunch participation rates. *JAMA Pediatr.* 2016;170(1):e153918-e153918.

97. Mansfield JL, Savaiano DA. Effect of school wellness policies and the Healthy, Hunger-Free Kids Act on food-consumption behaviors of students, 2006–2016: a systematic review. *Nutr Rev.* 2017;75(7):533-552.

98. Kenney EL, Barrett JL, Bleich SN, Ward ZJ, Cradock AL, Gortmaker SL. Impact of the Healthy, Hunger-Free Kids Act on Obesity Trends. *Health Aff.* 2020;39(7):1122-1129.

99. Kinderknecht K, Harris C, Jones-Smith J. Association of the Healthy, Hunger-Free Kids Act with dietary quality among children in the US National School Lunch Program. *JAMA.* 2020;324(4):359-368.

100. Centers for Disease Control and Prevention. *Local School Wellness Policies: Where Do They Stand and What Can You Do?* ERIC Clearinghouse; 2014.

101. Chriqui J, Resnick E, Schneider L, et al. School district wellness policies: Evaluating progress and potential for improving children's health five years after the federal mandate. Brief Report. Volume 3. *ERIC* 2013.

102. Centers for Disease Control and Prevention. School Health Index (SHI): Self-Assessment and Planning Guide. In: Atlanta, GA: Centers for Disease Control. Accessed September 1, 20121. www.cdc.gov/healthyschools/shi/index.htm

103. Dutra GF, Kaufmann CC, Pretto AD, Albernaz EP. Television viewing habits and their influence on physical activity and childhood overweight. *Jornal de Pediatria,* 2015;91(4):346-351.

104. Gortmaker SL, Must A, Sobol AM, Peterson K, Colditz GA, Dietz WH. Television viewing as a cause of increasing obesity among children in the United States, 1986-1990. *Arch Pediatr Adolesc Med.* 1996;150(4):356-362.

105. Andersen RE, Crespo CJ, Bartlett SJ, Cheskin LJ, Pratt M. Relationship of physical activity and television watching with body weight and level of fatness among children: results from the Third National Health and Nutrition Examination Survey. *JAMA*. 1998;279(12):938-942.

106. Bleakley A, Jordan AB, Hennessy M. The relationship between parents' and children's television viewing. *Pediatrics*. 2013;132(2):e364-e371.

107. Andreyeva T, Kelly IR, Harris JL. Exposure to food advertising on television: associations with children's fast food and soft drink consumption and obesity. *Econ Hum Biol*. 2011;9(3):221-233.

108. Story M, Neumark-Sztainer D, French S. Individual and environmental influences on adolescent eating behaviors. *J Am Diet Assoc*. 2002;102(suppl 3):S40-S51.

109. Bremer AA. Adolescent development. *Pediatr Ann*. 2012;41(4):145.

110. McNeely C, Blanchard J. *The teen years explained: A guide to healthy adolescent development*. Jayne Blanchard; 2010.

111. Sigman-Grant M. Strategies for counseling adolescents. *J Am Diet Assoc*. 2002;102(suppl 3):S32-S39.

112. Resnick MD, Chambliss SA, Blum RW. Health and risk behaviors of urban adolescent males involved in pregnancy. *Fam Soc*. 1993;74(6):366-374.

113. Story M, Resnick MD. Adolescents' views on food and nutrition. *J Nutr Educ*. 1986;18(4):188-192.

114. Johnson DS, Lino M. Teenages: employment and contributions to family spending. *Monthly Lab Rev*. 2000;123:15.

115. Channel One Network. Teen Fact Book. 1998.

116. Schürmann S, Kersting M, Alexy U. Vegetarian diets in children: a systematic review. *Eur J Nutr*. 2017;56(5):1797-1817.

117. Golden NH, Katzman DK, Sawyer SM, Ornstein RM. Position paper of the society for adolescent health and medicine: medical management of restrictive eating disorders in adolescents and young adults references. *J Adolesc Health*. 2015;56(1): 121-125.

118. Golden NH. The adolescent: vulnerable to develop an eating disorder and at high risk for long-term sequelae. *Ann N Y Acad Sci*. 1997;817(1):94-97.

119. Rohde P, Stice E, Marti CN. Development and predictive effects of eating disorder risk factors during adolescence: implications for prevention efforts. *Int J Eat Disord*. 2015;48(2): 187-198.

120. Manley AF. Physical activity and health: a report of the Surgeon General. 1996.

121. Holt K. Bright futures nutrition, pocket guide. *Am Acad Pediatrics*. 2011.

122. Piercy KL, Troiano RP, Ballard RM, et al. The physical activity guidelines for Americans. *JAMA*. 2018;320(19): 2020-2028.

123. Booth KM, Pinkston MM, Poston WSC. Obesity and the built environment. *J Am Diet Assoc*. 2005;105(5):110-117.

124. Lee SM, Burgeson CR, Fulton JE, Spain CG. Physical education and physical activity: results from the School Health Policies and Programs Study 2006. *J Sch Health*. 2007;77(8): 435-463.

125. Eisenberg ME, Olson RE, Neumark-Sztainer D, Story M, Bearinger LH. Correlations between family meals and psychosocial well-being among adolescents. *Arch Pediatr Adolesc Med*. 2004;158(8):792-796.

126. Gillman MW, Rifas-Shiman SL, Frazier AL, et al. Family dinner and diet quality among older children and adolescents. *Arch Fam Med*. 2000;9(3):235-240.

127. Allison DB, Matz PE, Pietrobelli A, Zannolli R, Faith MS. Genetic and environmental influences on obesity. In: *Primary and secondary preventive nutrition*. Springer; 2001:147-164.

128. Fisher JO, Birch LL. Restricting access to palatable foods affects children's behavioral response, food selection, and intake. *Am J Clin Nutr*. 1999;69(6):1264-1272.

129. Harris HA, Jansen E, Rossi T. 'It's not worth the fight': fathers' perceptions of family mealtime interactions, feeding practices and child eating behaviours. *Appetite*. 2020;150:104642.

130. Roess AA, Jacquier EF, Catellier DJ, et al. Food consumption patterns of infants and toddlers: findings from the Feeding Infants and Toddlers Study (FITS) 2016. *J Nutr*. 2018;148(suppl 3):1525S-1535S.

131. Briefel RR, Deming DM, Reidy KC. Parents' perceptions and adherence to children's diet and activity recommendations: the 2008 Feeding Infants and Toddlers Study. *Prev Chronic Dis*. 2015;12:E159.

132. Satter E. *Child of mine: Feeding with love and good sense*. Bull Publishing Company; 2012.

133. Satter E. *How to get your kid to eat: but not too much*. Bull Publishing Company; 2012.

134. Satter E. *Secrets of feeding a healthy family: how to eat, how to raise good eaters, how to cook*. Kelcy Press; 2008.

135. Drewnowski A, Specter SE. Poverty and obesity: the role of energy density and energy costs. *Am Journal Clin Nutr*. 2004;79(1):6-16.

136. Jones SJ, Jahns L, Laraia BA, Haughton B. Lower risk of overweight in school-aged food insecure girls who participate in food assistance: results from the panel study of income dynamics child development supplement. *Arch Pediatr Adoles Med*. 2003;157(8):780-784.

137. Gibson D. Long-term food stamp program participation is differentially related to overweight in young girls and boys. *J Nutr*. 2004;134(2):372-379.

138. Hudak KM, Racine EF. Do additional SNAP benefits matter for child weight? Evidence from the 2009 benefit increase. *Econ Hum Biol*. 2021;41:100966.

139. Williams PA, Cates SC, Blitstein JL, et al. Evaluating the impact of six Supplemental Nutrition Assistance Program Education Interventions on children's at-home diets. *Health Educ Behav*. 2015;42(3):329-338.

140. Ogden CL, Carroll MD, Fryar CD, Flegal KM. Prevalence of obesity among adults and youth: United States, 2011-2014. *NCHS Brief*. 2015;219:1-8.

141. Freedman DS, Khan LK, Serdula MK, Dietz WH, Srinivasan SR, Berenson GS. The relation of childhood BMI to adult adiposity: the Bogalusa Heart Study. *Pediatrics*. 2005;115(1): 22-27.

142. Berenson GS, Bogalusa Heart Study Research Group. Childhood risk factors predict adult risk associated with subclinical

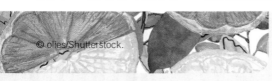
© olies/Shutterstock.

Learning Portfolio

cardiovascular disease: The Bogalusa Heart Study. *Am J Cardiol.* 2002;90(10, suppl 3):L3-L7.

143. Hill JO, Wyatt HR, Reed GW, Peters JC. Obesity and the environment: where do we go from here? *Science.* 2003;299(5608):853-855.

144. Gibson LY, Byrne SM, Blair E, Davis EA, Jacoby P, Zubrick SR. Clustering of psychosocial symptoms in overweight children. *Aust N Z J Psychiatry.* 2008;42(2):118-125.

145. Sahoo K, Sahoo B, Choudhury AK, Sofi NY, Kumar R, Bhadoria AS. Childhood obesity: causes and consequences. *J Fam Med Prim Care.* 2015;4(2):187-192.

146. Epstein LH, Wrotniak BH. Future directions for pediatric obesity treatment. *Obesity (Silver Spring, Md).* 2010;18(suppl 1):S8-S12.

147. Ogden CL, Carroll MD, Kit BK, Flegal KM. Prevalence of childhood and adult obesity in the United States, 2011-2012. *JAMA.* 2014;311(8):806-814.

148. Pratt CA, Loria CM, Arteaga SS, et al. A systematic review of obesity disparities research. *Am J Prev Med.* 2017;53(1):113-122.

149. Dietz WH. Overweight in childhood and adolescence. *N Engl J Med.* 2004;350(9):855-857.

150. Booth SL, Sallis JF, Ritenbaugh C, et al. Environmental and societal factors affect food choice and physical activity: rationale, influences, and leverage points. *Nutr Rev.* 2001;59(3):S21-S36.

151. Boone JE, Gordon-Larsen P, Adair LS, Popkin BM. Screen time and physical activity during adolescence: longitudinal effects on obesity in young adulthood. *Int J Behav Nutr Phys Act.* 2007;4(1):1-10.

152. Epstein LH, Gordy CC, Raynor HA, Beddome M, Kilanowski CK, Paluch R. Increasing fruit and vegetable intake and decreasing fat and sugar intake in families at risk for childhood obesity. *Obes Res.* 2001;9(3):171-178.

153. Fox H, McManus MA, Schmidt H. WIC reauthorization: opportunities for improving the nutritional status of women, infants, and children. *NHFP Background Paper.* 2003;1-35. 2017.

154. Kowaleski-Jones L, Duncan GJ. Effects of participation in the WIC program on birthweight: evidence from the national longitudinal survey of youth. *AmJ Pub Health.* 2002;92(5):799-804.

155. Kreider B, Pepper JV, Roy M. Identifying the effects of WIC on food insecurity among infants and children. *South Econ J.* 2016;82(4):1106-1122.

156. Conrey EJ, Frongillo EA, Dollahite JS, Griffin MR. Integrated program enhancements increased utilization of farmers' market nutrition program. *J Nutr.* 2003;133(6):1841-1844.

157. Woelfel ML, Abusabha R, Pruzek R, Stratton H, Chen SG, Edmunds LS. Barriers to the use of WIC services. *J AmDiet Assoc.* 2004;104(5):736-743.

158. Zimmer MC, Beaird J, Steeves EA. WIC participants' perspectives of facilitators and barriers to shopping with eWIC compared with paper vouchers. *J Nutr Edu Behav.* 2020;53(3):195-203.

159. Swensen AR, Harnack LJ, Ross JA. Nutritional assessment of pregnant women enrolled in the Special Supplemental Program for Women, Infants, and Children (WIC). *J Am Diet Assoc.* 2001;101(8):903-908.

160. Chaparro MP, Crespi CM, Anderson CE, Wang MC, Whaley SE. The 2009 special supplemental nutrition program for women, infants, and children (WIC) food package change and children's growth trajectories and obesity in Los Angeles County. *AmJ Clin Nutr.* 2019;109(5):1414-1421.

161. Rosenberg TJ, Alperen JK, Chiasson MA. Why do WIC participants fail to pick up their checks? An urban study in the wake of welfare reform. *A Journal Pub Health.* 2003;93(3):477-481.

162. Hanks AS, Gunther C, Lillard D, Scharff RL. From paper to plastic: understanding the impact of eWIC on WIC recipient behavior. *Food Policy.* 2019;83:83-91.

CHAPTER 10

The Importance of Community and Public Health Nutrition Programs in Preventing Disease and Promoting Adult Health

Marianella Herrera-Cuenca DSc, MD

(We would like to acknowledge the work of Judith Sharlin, PhD, RDN, in the past editions of Nutrition in Public Health.)

Learning Outcomes

AFTER STUDYING THIS CHAPTER AND REFLECTING ON THE CONTENTS, YOU SHOULD BE ABLE TO:

1. Identify the primary causes of death and disability in adults in the United States.
2. Describe primary, secondary, and tertiary levels of health prevention and health promotion and their relationship to nutrition program planning.
3. Identify risk factors for chronic diseases and their implication for nutrition.
4. Describe the dietary risk factors associated with the leading chronic diseases.
5. Discuss the common features of the dietary guidelines issued by the major U.S. health organizations.

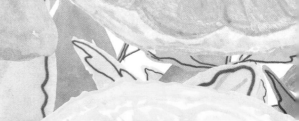

Nutrition Program Initiatives with the role of fostering behavior change toward food and nutrition and supporting caring practices.[1-7]

Prevention Those interventions that occur before the initial onset of disorder.

Chronic Disease Also known as noncommunicable disease; is not passed from person to person. It is of long duration and generally slow progression. The four main types of chronic diseases are cardiovascular, cancers, chronic respiratory diseases, and diabetes.

Pandemic Learning Opportunity

See http://www.cdc.gov/chronicdisease/ to learn about chronic disease in the United States and the impact of Covid-19.

Read more about food insecurity in Chapter 13.

Introduction

Growing scientific evidence reveals that healthy dietary intake and adequate nutrition status in adults contributes significantly to preventing illnesses and premature deaths in the United States.[8] Life expectancy has increased dramatically over the past century, and in 2018, the average life expectancy is 78.7 years.[9,10] Health and **nutrition programs** for adults aim at **prevention**, as well as improving quality of life. However, six of 10 adults have a **chronic disease** and four of 10 have two or more. Also, chronic diseases account for seven of every 10 deaths in the United States[11,12] The increasing cost of crisis medical care and the growing economic burden provide a cost-effective incentive for individuals and our nation to prevent chronic disease. Chronic diseases cost the United States 86% of the nation's healthcare cost. Despite this statistic, only 3% of the total annual healthcare expenditures in our nation were spent on prevention.[13] Nutrition interventions and policies target the factors related to adult health and aim to prevent chronic diseases that are the leading causes of death and disability.

Strong evidence has been arising in the past decades on the early origins of chronic diseases and the influence of maternal exposure to inadequate environmental conditions. Maternal pre-conceptional nutrition status as well as an inadequate weight gain during pregnancy are showing impact on the baby's and mother's future health, implying that adulthood health might be altered by early life conditions, particularly in utero, early infancy, and school years.[14]

In addition to all of the above, the global pandemic believed to initiate in Wuhan, China, in December of 2019, has had an impact on the US population's health as more than 6,800,000 cases have been reported, including older adults, who presented a higher incidence at the beginning of the pandemic and a median age of Covid-19 cases decline from 46 years in May of 2020 to 38 years in August. Besides the number of Covid-19 cases that are increasing, the economic consequences due to the measures of social isolation and stay-at-home messages impacted the income of families, as many businesses, enterprises, and other employment sources went into an economic turndown, which translated in lost jobs or diminished salaries for many Americans, thus increasing the levels of poverty and food insecurity in the country.[15] The decreased economy exacerbated the gaps along racial/ethnic and socioeconomic perimeters, with low-income Americans, Black, and Hispanic Americans, the most likely to get sick and die from COVID-19.[15]

Chronic Diseases: The Leading Causes of Death and Disability

To successfully create programs to promote health, longevity, and the quality of life, we must examine the leading causes of death and disability. Data from the National Center for Health Statistics (NCHS) show that chronic diseases were the leading causes of death in 2019 (See **Table 10–1**). Cardiovascular diseases and cancer account for 44.2% of all deaths in the United States, which means a decrease of 6% compared with 2013 data. More than 60% of chronic disease mortality can be attributed to lifestyle factors, such as diet, which can be modified.[16] A recent report on the health status of U.S. adults emphasized that increasing numbers of people still smoke, are physically inactive, and are overweight.[17,18] Researchers noted that approximately half of the deaths among U.S. adults could have been prevented.[19] These findings revealed that 400,000 deaths occur each

TABLE 10–1
Leading Causes of Death, United States, 2019

Data are for the United States
Number of deaths for leading causes of death

- Heart disease: 659,041
- Cancer: 599,601
- Accidents (unintentional injuries): 173,040
- Chronic lower respiratory diseases: 156,979
- Stroke (cerebrovascular diseases): 150,005
- Alzheimer's disease: 121,499
- Diabetes: 87,647
- Nephritis, nephrotic syndrome, and nephrosis: 51,565
- Influenza and pneumonia: 49,783
- Intentional self-harm (suicide): 47,511

Data from Mortality in the United States, 2019, data table for figure 2.

year due to poor diet and physical inactivity.[19] This number was found to be 20% less in a 2000 study.[20] It appears that the increasing trend of overweight and obesity will likely overtake tobacco as the leading preventable cause of mortality in the United States.[19] Although mortality rates from heart disease, stroke, and cancer have declined, behavioral changes have led to an increased prevalence of obesity and diabetes.[21,22] Dietary factors have been associated, during the last decades, with four of the 10 leading causes of death: coronary heart disease (CHD), some types of cancer, stroke, and type-2 diabetes.[23] The 2006 Surgeon General's report confirmed these findings: "For two out of three adult Americans who do not smoke and do not drink excessively, one personal choice seems to influence long-term health prospects more than any other, what we eat."[24]

Determinants of Health, Risk Factors, and Chronic Disease

Chronic diseases, although prevalent and costly, are among the most preventable. Research has identified a Health Promotion and Preventive Action model (HPA) for **risk factors**.[25] In this model, risk factor identification, reduction, modification, and education are related to human health and developmental stages.[25] Risk factors can be defined as those specific characteristics associated with an increased chance of developing a chronic disease. Risk factors that can be changed or modified, such as diet or physical activity, are under an individual's personal choices.

Healthy People (HP) 2030 provides the most recent **guidelines** and recommendations for specific health objectives and goals for the nation.[9] Initially, HP 2010 revealed that individual biological behaviors and environmental factors were responsible for approximately 70% of all premature deaths.[9] Biological factors such as age or gender are not modifiable. However, the leading causes of death are associated with dietary factors and sedentary behaviors, which are modifiable. Actually, the HP 2030 Leading Health indicators (LHIs) were selected and organized using a Health Determinants and Health Outcomes by Life Stages conceptual framework previously formulated. The Determinants of Health illustrate how individual biology and behaviors influence health through the individual's social and physical environments.[9] The HP 2020 statement similarly stated: "This approach is intended to draw attention to both: individual and societal determinants that affect the public's health and contribute to health disparities from infancy through old age, thereby highlighting strategic opportunities to

Strategy Tip

Viewing Table 10–1, how many diseases may be prevented by changing the diet?

Risk factor Can be defined as those specific characteristics associated with an increased chance of developing a chronic disease.

Guideline Information intended to advise people.

promote health and improve quality of life for all Americans." In summary, determinants of health consist of:

1. Health disparities: biological, social, economic, and environmental factors and their relationships
2. Health Across Life Stages: where LHIs are being examined using a life-stage perspective.[26]

Based on this history, HP 2030 includes sets data-driven objectives to improve health and well-being over the next decade. This approach comprises 355 core objectives that have 10-year targets and are associated with evidence-based interventions. These interventions will help track progress toward the achievements of the Healthy People vision, which is: "A society in which all people can achieve their full potential for health and well-being across the lifespan."[9]

Prevention Strategies

Health promotion and disease prevention provide complementary interventions to change health risk factors. Prevention efforts in public heath, community, and worksite settings are divided into three levels: primary prevention (health promotion), secondary prevention (risk appraisal and reduction), and tertiary prevention (treatment and rehabilitation).[27-29]

Primary Prevention: Health Promotion

Primary prevention **strategies**, or health promotion, encourage health-enhancing behaviors by giving individuals, families, and communities ways to reduce risk factors associated with disease and injury.[29] Risk factors include environmental, economic, social, and biological aspects. Good examples of primary prevention strategies include nutrition and weight management classes in a community center for adults, environmental changes to provide nutritious choices in a school cafeteria vending machine, and Fruits and Veggies More Matters campaigns to increase the availability of fresh fruits and vegetables from farmer's markets.[29] Primary prevention strategies seek to expand the positive potential of health.[30]

A holistic approach, embracing individual lifestyle factors; the environment; and economic, social, and political factors, can help communities and private-sector partners to achieve health promotion and disease prevention goals. Providing information, available on food labels and through health messages to the public, is one effective method. These messages encourage consumers to apply the U.S. Dietary Guidelines and MyPlate strategy[31] Dietary Reference Intakes, and the Dietary Guidelines Alliance's through the It's All About You campaigns.[32-34] Voluntary community and health organizations, the federal government, worksite programs, and schools can reach consumers daily to promote nutrition interventions.

The media remains an effective means of communicating nutrition issues to the public.[35] Programs to promote physical activity and fitness, good nutrition, and smoking cessation must be broadly accessible. Worksite nutrition-centered health promotion and disease prevention programs provide opportunities to harness social support and influence.[36]

Motivations should be provided for food processors and vendors, restaurant chefs, and school and worksite cafeteria managers to prepare and serve foods lower in fat, calories, and sodium. Finally, legislation and regulations can be ratified to endorse more complete food and nutrition labeling. Food labels that provide short, unequivocal, positive messages aimed at a single behavior prove beneficial to consumers.[37,38]

Strategy An evidence-based method or plan of action designed to achieve a particular goal.

Pandemic Learning Opportunity

What happened to the availability of farmer's markets during the pandemic? How did that affect health?

Healthy People 2030 outlines 355 measurable community and public health objectives that have 10-year targets and are associated with evidence-based interventions, with a small subset of 23 high-priority core objectives selected to drive action toward improving health and well-being.

TABLE 10-2
Healthy People 2030; Leading Health Indicators

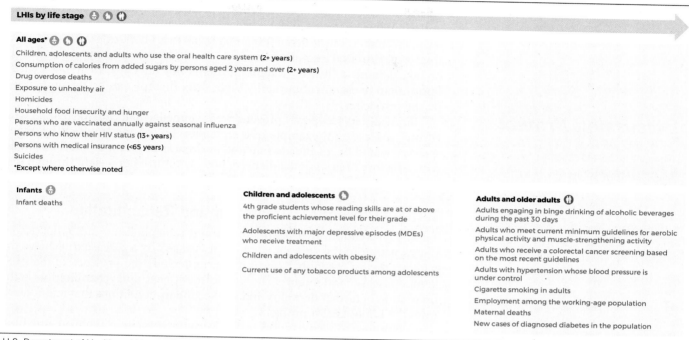

LHIs by life stage

All ages*
Children, adolescents, and adults who use the oral health care system (2+ years)
Consumption of calories from added sugars by persons aged 2 years and over (2+ years)
Drug overdose deaths
Exposure to unhealthy air
Homicides
Household food insecurity and hunger
Persons who are vaccinated annually against seasonal influenza
Persons who know their HIV status (13+ years)
Persons with medical insurance (<65 years)
Suicides
*Except where otherwise noted

Infants
Infant deaths

Children and adolescents
4th grade students whose reading skills are at or above the proficient achievement level for their grade
Adolescents with major depressive episodes (MDEs) who receive treatment
Children and adolescents with obesity
Current use of any tobacco products among adolescents

Adults and older adults
Adults engaging in binge drinking of alcoholic beverages during the past 30 days
Adults who meet current minimum guidelines for aerobic physical activity and muscle-strengthening activity
Adults who receive a colorectal cancer screening based on the most recent guidelines
Adults with hypertension whose blood pressure is under control
Cigarette smoking in adults
Employment among the working-age population
Maternal deaths
New cases of diagnosed diabetes in the population

U.S. Department of Health and Human Services, Leading Health Indicators. Retrieved from https://health.gov/healthypeople/objectives-and-data/leading-health-indicators

The HP 2030 objective topics include:

Health Conditions
Health Behaviors
Populations
Settings and Systems
Social Determinants of Health

The 23 smaller subsets of goals prioritized as per the health indicators can be viewed in **Table 10–2**.

It is essential that these objectives are disseminated and that the prevention strategies are translated into feasible actions for the population. In order to achieve that, HP 2030 has been updating the channels of dissemination of information and giving access to health promotion and education tips through the new virtual requirements, which include the availability of contents to be used in community, organizations and enterprises, schools, and other environments at no cost. These resources are best used in social media, organization's websites, and other forms of digital materials, and have specific instructions to increase engagements on the topics required to contribute to the health promotion. There is a call for regularly checking out messages from the National Health Observances (NHOs) on prioritized issues related to HP 2030 topics and objectives.

Secondary Prevention: Risk Appraisal and Risk Reduction

Secondary prevention includes risk appraisal and screening to emphasize early detection and diagnosis of disease.[25,28,29] Secondary prevention begins at the point where the pathology of a disease may occur. It encompasses diagnostic services that include screening, surveillance, and clinical examinations.[25] Screening strategies include follow-up education, counseling, and health referral. One model for secondary prevention involving screening is a cholesterol screening program for early detection of cardiovascular problems, such as elevated blood pressure, elevated blood cholesterol, and high glucose levels.[39,40] For people with an elevated blood cholesterol level, this means introducing "therapeutic lifestyle changes" such as reducing total and saturated fat in the diet, increasing physical activity, and reducing or maintaining a healthy weight. If this is not effective, or if low-density lipoprotein levels are abnormally high, drug therapy can be recommended by the physician.

Strategies in secondary prevention are aimed at self-care for people with chronic diseases. An example of a secondary prevention program involving self-care would be an educational and awareness program to teach a woman with a history of gestational diabetes how to control her weight through diet and exercise.[28,29]

Tertiary Prevention: Treatment and Rehabilitation

Tertiary prevention involves treatment and rehabilitation and is defined as the reduction in the amount of disability caused by a disease to achieve the highest level of function.[38] Tertiary factors include the presence of diabetes, kidney disease, and angina. The goal of treatment and rehabilitation is the prevention of further disability and any secondary conditions that might result from the initial health problem.

Examples of tertiary prevention programs include medical nutrition therapy (MNT) for people suffering from kidney disease, nutrition education about vitamin and mineral supplementation and feeding strategies to prevent further complications of wasting from HIV/AIDS, and cardiac rehabilitation through diet, exercise, and stress management. The ultimate goal of tertiary prevention is, through rehabilitation, to restore the individual to an "optimal" level of functioning, given the constraints of the disease.[29]

Early prevention: Developmental Origins of Health and Disease and Life Course Approach

The foundation for a healthy adulthood starts at a very early stage of life. Since Barker's first announcements of the theory of fetal programming, the evidence toward the initial statements: "The nourishment a baby receives from its mother and its exposure to infections after birth, determine its susceptibility to chronic diseases later in life,"[41] have been continually growing and gave name to the **Developmental Origins of Health and Disease (DOHaD)** field, which had shown that the environment in which the embryo, fetus, and young child grow and develop influences not only **life course** health and well-being but also the risk of later chronic noncommunicable diseases.[42]

Interestingly, the saving costs of early prevention are high, and the evidence toward the intergenerational risk of fetal programming of chronic diseases supports efforts to implement interventions as early as in adolescence. Ensuring that adolecscents are appropriately nourished, along with preventing them from developing harmful habits such as alcohol intake and smoking, and providing obstetric controls that encourage adequate nutrition and weight gain within the recommended guidelines is essential.[43]

Healthy People 2030 has strengthened maternal, infant, and children goals because taking care of these groups is caring for the next generation; therefore, it constitutes the baseline for early prevention of chronic diseases during adulthood and ameliorates both the cost of starting a life in poor health conditions and the early onset of chronic diseases during early adulthood.[44]

Discussion Prompt

Who would be best to educate clients about diet? Why? Is this service available?

Developmental Origin of Health and Disease A field of inquiry with the aim of identifying, quantifying, and evaluating strategies to modify prenatal and perinatal determinants of adverse adult health outcomes.

Life course approach The study of long-term effects on chronic disease risk of physical and social exposures during gestation, childhood, adolescence, young adulthood, and later adult life.

Also, the Special Supplemental Nutrition Program for Women, Infants, and Children (WIC) provides federal grants to states for supplemental foods, healthcare referrals, and nutrition education for low-income pregnant, breastfeeding, and nonbreastfeeding postpartum women. Also included are infants and children up to age 5 years who are found to be at nutritional risk, thus enhancing the well-being for these vulnerable groups.

Strategies such as monitoring the adequate weight gain during pregnancy, the reinforcement of exclusive breastfeeding practices, the sleeping hours during childhood, and smoking or not during the preconceptional period of father and mothers and during pregnancy are factors that are preventable. These are great contributors toward future health, thus requiring an effort to be included while making recommendations for early prevention of chronic diseases.[45]

Implications of Prevention Levels

Prevention levels are useful concepts to help set objectives for public health programs concerned with adult health in communities, worksites, and other settings. Recent findings underscore the need to emphasize population-based prevention programs.[46,47] As discussed earlier, research points to a holistic approach that aims at health, as well as prevention, when using this concept for public health programs. This approach was embraced in HP 2010, reinforced in HP2020 in terms of the nutrition and health objectives and strengthened in HP 2030 in its approach for early prevention and establishing the leading health indicators by life stage. The approach promoted and aligned the latest available evidence with efficient interventions that can be cost-effective.[9] For each goal, the holistic approach is addressed involving individual lifestyle factors, environmental factors, social and political issues, and access to quality healthcare.

Community and public health endeavors focus on primary or secondary prevention. It is important to choose the appropriate prevention level when planning a community or public health program. This is illustrated with two different approaches for handling CHD risk factors with one intended to reduce the prevalence of high blood pressure and the other to reduce obesity levels.

Research says that 90% of adult Americans have had their blood pressure measured in the past 2 years and could state whether it was normal or abnormally high.[48] According to the CDC, in 2018, nearly half a million deaths in the United States included hypertension as a primary or contributing cause. And, nearly half of adults in the United States (108 million, or 45%) have hypertension (defined as a systolic blood pressure ≥130 mm Hg or a diastolic blood pressure ≥80 mm Hg) or are taking medication for hypertension. Only approximately one in four adults (24%) with hypertension have their condition under control.[49-51] In addition, ethnic disparities exist for prevalence rates of high blood pressure, and African Americans in the United States have a greater prevalence of high blood pressure than Caucasians.[50] These data suggest that in order to reduce mortality from hypertension, secondary prevention strategies should be directed toward persons with hypertension (especially those with elevated systolic pressures), African Americans, and the elderly.

In contrast, Americans are aware of the growing obesity epidemic and the significance of elevated body mass index (BMI) (<30) for the risk of death and illness.[51] Americans understand the viability of lowering this risk factor associated with many obesity factors associated with chronic diseases. According to the CDC, obesity prevalence in the

Recent findings show that systolic (higher number) blood pressure is a more important predictor of heart disease than diastolic blood pressure, especially in the elderly.[51]

Strategy Tip

What factors contribute to high blood pressure? Who should be a medical team member to help clients with their diet?

Read more about obesity and cancer at: https://www.cdc.gov/obesity/data/adult.html

Read more about health programs at: https://www.ahealthieramerica.org/articles/let-s-move-84 and https://eatrightfoundation.org/why-it-matters/public-education/kids-eat-right/

Strategy Tip

Why should health insurers promote prevention programs? Should they hire dietitian/nutritionists?

U.S. Dietary Guidelines: https://www.dietaryguidelines.gov/sites/default/files/2020-12/Dietary_Guidelines_for_Americans_2020-2025.pdf

Dietary Guidelines of the American Heart Association: http:// www.americanheart.org/presenter.jhtml?identifier=851

American Cancer Society: http://www.cancer.org

American Institute for Cancer Research: http://www.aicr.org

Academy of Nutrition and Dietetics: http://www.eatright.org

Alternate Healthy Eating Index: http://www.hsph.harvard.edu/nutritionsource/pyramids.html

American Diabetes Association: http://www.diabetes.org The Obesity Society www.

USDA Choose MyPlate: http://www.choosemyplate.gov/MyPlate

United States was 42.4% in 2017–2018. Obesity-related conditions, often called comorbidities, include heart disease, stroke, type 2 diabetes, and certain types of cancer, which are some of the leading causes of preventable and premature death.[51]

Extensive data exist to substantiate that making lifestyle changes such as engaging in regular physical activity and healthy eating could, at the very least, halt the continued growth of the obesity epidemic.[51] One primary community and public prevention effort is called America on the Move,[52] a national initiative dedicated to helping individuals and communities become more physically active and to eat more healthfully. The program creates and supports an "integrated grassroots network" at the state level to build communities that support individual behavior changes. In addition, America on the Move involves public and private partnerships at the national, state, and local levels. It publicizes small behavioral changes, such as cutting 100 calories a day and taking 2,000 steps daily.

From the life course early-stage prevention, programs such as Let's Move,[53] now in alliance with a Healthier America, and the Academy of Nutrition and Dietetics' Foundation program Kids Eat Right[54] were introduced to improve the health of the next generation of American kids. Thus, instilling healthy lifestyle habits that should be introduced as early as possible because they are the foundation for a healthy adulthood.

Health promotion and chronic disease prevention programs should focus on coalition building between community-based nutrition and health professionals, government, local businesses, health agencies, and insurers.[29] In this rapidly changing healthcare environment, continued training and research in public health program development is crucial to provide evidence of the efficacy of health prevention and promotion.

All levels of prevention should be addressed when devising strategies for dietary behavior changes for chronic disease prevention. However, for some diseases, the nutrition strategy may prove similar at each prevention level. Weight reduction, for example, may prevent the onset of hypertension or be part of the treatment for type 2 diabetes. In the case of other diseases, such as cancer, nutrition strategies might vary with the prevention level.

Dietary Guidelines for Disease Prevention

Various health organizations and government agencies have issued dietary guidelines and recommendations based on current scientific evidence. Since 1989, several initiatives including the National Research Council and its published report, *Diet and Health: Implications for Reducing Chronic Disease Risk*, provided evidence for the relationship among all major chronic conditions and diet.[11] More recently, HP 2010, HP 2020, and continued by HP 2030 set forth a comprehensive health promotion and disease prevention program for the nation. HP 2030s comprehensive nutrition and weight status agenda includes health promotion to reduce chronic disease risk through the consumption of healthful diets, this time identifying the needs according to specific population groups.[55]

The Dietary Guidelines for Americans 2020–2025 confirm that approximately 74% of all American adults are overweight or obese. Adults ages 40–60 years have the highest rate of obesity (43%) of any age group with adults 60 years and older having a 41% rate of obesity. Approximately 18.2 million adults have coronary artery disease (first cause of death), about 11% of Americans have either type 1 or type 2 diabetes, and more than 1.3 million people are living with colorectal cancer. More women (17%) than men (5%) have osteoporosis.[56-60]

Besides translating science into succinct, food-based guidance that can be used by Americans to achieve a healthy and enjoyable diet, with a disease prevention focus, the new guidelines provide evolving recommendations as new evidence becomes available.[61] Now, a fundamental premise of the 2020–2025 Dietary Guidelines is that just about everyone, no matter their health status, can benefit from a healthier diet. The second focus is on consuming a healthy dietary pattern, as part of understanding that people will consume a combination of foods, therefore, the nutrient intake is part of a whole pattern rather than individual nutrients, foods, or foods groups in isolation. The third is the focus on a lifespan approach, which is an emphasis on following the appropriate food pattern for every life stage from infancy through older adulthood and provides specific recommendations according to the characteristics of each phase.[61]

As the recent history indicates, the U.S. Dietary Guidelines were assessed in terms of surveillance and research needs, especially related to risk for chronic diseases, such as cancer, cardiovascular diseases, and diabetes.[56] Different associations gave input on the Dietary Guidelines. This provided us with revised Dietary Guidelines. The American Heart Association (AHA) recommended greater emphasis on the diet as a whole and, specifically, to certain protective foods for chronic disease risk prevention.[57] The American Cancer Society and the American Institute for Cancer Research reinforced these guidelines and further emphasized eating foods from plant sources.[58] The Academy of Nutrition and Dietetics reiterated these health-promoting dietary guidelines and continued to be involved in update evidences.[59] The Alternate Healthy Eating Index (AHEI) suggested targeting food choices and nutrient intake associated with chronic disease risk.[60] The American Institute for Cancer Research stated: "Our research has shown that a diet that prevents cancer can also prevent other chronic diseases. . . the United States Department of Agriculture (USDA) and other major health organizations are now largely in agreement about specific Dietary Guidelines that protect overall health."[62]

The American Heart Association, the American Cancer Society, the American Diabetes Association, and the American Institute of Cancer Research concur with the new dietary recommendations.[62] In addition, the American Cancer Society, the American Diabetes Association, and the American Heart Association collaborated to work on health promotion and disease prevention.[62] In their collaborative efforts, these organizations are making unified health statements concerning the prevention of heart disease, cancer, diabetes, and related risk factors. These efforts, updated in recent publications, continue to support the following dietary patterns that may help reduce the risk of chronic diseases[62,63]:

- Consume a diet that emphasizes whole grains and legumes, vegetables, and fruits.
- Decrease saturated fat and dietary cholesterol; avoid trans fat; limit red meat and full-fat dairy products.
- Limit intake of foods and beverages high in added sugars.
- Limit overall intake of calories and engage in regular physical activity to maintain a healthy body weight.

The Dietary Guidelines for Americans 2021–2025, key recommendations reach even further and highlight the relevance of having a healthy eating pattern that includes:

- A variety of vegetables from all of the subgroups—dark green, red and orange, legumes (beans and peas), starchy, and other
- Fruits, especially whole fruits

- Grains, at least half of which are whole grains
- Fat-free or low-fat dairy, including milk, yogurt, cheese, and/or fortified soy beverages
- A variety of protein foods, including seafood, lean meats and poultry, eggs, legumes (beans and peas), and nuts, seeds, and soy products
- Oils, including vegetable oils and oils in food, such as seafood and nuts

Despite the evidence of the importance of diet to health, vegetable and fruit consumption among adults continues to be below recommended amounts. Historically, consumption of grains, fruits and vegetables has been below the recommendations. According to the U.S. Department of Agriculture's in 25-year-old research, the 1994–1996 Continuing Survey of Food Intakes by Individuals and the Food Guide Pyramid, only 3% of individuals at that time met four of the five recommendations for the intake of grains, fruits, vegetables, dairy products, and meats.[64,65]

More recently, although some improved, according to the CDC Morbidity and Mortality report during 2007–2010, 76% of Americans did not meet fruit intake recommendations and 87% did not meet vegetable intake recommendations.[66] The recent report on the 2021–2025 Dietary Guidelines continues to show that more than 80% of the population have dietary patterns that are low in vegetables, fruits, and dairy. With the update of the Dietary Guidelines for the Americans and the focus on healthy food patterns, the development of four key steps for achieving good nutrition for all Americans is described in **Table 10–3**.

TABLE 10–3
The Guidelines

Guideline 1: Follow a Healthy Dietary Pattern at every life stage:

- (Adults) A dietary pattern at the 2,000 calorie level should include daily or weekly amounts from food groups, subgroups, and components: Vegetables, fruits, grains, dairy, protein foods, oils and establish limit on calories for other uses (table).
- Explain the health benefits of a healthy pattern for improving health and reducing risk of diet-related chronic diseases.
- States that a healthy dietary pattern supports appropriate calorie levels, per individual needs, depending on a number of factors: age, sex, height, weight, level of physical activity, pregnancy, and lactation status.
- Follow key dietary principles: Meet nutritional needs primarily from foods and beverages, choose a variety of options from each food group and pay attention to portion size

---

Guideline 2: Customize and enjoy food and beverage choices to reflect personal preferences, cultural traditions, and budgetary considerations:

- Start with personal preferences, and start including a variety of foods as early as possible into day-to-day choices
- Incorporate cultural traditions
- Consider budget

Guideline 3: Focus on meeting food group needs with nutrient dense foods and beverages and stay within calorie limits:

- As substantial improvements are needed to reach recommended levels of intake on fruits, vegetables, dairy, and seafoods
- Ensuring consumption of dense nutrients in foods will improve the intake of micronutrients such as calcium and magnesium. Also, fiber can be improved by adopting a healthy dietary pattern

---

Guideline 4: Limit foods and beverages higher in added sugars, saturated fats, and sodium, and limit alcoholic beverages:

- Making nutrient-dense choices: one meal at a time
- Making healthy choices
- Paying attention to added sugars
- Limiting saturated fat intake to less than 10% of calories per day
- Limiting excessive sodium intake according to the Chronic Disease Risk Reduction levels defined by the National Academies of 2,300 mg/day for adults
- Alcoholic beverages: A strong statement made regarding alcoholic beverages are not part of the USDA Dietary Patterns, and that alcohol consumption increases the risks for some types of cancer and cardiovascular diseases.

Dietary Guidelines for Americans 2020–2025 Make Every Bite Count With the Dietary Guidelines Ninth Edition. Retrieved from https://www.dietaryguidelines.gov /sites/default/files/2020-12/Dietary_Guidelines_for_Americans_2020-2025.pdf, pp. ix–x; Accessed March 14, 2021.

The new Guidelines approach goes beyond a mere recommendation by promoting the understanding of the benefits of good nutrition at every stage of the life and aiming at focusing on the needs and requirements of each. These new guidelines are based on what people usually drink and eat, the dietary pattern, and how the parts of the pattern act synergistically to affect health, which as a result might better predict overall health status and disease risk than individual foods or nutrients. These recommendations have solid key messages.

These Dietary Guidelines revisions have been translated into MyPlate recommendations, which is a graphic way, illustrates the five foods groups that are key for a healthy diet using a place setting for a meal that includes: fruits, vegetables, grains, proteins, and dairy. This constitutes an easy way to remind people what are the healthy options to include on a daily basis, focusing on smart accessible food choices. See the MyPlate graphic in Chapter 1.

> See MyPlate at: https://myplate-prod
> .azureedge.net/sites/default/files/2020
> -12/MyPlate_blue_0.jpg

In summary, diverse health organizations stress the similarities in the dietary recommendations for reducing disease risk. These recommendations are to eat less saturated fat and trans fat; increase consumption of fruits, vegetables, whole grains, and legumes; limit added sugar and sodium; drink alcohol in moderation; and increase physical activity. By using clear terms, community and public health nutrition professionals can make the message easier for the public to understand, value, and implement.

Pandemic Learning Opportunity

These organizations have also moved toward making recommendations for providing guidelines to follow during the COVID-19 pandemic. The pandemic forced many Americans to be food insecure. One of the relevant initiatives that came out of the pandemic food access problems were the creation of healthy cooking starter kits for ensuring that families know how to best optimize their food resources while eating as healthy as possible.

Diet and Health: Nutrition Strategies, Health Determinants, and Risk Factors

Nutrition strategies are essential in the prevention and management of several chronic diseases and their risk factors. When developing a community or public health program, risk factor assessment needs to be addressed. The following criteria can be assessed:

- The risk factor must have a strong association with the development of a chronic disease (e.g., obesity and heart disease).
- The risk factor must affect a significant number of people.
- The risk factor must be modifiable, so it can be reduced or changed.
- The risk factor must have a modification that, when changed or reduced, results in decreased mortality.

Because many risk factors can be modified by healthy lifestyle changes, early recognition of the risk factors for chronic disease prevention is critical.

> Read more about needs assessment in Chapter 5.

Obesity

Rates of excessive weight and obesity are steadily growing in our country, reaching 42.4% in 2017–2018, with no significant differences between men and women among all adults or by age group.[59,63,67-70] The National Institutes of Health (NIH) Expert Panel uses BMI for defining overweight and obesity.[71] The cut-off point for overweight is a BMI of 25 kg/m^2. Obesity, defined as having a BMI of 30 kg/m^2, has doubled among adults since 1980. Extreme obesity (BMI of >40 kg/m^2) increased from 4.7% in 1999–2000 to 5.9% in 2003–2004.[72] The age-adjusted prevalence of overweight and obesity (BMI >25 kg/m^2) increased from 64.5% in 1999–2000 to 66.3% in 2003–2004. At the same time, obesity (BMI of 30 kg/m^2) increased from 30.5% to 34.3%.[68]

For the period of 2017–2018, the age-adjusted prevalence of severe obesity in adults was 9.2% and was higher in women than in men. Among adults, the prevalence of both obesity and severe obesity was highest in non-Hispanic black adults compared with other race Hispanic-origin groups, and from 1999–2000, the prevalence of both obesity and severe obesity increased among adults. Many diseases are associated with overweight and obesity, including CHD, stroke, high blood pressure, diabetes, arthritis-related disabilities, sleep apnea, gallbladder disease, and some cancers.[73]

The public health burden of overweight and obesity is overwhelming in terms of premature deaths and disability, lost productivity, and social stigmatization.[74] Medical expenses for obesity accounted for 9.1% of total U.S. medical expenditures in 1998 and may have reached as high as 92.6 billion dollars in 2002.[75] Another estimate places the total cost of obesity at $117 billion.[11] According to new estimates, in 2016, chronic diseases driven by the factor of obesity and overweight accounted for $480.7 billion in direct costs in the United States with an additional $1.24 trillion in indirect costs due to lost economic productivity. The total cost of chronic diseases due to obesity and overweight was $1.72 trillion equivalent to 9.3% of the US gross domestic product. In consequence, obesity is the greatest contributor to the burden of chronic diseases in the United States, accounting for 47.1% of the total cost of chronic diseases nationwide. There is a link between the higher prevalence of obesity and increased medical spending, so there is substantial benefit in addressing obesity from a prevention perspective.[76]

In addition, obesity rates are higher among certain population groups, such as Hispanic Americans, African Americans, Native Americans, and Pacific Islander American women.[69,73] Research has reported, however, that overweight has increased in all parts of the U.S. population.[77,78] The recent trend of overweight in the United States has become so severe that if it is not reversed in the next few years, poor diet and lack of physical exercise will likely become the leading preventable cause of mortality among adults.[19]

Many factors contribute to overweight and obesity. For each individual, metabolic and genetic factors, as well as behaviors affecting dietary intake and physical activity, contribute to being overweight. Cultural, environmental, and socioeconomic influences also play a role. Most overweight and obese individuals eat more calories from food than they expend through physical activity. As body weight increases, so does the prevalence of health risks in an individual. For this reason, encouraging obese individuals to adopt new eating and physical activity habits is of vital importance.

At the beginning of 2016, the Academy of Nutrition and Dietetics released it position statement related to: Interventions for the Treatment of Overweight and Obesity in Adults as follows: "Successful treatment of overweight ... are influenced by many factors; incorporating more than one level of the socioecological model and addressing several key factors in each level may be more successful than interventions targeting any one level and factor alone."[79]

Recently, a strong emphasis is being made on prevention of weight gain alongside the recommendations of weight loss. In its document, The Obesity Society stated that: Eradicating America's Obesity Epidemic in 2009[80] emphasized fighting obesity, not the obese, preventing the gaining of excess weight during childhood, promoting an awareness about the complexity of obesity, highlighting the elevated cost of being obese, as well as preventing weight gain on adults, and supporting research to improve the science behind recommendations.

Several initiatives have been on the rise to eradicate the obesity epidemic in America, including the different factors for successful lifestyle changes. A good example of community impact on prevention and management of weight loss can be found in the initiative of the University of Colorado through the Anschutz Health and Wellness Center. Collaboration among researchers, physicians, dietitians, and health practitioners helped: "Our goal is to create the nation's go-to research facility for wellness and integrated programs providing whole-person support."[80]

Visit http://www.anschutzwellness.com/ for more information about this community health wellness program.

Weight Management

The goals and outcomes of weight-management programs should be guided by an assessment of an individual's weight related to their height or body mass index (BMI) and health. The National Heart, Lung, and Blood Institute (NHLBI) guidelines recommend intervention for people who are overweight and have two or more risk factors associated with their weight.[81] Furthermore, according to the position papers of the Academy of Nutrition and Dietetics from the last decades, "Interventions for the treatment of overweight and obesity in adults, the appropriate weight management, assessment, monitor, and evaluation should incorporate the following areas[79,82,83]:

Food- and nutrition-related history

- Beliefs and attitudes, including food preferences and motivation
- Food environment, including access to fruits and vegetables
- Dietary behaviors, including eating out and screen time
- Diet experience, including food allergies and dieting history
- Medications and supplements
- Physical activity

Anthropometric measurements

- Height, weight, body mass index
- Waist circumference
- Weight history
- Body composition

Biochemical data, medical tests, and procedures

- Glucose and endocrine profile
- Lipid profile

Nutrition-focused physical findings

- Ability to communicate
- Affect
- Amputations
- Appetite

- Blood pressure
- Body language
- Heart rate

Client history

- Appropriateness of weight management in certain populations (such as eating disorders, pregnancy, receiving chemotherapy)
- Client and family medical and health history
- Social history, including living or housing situation and socioeconomic status

For an individual, the goal of a weight management program should focus on the prevention of weight gain as well as weight loss. This recommendation encourages individuals to adopt healthier lifestyles, such as increasing physical activity and choosing less calorically dense foods. With this approach, weight loss will lead to reductions of health risks.[84] A weight loss of as little as 10% can improve health risks associated with overweight and obesity.[85]

For effective weight management programs, a multidisciplinary team should be involved, including a physician, a dietitian/nutritionist, an exercise physiologist, and a behavioral therapist. Healthcare professionals ought to be especially dedicated and sensitive to the needs of overweight and obese individuals. It is appropriate to discuss realistic goals of weight loss and maintenance so that shared responsibility for weight management can develop between the provider and the individual. Goals might include the following:[84,70]

- Prevention or cessation of weight gain in an individual who is continuing to see an increase in his or her weight
- Progress in physical and emotional health
- Small, realistic weight losses achieved through sensible eating and exercise
- Improvements in eating, exercise, and any behaviors apart from weight loss

Establishing both short- and long-term treatment goals and documenting measures before implementing the weight management plan and after the individual has started on the plan are important parts of care. Positive behavior changes, other than absolute weight, should be rewarded as these can be very motivating.[71,72]

Physical activity is highly recommended as an essential part of a weight-management program. It is well established that to maintain weight loss, healthful dietary habits must be coupled with increased physical activity.[73] Physical activity contributes to weight loss not only by changing energy balance but also by positively changing body composition by increasing lean body mass. Exercise decreases the risk of chronic disease and improves mood and quality of life. Many experts believe that physical inactivity is responsible for the increasing prevalence of overweight and obesity in the United States.[74-76]

The biggest challenge in weight management is to maintain a healthy weight once it is achieved. It is essential to include physical activity in weight-loss programs because regular physical activity is one of the best predictors of weight maintenance.[77-86] Unfortunately, studies show that within 5 years, a majority of people regain the weight they have lost.[87] The National Institutes of Health (NIH) recommends that both dietary and physical activity changes need to be continued indefinitely for weight loss to be maintained.[87] A comprehensive lifestyle program that focuses on nutrition, exercise, cognitive behavioral changes, and medical monitoring has been shown to be most effective for long-term success.[88]

See these health recommendations at: https://www.niddk.nih.gov/health-information/weight-management/healthy-eating-physical-activity-for-life/health-tips-for-adults

---

Strategy Tip

Combining weight loss with regular physical activity reduces one's risk for chronic diseases such as heart disease and diabetes by reducing both blood cholesterol and blood glucose levels.

Due to the increased prevalence in overweight and obesity in the United States, weight management becomes crucial for primary prevention of many chronic diseases. It is the foundation of secondary and tertiary prevention of hypertension, high blood cholesterol, diabetes, arthritis, and some cancers. It is important for healthcare providers to lobby for public health policies that endorse the treatment and management of weight. Also, clients must be informed of the known healthy and positive outcomes achieved through weight management programs.

Cardiovascular Disease

Cardiovascular disease continues to be the nation's leading cause of death, accounting for more than 36% of all deaths in the United States. Despite a decline in heart-disease mortality, which is still one in four American adults, one person dies every 36 seconds, or more than 655,000 Americans die of cardiovascular disease each year, according to CDC updated data.[89] In addition, 18.2 million adults aged 20 and older have Coronary Artery Disease (CAD), and approximately two in 10 deaths from CAD occur in adults less than 65 years old. Three modifiable health behaviors—poor nutrition, lack of physical activity, and smoking—contribute greatly to the burden of heart disease.

Cardiovascular diseases include diseases of the heart and blood vessels: Coronary Heart Disease (CHD), stroke, and peripheral vascular diseases. CHD is the most common form of cardiovascular disease, and usually involves atherosclerosis and hypertension. Atherosclerosis is characterized by the build-up of plaques along the inner walls of the arteries, causing inadequate blood flow and leading to serious cardiovascular problems.

The consequences of cardiovascular disease are usually heart disease and stroke; these two diseases combined cause one death every 33 seconds.[11] About 61 million Americans live with the effects of heart disease and stroke. The annual cost of cardiovascular disease and stroke is estimated at $475 billion.[11] The death rate from cardiovascular disease fell by 17% in the last part of the 20th century; however, the number of deaths increased by 2.5% each year due to the growth and size of the population aged 65 years and older.[50] The decrease in the mortality rates due to cardiovascular disease is attributed to primary prevention (e.g., a decrease in dietary intake of saturated fat), secondary prevention (e.g., early detection and treatment of hypertension), and improved medical and surgical treatments.[90]

However, in 2013, the American Heart Association Update report stated that the adjusted population attributable fractions for cardiovascular disease (CVD) mortality were as follows: 40.6% (95% confidence interval [CI], 24.5–54.6) for high blood pressure; 13.7% (95% CI, 4.8–22.3) for smoking; 13.2% (95% CI, 3.5–29.2) for poor diet; 11.9% (95% CI, 1.3–22.3) for insufficient physical activity; and 8.8% (95% CI, 2.1–15.4) for abnormal glucose levels.

This means that in general, mortality and prevalence rates of cardiovascular disease could be improved by reducing the major risk factors: high blood pressure, high blood cholesterol, tobacco use, physical inactivity, and poor nutrition. Controlling one or more of these risk factors could have a major public health impact on our country.[90,91]

Hypertension

High blood pressure or hypertension remains a "silent killer" in the United States. In 2018, nearly half a million death in the United States included hypertension as a primary or contributing cause, and nearly half of adults in

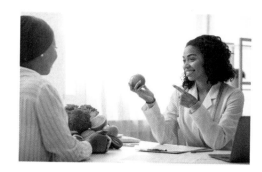

Weight loss counseling takes a slow and methodical process to learn and adapt to differing eating habits.
© Prostock-studio/Shutterstock.

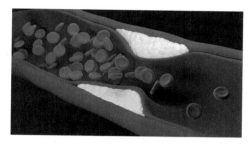

Plaque can fill the artery, blocking blood flow.
© MP Art/Shutterstock.

Confidence Interval (CI) relates to the value or number as stated probability of being included in it.

Read more about hypertension at: CDC High Blood Pressure https://www.cdc .gov/bloodpressure/facts.htm#:~:text =Nearly%20half%20of%20adults%20in ,are%20taking%20medication%20for %20hypertension.&text=Only%20about %201%20in%204,have%20their%20 condition%20under%20control.

the United States (108 million or 45%) have hypertension.[50] High blood pressure is a major independent risk factor for cardiovascular disease. Hypertension increases the risk of heart attack, heart failure, stroke, and kidney disease.[92] This is significant because heart disease and stroke are the first and third leading causes of death in the United States, respectively.[11]

In the latest classification of blood pressure for adults, normal blood pressure is considered to be 120/80 mm Hg and prehypertension is designated as 120–139 systolic or 80–89 mm Hg diastolic pressure.[92] High blood pressure for adults is defined as a systolic pressure of >140 mm Hg, or a diastolic pressure of >90 mm Hg. It has been determined some time ago that systolic blood pressure is a more important predictor of CHD in older adults than diastolic blood pressure.[93]

In **Figure 10–1**, the next graphic, a trend toward high blood pressure with increasing age can be observed according to data from National Health and Nutrition Examination Survey in 2017–2018 and shows the prevalence of high blood pressure in adults ≥18 years of age by age and sex.

The number of people who were able to control their high blood pressure from lifestyle changes and the use of antihypertensive drugs rose from about 16% in 1971–1972 to about 65% in 1988–1994.[94] The age-adjusted death rate attributed to hypertension rose by about 36.4% over the 1991–2001 decade, with the actual number of deaths increasing by 53%.[63] From 1995 to 2005, the death rate from high blood pressure increased by 23% and the actual number of deaths rose to 56.4%.[95] Among people with high blood

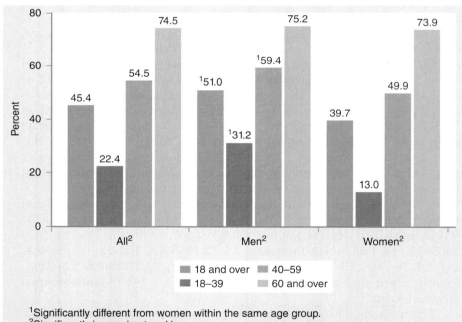

¹Significantly different from women within the same age group.
²Significantly increasing trend by age.
NOTES: Hypertension is defined as systolic blood pressure greater than or equal to 130 mmHg or diastolic blood pressure greater than or equal to 80 mmHg, or currently taking medication to lower blood pressure. Estimates for age group 18 and over are age adjusted by the direct method to the U.S. Census 2000 population using age groups 18–39, 40–59, and 60 and over. Crude estimates are 48.2% for all persons, 52.5% for men, and 44.0% for women.

FIGURE 10–1 Prevalence of Hypertension.

NCHS, National Health and Nutrition Examination Survey, 2017–2018. https://www.cdc.gov/nchs/products /databriefs/db364.htm

pressure, 69% are being treated, 45% have it under control, and 54.6% do not have their blood pressure under control.[95] Significant disparities exist among persons diagnosed with hypertension. For example, African Americans have high blood pressure at an earlier age, and in general, have higher blood pressures.[96] Twenty-two percent of Americans are unaware that they have hypertension.[95,97]

The latest guidelines for the treatment of hypertension are found in *The Seventh Report of the Joint National Committee on Prevention, Detection, Evaluation, and Treatment of High Blood Pressure*.[92] This report advocates major lifestyle modifications shown to lower blood pressure, enhance antihypertensive drug efficacy, and decrease cardiovascular risk. General lifestyle modifications include weight reduction for overweight or obese individuals with the goal for a BMI being 18.5–24.9.[98,99] The adoption of the Dietary Approaches to Stop Hypertension (DASH) eating plan,[96] reducing sodium intake,[100] increasing physical activity,[101] and moderating alcohol consumption assisted in this endeavor.[102,103] The DASH eating plan is a diet rich in calcium and potassium, consisting of fresh fruits, vegetables, and low-fat dairy products.[100,103] The DASH eating plan advocates a low sodium intake; intakes of 1,600 mg have been found to be as effective as single-drug therapy in lowering blood pressure.[100] Other specific lifestyle modifications include reducing sodium to 2,400 mg a day, engaging in regular aerobic physical activity at least 30 minutes a day (most days of the week), and limiting alcohol consumption (two drinks/day for men; 1 drink/day for women).[92] The Report's guidelines recommend these lifestyle modifications for all individuals.

There are several types of drugs for those who have not achieved the goal blood pressure; some individuals might require more than one drug to get their blood pressure under control.[104] First-line medication include: diuretics, angiotensin converting inhibitors, angiotensin receptors blockers, beta blockers, and calcium channel blockers. To include pharmacotherapy as a treatment alternative, physician referral and supervision is required.

Cholesterol

High blood cholesterol is one of the major independent risk factors for heart disease and stroke.[11] Modifying this risk factor is effective in reducing cardiovascular disease mortality. Animal, epidemiologic, and metabolic research show that having elevated blood cholesterol levels is associated with cardiovascular disease. Despite the available recommended dietary guidelines and medications, approximately 45% of Americans had in the past total blood cholesterol levels of ≥200 mg/dL and almost 33% have a low-density lipoprotein (LDL) cholesterol of ≥130 mg/dL.[11] Recent data show that between 1999–2000 and 2005–2006, mean serum total cholesterol levels in adults aged 20 and older declined from 204 mg/dL to 199 mg/dL.[105] According to recent data from the Centers for Disease Control and Prevention, nearly 29 million adult Americans have a total cholesterol level greater than 240 mg/dL or 10.5% in 2017–2018. The prevalence of low high-density lipoproteins (HDL) declined from 22.2% during 2007–2008 to 16% during 2017–2018.

Research from the 1980s showed that lowering high blood cholesterol significantly reduces the risk for heart attacks and reduces overall mortality rates. As a result, the National Cholesterol Education Program (NCEP) was launched in 1985.[106] Current guidelines recommend that all adults aged 20 or older have their blood cholesterol levels checked every 5 years as a preventive measure.[96] Nevertheless, over 80% of Americans who have high blood cholesterol do not have it under control.

Discussion Prompt

Brainstorm on some community and public health programs people could join to learn and lower their blood pressure. Be creative, as people need motivation to join.

Visit https://pubmed.ncbi.nlm.nih.gov /12748199/ for more information about the *Seventh Report of the Joint National Committee on Prevention, Detection, Evaluation, and Treatment of High Blood Pressure*. And https://www.nhlbi.nih.gov /health-topics/dash-eating-plan to learn about the DASH eating plan.

Strategy Tip

A typical food intake in the United States, complete with convenience and fast foods, may provide 10,000–20,000 mg of sodium per day!

Strategy Tip

LDL represents the unwanted cholesterol that clogs arteries, while HDL represents the good cholesterol usually raised by aerobic exercise.

In 2001, the NCEP released updated clinical guidelines in its report of the Expert Panel on the Detection, Evaluation and Treatment of High Blood Cholesterol in Adults, referred to as the Adult Treatment Panel (ATP) III.[107] This report updated the recommendations made in ATP II and I for people with high blood cholesterol levels, and reinforces findings from studies that confirm elevated LDL cholesterol to be a major cause of CHD. The guidelines in ATP III focus on LDL-lowering cholesterol strategies and on primary prevention in persons with multiple risk factors.[108] In 2004, an update was added to the NCEP guidelines on cholesterol management that advised physicians to consider new, more intensive medical treatments, such as statin drugs for people at high and moderately high risk for a heart attack.[109]

The ATP III report recommends a complete lipoprotein profile that includes total cholesterol, LDL cholesterol, HDL cholesterol, and triglycerides as the preferred test rather than screening for total cholesterol and HDLs alone (See **Table 10–4**). For LDL-lowering therapy, a person's risk status needs to be assessed based on multiple risk factors including cigarette smoking, hypertension, low HDL, family history of premature CHD, and age.

Diabetes is considered a CHD equivalent in assessing a person's risk. In addition, the current guidelines use the Framingham scoring projections of 10-year absolute CHD risk to identify people who need more intensive therapy and those with multiple metabolic risk factors. NCEP[109] defines high-risk patients as those who have CHD, diabetes, or multiple risk factors, such as hypertension or smoking, which give them a greater than 20% chance of having a heart attack within 10 years. Very high-risk patients are those who have cardiovascular disease together with either multiple risk factors (especially diabetes), or badly controlled risk factors (e.g., smoking), or metabolic syndrome (a constellation of risk factors associated with obesity). For moderately high-risk and high-risk persons, the ATP III report and

TABLE 10–4
ATP III Classification of LDL, Total, and HDL Cholesterol (mg/dL)

LDL Cholesterol—Primary Target of Therapy	
<100	Optimal
100–129	Near optimal/above optimal
130–159	Borderline high
160–189	High
≥190	Very high
Total Cholesterol	
<200	Desirable
200–239	Borderline high
≥240	High
HDL Cholesterol	
<40	Low
≥60	High

National Cholesterol Education Program. National Institute of Health. National Heart, Lung and Blood Institute. ATP III Guidelines At-A-Glance Quick Desk Reference. Available at: http://www.nhlbi.nih.gov/files/docs/guidelines/atglance.pdf

update recommend drug therapy in addition to therapeutic lifestyle changes (TLC), which include intensive use of nutrition, weight control, and physical activity.[108,110]

The specific parts of TLC include the following: reducing intakes of saturated fat to 7% of total calories and decreasing cholesterol to 200 mg per day. Total fat from calories can be in the 25–35% range, as long as saturated and trans-fatty acids are kept low. Individuals are encouraged to use plant stanols and sterols in their diet (2 g/day). Small amounts of plant sterols, or phytosterols occur naturally in pine trees and foods like soybeans, nuts, grains, and oils. Increasing soluble fiber to 10 to 25 g/day is also recommended with weight reduction and increased physical activity. Because overweight and obesity are considered major underlying risk factors for CHD, weight reduction enhances LDL-lowering interventions.

In comparing the recommendations set forth in the ATP III report with the more recent updates, more intensive treatment options are delineated for very high-risk individuals. For high-risk patients, the goal in both reports remains an LDL level of 100 mg/dL; for very high-risk patients, a therapeutic option is to treat with statins to lower levels to 70 mg/dL. The update lowers the threshold for drug therapy to an LDL of 100 mg/dL and recommends drug therapy for those high-risk people whose LDL is 100 to 129 mg/dL.[106-110]

According to ATP III, for moderately high-risk persons, the LDL treatment goal is 130 mg/dL and drug therapy is recommended if LDL levels are 130 mg/dL. In the update, there is a therapeutic option to set the treatment goal at LDL 100 mg/dL and to use statin drug therapy if LDL is 100 to 129 mg/dL to reach the goal. In the update, when LDL drug therapy is used, it is advised that enough medication be used to achieve at least a 30–40% reduction in LDL levels. In both reports, anyone with LDL above the goal is a candidate for Therapeutic Lifestyle Changes (TLC). In the update, any person at high or moderately high risk who has lifestyle-related risk factors should follow TLC, regardless of LDL level.[108,110]

As individuals learn about their risk factors and begin TLC, more dietitians/nutritionists will be asked to help people make necessary dietary changes. ATP III guidelines recommend that physicians refer individuals to dietitians for medical nutrition therapy.[108] At all stages in the model of TLC, the referral to a dietitian/nutritionist is recommended. This challenges community and public health providers to provide diet and exercise recommendations that will make a difference to those with elevated blood cholesterol levels. Dietitians/nutritionists also need to consider prevailing eating and ethnic habits when counseling people to lower blood cholesterol levels.

In terms of adhering to the ATP III protocol guidelines (and the update), patients and healthcare providers are key players in realizing the benefits of cholesterol-lowering and attaining the highest possible levels of CHD risk reduction. Both screening for risk factors and compliance in adopting the lipid-lowering guidelines are essential; in reality, fewer than 50% of those persons eligible for meeting the criteria actually receive treatment.[108]

Physical Activity

Research demonstrates that virtually all individuals benefit from regular physical activity. In spite of progress in physical activity prevalence, in 2018, more than 45% of American adults were not meeting the physical activity recommendations.[111] According to recent research, the prevalence of regular, no leisure-time physical activity among adults is 15%, and this estimate ranged from 17.3–47.7%.[68] Inactivity increases with age and is more common among women than men. Also, those with lower incomes and less

---

Discussion Prompt

Look up the cholesterol content of some animal source foods, such as eggs and beef. How do food staples relate to the cholesterol levels found in Americans?

Discussion Prompt

The decision to go on drug therapy for high LDL levels is dependent on a multitude of risk factors and is decided between the physician and the patient. Discuss how many people in your family are taking cholesterol-lowering drugs. How does their diet affect their cholesterol levels?

Statin drugs: These lower blood cholesterol by inhibiting 3-hydroxy-3-methylglutaryl coenzyme A reductase (HMG-CoA reductase), a liver enzyme that is responsible for producing cholesterol.

> Read more about physical activity and health at: https://www.cdc.gov/physicalactivity/downloads/trends-in-the-prevalence-of-physical-activity-508.pdf and https://www.cdc.gov/physicalactivity/data/inactivity-prevalence-maps/index.html

education exercise less than those with higher incomes or education.[111] Physical inactivity thus is a prevalent risk factor in the United States. People who are sedentary are almost twice as likely to develop CHD as people who engage in regular physical activity.[109] The risk imposed by physical inactivity is almost as high as other well-known CHD risk factors, such as high blood cholesterol, high blood pressure, or smoking.[109,111] Even moderate physical activity produces significant health benefits, such as a decreased risk of CHD.[112] Research shows that moderate physical activity, such as walking 30 minutes a day five times a week, is more likely to be adopted and maintained than vigorous activity.[113]

There are many health benefits to be gained from regular physical activity. It enhances cardiovascular function, reduces very low-density lipoprotein (VLDL) levels, raises HDL cholesterol, and can lower LDL cholesterol levels.[108] Physical activity lowers blood pressure and reduces insulin resistance. Overall, physical activity improves muscle function, cardiovascular function, and physical performance, and aids in weight management.[111] Dietitians/nutritionists should become aware of the different types of physical activity, especially moderate levels of activity, that can lower an individual's risk for cardiovascular disease.

Without a doubt, physical activity is part of the equation of maintaining an adequate weight, not only because of its role affecting energy's expenditure but also how it affects the active regulation of energy balance, including the brain circuitry that participates in the regulation of food intake.[114] In addition, physical activity is not only important for weight loss but it is also relevant for maintaining the lost weight. There are several studies that support the key role of physical activity regarding this issue.[113]

For increasing physical activity, taking into account complex behaviors and interventions is needed, including individual motivation, peer groups and families, institutions such as workplaces and schools, community resources, and policies and media. It is also important to mention an example of federal transportation policies that have implications for physical activity: The Safe, Affordable, Flexible, Efficient Transportation Equity Act: A Legacy for Users or SAFETEA-LU; which not only promoted safe ways for general transportation but also for improving physical activity, particularly for school children through the Safe Routes to School through the development of safe infrastructure so they can walk or bicycle to school. Another way in which this program is helping to improve levels of physical activity in adults is through the Work Zone Safety that aims to provide safe ways for adults to walk or cycle to their workplace or do their errands at their community. It should be noted that Safe Routes to School is being evaluated for its impact on physical activity as well as on BMI and social factors.[114]

Smoking

Currently, smoking has declined from 20.9% (nearly 21 of every 100 adults) in 2005 to 14% (14 of every 100 adults) in 2019, and the proportion of ever smokers who have quit has increased. This is an estimated of 34.1 million American adults smoking cigarettes and more than 16 million living with a smoking-related disease.

Cigarette smoking is responsible for more than 480,000 deaths each year, including deaths from secondhand smoke; it is the single largest preventable cause of death and disease among U.S. adults.[115] Public health professionals, concerned about the risk factors for cardiovascular disease, need to discuss smoking with clients because it is a leading risk factor. Of the estimated 12 million deaths from smoking, almost half (5.5 million) are deaths from cardiovascular diseases.[109] An estimated 1.1 million Americans

> Read more about smoking and health at: https://www.cdc.gov/tobacco/data_statistics/fact_sheets/adult_data/cig_smoking/index.htm#:~:text=In%202019%2C%20nearly%2014%20of,with%20a%20smoking%2Drelated%20disease

had a new or recurrent heart attack because of smoking. Cigarette smoking results in a two- to threefold risk of dying from coronary heart disease.[116] Smoking-related CHD may also contribute to congestive heart failure, causing 4.6 million people to suffer from this disease.[116] Smoking approximately doubles a person's risk of stroke, which is the third-leading cause of death in the United States. However, the risk of stroke decreases when an individual stops smoking. Nonsmokers exposed to secondary smoke increase their risk of heart disease by 25–30%.[116]

Smoking cessation is also effective in preventing heart disease. In fact, after just 1 year of smoking abstinence, people who quit smoking have a 50% lower risk of death from CHD than those who continue to smoke.[116] Studies have shown that secondhand smoke exposure causes heart disease among adults, with an estimated 33,951 deaths each year.[116-118]

Smoking is a modifiable risk factor, and its modification is effective in preventing cardiovascular disease mortality. Smoking cessation is particularly important in people with other cardiovascular risk factors such as high blood pressure and elevated blood cholesterol, since these risk factors work synergistically. Cigarette smoking is also a risk factor for other leading causes of death and disability, including several kinds of cancer and chronic lung diseases.[116]

Trends

Despite the progress made in decreasing premature heart disease mortality rate among adults in the United States aged 25–64 years by 70% since 1968, the rate has been stagnant from 2011 on and in 2017 still accounted for almost one in five of all deaths among this age group. With important prevalence on risk factors such as hypertension, high cholesterol, diabetes, physical inactivity, a proportion of smoking adults and unhealthy dietary patterns, described earlier in this chapter, the public health concern still exists and programs and guidelines continue to exhort the authorities, organizations, and population to take good action toward wellness.

Results from epidemiologic studies suggest that diets rich in fruits, vegetables, whole grains, and low-fat dairy foods are associated with a lower risk of mortality from many chronic diseases, including heart disease.[60] This nutritional pattern is supported by all of the major health organizations. Nevertheless, a large gap remains between recommended dietary patterns and what U.S. adults actually eat. Only about one-fourth of U.S. adults eat the recommended five or more servings of fruits and vegetables each day.[11]

Cancer

Cancer is an umbrella term used to describe a large group of diseases characterized by uncontrolled growth and spread of abnormal cells.[64] Cancer is the second leading cause of death in the United States, causing one in every four deaths. In 2020, an estimated 1,806,590 of new cases would have been diagnosed with 606,520 Americans dying from this disease.[11] The most common cancer (according to the estimated new cases in 2020) are breast cancer, lung and bronchus cancer, prostate cancer, colon and rectum cancer, melanoma of the skin, bladder cancer, non-Hodgkin lymphoma, kidney and renal pelvis cancer, endometrial cancer, leukemia, pancreatic cancer, thyroid cancer, and liver cancer. According to the American Cancer Society, about one-third of cancer deaths are preventable and are attributed to dietary factors, physical inactivity, overweight, or obesity.[64] For U.S. adults who don't smoke, dietary choices and physical activity are the most modifiable determinants

Pandemic Learning Opportunity

With limited funds for food supplies occurring in the pandemic, discuss the consumption level of fruits and vegetables.

of cancer risk. All cancers caused by cigarettes and heavy use of alcohol can be prevented.[64]

The death rate from cancer and the total number of people who develop or die from cancer each year continues to increase because of our aging population.[119-123] The overall decrease in death rates from cancer is due to a decline in smoking and more effective detection and screening. The recent decrease in deaths from breast cancer in Caucasian women, for example, is due to a greater use of breast screening in regular medical care. Cancer death rates vary by gender, race, and ethnicity. For example, African Americans are more likely to die from cancer than Caucasians.[124] However, by 2040, the number of cases per year is expected to rise to 29.5 million and the number of cancer-related deaths to 16.4 million.

Although inherited genes play a significant role in cancer risk, they only explain part of all cancer incidences.[64] Most of the variation in cancer incidence cannot be explained by inherited factors. The predominant causes of cancer are external factors such as cigarette smoking, diet or nutrition, weight, and physical activity.[64,124] These factors act to modify the risk of cancer at all stages. It is estimated that more than 50% of all cancers could be prevented through dietary improvements, such as reducing total fat and increasing fruit and vegetable consumption, and smoking cessation.[116,125] Doll and Peto[126] estimated that approximately 10–70% of deaths from cancer were attributable to diet. The science of nutrition and cancer is evolving but still is not as developed as that of diet and cardiovascular disease. Many large-scale studies are currently underway to further elucidate the relationship between various nutrients and cancer.[127] Future research points to the areas of diet and gene interactions and biomarkers for cancer will advance our understanding in this area.[128]

Current dietary recommendations are based on evidence from the American Cancer Society, the American Institute of Cancer Research/World Cancer Research Fund, and the Harvard Cancer Prevention Study.[64,129,130] The American Cancer Society updated its guidelines on nutrition and physical activity after reviewing current scientific evidence.[131] In general, the current dietary guidelines encourage the consumption of plant-based diets without relying on processed foods. The guidelines endorse eating a healthy dietary pattern that promotes healthy weight control along with physical activity.[64,130] For cancer prevention, the ACS recommends that individuals eat five or more servings of fruits and vegetables a day. Fruit and vegetable consumption may protect against cancers of the mouth and pharynx, esophagus, lung, stomach, colon, and rectum.[132] Specifically, nutrition and food scientists agree on the following recommendations to lower cancer risk[64,133]:

- Eat a plant-based diet that includes a wide variety of fruits, vegetables, whole grains, beans, and legumes. The recommendation is to choose whole grains over refined sources and eat three to five servings of vegetables and two to four servings of fruits per day.
- Eat less fat from all food sources.
- Limit excess calories and maintain a healthful weight throughout life. Eat a sound diet and incorporate moderate or vigorous physical activity 5 days a week or more to further reduce risks of cancer.
- If you drink alcohol, do so in moderation.

Nutrition supplements are not universally recommended for cancer prevention. Instead, the cancer-prevention benefits of diet are considered among the best due to the interactions of many vitamins, minerals, and other plant-derived substances naturally occurring in foods.[64,129,132] However, the possible benefits of supplemental folate, calcium, and selenium are noted.[64,131] By eating whole foods and following the cancer-prevention dietary recommendations along with physical activity, the protection of the body's cells may occur during the initiation, promotion, and progression stages of cancer. These food substances may repair damage that has already occurred in cells. Some studies suggest that individuals do not need to be concerned about the pesticide residues on fruits and vegetables, because the benefits of eating fruits and vegetables far outweigh any potential risk.[129] More long-term studies may help to confirm this definitively.

The study of diet and cancer prevention is relatively new. Dietitians and other public healthcare professionals need to stay abreast of these discoveries in order to give appropriate guidance to individuals at risk. The basis of MNT should include those recommendations set forth by the American Cancer Society and the World Cancer Research Fund/American Institute for Cancer Research.[64,130,132]

> Read more about diet and cancer at: https://www.cdc.gov/cancer/dcpc /prevention/other.htm

Diabetes

Diabetes is a serious, costly, and increasingly common chronic disease that poses a significant public health challenge. In 2019 , diabetes was the 8th leading cause of death in the United States.[133] In 2018, 34.2 million Americans had diabetes, of which 26.8 million or 10.5% of the population have been diagnosed and 7.3 millions of these people were undiagnosed.[11] Type 2 diabetes used to be called adult-onset diabetes and may account for approximately 90% to 95% of all diagnosed cases of diabetes.[134] The total prevalence of diabetes in the United States is expected to more than double from 2005 to 2050: from 5.6% to 12%.[135] By 2050, an estimated 29 million Americans are expected to have been diagnosed with diabetes. The increase in the number of cases has been particularly high within certain ethnic and racial groups in the United States.[136]

Medical complications of type 2 diabetes include heart disease, kidney failure, leg and foot amputations, and blindness. Diabetes is the leading cause of new cases of blindness among adults aged 18–64 years and crude data for 2018 showed that 11.7% reported vision disability, including blindness.[11] The majority of the deaths caused by diabetes are due to diabetes-associated cardiovascular disease. The presence of diabetes in adults is associated with a two- to fourfold increase in CHD compared with nondiabetic adults. Almost three-quarters of adults with diabetes have hypertension.[11] Diabetes is the cause of 44% of end-stage renal disease cases, and for the 2013–2016 period, 57.0% of adults diagnosed with diabetes had chronic kidney disease, of which over half (52.5%) had moderate to severe chronic kidney disease (stages 3 or 4). Severe forms of nervous system damage occur in 60–70% of diabetic adults. Approximately 60% of all nontraumatic amputations in the United States occur in people with diabetes.[137] Periodontal or gum disease is also more common among diabetics. As a result, diabetes is a costly disease, with the total attributable costs (direct and indirect) estimated at $237 billion in 2017, and between 2012 and 2017, excess medical costs per person associated with diabetes increases from $8,417 to 9,601.[137,138]

Type 2 diabetes is associated with the following factors:

- *Age:* Diabetes is most common in people over 60 years of age; however, earlier onset has been seen recently.[137]
- *Ethnicity:* Deaths from diabetes are twice as high for African Americans as for Caucasians; Native Americans, Hispanic

Americans, and certain Pacific Islander American and Asian American populations also have higher rates.[135]

- *Genetics and family history:* Genetic markers that indicate a greater risk for type 2 diabetes have been identified.
- *Obesity:* The increased prevalence of obesity among adults is positively associated with the increased rates of diabetes.[138,139] Data from clinical trials strongly support the potential of moderate weight loss to reduce the risk of type 2 diabetes.[140]
- *History of gestational diabetes in women:* Gestational diabetes is a form of glucose intolerance that develops in some women during pregnancy. Obesity is associated with gestational diabetes. Women with a family history of gestational diabetes and Hispanic American and African American women are at increased risk.[141]
- *Impaired glucose metabolism:* People with prediabetes, or who are at increased risk of developing diabetes, have impaired fasting blood glucose. Research studies suggest that weight loss and increased physical activity among people with prediabetes may return glucose levels to normal and prevent the onset of diabetes.[136]
- *Physical inactivity:* If you are at higher risk and fairly inactive, or exercise fewer than three times a week, you are more likely to develop type 2 diabetes.

Read more about diabetes at: https://www.cdc.gov/nchs/products/databriefs/db395.htm

In the United States, recent lifestyle changes such as decreased physical activity and increased energy consumption, which contribute to the increased prevalence rates of obesity, are also strong risk factors for diabetes.[140] On the other hand, positive lifestyle changes such as diet, weight loss of 5–7%, and moderate-intensity physical activity (e.g., walking 30 minutes a day) can delay the onset of diabetes. The Diabetes Prevention Program,[141] a major, large-scale study of over 3,000 people at high risk for developing diabetes, confirmed this, and found a 58% reduction in the development of diabetes over a 3-year period. The findings from this study, sponsored by the NIH, showed that exercise, a healthy diet, and weight loss can reduce the risk of developing diabetes by as much as 71% in high-risk individuals.[140,141]

Medical nutrition therapy is an essential part of diabetes management for adults. Its objectives include[141]:

- Attaining and maintaining optimal metabolic outcomes including normalizing blood glucose levels, maintaining a lipid profile that reduces vascular disease risk, and normalizing blood pressure levels
- Preventing, delaying, and treating the onset complications by modifying nutrient intake and lifestyle to prevent and treat obesity, cardiovascular disease, hypertension, and nephropathy
- Optimizing health through sensible food choices and physical activity
- Addressing personal and cultural preferences as well as lifestyle factors, including a person's willingness to change, when determining individual nutritional needs

In terms of specific nutrients and dietary recommendations for type 2 diabetes, studies in healthy subjects and those at risk for type 2 diabetes support the importance of including foods containing complex carbohydrates in the diet, particularly those from whole grains, fruits, vegetables, and low-fat milk.[141] Reduced intake of total fat, especially saturated fat, may reduce the risk of diabetes.

Taking into account that the increase of type 2 diabetes is closely linked to the rise in obesity, it is important to coordinate efforts to start prevention as early as possible. Recent research has been emphasizing the relevance of early prevention as early as during pregnancy, first to prevent excessive gestational weight gain, gestational diabetes, and its consequences including fetal macrosomia in those women who may be at risk. Also, the first years of life have a crucial impact on the developing of adequate neuroendocrine signals that will impact the appetite-satiety regulatory axis.[142]

Pregnancy is a period in which women are susceptible to introduce changes into their routines in order to benefit their babies; healthcare control frequency is higher, so contacts between healthcare providers can be an excellent window of opportunities for prevention. If these changes and recommendations are maintained in the postnatal period, a big step toward breaking intergenerational cycles of obesity and type 2 diabetes can be taken.[143]

During the first 3 years of life, exclusive breastfeeding and introduction of the right foods at the right time for a proper weaning period will establish an adequate metabolic environment that will promote the future health of the individual.[14]

As stated by the American Diabetes Association in its Standards of Medical Care in Diabetes-2016,[144] strategies for improving care related to lifestyle changes and prevention of diabetes complications should:

1. Optimize provider and team behavior in order to prioritize timely and appropriate intensification of lifestyle and/or pharmacologic therapy for patients who have not achieved beneficial levels of glucose, blood pressure or lipid control.
2. Support patient behavior change: which includes a systematic approach to supporting patients' behavior change efforts, including healthy lifestyle choices, disease self-management, and prevention of diabetes complications.
3. Change the care system to ensure the best high-quality care, as basing care on evidence-based guidelines, activating and educating patients, expanding the role of teams to implement more intensive care disease management strategies and identifying/developing/engaging community resources and **public policy** that support healthy lifestyles are among the key changes proposed.[144]

Programs and initiatives such as HP 2030 include strategies at the worksite; community-level and individual management of diabetes. Also, the maternal, infant, and child component includes diabetes to identify those individuals at risk at early stages and the goal of reducing the annual number of new cases of diagnosed diabetes in the population testing for diabetes has been strengthened to avoid the associated complications. On the other hand, the National Diabetes Program includes counseling programs that intend to change harmful behaviors into healthier ones. Through attendance in group sessions of people with similar goals and motivation, people are required to attend weekly sessions during the first 6 months and keep attendance at least once bi-weekly during the second 6 months. The activities and educational sessions include the promotion of physical activity.

In terms of diabetes prevention, the Diabetes Prevention Research Group conducted a study in 3,243 individuals with prediabetes and were randomly assigned to one of three groups: lifestyle intervention, drug intervention, and drug placebo, to check the effectiveness of the interventions proposed by the group. These include the goals of losing 7% of the body weight and engaging in the nationally recommended 150 minutes per week of moderate, intense

Discussion Prompt

What kinds of programs and which personnel would be key in a community or public health program to assist in making lifestyle changes for clients?

Policy Rule, guideline, or practice established by an elected or appointed authority, administration, or management. Policy interventions targeting communities and organizations have a much greater potential impact or reach than individual or interpersonal/group interventions.

physical activity. Over the course of the 3-year study, all participants were randomized to the lifestyle interventions group, reporting significantly greater physical activity levels relative to the other groups; had significantly greater weight loss; and showed a 58% greater decrease in diabetes incidence relative to the placebo group.[144]

In summary, lifestyle changes such as reduced energy intake, increased physical activity, and nutrition education (with the goal of promoting weight loss) represent essential aspects of type 2 diabetes management for adults. HP 2030[136] discusses the challenges of diabetes and the preventive interventions aimed at them: primary prevention, screening and early diagnosis, access, and quality of care. This includes secondary and tertiary prevention, such as glucose control and decreasing complications from diabetes.[137] As dietitians/nutritionists, public health professionals, and educators, many opportunities exist to contribute to the effective management of diabetes.

Osteoporosis

As an individual grows, bones develop and become larger, heavier, and denser. At approximately age 30 years, peak bone mass is achieved in both men and women. After this time period, adults begin to lose bone mass, and this continues as they get older. Osteoporosis (i.e., porous bone disease) develops when bone loss reaches the point of causing fractures under common, everyday stresses. Due to increased bone fragility, there is a greater susceptibility to fractures of the hip, spine, and wrist. Both men and women suffer from osteoporosis.[145]

Osteoporosis currently affects 44 million Americans, or 55% of people aged 50 and older; 68% of women over 50 have the disease.[146,147] These rates correspond to one in two women and one in four men (aged >50 years) who will experience an osteoporosis-related fracture in their lifetime.[146]

In the United States, about one in 10 people ages 50 years and older have osteoporosis. The percent of men 65 years and older with osteoporosis of the femur neck or lumbar spine is 5.1%; whereas women 65 years and older with the same disease is 24.5%. The National Osteoporosis Foundation (NOF) announced in 2018 that approximately 10.2 million adults in the United States had osteoporosis with an additional 43.2 million having low bone mass.[147]

Osteoporosis causes significant disability with important economic consequences, costing about $19 billion each year in direct expenditures (hospitals and nursing homes).[148] By 2025, experts predict that these costs will rise to about 25.3 billion.[148] Of the 2 million fractures occurring each year due to osteoporosis, over 300,000 are hip fractures, 547,000 are vertebral fractures, and 450,000 are wrist fractures. Of the 300,000 annual hip fractures, 24% result in death following complications from the fracture.[147]

Osteoporosis is often called the "silent disease" because it can occur without any overt symptoms. The technical standard for measuring bone mineral density is dual-energy x-ray absorptiometry (DXA). A low–bone-mass density is a strong predictor of fracture risk.[147] Bone density tests can detect osteoporosis before a fracture occurs and they can serve as a predictor for future fracture risks.

The chances of developing osteoporosis are greatest in white women beyond menopause. Women have less bone tissue and lose bone more easily than men due to the hormonal changes involved in menopause. Those individuals who have a low dietary intake of calcium and vitamin D over a lifetime, and who are physically inactive, cigarette smokers, excessive alcohol drinkers, thin and small-framed, and who have a family history of

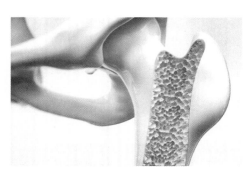

The bone weakens with osteoporosis.

© Crevis/Shutterstock.

osteoporosis are at increased risk.[146,147] White and Asian American women are at highest risk, whereas African American and Hispanic American women have lower risks.[147] Excessive intake of protein, sodium, and caffeine also contribute to being at risk for osteoporosis. Anorexia nervosa, the use of certain medications, and low testosterone levels in men are risk factors for osteoporosis.

Given this context, HP 2030 focuses on preventing and treating this disease, improving testing and aiming at reducing hip fractures on those who already have the disease. The five factors that can be modified to prevent osteoporosis are: 1) a diet rich in calcium and vitamin D; 2) weight-bearing exercise; 3) a healthy lifestyle that excludes smoking and excessive alcohol intake; 4) routine bone-density measurements; and 5) the use of medication, when appropriate.[148]

Nutrition is an important modifiable risk factor in terms of both bone health and the prevention and treatment of osteoporosis. An adequate amount of calcium and vitamin D contributes significantly to bone health. Low calcium and vitamin D intakes are associated with low bone mass, rapid bone loss, and high fracture rates.[149] Bone is a living, growing tissue, and 99% of the body's calcium is found in bone. Throughout one's lifetime, bone formation and resorption occur. This process, which is known as *bone turnover*, is responsive to dietary calcium regardless of age. Dietary calcium works to strengthen bone by suppressing bone resorption and parathyroid hormone.[149]

According to the *NIH Consensus Statement on Osteoporosis*,[148] calcium is the most important nutrient for the prevention of osteoporosis. Actual calcium intakes for most of the U.S. population, however, are considerably lower than the current Dietary Reference Intakes (DRI).[149] Many studies have shown that adult skeletal health is improved by increasing dairy foods or calcium intake in the diet.[149] The DASH diet, used to treat hypertension, is a low-fat diet, rich in calcium, that has been shown to reduce bone turnover and reduce the risk of osteoporosis.[99] Calcium requirements can be met with low-fat dairy products; however, low consumption of milk and other dairy products in the U.S. diet is mainly responsible for low calcium intakes among U.S. adults.[145-148] Other foods contain calcium, such as dark leafy greens, but these usually provide less calcium per serving than milk, and most Americans do not eat these vegetables often. For individuals who do not consume enough calcium in their diets, calcium supplements are recommended.

Vitamin D also plays an important role in calcium absorption and bone health. Vitamin D is a major determinant of intestinal calcium absorption. When skin is exposed to sunlight, the body synthesizes vitamin D. However, studies show decreased production of vitamin D in the elderly and individuals who are housebound, especially in the winter months.[146] Due to inadequate intake of vitamin D in a high proportion of older adults, the most recent DRIs have increased the vitamin D requirements for people 50 years and older.[148] Low-fat and nonfat milk, excellent sources of calcium, are fortified with 100 IU of vitamin D per serving.

In conclusion, osteoporosis is a serious public health disease and is largely preventable. Starting early in life, both females and males should be advised on how to incorporate sources of calcium into their diets. The use of low-fat and nonfat dairy foods should be recommended, and if persons cannot consume dairy products, other food sources and calcium supplements are necessary. Adequate vitamin D intake needs to be addressed as well. Community and public health dietitians/nutritionists should encourage individuals to participate regularly in physical activity. Modifiable lifestyle factors should be discussed to promote bone health throughout life.

Strategy Tip

Brainstorm on what a community or public health program should include in an osteoporosis prevention program.

Chronic Kidney Disease

Chronic Kidney Disease (CKD) constitutes any condition that causes reduced kidney function over a period of time and is present when a patient's glomerular filtration rate remains below 60 milliliters per minute for more than 3 months or when a patient's urine albumin-to-creatinine ratio is over 30 milligrams (mg) of albumin for each gram (g) of creatinine (30 mg/g).

Diabetes and high blood pressure are the two leading causes of CKD in the United States and diabetes is the most common cause of kidney failure.[150] Results from the Diabetes Prevention Program funded by the National Institute of Diabetes and Digestive and Kidney Diseases (NIDDK) show that moderate exercise, a healthier diet and weight reduction can prevent the development of type 2 diabetes in individuals at risk.[150] This is consistent with every other noncommunicable disease previously mentioned in this chapter, and these lifestyle guidelines are consistent with the Chronic Kidney Disease HP 2030 objectives.[151] According to CDC data for 2019, 15% of U.S. adults or 37 million people are estimated to have CKD. Most (9 in 10) adults with CKD do not know they have it and one in two people with very low kidney function, who are not on dialysis, do not know they have CKD.

CKD is a complex stage of the disease that has negative consequences for health, as people with no CKD are more likely than people with stage 3–5 CKD to be alive 1 year after a heart attack. In terms of prevention, controlling high blood pressure, blood glucose, keeping cholesterol in the target range, weight loss as needed, stopping smoking and taking drug therapy, if indicated, are the NIDDKD recommendations. Once again, healthy food choices and becoming physically active are important steps toward slowing or stopping the progression of CKD. Additionally, a person's lifestyle can decrease or increase the chances of developing diabetes, dyslipidemia, obesity, and high blood pressure, thus increasing the risk for CKD.[151]

The National Kidney Disease Education Program (NKDEP) has developed several tools for screening patients for education and prevention of acquiring CKD once a person has been diagnosed with diabetes, high blood pressure, or both, including educational sessions, testing for kidney disease, promoting patient self-management, and referral to a dietitian/nutritionist who can adjust portions and give orientation on food choices, including sodium levels to be consumed according to the level of kidney disease.[152] Some of the specific dietary recommendations that government agencies support are:

- Buy fresh food more often. Sodium (a part of salt) is added to many packaged foods and should be avoided.
- Use spices, herbs, and sodium-free seasonings in place of salt.
- Check the Nutrition Facts label on food packages for sodium. A Daily Value of 20% or more means the food is high in sodium.
- Try lower-sodium versions of frozen dinners and other convenience foods.
- Rinse with water or avoid canned vegetables, beans, meats, and fish.
- Eat small portions of protein foods.

CKD is a complex management situation. Focusing on persons at risk should be the top priority to avoid costly treatments and encouraging lifestyles. Change is key for achieving reductions in prevalence of CKD, particularly in Americans older than 60.[152]

Acquired Immune Deficiency Syndrome (AIDS)

In 1981, a new infectious disease, acquired immune deficiency syndrome (AIDS), was first identified in the United States. A few years later, human immunodeficiency virus (HIV) was identified as the viral agent that causes AIDS. HIV/AIDS has affected almost every ethnic, socioeconomic, and age group in the United States.[153]

AIDS, a deadly disease, is the end-stage of HIV infection. The infection progresses to overwhelm the immune system and leaves individuals defenseless against numerous other infections and diseases. HIV is spread through direct contact with contaminated body fluids, sexual relations, direct blood contact, or from mother to infant. In 1996, death rates from AIDS in the United States declined for the first time.[153] Nevertheless, HIV/AIDS remains a significant cause of illness, disability, and death in the United States. According to the Centers for Disease Control and Prevention (CDC)[154] death rates have dropped dramatically in the United States due to the introduction of antiretroviral therapies.[154]

Health complications for people with HIV/AIDS are immune dysfunction and its associated complications, which include malnutrition and wasting. HIV targets the immune system, rendering an individual susceptible to infections and disease. The CDC defines the AIDS-related wasting syndrome as a 10% weight loss in a 6-month period accompanied by diarrhea or fever for more than 30 days.[153] Malnutrition and its complications can reduce one's tolerance to medications and other therapies. Malnutrition occurs in the form of tissue wasting, fat accumulation, increased lipid levels, and risk of other chronic diseases. The Academy of Nutrition and Dietetics Association's (AND) Position Paper[155] strongly supports nutrition evaluation and medical nutrition therapy as parts of the ongoing health care of HIV-infected individuals. In terms of medical nutrition therapy, this includes early assessment and treatment of nutrient deficiencies, the maintenance and restoration of lean body mass, and continued support for performing daily activities and maintaining quality of life. According to AND, nutrition education and guidance should incorporate the following aspects[155]:

- Healthful eating principles
- Water and food safety issues
- Perinatal and breastfeeding issues
- Nutrition management for symptoms such as anorexia, swallowing problems, and diarrhea
- Food–medicine interactions
- Psychosocial and economic issues
- Alternative feeding methods (supplementation, tube feeding, or parenteral nutrition)
- Additional therapies, including physical activity and disease management
- Guidelines for evaluating nutrition information, diet claims, and individual mineral and vitamin supplementation
- Strategies for treatment of altered fat metabolism
- Food insecurity risk
- Changes in body composition
- Biochemical indices
- Clinical indicators of comorbid disease

Pandemic Learning Opportunity

Those persons with immune-suppressive conditions were at a higher risk during Covid-19.

Although the side effects from antiretroviral therapy regimens are less prevalent now, micronutrient deficiencies and chronic anemia remain

The maintenance and restoration of nutrition stores are interrelated with recommended medical therapies for those with HIV/AIDS; therefore, it is essential that a public health dietitian/nutritionist be an active participant in the healthcare team to provide optimal medical nutrition therapy.

COVID-19 Community and Public Health Implications

As the impact of the Covid-19 pandemic and the economic turndown have been important all over the population, it is particularly more difficult among Blacks, Latinos, Indigenous, and immigrant households. At the beginning of 2021, results from the Household Pulse Survey showed that approximately 24 million adults (11% of adults in the United States) reported that their household sometimes or often didn't have enough food to eat in the last 7 days. This is far above the prepandemic rate given by the USDA showing 3.4% of adults having food supply difficulties. Included in the US pandemic response were vaccinations, unemployment benefits, welfare or temporary assistance for needy families (TANF), food stamps, Medicaid, and children's health insurance program (CHIP).

Read more about food insecurity in Chapter 13.

significant nutritional risk for the population living with HIV. Monitoring the co-existence of other infectious diseases will be useful to implement the adequate nutrition intervention in these clients.

Strong evidence says that nutrition is related to immunity and that poorly nourished individuals are at greater risk for infectious diseases including viral infections. Thus, maintaining an adequate diet is recommended by MyPlate, or Healthy Eating Plate, that emphasize fruits, vegetables, whole grains, legumes and nuts, with a moderate consumption of fish, dairy foods, and poultry. There should be a limited intake of red and processed meat and refined carbohydrates and sugar.

People with chronic, noncommunicable diseases have an increased risk for complications when infected by the Covid-19 virus. Initial data pointed to older adults and those with cardiovascular diseases, diabetes, respiratory or kidney disease, with increasing evidence of obesity to be linked to more severe COVID-19 and death.

Now, with the Covid-19 challenges in food security and increasing poverty, rethinking strategies to compensate the population's needs are key issues and planning for access to the wellness programs through the national territory to provide the tools, strategies, and care that evidence have reported to be the best are more relevant than ever.

Summary

While there is improvement in understanding chronic disease etiology and its complications over the health status, a huge number of Americans are still exposed to the consequences of these diseases. There are many benefits of adopting a healthy lifestyle including an adequate diet, performing physical activity and not smoking are major contributors to the prevention of obesity, type 2 diabetes, cancer, and cardiovascular diseases. The impact of introducing healthy habits as early as possible is an efficient way of reducing the elevated psychological, physical, and economic cost of the disabilities caused by the progression of these diseases.

Programs for prevention have been developed by community and public health programs with the aim of reducing the burden of chronic diseases in the United States. These programs include those designed to address specific topics and objectives for actions that will prevent or ameliorate health conditions on those that are exposed to the risk factors. Food provisional programs aim to supplement those vulnerable groups in disadvantaged situations, promoting early impact to the young; thus, hoping to guarantee future health and minimizing the effects of starting life in poor conditions. Community and public health outreach have provided components of a healthy lifestyle including nutrition, physical activity, and stress management. These programs were made modifiable through efficient cost interventions and through efforts to promote changes to the population's habits.

Learning Portfolio

© olies/Shutterstock.

Issues for Discussion

1. What would you propose should be incorporated into community and public health programs that focus on nutrition as an important preventive factor in illness, disability, and death?
2. What advice would you give to the individual in the community in regard to preventing chronic disease risk factors such as obesity, physical inactivity, and smoking in order to reduce society's financial burden?
3. In the context of the COVID-19 pandemic, what would your primary action be toward guaranteeing food access?

Practical Activities

1. Look up a primary care facility in your community on the Internet and list the nutritional services available. Do you think they are adequate?
2. Look up nutritional volunteer educational activities on the Internet. Report your findings.
3. Check the educational activities related to health within your University and compile a list of what is being offered. Are there services that you would include? Eliminate?
4. Check on digital resources that complement interventions on nutrition and health programs. What are they?

Key Terms

	page
Nutrition Program	306
Prevention	306
Chronic Disease	306
Risk factor	307
Guideline	307
Strategy	308
Developmental Origin of Health and Disease	310
Life course approach	310
Policy	329

Case Study: Building a Community Health Team

You have been made the director of a new community health team in a town that has not had one before.

1. What programs might you consider researching after reading this chapter? What staff might you need for each program?

Case Study: Community and Public Health Nutrition During Covid-19

You are a community dietitian/nutritionist working in a low-income, small, rural town and are reviewing your town's nutritional status during the Covid-19 pandemic. From collected data you find both obese (42%) and undernourished adults (15%).

1. What elements for intervention should be taken into account?
2. What nutrition community interventions would you recommend?
3. What is your higher risk group for getting infected by the virus?

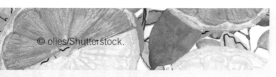
© olies/Shutterstock.

Learning Portfolio

Resources

1. U.S. Dietary Guidelines: http://www.health.gov/2020/dietaryguidelines/
2. Dietary Guidelines of the American Heart Association: http://www.americanheart.org/presenter.jhtml?identifier=851
3. American Cancer Society: http://www.cancer.org
4. American Institute for Cancer Research: http://www.aicr.org
5. Academy of Nutrition and Dietetics:http://www.eatright.org
6. Alternate Healthy Eating Index: http://www.hsph.harvard.edu/nutritionsource/pyramids.html
7. American Diabetes Association: http://www.diabetes.org The Obesity Society www.
8. USDA Choose MyPlate http://www.choosemyplate.gov/MyPlate

References

1. Engle PL, Pelto GH. The Responsive feeding: implications for policy and program implementation. *J Nutr*. 2011;141(3):508-511. https://doi.org/10.3945/jn.110.130039
2. UNICEF (United Nations Children's Fund). 2020. *Nutrition, for every child: UNICEF Nutrition Strategy 2020–2030*. UNICEF, New York. Accessed January 25, 2021. https://www.unicef.org/media/92031/file/UNICEF%20Nutrition%20Strategy%202020-2030.pdf
3. Vermont Department of Health. 2016. *What is Prevention?* Accessed January 6, 2021. http://healthvermont.gov/adap/prevention/prevention_fact.aspx
4. Academy of Nutrition and Dietetics. International Dietetics & Nutrition Terminology (IDNT) Reference Manual. *Standardized Language for the Nutrition Care Process*. 4th Edition. Chicago, IL; 2013;403-410.
5. World Health Organization. *Noncommunicable diseases*. 2020. Accessed January 30, 2021. https://www.who.int/health-topics/noncommunicable-diseases#tab=tab_1
6. Gillman MW, Blaisdell CJ. Environmental influences on Child Health Outcomes, a research program of the National Institutes of Health. *Curr Opin Pediatr*. 2018;30(2):260-262. doi: 10.1097/MOP.0000000000000600
7. Ben-Shlomo Y, Cooper R, Kuh D. The last two decades of life course epidemiology, and its relevance for research on ageing. *Int J Epidemiol*. 2016;45(4):973-988. doi: 10.1093/ije/dyw096
8. Carlson A, Frazão E. Food costs, diet quality and energy balance in the United States. *Physiol Behav*. 2014;134:20-31. doi: 10.1016/j.physbeh.2014.03.001
9. Institute of Medicine (US). How far have we come in reducing health disparities? Progress since 2000: workshop summary. Washington (DC): National Academies Press (US); 2012. Accessed December 12, 2012. https://www.ncbi.nlm.nih.gov/books/NBK114239/
10. Centers for Disease Control and Prevention. *FastStats: Life Expectancy 2018*. Accessed January 26, 2021. http://www.cdc.gov/nchs/fastats/life-expectancy.htm
11. McRobbie MA, Kolbe LJ. The academy's pivotal role in supporting public-private partnerships to prevent chronic diseases. *Prev Chronic Dis*. 2009;6(2):A73.
12. Centers for Disease Control and Prevention. *National Vital Statistics Reports. United States Life Tables*. 2018;69:2. Accessed January 13, 2021. https://www.cdc.gov/nchs/data/nvsr/nvsr69/nvsr69-12-508.pdf
13. Centers for Disease Control and Prevention, National Center for Health Statistics. Effectiveness in disease and injury prevention; estimated national spending on prevention. U.S., 1988. *MMWR Morbid Mortal Wkly Rep*. 1992;41:529-531.
14. Gillman MW, Ludwig DS. How early should obesity prevention start? *N Engl J Med*. 2013;369:2173-2175.
15. Wolfson JA, Leung CW. Food insecurity during COVID-19: an acute crisis with long-term health implications. *Am J Pub Health*. 2020;110(12):1763-1765. https://doi.org/10.2105/AJPH.2020.305953
16. Lichtenstein AH, Appel LJ, Brands M., et al. Diet and lifestyle recommendations revision 2006: a scientific statement from the American Heart Association Nutrition Committee. *Circulation*. 2006;114(1):82-96. [Published correction appears in Circulation. 2006 Dec 5;114(23):e629] [Published correction appears in Circulation. 2006 Jul 4;114(1):e27]. doi: 10.1161/CIRCULATIONAHA.106.176158
17. National Center for Health Statistics. *Health, U.S., 2003*. Washington, DC: U.S. Government Printing Office; 2003. Accessed January 4, 2004. https://www.cdc.gov/nchs/surveys.htm#tabs-1-4
18. Remington PL, Brownson RC, Fifty years of progress in chronic disease epidemiology and control. *Morbidity and Mortality Weekly Report*. 2011;60(4):70-77.
19. Mokdad AH, Marks JS, Stroup DF, Gerberding JL. Actual causes of death in the United States, 2000. *JAMA*. 2004;291(10):1238-1245.
20. Mokdad AH, Marks JS, Stroup DF, Gerberding JL. Correction: actual causes of death in the United States, 2000. *JAMA*. 2005;293(3):293-294. doi: 10.1001/jama.293.3.293
21. U.S. Department of Health and Human Services, Centers for Disease Control and Prevention. National Center for Health Statistics. Health, United States, 2018. Hyattsville, MD; 2019. https://www.cdc.gov/nchs/data/hus/hus18.pdf
22. Koplan JP, Dietz WH. Caloric imbalance and public health policy. *JAMA*. 1999;282(16):1579-1581.
23. Kochanek KD, Xu J, Arias E. Mortality in the United States, 2019. *NCHS Data Brief*. 2020;395:2-8. https://www.cdc.gov/nchs/data/databriefs/db395-H.pdf
24. Centers for Disease Control and Prevention (US), National Center for Chronic Disease Prevention and Health Promotion (US), Office on Smoking and Health (US). *How Tobacco Smoke Causes Disease: The Biology and Behavioral Basis for Smoking-Attributable Disease: A Report of the Surgeon General*. Atlanta (GA): Centers for Disease Control and Prevention (US);

2010. Accessed February 26, 2021. https://www.ncbi.nlm.nih.gov/books/NBK53017/

25. Elo SL, Caltrop JB. Health promotive action and preventive action model (HPA model) for the classification of health-care services in public health nursing. *Scand J Public Health.* 2002;30(3):200-208.

26. U.S. Department of Health and Human Services. Healthy People. 2020. *Leading Health Indicators Development and Framework.* Accessed February 26, 2021. http://www.healthypeople.gov/2020/leading-health-indicators/Leading-Health-Indicators-Development-and-Framework

27. Edelstein S, ed. *Nutrition in public health.* 4th ed. Jones & Bartlett Learning; 2018.

28. Shamansky SL, Clausen CL. Levels of prevention: examination of the concept. *Nurs Outlook.* 1980;28(2):104-108.

29. Fitzgerald N, Morgan KT, Slawson DL. Practice paper of the Academy of Nutrition and Dietetics abstract: the role of nutrition in health promotion and chronic disease prevention. *J Acad Nutr Diet.* 2013;113(7):983. doi: 10.1016/j.jand.2013.05.007

30. Hu FB, Staija A, Rimm EB, et al. Diet assessment methods in the nurses' health studies and contribution to evidence-based nutritional policies and guidelines. *Am J Public Health.* 2016;106(9):1567-1572.

31. US Department of agriculture. MyPlate.gov. *MyPlate Kitchen 2020.* Accessed February 7, 2021. https://www.myplate.gov/myplate-kitchen

32. Dietary Guidelines Advisory Committee. *Scientific Report of the 2020 Dietary Guidelines Advisory Committee: Advisory Report to the Secretary of Agriculture and the Secretary of Health and Human Services.* Washington, DC: U.S. Department of Agriculture, Agricultural Research Service; 2020. Accessed February 2, 2021. https://www.dietaryguidelines.gov/2020-advisory-committee-report

33. U.S. Departments of Agriculture and Health and Human Services. *Nutrition and Your Health: Dietary Guidelines for America.* 5th ed. Home and Garden Bulletin, No.232. Washington, DC: U.S. Departments of Agriculture, Health and Human Services. 2000. https://www.dietaryguidelines.gov/sites/default/files/2019-05/2000%20Dietary%20Guidelines%20for%20Americans.pdf

34. U.S. Department of Agriculture and U.S. Department of Health and Human Services. Dietary Guidelines for Americans, 2020-2025. 9th Edition. Accessed December 7, 2020. https://www.dietaryguidelines.gov/resources/2020-2025-dietary-guidelines-online-materials

35. Nitzke S, Freeland-Graves J. American Dietetic Association, Olendzki BC. Position of the American Dietetic Association: total diet approach to communicating food and nutrition information. *J Am Diet Assoc.* 2007;107(7):1224-1232. doi: 10.1016/j.jada.2007.05.02

36. American Dietetic Association and the Office of Disease Prevention and Health Promotion, Public Health Service, U.S. Department of Health and Human Services. *Worksite Nutrition; A Guide to Planning, Implementation, and Evaluation,* 2nd ed. Chicago, IL: American Dietetic Association; 1993.

37. Campbell IH, Rudan I. Effective approaches to public engagement with global health topics. *J Glob Health.* 2020;10(1):01040901. doi: 10.7189/jogh.10.010901

38. Murdaugh CL, Parsons M, Pender NJ. *Health Promotion in Nursing Practice.* 8th ed. Mexico, Bogotá: Pearson; 2019. https://research.usc.edu.au/discovery/fulldisplay?vid=61USC_INST:ResearchRepository&docid=alma99258105202621&lang=en&context=SP

39. HealthyPeople.gov. 2030 *Topics and Objectives.* Accessed January 26, 2021. https://health.gov/healthypeople

40. Eckel RH, Kris-Etherton P, Lichtenstein AH, et al. Americans' awareness, knowledge, and behaviors regarding fats: 2006-2007. *J Am Diet Assoc.* 2009;109(2):288-296. doi: 10.1016/j.jada.2008.10.048

41. Barker DJP. *Mothers, babies and disease in later life.* 2nd ed. New York: Churchill Livingstone; 1998.

42. International Society for Developmental Origins of Health and Disease. *The Cape Town Manifesto* 2015. Accessed January 7, 2016. https://dohadsoc.org/wp-content/uploads/2015/11/DOHaD-Society-Manifesto-Nov-17-2015.pdf

43. Alderman H. The economic cost of a poor start to life. *J Dev Origins Health Dis.* 2010;1(1):19-25.

44. USDA Food and Nutrition Service. 2020. *Women, Infants and Children (WIC).* Accessed January 7, 2021. https://www.fns.usda.gov/wic

45. Wimbush FB, Peters RM. Identification of cardiovascular risk: use of a cardiovascular-specific genogram. *Public Health Nurs.* 2000;17(3):148-154.

46. Krantz MJ, Beaty B, Coronel-Mockler S, Leeman-Castillo B, Fletcher K, Estacio RO. Reduction in cardiovascular risk among Latino participants in a community-based intervention linked with clinical care. *Am J Prevent Med.* 2017;53(2):e71-e75.

47. U.S. Department of Health and Human Services, Centers for Disease Control and Prevention, National Center for Health Statistics. *National Health Interview Survey (NHIS);* 2003. https://www.cdc.gov/nchs/nhis/about_nhis.htm

48. Shlisky J, Bloom DE, Beaudreault AR, et al. Nutritional considerations for healthy aging and reduction in age-related chronic disease. *Adv Nutr.* 2017;8(1):17-26. doi: 10.3945/an.116.013474

49. U.S. Department of Health and Human Services. National Heart, Lung, and Blood Institute (NHLBI). *National High Blood Pressure Education Program.* Accessed February 20, 2016. https://www.nhlbi.nih.gov/files/docs/resources/heart/hbp_salt.pdf

50. Centers for Disease Control and Prevention, National Center for Chronic Disease Prevention and Health Promotion, (NCCDPHP). *Heart Disease and Stroke: CDC works to prevent heart disease and stroke and promote heart health.* 2020. https://www.cdc.gov/chronicdisease/resources/publications/factsheets/heart-disease-stroke.htm; https://www.cdc.gov/chronicdisease/resources/publications/aag.htm

51. Manson JE, Bassuk SS.). Invited commentary: the Framingham Offspring Study—a pioneering investigation into familial aggregation of cardiovascular risk. *Am J Epidemiol.* 2017;185(11):1103-1108. doi: 10.1093/aje/kwx068 https://academic.oup.com/aje/article/185/11/1103/3849390?login=true

52. America on the Move. Accessed September 1, 2021. https://letsmove.obamawhitehouse.archives.gov/about

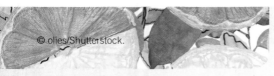
© olies/Shutterstock.

Learning Portfolio

53. LetsMove.gov. 2010. *LetsMove*. Accessed January 7, 2021. http://www.letsmove.gov/

54. Academy of Nutrition and Dietetics. Eat Right. *Kids Eat Right*. 2010. Accessed January 7, 2021. http://www.eatright.org/resources/for-kids/

55. Schulze MB, Martínez-González MA, Fung TT, Lichtenstein AH, Forouhi NG. Food based dietary patterns and chronic disease prevention. *BMJ*. 2018;361:k2396. Accessed January 7, 2021. https://www.bmj.com/content/361/bmj.k2396.long

56. The dietary guidelines: surveillance issues and research needs. (Supplement: AICR 11th Annual Research Conference on Diet, Nutrition and Cancer). *J Nutr*. 2001;131(suppl 2): S3154-S3155.

57. Carson J.A.S, Lichtenstein AH, Anderson CAM, et al. Dietary cholesterol and cardiovascular risk: a science advisory from the American Heart Association. *Circulation*. 2020;141(3): e39-e53.

58. American Institute for Cancer Research. Accessed April 22, 2019. http://www.aicr.org

59. Position of The American Dietetic Association and the Dietitians of Canada: nutrition and women's health. *J Am Diet Assoc*. 2004;104(6):984-1001.

60. Reedy J, Krebs-Smith SM, Miller PE, et al.). Higher diet quality is associated with decreased risk of all-cause, cardiovascular disease, and cancer mortality among older adults. *J Nutr*. 2014;144(6):881-889. doi: 10.3945/jn.113.189407

61. DietaryGuidelines.gov. The dietary guidelines for Americans. Accessed January 7, 2021. https://www.dietaryguidelines.gov/sites/default/files/2020-12/Dietary_Guidelines_for_Americans_2020-2025.pdf

62. Han L, You D, Ma W, et al. National trends in American Heart Association revised life's simple 7 metrics associated with risk of mortality Among US adults. *JAMA Netw Open*. 2019;2(10):e1913131. doi: 10.1001/jamanetworkopen.2019.13131

63. Yanping L, Schoufour J, Wang DD, et al. Healthy lifestyle and life expectancy free of cancer, cardiovascular disease, and type 2 diabetes: prospective cohort study. *BMJ*. 2020; 368:l6669.

64. American Cancer Society. Cancer Facts & Figures 2021. Atlanta, GA; 2021. Accessed January 7, 2021. https://www.cancer.org/research/cancer-facts-statistics/all-cancer-facts-figures/cancer-facts-figure-2021.html#:~:text=The%20Facts%20%26%20Figures%20annual%20report,incidence%2C%20mortality%2C%20and%20survival%20statistics

65. U.S. Department of Agriculture. *Food Consumption and Nutrient Intakes*. Washington, DC: USDA; 2014. Accessed January 7, 2021. https://www.ers.usda.gov/data-products/food-consumption-and-nutrient-intakes/

66. Moore LV, Thompson FE. *Adults Meeting Fruit and Vegetable Intake Recommendations - United States.2013. Morbidity and Mortality Weekly Report*. 2015;64(26):709-713. Accessed January 7, 2021. http://www.cdc.gov/mmwr/preview/mmwrhtml/mm6426a1.htm

67. U.S. Department of Agriculture. *News release: scientific update of food guidance presented to the Dietary Guidelines Committee*. Accessed January 7, 2021. https://www.usda.gov/media/press-releases/2020/07/15/usda-posts-2020-dietary-guidelines-advisory-committees-final-report

68. Hales CM, Carroll MD, Fryar CD, Ogden CL. Prevalence of obesity and severe obesity among adults: United States, 2017–2018. 2020. Accessed January 7, 2021. https://www.cdc.gov/nchs/products/databriefs/db360.htm

69. Ogden CL, Carroll MD, Kit BK, Flegal KM. Prevalence of childhood and adult obesity in the United States, 2011-2012. *JAMA*. 2014;311(8):806-814. doi: 10.1001/jama.2014.732

70. U.S. Department of Health and Human Services (USDHHS), Centers for Disease Control and Prevention (CDC), Division of Nutrition, Physical Activity, and Obesity. Adult Obesity Facts. Accessed January 10, 2021. http://www.cdc.gov/obesity/data/adult.html

71. Wharton S, Lau DCW, Vallis M, et al. Obesity in adults: a clinical practice guideline. *CMAJ*. 2020;192(31):E875-E891. doi: 10.1503/cmaj.191707. https://www.cmaj.ca/obesity

72. Hales CM, Fryar CD, Carroll MD, Freedman DS, Ogden CL. Trends in obesity and severe obesity prevalence in US youth and adults by sex and age, 2007-2008 to 2015-2016. *JAMA*. 2018;319(16):1723-1725. doi: 10.1001/jama.2018.3060

73. U.S. Department of Health and Human Services. Healthy People 2030. Accessed January 7, 2021. https://health.gov/healthypeople

74. Office of the Surgeon General (US). The Surgeon General's vision for a healthy and fit nation. Background on Obesity. Rockville (MD): Office of the Surgeon General (US); 2010. Accessed January 7, 2021. https://www.ncbi.nlm.nih.gov/books/NBK44656/

75. Bozzi DG, Hersch Nicholas L. A causal estimate of long-term health care spending attributable to body mass index among adults. *Econ Hum Biol*. 2021;41:100985.

76. Finkelstein EA, Trogdon JG, Cohen JN, Dietz W. Annual medical spending attributable to obesity: payer-and service-specific estimates. *Health Aff*. 2009;28(5 suppl 1):w822-w831.

77. Chobot A, Górowska-Kowolik K, Sokolowska M, Jarosz-Chobot P. Obesity and diabetes—not only a simple link between two epidemics. *Diabet Metab Res Rev*. 2018;34(7):e3042.

78. Al-Goblan AS, Al-Alfi MA, Khan MZ. Mechanism linking diabetes mellitus and obesity. *Diabet Metab Syndr Obes*. 2014;7: 587-591. doi: 10.2147/DMSO.S67400

79. Raynor HA, Champagne CM. Position of the Academy of Nutrition and Dietetics: Interventions for the treatment of overweight and obesity in adults. *Acad Nutr Diet*. 2016;116(1):129-147. Accessed January 7, 2021. http://dx.doi.org/10.1016/j.jand.2015.10.031

80. The Obesity Society. *Eradicating America's Obesity Epidemic, August 2009*. 2010. Accessed January 7, 2021. https://www.washingtontimes.com/news/2009/aug/16/solutions-eradicating-americas-obesity-epidemic/

81. Ezzati M. Excess weight and multimorbidity: putting people's health experience in risk factor epidemiology. *Lancet Public Health*. 2017;2(6):e252-e253.

82. Chan RSM, Woo J. Prevention of overweight and obesity: how effective is the current public health approach. *Int J Environ Res Public Health*. 2010;7(3):765-783.

83. Kassirer JP, Angell M. Losing weight—an ill-fated New Year's resolution. *N Eng J Med.* 1998;338:52-54.

84. Hansen AR., Rustin C, Opoku S, Shevatekar G, Jones J, Zhang J. Trends in US adults with overweight and obesity reporting being notified by doctors about body weight status, 1999 – 2016. *Nutr Metab Cardiovasc Dis.* doi: 10.1016/j.numecd.2020.01.002

85. Secor, M. Exercise and obesity: the role of exe rise in prevention, weight loss, and maintenance of weight loss. *J Am Assoc Nurse Pract.* 2020;32(7):530-537. doi: 10.1097/JXX.0000000000000452

86. NIH Technology Assessment Conference Panel. Methods for voluntary weight loss and control. *Ann Intern Med.* 1993;119:764-770.

87. Jeffrey RW, Epstein LH, Wilson GT, et al. Long-term maintenance of weight-loss: current status. *Health Psychol.* 2000;19(1, suppl):5-16. https://doi.org/10.1037/0278-6133.19.Suppl1.5

88. U.S. Department of Health and Human Services (USDHHS), Centers for Disease Control and Prevention (CDC), Heart Disease. *Heart Disease Facts.* Accessed January 10, 2015. https://www.cdc.gov/heartdisease/facts.htm

89. American Heart Association. *Heart Disease and Stroke Statistics: 2009 Update.* Dallas, TX: American Heart Association; 2009. https://www.cdc.gov/heartdisease/facts.htm

90. Go AS, Mozaffarian D, Roger VL, et al. Heart disease and stroke statistics—2013 update. A report from the American Heart Association. *Circulation.* 2013;127(1):e6-e245. doi: 10.1161/CIR.0b013e31828124ad

91. U.S. Department of Health and Human Services, NIH, NHLBI, NHBPEP, JCN 7 Express. *The Seventh Report of the Joint National Committee on Prevention, Detection, Evaluation, and Treatment of High Blood Pressure.* NIH Pub. No. 03–5233. Bethesda MD, National Institutes of Health; 2003.

92. American Heart Association, 2012. *Heart Disease and Stroke Statistics-2013* Update. American Heart Association, 12, e6-e245. Accessed January 7, 2021. http://circ.ahajournals.org/content/127/1/e6

93. National Institutes of Health Heart, Lung, and Blood Institute. *Morbidity and Mortality: 2012 Chartbook on Cardiovascular, Lung, and Blood Diseases.* Bethesda, MD: Public Health Service, National Institutes of Health, NHLBI; 2012. https://www.nhlbi.nih.gov/files/docs/research/2012_ChartBook_508.pdf

94. American Heart Association. 2021 Heart disease and stroke statistics update fact sheet at-a-glance. 2021. https://www.heart.org/-/media/phd-files-2/science-news/2/2021-heart-and-stroke-stat-update/2021_heart_disease_and_stroke_statistics_update_fact_sheet_at_a_glance.pdf?la=en

95. U.S. Department of Health and Human Services. *Healthy People 2010: Understanding and Improving Health,* 2nd ed. Washington, DC: U.S. DHHS; 2000; Chapter 12-Heart Disease and Stroke: 12-3–12-33.

96. National Heart, Lung, and Blood Institute (NHLBI). *Keep High Blood Pressure Under Control.* Accessed September 1, 2021. https://www.nhlbi.nih.gov/education/high-blood-pressure

97. The Trials of Hypertension Prevention Collaborative Research Group. Effects of weight-loss and sodium reduction intervention on blood pressure and hypertension incidence in overweight people with high-normal blood pressure: The Trials of Hypertension Prevention, Phase II. *Arch Intern Med.* 1997;157:657-667.

98. He J, Whelton PK, Appel LJ, Charleston J, Klag MJ. Long-term effects of weight-loss and dietary sodium reduction on incidence of hypertension. *Hypertension.* 2000;35:544-549.

99. Sacks FM, Svetkey LP, Vollmer WM, et al. Effects on blood pressure of reduced dietary sodium and Dietary Approaches to Stop Hypertension (DASH) diet. *N Engl J Med.* 2001;344:3-10.

100. Chobanian AV, Hill M. National Heart, Lung, and Blood Institute Workshop on Sodium and Blood Pressure: a critical review of current scientific evidence. *Hypertension.* 2000;35:858-863.

101. Whelton SP, Chin A, Xin X, He J. Effect of aerobic exercise on blood pressure: a meta-analysis of randomized, controlled trials. *Ann Intern Med.* 2002;136:493-503.

102. Xin X, He J, Frontini MG, Ogden LG, Motsamai OI, Whelton PK. Effects of alcohol reduction on blood pressure. A meta-analysis of randomized controlled trials. *Hypertension.* 2001;38:1112-1117.

103. Vollmer WM, Sacks FM, Ard J, et al. Effects of diet and sodium intake on blood pressure: subgroup analysis of the DASH-Sodium Trial. *Ann Intern Med.* 2001;135:1019-1028.

104. Nguyen Q, Dominguez J, Nguyen L, Gullapalli N. Hypertension management: an update. Am *Health Drug Benefits.* 2010;3(1):47-56.

105. National Center for Health Statistics (NCHS). High serum total cholesterol—an indicator for monitoring cholesterol -lowering efforts; U.S. adults, 2005-06. *NCHS Data Brief.* 2007;2.

106. Cleeman JI, Lenfant C. The National Cholesterol Education Program: progress and prospects. *JAMA.* 1998;280(24):2099-2104.

107. U.S. Department of Health and Human Services, NHLBI. *National Cholesterol Education Program, Third Report of the Expert Panel on the Detection, Evaluation, and Treatment of High Blood Cholesterol in Adults (Adult Treatment Panel III).* NIH Pub. No. 01–367. Bethesda, MD: National Institutes of Health; 2001.

108. U.S. Department of Health and Human Services. *Healthy People 2010: Understanding and Improving Health,* 2nd ed. Washington, DC: U.S. DHHS; 2000: 22-Physical activity and fitness. Bethesda, MD; Chapt 22: 22-3–22-36.

109. Grundy SM, Cleeman JI, Bairey Merz CN, et al. Implications of recent clinical trials for the National Cholesterol Education Program Adult Treatment Panel III Guidelines. *Circulation.* 2004;44(3):720-732.

110. U.S. Department of Health and Human Services. *Physical activity and health: a report of the Surgeon General, 1996.* Atlanta, GA: Centers for Disease Control and Prevention, National Center for Chronic Disease Prevention and Health Promotion; 1996.

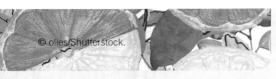
© olies/Shutterstock.

Learning Portfolio

111. NIH Consensus Development Panel on Physical Activity and Cardiovascular Health. Physical activity and cardiovascular health. *JAMA*. 1996;276:241-246.

112. Pate RR, Pratt M, Blair SN, et al. Physical activity and public health: a recommendation from the Centers for Disease Control and Prevention and the American College of Sports Medicine. *JAMA*. 1995;273:402-407.

113. Leslie Pray Rapporteur, Roundtable on Obesity Solutions; Food and Nutrition Board; Institute of Medicine. Physical activity: moving toward obesity solutions: workshop summary. The National Academy Press. Washington, DC, 2015.

114. U.S Department of Transportation. Federal Highway Administration. *A Summary of Highway Provisions in SAFETEA-LU*. 2005. Accessed January 11, 2021. http://www.fhwa.dot.gov/safetealu/summary.htm

115. U.S. Department of Health and Human Services. The health consequences of involuntary exposure to tobacco smoke: a report of the Surgeon General; 2006. Accessed April 22, 2021. http://www.surgeongeneral.gov/library/secondhandsmoke/

116. U.S. Department of Health and Human Services. *The Health Benefits of Smoking Cessation: A Report of the Surgeon General, 1990*. Atlanta, GA: U.S. DHHS, CDC, Center for Chronic Disease Prevention and Health Promotion, Office on Smoking and Health; 1990.

117. Glantz SA, Parmely WW. Passive smoking and heart disease: mechanisms and risk. *JAMA*. 1995;273:1047-1053.

118. Centers for Disease Control and Prevention. Decline in deaths from heart disease and stroke—United States, 1990–1999. *MMWR Morbid Mortal Wkly Rep*. 1999;48(30):649-680.

119. Serdula MK, Gillespie C, Kettel-Khan L, Farris R, Seymour J, Denny C. Trends in fruit and vegetable consumption among adults in the United States: Behavioral Risk Factor Surveillance System, 1994–2000. *Am J Public Health*. 2004;94(6):1014-1018.

120. Ernst ND, Sempos ST, Briefel RR, Clark MB. Consistency between U.S. dietary fat intake and serum total cholesterol concentrations; the National Health and Nutrition Examination Surveys. *Am J Clin Nutr*. 1997;66(4):965S-972S.

121. Ries L, Eisner M, Kosary C, et al. *SEER: Cancer Statistics Review, 1975–2000*. National Cancer Institute; 2003.

122. Stewart SL, King JB, Thompson TD, Friedman C, Wingo P. Cancer mortality surveillance—United States, 1990-2000. *MMWR Surveill Summ*. 2004;53(3):1-108.

123. Key TJ, Allen NE, Spencer EA, Travis RC. The effect of diet on risk of cancer. *Lancet*. 2002;360(9336):861-868.

124. Willett, W. Diet and nutrition. In: Schottenfield D., Frammeni JF Jr, eds. *Cancer Epidemiology and Prevention*, 2nd ed. New York: Oxford University Press; 1996:438-461.

125. Doll R, Peto R. The causes of cancer: qualitative estimates of avoidable risks of cancer in the United States today. *J Natl Cancer Inst*. 1981;66(6):1192-1308.

126. McGinnis JM, Forge WH. Actual causes of death in the United States. *JAMA*. 1993;270(18):2207-2212.

127. Mandelson MT, Oestreicher N, Porter PL, et al. Breast density as a predictor of mammographic detection: comparison of interval- and screen-detected cancers. *J Natl Canc Inst*. 2000;92(13):1081-1087.

128. American Institute of Cancer Research. Accessed March 1, 2021. http://www.aicr.org

129. FANSA. Statement on diet and cancer prevention in the United States. Accessed July 7, 2009. http://www.eatright.org

130. Byers T, Nestle M, McTiernan A, et al. American Cancer Society guidelines on nutrition and physical activity for cancer prevention: reducing the risk of cancer with healthy food choices and physical activity. *CA Cancer J Clin*. 2002;52(2):92-119.

131. American Cancer Society (ACS). Cancer Statistics 2009. Atlanta, GA: ACS; 2009.

132. National Vital Statistics Report. *Deaths: Preliminary data for 2004*. November 20, 2007.

133. National Institutes of Health, National Institute of Diabetes and Digestive and Kidney Diseases. Diabetes Prevention Program. Accessed Septemember 1, 2021. https://www.niddk.nih.gov/about-niddk/research-areas/diabetes/diabetes-prevention-program-dpp

134. Narayan KM, Boyle JP, Geiss LS, et al. Impact of recent increase on incidence on future diabetes burden U.S., 2005–2050. *Diabetes Care*. 2006;29(9):2114-2116.

135. Centers for Disease Control and Prevention. *National Diabetes Fact Sheet: General Information and National Estimates on Diabetes in the U.S., 2003*, revised ed. Atlanta, GA: U.S. Dept. of Health and Human Services, Centers for Disease Control and Prevention; 2004.

136. U.S. Department of Health and Human Services. *Healthy People 2010: Understanding and Improving Health*. 2nd ed. Washington, DC: U.S. DHHS; 2000;3-34–5-35.

137. National Institute of Diabetes, Digestive and Kidney Diseases (NIDDK). *National Diabetes Statistics, 2020*. Accessed April 22, 2021. https://www.niddk.nih.gov/health-information/health-statistics/diabetes-statistics

138. Mokdad AH, Ford ES, Bowman BA, et al. Diabetes trends in the U.S.: 1990-1998. *Diabetes Care*. 2000;23(9):1278-1283.

139. Diabetes Prevention Program Research Group. Reduction in the incidence of type 2 diabetes with lifestyle intervention or metformin. *N Engl J Med*. 2002;346:393-403.

140. Center for Disease Control and Prevention. *National Diabetes Prevention Program*. 2016. Accessed January 11, 2021. http://www.cdc.gov/diabetes/prevention/index.html

141. American Diabetes Association. Nutrition principles and recommendations in diabetes. *Diabetes Care*. 2004;27:S36.

142. Koletzko B, Brands B, Poston L, Godfrey K, Demmelmair H. Early nutrition programming of long-term health. *Proc Nutr Soc*. 2012;71(3):371-378. doi: 10.1017/S0029665112000596

143. Pollard TM, Rousham EK, Colls R. Intergenerational and family approaches to obesity and related conditions. *Ann Hum Biol*. 2011;38(4):385-389.

144. American Diabetes Association. Standards of Medical Care in Diabetes—2016 Diabetes Care 2016;39(suppl 1):S1-S2. doi: 10.2337/dc16-S001

145. National Institutes of Health. *Osteoporosis and Related Bone Diseases, National Resource Center, 2008*. Accessed April 22, 2010. http://www.niams.nih.gov/Health_Info/Bone/. National Osteoporosis Foundation. *Osteoporosis, Disease Statistics,*

2004. Accessed April 22, 2010. http://www.nof.org/aboutnof /founding.htm

146. National Institutes of Health Consensus Development Panel on Osteoporosis. Osteoporosis prevention, diagnosis, and therapy. *JAMA*. 2001;285(6):785-795.

147. Heany RP. The importance of calcium intake for lifelong skeletal health. *Calcif Tissue Int*. 2002;70:70-73.

148. Standing Committee on the Scientific Evaluation of Dietary Reference Intakes. Food and Nutrition Board, Institutes of Medicine. *Dietary Reference Intakes for Calcium, Phosphorus, Magnesium, Vitamin D, and Fluoride*. Washington, DC: National Academy Press; 1999.

149. Let's Eat Healthy. Milk. Accessed September 1, 2021. https://www.healthyeating.org/nutrition-topics/milk-dairy/dairy -foods/milk

150. U.S. Department of Health and Human Services. National Institute of Diabetes and Digestive and Kidney Diseases. 2020. *Chronic Kidney Disease*. Accessed September 1, 2021. https://www.niddk.nih.gov/health-information/kidney-disease /chronic-kidney-disease-ckd

151. U.S. Office of Disease Prevention and Health Promotion. HealthyPeople.gov. 2020. *Chronic Kidney Disease*. Accessed January 3, 2021. http://www.healthypeople.gov/2020/topics -objectives/topic/chronic-kidney-disease

152. U.S. Department of Health and Human Services. National Institute of Diabetes and Digestive and Kidney Diseases. Chronic kidney diseases prevention. Accessed January 3, 2021. http://www.niddk.nih.gov/health-information/health -communication-programs/nkdep/Pages/default.aspx

153. Centers for Disease Control and Prevention. HIV Prevalence estimate—US, 2006. *MMWR Morbid Mortal Wkly Rep*. 2008;57(39):1073-1076.

154. U.S. Department of Health and Human Services. *Healthy People 2010: Understanding and Improving Health*. 2nd ed. Washington, DC: U.S. DHHS; 2000. Chapter 13, HIV: 13-3–13-27.

155. Position of the American Dietetic Association and Dietitians of Canada. Nutrition intervention in the care of persons with human immunodeficiency virus infection. *J Am Diet Assoc*. 2000;100:708-717.

CHAPTER 11

Promoting Older Adult Nutrition

Shirley Y. Chao, PhD, RDN, LDN, FAND

Amy Sheeley, PhD, RDN

(We acknowledge the work of Andrea T.K. Roche, MS, RDN, LDN; Joseph M. Carlin, MS, RDN, LDN, FADA; Stacey Chappa, RDN; Shirley Chao, PhD, RDN, LDN, FAN; and Sari Edelstein, PhD, RDN, for their work on past editions of Nutrition in Public Health.)

Learning Outcomes

AFTER STUDYING THIS CHAPTER AND REFLECTING ON THE CONTENTS, YOU SHOULD BE ABLE TO:

1. Describe how the number of older Americans is growing due to improvements in health care and nutrition.
2. Describe the demographic characteristics of the older adult population, including the baby boomer population.
3. Discuss the wellness concerns of older adults, especially in terms of nutritional needs, screening, assessment, and current recommendations.
4. Identify how community and public health initiatives have and can best address these wellness concerns.

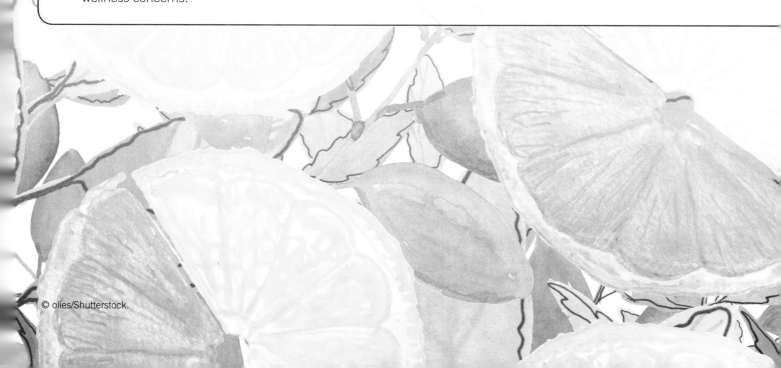

Introduction

The importance of nutrition throughout the lifecycle cannot be refuted; however, recognizing the differences in nutritional needs during the specific times of growth, development, and aging is becoming increasingly more appreciated and understood. This is especially important with the rapid growth of the older adult population, stratified by the U.S. Census Bureau as the "young old," those aged 65 to 74; the "old," those aged 75 to 84; and the "oldest old," those aged 85 or older. In 2017, there were an estimated 92,000 centenarians, and by 2050, this number is expected to rise to 386,000.[1]

Although it is known that energy needs decrease with age, much less is known about specific needs of various nutrients and minerals for these different segments of older adult populations. Identifying these nutritional differences as our society continues to live longer and longer is becoming ever more important.

This chapter provides an overview of the growing American adult population, nutritional needs and concerns, screening and assessment methods, and the various ways in which community and public health initiatives have and can continue to address these ever-evolving wellness concerns.

The Older Population and Improvements in Health and Nutrition

The second half of the 20th century was a time when Americans began to take notice of the ever-growing population of older people around them. While the total population of the United States grew from 150 million to an estimated 328 million from 1950 to 2019 (more than doubling in size), the population of those 65 years and older grew rapidly, as well, representing approximately 16% of the total population.[1,2] Even more impressive was the growth in the population over 75 years of age, which increased from 4–6.8% of the population.

During the first half of the 20th century, improvements in the prevention and control of infectious diseases had a profound effect on increasing life expectancy. After 1950, improvements in nutrition, housing, hygiene, and medical care contributed to a longer life span. Life expectancy at birth increased for men from 48 years in 1901 to 76.1 years of age in 2017; for women, the increases were even more impressive, from 51 to almost 81 years of age.[3] The life expectancy of those in other countries, particularly Japan, holds out hope that longevity can be increased even more in the United States.

One of the major reasons why people are living longer is due to decreases in mortality caused by heart disease, stroke, and unintentional injuries. Government statistics reveal that although heart disease is still the leading cause of death in the United States, the death rate from heart disease decreased by 40% from 1980 to 2017. The death rate from stroke declined during the same period.[4] Both of these diseases are closely associated with high blood pressure, high cholesterol, lack of physical activity, and obesity. Health promotion initiatives, healthier lifestyles, and exercise programs offer the potential of increasing life expectancy.

The aging of the population has important consequences to the health and well-being of all Americans. Not only will it put increased demands upon the healthcare system but at the community level there will also be a similar demand for a full range of services, including nutrition services.

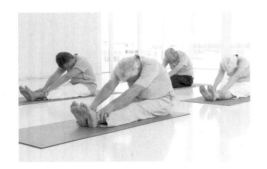

Healthier lifestyles have extended the lives of older adults.

© PedroMatos/Shutterstock.

Strategy Tip

Health professionals educated on geriatric care will be in higher demand as older Americans live longer.

Characteristics and Demographics of the Older Adult Population

Older adults in the United States are living longer, healthier, and more functionally fit lives than ever before. Those born today can expect to live an average of 78.6 years, an increase of approximately 30 years in the twentieth century. Between 2016 and 2035, the over-65 population will grow to nearly 78 million people, and that number is expected to increase to 89 million by 2055.[2] The fastest growing segment of the older populations is composed of those 85 and older and is expected to increase from 6.7 million to approximately 9 million by the year 2030. More than 70% of older men are married, whereas only 44% of older women are married, in part due to the fact that women tend to live longer than men.[5] This has implications in that approximately 44% of women over 75 live alone.[5] Members of older adult minority groups are also on the rise. In 2016, 39% of persons 65 or older were members of racial or ethnic minority populations: 12% were African Americans (not Hispanic); 5.4% were Asian or Pacific Islander (not Hispanic); 0.7% were Native American (not Hispanic); 0.2% were Native Hawaiian/Pacific Islander, (not Hispanic); and 2.4% of persons 65 or older identified themselves as being of two or more races. Persons of Hispanic origin (who may be of any race) represented 18% of the older population.[6]

Baby Boomers

Interestingly enough, one-third of the United States' population is composed of **baby boomers**, defined as those born between 1946 and 1964. During these decades, the population jumped in number, allowing relative prosperity. This gave individuals opportunities to achieve education levels beyond their prior generations and to live in a world with major advances in medical science and technology.[7] The initial wave of this cohort has entered the retirement years and is facing the demands of aging. A literature review suggests that these persons have specific characteristics, needs, and demands other than the elderly population served by the public health community in the past.[7,8] Taking into account the research on education level, family complexity, diversity, income, and health conditions, major needs for these boomers have begun to surface. To sum up current research simply, the baby boomers' needs center on quality of life.

Aging is a multidimensional process influenced by health, desires, family roles, and productivity. Sensitivity to family dynamics and diversity are important considerations when serving baby boomers. The well-being of the boomer generation encompasses screening, assessment, diet, supplement usage, exercise, sexual vitality, pain management, management of health, and living conditions. Boomers acquire health information through education by healthcare providers, academia, public health programs, and increasingly, the Internet. Health care must integrate alternative and traditional medicine, as long-term care is moving from a traditional medical model toward a holistic approach. To ensure quality of life and overall wellness of boomers, their needs must be addressed and met. This responsibly falls on the community at large, which is comprised of the private, public, government/regulatory, and academic/research sectors.

Growing up after World War II, baby boomers were better educated and better paid than previous American generations. Boomers are becoming our nation's elders; the youngest baby boomer turned 56 years old in 2020 while the oldest is age 74.

Baby Boomers One-third of the United States' population is composed of baby boomers, defined as older adults born between 1946 and 1964.

Baby boomers are those persons born between the years 1946 and 1964. There are currently 73 million baby boomers in the United States. https://www.census.gov/library/stories/2019/12/by-2030-all-baby-boomers-will-be-age-65-or-older.html

TABLE 11-1
Characteristics of the Boomer Generation

Characteristic	Definition
Heritage and family structure	More ethnically diverse than generations before them. Have fewer children than their parents' generation. Have higher rates of divorce and remarriage than their parents' generation. Grandparents are often raising grandchildren. More formal education than previous generations of senior citizens.
Income (median or household)	Higher median family and household incomes than previous generations of senior citizens (although the cost of living is much higher today than it was 20–40 years ago).
Employment	Longer working hours than their parents' generation and more women employed outside of the home.
Health condition	Much more likely to smoke, be overweight, and have a sedentary lifestyle than their parents' generation. Sedentary lifestyle is a risk factor for heart disease, cancer, and diabetes.

Boomers have different characteristics, needs, and demands than the elderly population currently served by the community sectors. Boomers' heritage and family structure, formal education, income, employment, and health conditions are different from that of most of today's elders. Assessing the characteristics of boomers' needs and demands provides a portrait of who they are (**Table 11–1**).

As stated previously, the general needs of boomers center on maintaining the quality of their lives. **Health-related quality of life** is a scientific concept that describes a person's perception of their health, well-being, and ability to function. Aging is a multidimensional process characterized by biological changes, evolving wants and needs, family roles, and productivity.[9]

Health-related quality of life A scientific concept that describes a person's perception of their health, well-being, and ability to function.

Unique Features of Baby Boomers

Boomers have complex family structures and greater diversity than previous generations. Family dynamics are an important consideration when working with boomers. Many are still caring for their elderly parents. Due to the high divorce rate and number of single parents, boomers may also be caring for their grandchildren.[10] In a 2014 American Community Survey, data stated that approximately 7 million grandparents had grandchildren living with them, and about 34% of these people reported being the primary caregiver of their grandchildren. Therefore, public health programs must appeal to dynamic families. Community and public health professionals also need to customize and adjust existing programs, materials, and means of communication to fit the demographic diversity of age, language, and ethnic culture of the boomer population.[7] It is important to have culturally sensitive and knowledgeable workers on staff to best serve this population.

Boomers have more formal education than their elders. According to the 2016 American Community Survey, 83% of people over 60 years of age graduated from high school, compared with only 65% in 2000. Approximately 27% of people over age 64 have a bachelor's degree or higher, compared with 15% in 2000.[5] The average household income for boomers is $78,000 annually[11]. Boomers are expected to retire later in life and slowly shift from full-time employment to retirement. For them, jobs provide a source of income, add meaning to life, and may prevent social isolation. By creating new identities and roles, boomer women are becoming a strong force in the workplace. Women, as a whole, contribute about 42% of all household income.[6]

Educational Demands of Older Adults

Older adults have a need for health education through many sources, as stated previously. The academic sector must continue to conduct research and publish results of trials and studies relevant to this population. Older adults are increasingly utilizing the Internet and apps to find health information.[12]

More public health programs that promote the health and well-being of seniors through education are needed. Preventative health measures need to be taken to reduce the prevalence of chronic, preventable diseases in the boomer population. Community and public health classes on diet and physical activity should be given that discuss the relationship between lifestyle behaviors and the development of heart disease, cancer, obesity, and diabetes. Smoking cessation programs can be initiated for boomers. A discussion of sexually transmitted diseases (STDs) is also a newer topic for this age group.

Community and public health programs also need to address the accuracy of health information provided by the media. Trained, knowledgeable professionals who are familiar with various nutritional supplements and their claims are needed to assist boomers in making informed, smart decisions. Boomers must be careful when purchasing and taking supplements because of possible prescription drug–nutrient interactions and reactions. Independent companies are needed to test health claims for products marketed to the public, which will help consumers and healthcare professionals to evaluate their health, wellness, and nutritional needs more effectively. In 2007, the FDA adopted more strict regulations that require manufacturers of dietary supplements to use **Good Manufacturing Practices**, which include quality and purity testing. Some companies even provide approval seals on their products to signify passage of laboratory tests for potency, purity, and freedom from harmful contaminants, such as the **U.S. Pharmacopeia Dietary Supplement Verification Program**, a voluntary testing and auditing program that ensures the safe manufacture of dietary supplements.[13]

In 2003, the FDA launched a grading system for products with health claims, with letters ranging from A to D. Products with health claims can now be supported with various degrees of scientific agreement. For example, grade A indicates that the health claim meets the significant scientific agreement standard, whereas grade D means that very limited and preliminary scientific research has been done, suggesting that the FDA concludes that there is little evidence supporting this claim.[14] Of course, because many of these products are not regulated as a drug, many manufacturers do not adhere to those standards to market their products.

Because many older adults seek health information through magazines, newspapers, and the Internet, they need to be educated on which sources are accurate and credible. More than 80% of people who are online access health information.[15] According to a recent study, only 38% of US adults reported accessing health information on the Internet without frustration.[16] It would be helpful if boomers were knowledgeable about peer-reviewed journal articles and able to distinguish between quality research designs and studies and those with false or misleading claims.

State of Health of Older Adult Population

The most recent data conclude that the leading causes of death in the United States are heart disease, cancer, accidents, respiratory diseases, stroke, Alzheimer's disease, diabetes mellitus, influenza and pneumonia, kidney

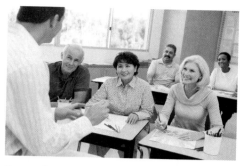

Many seniors are enrolling in educational-based classes.

© Monkey Business Images/Shutterstock.

Sexually transmitted diseases (STDs) can refer to other diseases besides HIV and AIDS, such as syphilis, gonorrhea, chlamydia, genital herpes, genital warts, hepatitis (A, B, and C), and nonspecific urethritis.

Good Manufacturing Practices The U.S. Food and Drug Administration (FDA) adopted stringent regulations that require manufacturers of dietary supplements to use quality and purity testing.

U.S. Pharmacopeia Dietary Supplement Verification Program A voluntary testing and auditing program that ensures the safe manufacture of dietary supplements providing approval seals on products to signify passage of laboratory tests for potency, purity, and freedom from harmful contaminants.

Strategy Tip

It is important for dietitians to be educated in safe supplements and drug-nutrient reactions to assist in answering the questions of seniors and others.

Discussion Prompt

What kinds of peer-reviewed journals are acceptable to rely upon for accurate information?

failure, and intentional self-harm.[17] Heart disease and cancer accounted for over one-half of all deaths, when combined.[17] Tobacco use, lack of physical activity, and poor nutrition are major contributors to heart disease and cancer.[18] Obesity and lack of physical activity are risk factors for developing type 2 diabetes. An estimated 34 million persons (13%) aged 18 years and older had either been diagnosed with diabetes or had undiagnosed diabetes. Diabetes is also the leading cause of kidney failure. More than 270,000 deaths and 130,000 lower-limb amputations occur annually due to diabetes.[19] Behavior modification through diet and exercise, as well as smoking cessation, can decrease the prevalence of heart disease, cancer, and diabetes. One in every five deaths is caused by tobacco.[20] Smokers who die of tobacco-related usage lose approximately 10 years of expected life.[20] In 2014, the Centers for Disease Control and Prevention (CDC) reported that cigarette smoking and exposure to secondhand smoke resulted in an estimated 480,000 deaths. About 14% of American adults, or about 34 million, smoke.[21] Elderly smokers who quit can obtain significant health benefits and risk reduction of death, which justifies the need for smoking cessation programs. Arthritis and back pain are other health conditions that affect quality of life and functionality. Some arthritis and back pain may be attributed to carrying excess body weight.

Several factors have contributed to the surge in weight among U.S. adults. Boomers value generous portion sizes and value, because they grew up at the same time that the fast-food industry was created. Convenience foods were introduced as well as meal replacement drinks and bars to accommodate the busy lifestyles of boomers. Fast food and snacks replaced home-cooked meals. Also, boomers adopted a sedentary lifestyle. Approximately 71% of Americans aged 20 and over are overweight including obesity.[22] The Behavioral Risk Factor Surveillance System revealed that 23 states had adult obesity rates between 30–34% and 12 states had obesity rates greater than 35%.[23] If the trends of overweight and obesity continue to rise, it is projected by 2030 that 50% of adults will be obese and one in four adults will have severe obesity (BMI >35).[24] It should also be noted that as female baby boomers crawl toward menopause and retirement, eating disorders among this age group have started to rise.

Approximately 75% of adults report engaging in some level of physical activity. Seventy-six percent of adults, however, did not achieve the recommended amount of aerobic and muscle-strengthening physical activities during leisure time.[25]

Arthritis is one of the most prevalent diseases in the United States and affects 54 million people. Arthritis limits the boomer's ability to be mobile and perform **activities of daily living (ADLs)** as well as **instrumental activities of daily living** (such as preparing meals and housekeeping), without assistance. The ability to function is a component of quality of life. Arthritis and other rheumatic conditions are a leading cause of work disability among US adults.[26] Arthritis limits the activities of 23.7 million US adults.[27] By 2040, an estimated 78 million (26%) adults in the United States aged 18 years or older are projected to have arthritis.[28] Low back pain is also prevalent among Americans. According to the American Academy of Orthopedic Surgeons, almost everyone will experience back pain at some time in their life.

In the United States, elderly people of all ethnicities are experiencing a proportionately greater rate of new AIDS cases than any other age group. In 2012, there were approximately 1.2 million persons living with AIDS in the United States. Older adults (55 years and older) accounted for approximately one-fourth of all cases.[29] Public health educational materials and risk reduction are needed to halt HIV/AIDS infection among older adults.

> Pandemic Learning Opportunity: Covid-19 changed the list for leading causes of death in seniors in 2021. Why were seniors so vulnerable?

Pandemic Learning Opportunity

Obese persons were more vulnerable to Covid-19 demise. Why are seniors more vulnerable?

Activities of Daily Living (ADLs)
Activities such as bathing, dressing, grooming, transferring from bed or chair, going to the bathroom (toileting), and feeding oneself.

Instrumental Activities of Daily Living Activities such as food preparation, use of telephone, housekeeping, laundry, use of transportation, responsibility for medication, managing money, and shopping.

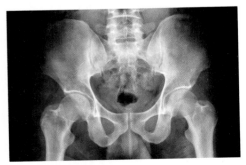

Arthritis can limit mobility and, therefore, exercise in older adults.

© Puwadol Jaturawutthichai/Shutterstock.

Health Insurance and Screening

Today's aging population is in need of a comprehensive health package that meets their nutritional and physical needs by integrating medically sound alternative and traditional medicine. Vitamins, supplements, pharmaceuticals, hormone therapies, and other anti-aging substances proliferate in the marketplace and are widely used by this population. For example, supplements and homeopathic remedies are used to manage nutritional status and pain. It is estimated that consumers spend approximately $30 billion on complementary or integrative medicine in the course of 1 year.[30]

In 2012, Americans spent more than $12 billion on vitamin, herbal, and other supplements, less than one-quarter of the amount spent on prescription drugs.[30] Thus, employers and health maintenance organizations (HMOs) should offer comprehensive health programs that include medically recognized homeopathic and complementary services. These services can be included in a health package that should contain screening, education and private consulting, and intervention.

Screening efforts for breast cancer, colorectal cancer, cervical cancer, high blood pressure, arthritis, cholesterol levels, and diabetes mellitus are crucial for the boomer population and need to be continued as a part of traditional medicine as they age. Screening by health professionals must also include nutritional intakes, eating patterns, supplement usage, physical activity patterns, and preferred modes of exercise. During this process, health professionals should also inquire about the boomer's interests or participation in alternative medicine therapies.

Once screening is completed, education through private consultation may be needed. Older adults may want to have several meetings with dietitians and/or personal trainers to improve their general condition and adopt a healthier lifestyle. Interventions can be developed through these private consultations.

Aging-In-Place

A new concept has emerged, called **aging-in-place**, which describes how a growing number of aging adults prefer to grow old at home.[31] Housing trends are shifting toward senior-friendly communities that encourage independent living rather than moving into institutions like nursing homes. Smart home technology assists this population by providing emergency assistance, fall prevention/detection, reminder systems, medication administration, and assistance for those with hearing, visual, or cognitive impairments.[32] Technological advances such as robots that serve as companions and assistants around the house will also likely become more popular, especially for the Boomer generation.[32]

Wellness Screening and Interventions

Screening and intervention efforts for older adults include identifying and cultivating healthy nutrition behaviors as well as appealing modes of exercise.

Screening

A widely used tool that has been validated for identifying malnutrition in the older population is the **Mini Nutritional Assessment (MNA)**.[33] In addition to a BMI assessment or calf circumference when BMI is not possible, this tool includes six questions assessing food intake in the past 3 months, weight loss in the past 3 months, mobility, psychological stress or acute disease, and neuropsychological problems.

Strategy Tip

Health professionals should be open to learn about alternate medicine therapies but rely on scientific data for conformation of use.

Homeopathic remedies may include chiropractic, massage, vitamins, yoga, herbals, hypnosis, acupuncture, and many other complementary therapies.

Aging-in-Place A concept that describes how a growing number of aging adults prefer to grow old at home.

Mini Nutritional Assessment (MNA) A validated nutrition screening and assessment tool that can identify geriatric patients aged 65 and above who are malnourished or at risk of malnutrition.

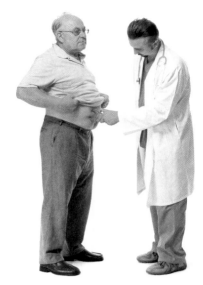

A skin-fold thickness exam is just one parameter used to assess muscle mass in seniors.

© Kurhan/Shutterstock.

Nutrition-Focused Physical Exam A physical exam used to accurately identify and grade malnutrition by identifying fat loss, muscle loss, and/or edematous conditions associated with or affecting nutrition status.

Prebiotics Substances that induce the growth or activity of microorganisms (e.g., bacteria and fungi) that contribute to the well-being of their host.

Probiotics A preparation (such as a dietary supplement) containing live bacteria that is taken orally to restore beneficial bacteria to the body.

Some physical assessment measures are simply not possible, nor accurate with older adults, especially due to physical and metabolic changes. For example, as individuals age, BMI loses accuracy as fat mass increases and height decreases due to vertebral compression.[34] In addition, height cannot be accurately obtained in those who are unable to stand up straight, those who are bedridden, those with spinal deformations, and those with osteoporosis. To remedy this, arm span or knee measurements may provide greater anthropometric measurements. Body composition measures may also bear little accuracy. For example, skin-fold thickness and mid-arm circumference are used to detect changes in body fat but are limited in this population to distinguish between changes in fat and muscle mass due to loss of elasticity and increased compressibility of aging skin. As the field of dietetics expands, the **Nutrition-Focused Physical Exam** may prove to provide the greatest accuracy in this population especially. Read more about the Nutrition-Focused Physical Exam at https://www.eatright.org/food/nutrition/healthy-eating /what-is-the-nutrition-focused-physical-exam

Nutrition

Nutrition requirements and recommendations change as we get older due to the aging effects of absorption, use, and excretion of nutrients.[35] The most recent dietary reference intakes (DRIs) categorize older populations into two separate groups: ages 50–70 and 71 and older. The Healthy Eating Index for older Americans, recommends an increase in whole grains, dark green and orange vegetables, legumes, and low-fat milk, as well as an increase in nutrient-dense foods that are low in solid fats and free of added sugars and low in sodium and saturated fat. There is also evidence that older individuals tend to have low intakes of protein, calories, total fat, fiber, calcium, magnesium, zinc, copper, folate, and vitamins B_{12}, C, E, and D.[36,37]

A challenge for the dietitian is to teach older adults proper, balanced nutrition and motivate them to make changes in their lifestyles. A top trend of Americans is consuming functional foods, that is, nutrient-enhanced, fortified foods as well as nutraceuticals and phytochemicals. People want to manage their health through the foods they eat and make selections based on health benefits. Instead of focusing on components of food, dietitians may need to focus on the benefits of eating certain foods.

Supplements, as discussed earlier, are another intervention. Supplement use is especially prevalent among baby boomers. According to NHANES data, 70% of those 60 years and older reported using vitamins and supplements.[38] Consumers spend billions on vitamins and minerals each year. The most frequently used products reported by older adults were multivitamin or mineral supplements, vitamin D, and omega-3 fatty acids.[38]

Prebiotics and **probiotics** are also gaining popularity. Prebiotics are substances that promote the growth or activity of a limited number of bacterial species in the gut. Prebiotics produce short-chain fatty acids that are critical to gut integrity, immune system functioning, calcium absorption, and cholesterol maintenance. Probiotics are live organisms that confer a health effect on the host.[39] Probiotics can be used to fight common female health problems such as urinary tract and vaginal infections. Some studies have shown the lactobacillus GG strain helps manage Crohn's disease and irritable bowel syndrome.[40] Lactobacillus is a very common probiotic found in yogurt consumed in the United States.[41] Dairy products are often supplemented with probiotics because they buffer stomach acid and increase the chance that the bacteria will survive.

Furthermore, older adults may be at nutritional risk because of the greater burden of comorbid illnesses coupled with the common physiological changes due to aging. Because of the impact of coexisting disease on overall nutritive status, a comprehensive, multidisciplinary approach is helpful in addressing all contributing factors in the diagnosis and treatment of compromised nutritional health in the elderly. The following checklist may serve as a preliminary guide to ensuring adequate nutrition among elderly patients:

- Multivitamin supplements are often recommended for older adults, especially those whose daily caloric intake is less than 1,500 kcal/day.
- Advise older adults about nutrient-dense food choices when appropriate.
- Investigate body weight losses of 4% or more.
- Nutritional supplements are recommended for at-risk elderly who have suffered fractures or are at risk for osteoporosis.
- Calcium and vitamin D supplementation have been shown to reduce hip fracture rates and are often recommended for patients over 65 years of age.
- Advise older adults on the merits of whole grains, fruits, and vegetables.
- Consider referrals to other health professionals such as speech and language pathologists, homecare or visiting nurse services, or other specialized geriatric services available in the community.

With that being said, nutrition care for our aging populations is not only about disease management or medical nutrition therapy (MNT) but has broadened with a stronger focus on healthy lifestyles and disease prevention. It is never too late to emphasize nutrition for health promotion and disease prevention.

Physical Activity

Without increased emphasis on better diets and more physical activity at all ages, healthcare expenditures will rise immensely as our population ages. Programs, classes, and facilities are needed that will attract older adults to engage in physical fitness. Needs assessment and surveys can articulate where the individual's interests lie and can help frame programs. In adults, regular physical activity has been associated with decreased risk of coronary heart disease, obesity, type 2 diabetes, osteoporosis, and postendometrial cancer. Physical activity has also been associated with increased longevity and lower rates of disability.[42]

Both the cardiovascular and resistance type of exercise can help maintain the muscle masses of aging adults. Encouraging strength training for both men and women is important. Circuit training that combines cardiovascular fitness and resistance training is popular among older adults. All older adults need to know about how to train prior to exercise, as the most common injuries affecting aging athletes include: ankle and knee sprains; strains in the hamstring, calf, and back muscles; rotator-cuff tendonitis; tennis elbow; stress fractures; and heel spurs.[43] Health professionals also need to encourage regular activity and discourage "weekend warriors." Poor conditioning and stiff bones and muscles in older adults may increase their risk for injuries.

America is a market-driven country, and older adults want to choose which services and products to purchase. Wellness programs need to be affordable and managed by credible, educated professionals. Such programs need to be located near the consumers' homes in order to be accessible, and they must have flexible hours to accommodate work schedules and family commitments. Programs that can be done at home are also becoming increasingly popular, especially after closures caused by Covid-19.[44] Finally, programs need to be diverse in order to adapt to each individual's demands. Older adults of

Discussion Prompt

Why should the registered dietitian be advised to be the medical practitioner to give medical nutrition therapy advice?

Food insecurity A term used to convey the idea that the availability of nutritionally adequate and safe foods or the ability to acquire acceptable foods in socially acceptable ways is limited or uncertain.

varying ages and skill levels need a variety of gym options, the choice of meeting with a dietitian or personal trainer, and the option of utilizing medically recognized homeopathic remedies. Dietitians need to package their materials differently to appeal to the different segments of older adults to be successful in establishing healthy eating habits. Time is a crucial factor, especially for many older adults, who need an effective workout in a short amount of time. Older adults are not only seeking physical benefits from exercise but also mind/spirit benefits. This reflects the shift from traditional, Western health care to a more integrative, holistic model.

Nutrition Support Services for Older Adults

The aging of the population has and will continue to put increased demands upon the healthcare system and similarly at the community level there. Prior to the 1970s, older Americans were more likely to be classified as living in poverty than any other age group. With the availability of inflation-adjusted government social insurance programs, Social Security, Supplemental Security Income, and nutrition intervention programs such as Supplemental Nutrition Assistance Programs (SNAP) and the Elderly Nutrition Program, the poverty rate for older Americans declined rapidly from approximately 30% in 1970 to approximately 9.2% in 2017.[45]

One method of assessing food and nutrition problems in the community is the concept of "food insecurity." **Food insecurity** is a term used to convey the idea that the "availability of nutritionally adequate and safe foods or the ability to acquire acceptable foods in socially acceptable ways is limited or uncertain."[45] Among those who experience food insecurity can be people who suffer from true hunger, which is defined as the "uneasy or painful sensation caused by a lack of food."[46] The ideal is to ensure that all older Americans are food secure, meaning that throughout the year, they have "access, at all times, to enough food for an active, healthy life."[46] A household food security study conducted by the U.S. Department of Agriculture in 2019 found that the prevalence rate for food insecurity in households with elderly persons was 7.2%. This increased to 8.7% for elderly persons living alone.[47] The idea of food insecurity, and the more precise definition of hunger, are major improvements over the vague and difficult-to-define term malnutrition, both under- and overmalnutrition, which was popular for most of the 20th century. Read more about food insecurity in all ages of the U.S. population in Chapter 13.

Feeding America's Elderly

On March 27, 1972, Congress passed Public Law 92-258, adding a new Title VII to the Older Americans Act (OAA), establishing a permanent program to provide life-saving meals to the elderly. Even though the new Elderly Nutrition Program (ENP) had bipartisan support in Congress, it was held hostage when the appropriation bill, which provided funding for the new title, was attached to the "Cease Fire in Cambodia Bombing Bill," and was repeatedly vetoed by the President. During the summer of 1973, the funds were finally released to the states. Almost overnight, thousands of community centers opened their doors to the elderly and began the process of delivering meals to older people's homes.

At that time, the law specified that meals were to be served in a congregate setting for socialization purposes and were to be delivered to the homes of those with serious mobility problems. Justification for this new program grew out of the social activism that paralleled America's soul searching during the 1960s, which was at the height of this country's involvement in the

Vietnam War and the Civil Rights movement. Providing nutritious meals to America's elderly was viewed as one of the many corrective actions society needed to take to provide for a more just America. Ending the Vietnam War and providing justice for African Americans were similar goals. The elderly was not the only group in society to be singled out for nutrition intervention programs. Both the U.S. Department of Agriculture's Supplemental Nutrition Assistance Program (SNAP, formerly the Food Stamps Program) and Commodity Foods Distribution programs were expanded and the Supplemental Nutrition Program for Women, Infants and Children (WIC) were initiated.

Following the implementation of these new nutrition intervention programs, the United States became acutely aware of its domestic hunger issues. SNAP grew. It had an average monthly participation of 1.5 million elderly households in 1998, spending approximately $1 billion in benefits for these households.[48]

The idea that would eventually result in the federal government promoting and financing a nutrition program for the elderly started to take shape shortly after World War II. In 1954, a group of women in a Philadelphia neighborhood decided to pack sandwiches in brown paper bags and deliver them to elderly "shut-ins." Newspaper accounts of the efforts of these "angels" delivering "meals on wheels" captured the imagination of America. As the story was repeated across the nation in newspaper accounts, women in other communities began to copy the Philadelphia angels. A survey conducted at the request of the federal government in 1971 counted 311 of these "meals on wheels" programs. Some programs served as few as 10 people a day while others served over 100. No one knows where the women got the original idea for this successful program. We know that in London during World War II, efforts were made by relief groups to deliver meals to older people trapped by the blitz. It is possible that these Philadelphia women may have heard about these British efforts from their soldier husbands stationed in London during the war.[49]

Before these small efforts to deliver meals to the homebound were created, formal programs to protect the nutritional well-being of the elderly did not exist. It was believed at that time that the needs of older people were being met at home by their families. Forgotten were the tremendous sociological changes that had occurred during the 20th century, particularly after World War II. Children were moving to take jobs a considerable distance away from their parents and grandparents. Furthermore, many older people, particularly women, found themselves living alone after the premature death of a husband. With decreased economic resources to provide for their health and well-being, a large number of older people suffered from food insecurity. When faced with the decision of whether to spend their scarce resources on food, prescription drugs, rent, or utilities, they chose to pay the rent. As their numbers grew, their desperate situation could no longer be ignored. In retrospect, it would not be unreasonable to conclude that prior to the establishment of elderly nutrition programs, many older people suffered from high mortality and morbidity rates because of the lack of proper nutrition.

In the late 1960s, the health and nutrition-related problems of the elderly came to the attention of Congress, particularly the Senate Select Committee on Nutrition and Human Needs chaired by Senator George McGovern. This committee held some of the first hearings ever on the nutritional problems associated with aging in America. These hearings were just one of several defining events during the 1960s that focused attention on the nutritional needs of America's older adults. In 1968, Congress authorized President Johnson to fund several demonstration programs to investigate the extent of the problem and test methods for delivering nutritional resources to the elderly.

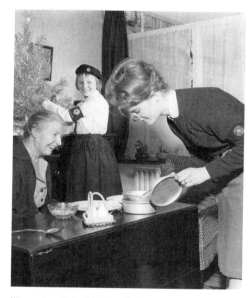

Women in a Philadelphia neighborhood decided to pack sandwiches and deliver them to elderly "shut-ins." Newspaper accounts of the efforts of these "angels" delivering "meals on wheels."

Courtesy of Red Cross.

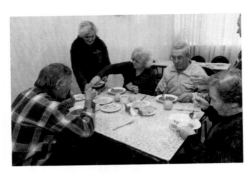

Seniors can come to congregate meals, now called Senior Centers in some areas.

© De Visu/Shutterstock.

Congregate Meals Meals provided in-group settings.

More information about the Older Americans Act is available at: https://acl.gov/programs /health-wellness/nutrition-services.

The idea for a federally supported nutrition program specifically targeting the elderly began taking root during the 1961 White House Conference on Aging. The deciding event during this turbulent period were the negative findings that came from the USDA's 1965 National Food Study on Food Consumption and Dietary Level. This study produced the shocking finding that as many as 6 to 8 million older persons might have deficient diets. These troubling statistics resulted in the creation of a task force on nutrition to develop both administrative and legislative recommendations for correcting the problem.

This task force decided to spend $2 million yearly for 3 years on demonstrations and to collect data in a systematic way concerning the nutrition needs of the elderly. These early demonstration programs tested two potential models for providing meals to older people: home-delivered meals and meals provided in group settings, called **congregate meals**. The home-delivered meals model was clearly designed with existing community meals-on-wheels programs in mind. The congregate program took as its model programs operated in the Jewish settlement houses located in the lower east side of Manhattan.[50]

By the time the White House Conference on Nutrition and Human Needs was held in 1969, the idea for a federally supported nutrition program for the elderly had the backing of federal policymakers. At the 1971 White House Conference on Aging, solid information from the many Title IV demonstration programs was available. By this time, a set of shared principles about the urgent need to respond to the nutritional needs of the elderly existed within the professional nutrition community and among political leaders. These values were incorporated into the OAA and to this day continue to serve as the basic justification for Congress and the administration to continue to support the program. These fundamental principles, as written into the OAA, declare that:

> . . . the purpose of the new nutrition program is to meet the acute need for a national policy which: provides older Americans, particularly those with low incomes, with low cost, nutritionally sound meals served in strategically located centers such as schools, churches, community centers, senior citizen centers, and other public or private facilities where they can obtain other social and rehabilitative services. Besides promoting better health among the older segment of the population through improved nutrition, such a program is aimed at reducing the isolation of old age, offering older Americans the opportunity to live their remaining years in dignity.

When the above statement was written, it was not envisioned that home-delivered meals would be a major part of the program. In the beginning, federal regulations required that state plans ensure that nutrition programs "provide home-delivered meals where necessary and feasible to meet the needs of target group eligible individuals who are homebound."[51,52] There was a perception, at least at the federal level, that private meals-on-wheels programs would continue to grow parallel with the OAA home-delivered meals component. Because of this perception, home-delivered meals were capped, and the total number of meals served that way could not exceed 10% of the total meals served in the state. It was assumed that independent meals-on-wheels providers had the capacity to expand and would want to remain independent of the federally funded programs.

This assumption was unfounded, and meals-on-wheels programs soon petitioned the states to be designated as the local service provider. They aggressively pursued federal funding to expand their programs. A few did remain independent, at least for a time, and continued to use the designation meals-on-wheels to distinguish themselves from the rapidly expanding federal home-delivered meals programs.

It soon became clear that the policy restricting home-delivered meals to 10% was unworkable. It was raised incrementally over the first couple of years by the Administration on Aging (AoA), now the Administration on Community Living (ACL), until Congress intervened in 1978 to amend the OAA, eliminating Title VII. The new amendments created the nutrition program anew, providing separate funding for congregate and home-delivered meals.

That separation continues to be in effect, with home-delivered meals representing almost 66% of all meals served. Clearly, the United States' expanding population of very frail elderly homebound is vulnerable and at great nutritional risk. Today, home-delivered meals and meals-on-wheels programs are different names for the same program.

In their yearly budget requests to Congress, the AoA has put the following clear and convincing reasons forward as to why home-delivered meals should continue to exist and even expand. A home-delivered meal:

- "[Is] the first in-home service that an older adult receives . . ."
- "Serves as a primary access point for all other in-home services."
- "Improves participant nutrient intake, decreases food insecurity, increases social interaction, and decreases social isolation, contributing to improved quality of life."
- "Play[s] an important role in the treatment, management, and delay of chronic disease and disease-related disability."
- "Provides an essential service to many caregivers by helping them maintain their own health and continued functionality."
- "Assists in decreasing the risk of complications associated with acute and chronic disease and contributes to improvements in quality of life."
- In summary, the home-delivered meal program "is a smart, cost-effective investment of public funds."

Factors that Promote Program Success

Over the past almost 50years, the Elderly Nutrition Program, also called the Older Americans Nutrition Program, has been viewed as a resounding success for many reasons. First, it set out to do exactly what it was charged to accomplish and had a positive and lasting nutritional impact on those who participated in the program. Second, states, area agencies on aging, and local service providers did not rely solely upon federal funding to support the program. In addition to participant donations, service providers tapped into their state legislatures for additional funding and received financial support from cities and towns in which the programs operated. To supplement these funds, programs turned to fundraising and the use of in-kind resources including facilities, and developed one of the most extensive and effective volunteer efforts in the country. In short, this program became successful because of the hundreds of thousands of volunteers who daily perform labor-intensive tasks, such as delivering hot meals to the homes of the isolated elderly.

Another reason for the success of the program, which seldom gets full credit today, is the careful planning that went into its design and implementation. These carefully planned steps ensured the stability and longevity of the program. These steps can serve as a textbook case study of how to implement a complicated nutrition intervention program.

The Elderly Nutrition Program can be found on the Administration for Community Living (ACL) website at https://acl.gov /programs/health-wellness/nutrition -services

AoA put in place an administrative structure, detailed policies and procedures, and a training strategy that effectively ensured that all providers of this new and unproven program had the knowledge and skills to operate a successful program. Even before the first meals were served, AoA had authored a carefully thought-out set of regulations, policies, and a comprehensive training manual.

In 1993, Florida International University, with funding primarily from the US Administration on Aging, assists Older Americans Act Nutrition Programs established National Resource Center on Nutrition, Physical Activities and Aging, and headed by Dr. Nancy Wellman and Dr. Dian Weddle.[53] The Center promotes active, healthy aging by working to reduce nutrition risk among older adults, especially minorities with health disparities. The goals are to support quality of life, improve functionality, promote independence, and decrease early nursing home admissions and hospitalizations through better nutrition. Since 2011, Meals on Wheels America has hosted the National Resource Center on Nutrition and Aging (NRCNA)[54] as part of a cooperative agreement with the Administration for Community Living (ACL) ending on December 31, 2020. The NRCNA's purpose is to build the capacity of senior nutrition programs funded by the Older Americans Act (OAA) to provide high-quality, person-centered services, and to assist ACL and stakeholders to identify current and emerging issues and opportunities to enhance program sustainability and resiliency.

Behind the backbone of this strong administrative structure, training, and technical assistance was the law itself, which provided straightforward guidance to the states on how to implement this program. It was clear from the language in the law that Congress expected the meals to be nutritious. Each meal had to contain one-third of the Recommended Dietary Allowances (RDAs), a reasonable target, given that very little was known about the nutritional needs of older persons at that time (Note that the RDAs have now been replaced with the Dietary Reference Intakes). When the program was first created, there was a strong belief that meals should be hot at the time of service, a concession to those older people and professional dietitians/ nutritionists who wanted to set the quality bar as high as possible. Older people, consulted in the 1970s about the design of the program, had vivid memories of the worldwide economic slump lasting from 1929 to 1939, and did not want to participate in a program that would be demeaning or humiliating. They did not want a meal that could in any way be interpreted as "being on the dole." They wanted to sit down to a "hot meal." This program was not to become a soup-and-sandwich program, which was common during the Great Depression!

Considerable thought was given to the delicate issue of how much participants should contribute to the cost of these meals. Some elderly people clearly had the resources to pay for these meals while others, just as clearly, did not. The solution to this dilemma was to install a donation system; participants could determine for themselves what they considered fair. Furthermore, this donation system was to be implemented in a way that protected the confidentiality and dignity of the participant. The decision not to charge older people for their meals has contributed in large measure to the success of the program.

The genius of this program lies in part in the simplicity of the legislation and accompanying regulations, which advocate for the needs of the elderly while promoting objectives that respect older people's needs for independence.

Like any law, it was not designed without flaws. As originally written, only hot meals could be served, and each meal had to meet one-third of the RDAs. In 1978, the law was amended to permit other than hot meals to be served, but they still had to meet the strict one-third RDA requirement. In 1990, the law was amended again to permit programs to offer a two-meals-a-day program, as long as the two meals combined equaled two-thirds of the RDA. Similarly, if three meals were served, the combined meals had to equal 100% of the RDA. These two changes, although not minor, attest to how well the program was designed in the beginning. These examples also demonstrate three truths: First, it is difficult, if not impossible, to write a flawless law because not all variables can be anticipated. Second, when writing legislation, extreme care needs to be taken because once something is put in the law, it might take years to make a correction. Third, all programs need to be monitored and periodically evaluated to ensure that the program is doing what it is supposed to do. Changing policy, procedures, or even the law itself may be necessary to put the program back on track. The simplicity of the nutrition provisions in the OAA has afforded both AoA and the states maximum flexibility on administering this program.

Meals are provided in a variety of settings, such as senior centers, senior housing facilities, schools, and church basements. Some meals are cooked on site; others are prepared in central commissaries and delivered to meal sites. In most cases, meals are prepared under contract with large food service management companies. A growing number of service providers have turned to frozen preplated meals, not only for home-delivered meals but also for congregate participants. More than half of the OAA annual budget supports the program, which provides approximately 250 million meals annually, with approximately 60% home-delivered and 40% congregate. Almost half of the programs have waiting lists.[40]

Program Evaluation

The importance of program evaluation and public health initiatives cannot be overlooked; therefore, the question must be asked: Did the Elderly Nutrition Program accomplish what it set out to accomplish? Between 1993 and 1995, AoA funded a nationwide evaluation of the Elderly Nutrition Program (ENP) as required under the OAO of 1965 when it was amended in 1992.[41] The legislation specified 19 areas for evaluation, with emphasis on the following:

- ENP's effects on participants' nutrition and socialization, compared with a similar population that does not participate in congregate or home-delivered meal programs.
- Is the program targeted to those who need the services most?
- How efficiently and effectively are services administered and delivered?
- What funds are available, and how are they allocated to service providers?

Mathematica Policy Research, Inc. was the contractor for the evaluation. It found that both congregate and homebound ENP participants, when compared with the overall U.S. population of 60 years of age and older, were: 1) older by 4 to 6 years; 2) more than two-thirds female (69%); 3) lived alone; and 4) were more likely to be impoverished.[42]

For almost all of the nutrients studied, both congregate and home-delivered meals supplied well over one-third of participants' daily intake. Many meals provided 40–50% of the RDAs. As to what the participants thought about the meals, about two-thirds of both congregate and

Discussion Prompt
_____

Which health professionals are best qualified to plan the delivered meals that must meet strict nutrient guidelines? Why?

home-delivered participants described themselves as being "very satis-fied" with the taste of the food. The Mathematica team summed up their findings as follows:

> "The ENP serves highly vulnerable people with characteristics that tend to put them at increased health and nutritional risk. ENP participants tend to be older, poorer, more likely to be members of racial or ethnic minorities, and more likely to live alone, compared with the overall population in the United States age 60 and older. Participants are also more likely to be in poor health, to have greater difficulty performing everyday tasks, and to have relatively high nutritional risk."[43]

The 1990s evaluation found that the program is serving the target population. This information is critical to the future of the program because it demonstrates that the ENP program is doing exactly what it set out to do. Large-scale public health programs that do what they are designed to do, and do it efficiently and effectively, are more likely to be successful in attracting future funding.

Because comprehensive evaluation research is expensive, AoA has used a number of tested performance measurement surveys to get a snapshot of how recipients of services rate the service, whether services are effectively targeted to vulnerable individuals, and whether services help older persons to maintain their independence and avoid premature institutionalization. AoA's 2003 Annual Report[44] shared the results on this survey with the aging network.

Even as far back as 2003, AoA found that home-delivered nutrition services "are effectively targeted to vulnerable populations." They found that 59% of respondents lived alone, 69% were 75 years of age or over, and 79% had difficulty with at least one activity of daily living (ADL), such as eating.

One element, critical to the success of the home-delivered meals program, is how well the participants like their meals. If the meals are either not consumed or only half eaten, no benefit is derived. This can be observed directly at congregate sites, but direct observation of eating patterns in the home of participants is difficult. In addition, delivering hot and tasty meals to people's homes has always been a major logistical and quality challenge. Despite the many difficulties in delivering these meals, 94% of respondents surveyed said that they liked the meal; 91% reported that meals almost always arrive when expected.

Since the early 1990s, nutrition programs have been using the *Determine Your Nutritional Health*[45] checklist as a tool to see to what degree participants are at nutritional risk. The survey found that 73% of respondents were at high nutritional risk. This statistic sounds realistic when 62% of respondents are reporting that the typical home-delivered meal provides one-half or more of their daily food intake. Twenty-five percent of respondents said that they did not always have enough money or food stamps to buy food. Clearly, food insecurity is a major problem among this vulnerable population.

When congregate meal participants were surveyed, 64% were 75 years or older and 56% lived alone. As for the quality of the meals, 92% of respondents said they were satisfied with the taste of the food, and 97% were satisfied with the temperature of the food.

When the congregate meals program was designed in the early 1970s, socialization opportunities for participants were one of the primary goals. The importance of socialization as a health factor was highlighted in a major

Find the *Determine Your Nutritional Health Checklist* at: http://www.dhs.gov.vi/home/documents/DetermineNutritionChecklist.pdf.

study published in *Science*.[46] After examining the literature on the subject, House et al., found that:

> ... social relationships, or the relative lack thereof, constitute a major risk factor for health—rivaling the effects of well-established health risk factors such as cigarette smoking, blood pressure, blood lipids, obesity, and physical activity.[46]

AoA's survey found that 96% of respondents like to visit with friends at the site; 73% like to participate in activities at the meal site; and 60% reported that their social opportunities have increased since they started receiving congregate nutrition services. Over the life of the ENP program, all formal and less formal evaluations have found the same results; the program does exactly what it was designed to do.

The Mathematica evaluation is trusted by many as the gold standard of the OAA nutrition program. Many other evaluations were done by ACL and found almost the same outcome as in 2003. Currently, ACL has an annual evaluation plan, which includes the evaluation activities the agency plans. Each annual plan describes the systematic collection and analysis of information about the characteristics and outcomes of programs, projects, and processes as a basis for judgments, to improve effectiveness, and/or inform decision makers about current and future activities.[55,56]

Other Community and Public Health Nutrition Interventions

As America's consciousness of the needs of older people grew, old programs were redesigned, others scaled back, and new programs implemented to meet the nutritional needs of older adults. The government appropriates about $1 billion annually for all food and nutrition intervention programs for older adults.[47] The largest of these is AoA's Older Americans Nutrition Program. Although AoA's program may be the most visible nutrition intervention in the public's mind, it is not the only federal program designed to improve the nutritional well-being of older persons. Other federal interventions include Supplemental Nutrition Assistance Programs, Commodity Supplemental Food Program, Child and Adult Care Food Program, Farmers' Market Nutrition Program, waivers under the Medicaid program, and Medical Nutrition Therapy (MNT) for Medicare beneficiaries. Nutrition education activities carried out in the various states, under the Cooperative Extension Service, can also be added to this list. (Medicare and the other government programs are also discussed in subsequent chapters.)[57]

Supplemental Nutrition Assistance Program

By far the largest of these programs in both numbers of participants and cost is the Supplemental Nutrition Assistance Program (SNAP) administered by the U.S. Department of Agriculture (USDA). The program provides older people with electronic benefit transfer cards (EBT) that can be used to purchase food items at retail stores. The purpose of the program is to assist low-income families, including the elderly, to buy food that is nutritionally adequate.[48]

The Commodity Supplemental Food Program

The Commodity Supplemental Food Program (CSFP) provides packaged food (e.g., juice, powdered milk, canned vegetables, and cheese) to low-income participants, including older persons. Older persons must have a household income at or below 130% of the poverty level. In fiscal year 2019, CSFP served about 736,110 low-income people each month; it is the only USDA nutrition program that provides monthly food assistance specially targeted to low-income seniors,[49] The majority of participants are older adults.[58] Only 33 states and two Native American reservations participate in the program.[51]

The Child and Adult Care Food Program

The Child and Adult Care Food Program (CACFP) serves any person 60 years of age or older, and any person 18 years of age or older who also has a functional impairment and attends a nonresidential daycare facility. The program provides meal reimbursements to the daycare facility, if licensed or approved by the state. According to FY 2020 Food and Nutrition Services annual report, the CACFP programs have 62 million Adult Day Care Centers nationwide.[59]

Seniors Farmer's Market Nutrition Program

In 2000, the USDA created the Seniors Farmers' Market Nutrition Program (SFMNP) to improve nutrition and food security among low-income senior citizens by helping them to purchase more fresh fruits and vegetables at farmers' markets.[53] This program is modeled after the Market Coupon Program developed by the Massachusetts Department of Food and Agriculture in 1986, which had as its focus participants in the WIC program. Seniors at nutritional risk were added in 1987.[54]

This program provides coupons to low-income seniors, which can be exchanged for eligible foods at farmers' markets, roadside stands, and community-supported agriculture programs. Besides providing fresh and nutritious foods for the elderly, the program is also designed to increase the domestic consumption of agricultural commodities and to help expand the network of farmers' markets. Fifteen million dollars in direct funding is available to the states each year. About 835,795 older people were served in fiscal year 2013.[55] Read more about Farmer's Market Coupons for Seniors at http://www.fns.usda.gov/sfmnp/senior-farmers-market-nutrition -program-sfmnp.

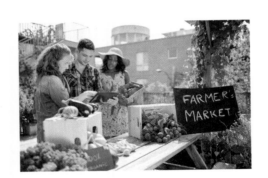
Farm to table foods are available at Farmer's Markets.
© AYA images/Shutterstock.

Medicaid & Nutrition Services

Currently, nutrition services are not a core Medicaid service. However, it must be made clear that many older persons who are eligible for nursing home placement may not be able to shop for food, store food safely, or plan and prepare regular, nutritious meals. Only 38 states include meals or nutrition services among the many benefits available through Medicaid waivers, such as home-delivered meals, nutrition risk-reduction counseling, and nutrition supplements as appropriate. A strong argument can be made to fund all or some nutrition services, including meals, based on health and nutrition risk criteria.

The Future

America's aging adult population has different health needs and demands from the elderly population being served in prior decades. These differences, due to increased longevity, will produce health needs related to a higher incidence of arthritis, obesity, and diabetes. Today's older adults will demand more medical education and intervention than past generations. In addition, it is impossible to predict how the federally funded nutrition program for the elderly will evolve in the future, but certainly it will change. Those familiar with the program anticipate that issues centered around wellness, lifestyle, health promotion, nutrition education, and exercise will become more important among today's aging population as they try to stay healthy and fit for as long as possible.

Evidence-Based/Self-Management

Title III-D of the OAA was established in 1987. It provides grants to states and territories for programs that support healthy lifestyles for health promotion and disease prevention.

Since 2003, the aging services network has been moving toward implementing evidence-based nutrition and health promotion programs. One of the commonly known programs is the Chronic Disease Self-management program, which is designed by Stanford University researcher Kay Lorig.[60] It is both an educational and support program designed to help older Americans take control of their nutritional health. The program stresses self-management strategies using behavior modification approaches. In FY 2012, Congressional appropriations law included, for the first time, an evidence-based requirement related to Title III-D funds. The grants are distributed to community organizations, research universities, local councils on aging, and healthcare providers. It expanded the nutrition wellness education to a broader senior population.

Internet/Social Media Learning

Another opportunity that holds promise for improving the health of seniors is the Internet. Although older adults have lagged behind younger adults in their adoption, a clear majority (67%) of today's older adults use the Internet, while 42% own smartphones. Today, 34% of Americans aged 65 and up say they use social networking sites like Facebook or Twitter.[61,62] Social media and online resources are a good way to reach both seniors as well as their family members and caregivers. A survey of seniors who use the Internet, released in 2015 by the Kaiser Family Foundation, found that topics related to prescription drugs were the most popular issue, followed by searches for information on nutrition, exercise or weight control, cancer, heart disease, and arthritis. This survey found that seniors say that they consider email and the Internet an important part of their lives that "they wouldn't want to do without."[63] In addition, seniors are accessing more telehealth services, especially since the COVID-19 pandemic.

With the rapid growth of the population of older adults in the United States, a need to increase wellness services and expand the nutrition data currently available for these individuals has evolved. The future of the Older Americans Nutrition Program, other federally supported nutrition programs, and the increase in Medicare and Medicaid coverage for nutrition services can be expected to be a valuable part of this nation's "safety net" for ensuring the independence, health, and longevity of America's aging population. To ensure that these initiatives are efficient and effective, nutrition professionals at all levels: federal, state, and community, must continually assess the nutritional needs of the elderly, modify the programs and best practices to meet those needs, and with periodic evaluation, determine whether desired outcomes are met. If these tried-and-true methods are followed, there is no reason why all Americans cannot grow old, knowing that there is a system in place to meet their nutritional needs when they need it.

Summary

The aging of the population has important consequences to the health and well-being of all Americans. Not only will it put increased demands upon the health care system, but at the community level, there will be a similar demand for a full range of services, including nutrition services. A greater understanding of the different nutritional needs throughout the various segments of these different age groups is becoming ever more appreciated and understood.[63] An increase in research to identify these specific nutritional requirements and differences as our society continues to live longer and longer is gaining increased merit. This will also include greater attention to novel screening and assessment methods and continual improvements in community and public health initiatives to address the ever-evolving wellness concerns of America's older adults.

Learning Portfolio

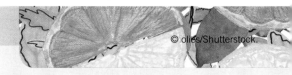

© olies/Shutterstock.

Issues for Discussion

1. Given that there are more and more demands made on the community and public health system, do you think that meeting the baby boomer demands is feasible?
2. Make suggestions as to how the community and public health system can meet the demands of an ever-aging population.
3. Compare a nutrition program that is available in another country (research) to the present nutrition program for elders in the United States. What are the similarities and differences?
4. Discuss the ethical implications of a government-funded nutrition program for the elderly.
5. Discuss possible improvements for future nutrition programs for the great number of elders the United States will experience.
6. Discuss the importance of evaluation in terms of the success and dissemination of public health initiatives.

Practical Activities

1. Discuss in detail the various components of a thorough nutrition assessment for older adults. Research specific differences between the "young old," those aged 65 to 74; the "old," those aged 75 to 84; and the "oldest old," those aged 85 or older.
2. Research unique concerns that might arise for nutrition professionals regarding nutrition care for **supercentenarians**.
3. Describe the physiologic, environmental, socioeconomic, and psychological factors that influence the nutrition status of older adults. Explore different solutions for addressing the related nutritional needs.
4. Develop a worksite wellness program specifically designed for baby boomers.

Key Terms

	page
Baby Boomers	345
Health-related quality of life	346
Good Manufacturing Practices	347
U.S. Pharmacopeia Dietary Supplement Verification Program	347
Activities of Daily Living (ADLs)	348
Instrumental Activities of Daily Living	348
Aging-in-Place	349
Mini Nutritional Assessment (MNA)	349
Nutrition-Focused Physical Exam	350
Prebiotics	350
Probiotics	350
Food insecurity	352
Congregate Meals	354
Supercentenarians	363

Supercentenarians The classification of the older adult population over the age of 110.

Case Study: Meals on Wheels

Sergio is a 69-year-old veteran who lives alone. He was referred to Meals-on-Wheels through a hospital discharge meals program because he was very underweight and unable to gain weight. Sergio was on oxygen continuously due to chronic obstructive pulmonary disease (COPD). His initial assessment yielded a nutrition risk score of 11 out of 19, with a score of 6 considered high nutrition risk. Sergio was placed on the Meals-on-Wheels program, which included a daily telephone reassurance call to check on him and monthly nutrition education. However, due to Sergio's poor health, he needed more than just a meal. A dietitian helped Sergio with a diet plan to gain weight and recommended that he use a nutrition supplement (which he likely cannot afford). He currently receives $967 a month from Social Security Income—an income only $60 more a month than the poverty level.

- What are the main challenges and obstacles that Sergio faces?
- What type of meal plan would be appropriate for Sergio?
- Are there any other services that he is eligible for and that the RD could refer him to? Propose possible solutions for Sergio, supporting access to food and adequate nutrition. Include federally funded food assistance programs that he is eligible for based on his socioeconomic status. If applicable, include community outreach programs supported by local agencies.
- Describe any limitations of the proposed solutions.
- Is there any information that the RD does not have readily available that needs to be uncovered to help Sergio move forward?

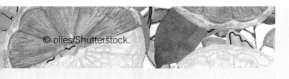
© olies/Shutterstock.

Learning Portfolio

Case Study: Nutrition Counseling for Older Adults

Mrs. Smith is an 87-year-old widow who lives alone and her daughter is her sole caregiver. She has had a poor appetite and has been losing weight (unknown amount). Her daughter helps with her food shopping but Mrs. Smith doesn't feel much like cooking. She is able to go out with assistance but isn't able to drive a car, which makes her feel isolated.

Diagnoses: HTN, high cholesterol

Risk: Malnutrition Screening Tool (MST)[1] = 2 FRAIL Scale[2] = 2

Height: 5'3" Current Weight: 101#

If you are the nutritionist asked to conduct home nutrition counseling:

1. What other information might you ask for?

2. What recommendations might you make?

At the six-month follow-up, Mrs. Smith reported that she had gained weight and was really enjoying eating at the meal site and making new friends. Since the arrival of the Covid-19 pandemic; however, it is impossible for her to attend activities at the meal site, making her feel isolated. In addition, it has not been safe for her daughter to visit, although she does call more often. Mrs. Smith is also unable to pick up the grab-and-go meals at the meal site so she was switched to home delivered meals. The driver rings the bell and leaves the meal at the door.

3. What are Mrs. Smith's new risks and what suggestions do you have for her?

Online Resources

1. Administration on aging: http://www.aoa.gov
2. American Association of Retired Persons: http://aarp.org
3. American Geriatrics Society: http://americangeriatrics.org
4. Centers for Medicare and Medicaid Services: http://cms.hhs.gov/
5. Meals on Wheels Association of America: https://www.mealsonwheelsamerica.org/
6. Mini Nutritional Assessment: https://www.mnaelderly.com/forms/mini/mna_mini_english.pdf
7. National Association of Nutrition and Aging Services Programs: http://www.nanasp.org
8. National Institute on Aging: https://www.nia.nih.gov/
9. National Institutes of Health Seniors Health: https://www.nia.nih.gov/health
10. Older Americans Act Nutrition Program: https://acl.gov/sites/default/files/news%202017-03/OAA-Nutrition_Programs_Fact_Sheet.pdf.
11. U.S. Food and Drug Administration – Food Safety for Older Adults: https://www.fda.gov/media/83744/download

References

1. The United States Census Bureau, Population Division. *Projected Age Groups and Sex Composition of the Population: Main Projections Series for the United States, 2017-2060.* Accessed June 26, 2020. https://www.census.gov/data/tables/2017/demo/popproj/2017-summary-tables.html
2. The United States Census Bureau, Population Division. National Population by Characteristics: 2010-2019: Population Estimates by Age (18+): July 1, 2019. Accessed June 14, 2020. https://www.census.gov/data/tables/time-series/demo/popest/2010s-national-detail.html
3. Centers for Disease Control and Prevention, National Center for Health Statistics, Division of Analysis and Epidemiology. Life expectancy at birth, at age 65, and at age 75, by sex, race, and Hispanic origin: United States, selected years 1900–2017. Accessed July 6, 2019. https://www.cdc.gov/nchs/hus/contents2018.htm?search=Life_expectancy
4. Centers for Disease Control and Prevention, National Center for Health Statistics: Health, United States, 2018 – Data Finder. Age-adjusted death rates for selected causes of death, by sex, race, and Hispanic origin: United States, selected years

1950–2017. Accessed November 2, 2018. https://www.cdc
.gov/nchs/data/hus/2018/005.pdf

5. U.S. Department of Health and Human Services Administration for Community Living, Administration on Aging (AoA). 2018 Profile of Older Americans. Accessed October 12, 2018. https://acl.gov/sites/default/files/Aging%20and%20
Disability%20in%20America/2018OlderAmericansProfile.pdf

6. Roberts AW, Ogunwole SU, Blakeslee L, Rabe MA. The population 65 years and older in the United States: 2016. *American Community Survey Reports.* 2018;ACS-38:1-25. https://www.census.gov/content/dam/Census/library
/publications/2018/acs/ACS-38.pdf

7. Centers for Disease Control and Prevention, Strategic and Proactive Communication Branch. Audience Insights: Communicating to Boomers. https://www.cdc.gov/health
communication/pdf/audience/audienceinsight_boomers.pdf

8. Kahana E, Kahana B. Baby boomers' expectations of health and medicine. *AMA J Ethics.* 2014;16(5):380-384. https://journalofethics.ama-assn.org/article/baby-boomers
-expectations-health-and-medicine/2014-05

9. van Leeuwen KM, van Loon MS, van Nes FA, et al. What does quality of life mean to older adults? A thematic synthesis. *PloS ONE.* 2019;14(3):e0213263. https://doi.org/10.1371
/journal.pone.0213263

10. The United States Census Bureau. Grandparents and grandchildren. Accessed September 09, 2016. https://www.census
.gov/newsroom/blogs/random-samplings/2016/09
/grandparents-and-grandchildren.html

11. The United States Census Bureau. Income and poverty in the United States: 2017. Accessed September 12, 2018. https://www.census.gov/library/publications/2018/demo/p60
-263.html

12. Tennant B, Stellefson M, Dodd V, et al. eHealth literacy and Web 2.0 health information seeking behaviors among baby boomers and older adults. *J Med Internet Res.* 2015;17(3):e70.

13. U.S. Pharmacopeia Dietary Supplement Verification Program, 2020. https://www.usp.org/services/verification
-services?language_content_entity=en

14. U.S. Food and Drug Administration. Guidance for industry: evidence-based review system for the Scientific Evaluation of Health Claims. Accessed January 2, 2009. https://www.fda
.gov/regulatory-information/search-fda-guidance-documents
/guidance-industry-evidence-based-review-system-scientific
-evaluation-health-claims

15. Fox S. The social life of health information, 2011. Pew Research Center. Accessed December 7, 2020. https://www.pewresearch
.org/internet/wp-content/uploads/sites/9/media/Files
/Reports/2011/PIP_Social_Life_of_Health_Info.pdf

16. Finney Rutten LJ, Blake KD, Greenberg-Worisek AJ, Allen SV, Moser RP, Hesse BW. Online health information seeking among US adults: measuring progress toward a Healthy People 2020 objective. *Public Health Reports.* 2019;134(6):617-625.

17. Xu JQ, Murphy SL, Kochanek KD, Arias E. Mortality in the United States, 2018. NCHS Data Brief, no 355. Hyattsville, MD: National Center for Health Statistics. 2020.

18. Bauer UE, Briss PA, Goodman RA, Bowman BA. Prevention of chronic disease in the 21st century: elimination of the leading preventable causes of premature death and disability in the USA. *Lancet.* 2014;384(9937):45-52.

19. Centers for Disease Control and Prevention. National diabetes statistics report, 2020. Atlanta, GA: Centers for Disease Control and Prevention, U.S. Dept. of Health and Human Services; 2020.

20. U.S. Department of Health and Human Services. The health consequences of smoking—50 years of progress: A report of the Surgeon General, 2014 U.S. Department of Health and Human Services, Atlanta, GA: Department of Health and Human Services, Centers for Disease Control and Prevention, National Center for Chronic Disease Prevention and Health Promotion, Office on Smoking and Health, 2014. Accessed December 7, 2020. https://onlinelibrary.wiley.com/doi
/abs/10.1111/dar.12309

21. Cornelius ME, Wang TW, Jamal A, Loretan C, Neff LJ. Tobacco product use among adults — United States, 2019. *MMWR Morbidity and Mortality Weekly Report.* 2020;69(46): 1736-1742. Accessed December 7, 2020. https://www.ncbi
.nlm.nih.gov/pmc/articles/PMC7676638/

22. Centers for Disease Control and Prevention, National Center for Health Statistics: Health, United States, 2018 – Data Finder. Table 21. Selected health conditions and risk factors, by age: United States, selected years 1988–1994 through 2015–2016. Accessed May 17, 2019. https://www.cdc.gov/nchs/data
/hus/2018/021.pdf

23. Centers for Disease Control and Prevention. Adult obesity prevalence maps: 2019. Accessed December 8, 2020. https://www.cdc.gov/obesity/data/prevalence-maps.html#
Resources

24. Ward ZJ, Bleich SN, Cradock AL, et al. Projected U.S. state-level prevalence of adult obesity and severe obesity. *N Engl J Med.* 2019;381:2440-2450.

25. Centers for Disease Control and Prevention, National Center for Health Statistics. Early release of selected estimates based on data from the 2018 National Health Interview Survey. Accessed December 8, 2020. https://www.cdc.gov/nchs/nhis/releases
/released201905.htm#7a

26. Theis KA, Roblin D, Helmick CG, Luo R. Prevalence and causes of work disability among working-age U.S. adults: 2011–2013, NHIS. *Disabil Health J.* 2018;11(1):108-115

27. Barbour KE, Helmick CG, Boring MA, Brady TJ. Vital signs: prevalence of doctor-diagnosed arthritis and arthritis-attributable activity limitation—United States, 2013–2015. *MMWR Morb Mortal Wkly Rep.* 2017;66(9):246-253.

28. Hootman JM, Helmick CG, Barbour KE, Theis KA, Boring MA. Updated projected prevalence of self-reported doctor-diagnosed arthritis and arthritis-attributable activity limitation among US adults, 2015–2040. *Arthritis Rheumatol.* 2016; 68(7):1582-1587.

29. Centers for Disease Control and Prevention. Diagnoses of HIV infection in the United States and dependent areas, 2014. HIV Surveillance Report 2015;26.

30. Nahin RL, Barnes PM, Stussman BJ. Expenditures on complementary health approaches: United States, 2012. *National Health Statistics Reports.* Hyattsville, MD: National Center for Health Statistics. 2016;95:1-12.

31. Rosenwohl-Mack A, Schumacher K, Fang M-L, Fukuoka Y. Experiences of aging in place in the United States: protocol

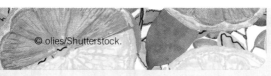
© olies/Shutterstock.

Learning Portfolio

for a systematic review and meta-ethnography of qualitative studies. *Syst Rev*. 2018;7(1):155.

32. Pruchno R. Technology and aging: an evolving partnership. *Gerontologist*. 2019;59(1):1-5.

33. Cereda E, Pedrolli C, Klersy C, et al. Nutritional status in older persons according to healthcare setting: a systematic review and meta-analysis of prevalence data using MNA®. *Clin Nutr*. 2016;35(6):1282-1290.

34. Engelheart S, Brummer R. Assessment of nutritional status in the elderly: a proposed function-driven model. *Food Nutr Res*. 2018;62(10.29219):1366. doi: 10.29219/fnr.v62.1366

35. Amarya S, Singh K, Sabharwal M. Changes during aging and their association with malnutrition. *J Clin Gerontol Geriatr*. 2015;6(3):78-84.

36. Krok-Schoen JL, Archdeacon Price A, Luo M. Low dietary protein intakes and associated dietary patterns and functional limitations in an aging population: a NHANES analysis. *J Nutr Health Aging*. 2019;23338-347.

37. Kaur D, Rasane P, Singh J, et al. Nutritional interventions for elderly and considerations for the development of geriatric foods. *Curr Aging Sci*. 2019;12(1):15-27.

38. Gahche JJ, Bailey RL, Potischman N, Dwyer JT. Dietary supplement use was very high among older adults in the United States in 2011–2014. *J Nutr*. 2017;147(10):1968-1976.

39. Sanders ME, Merenstein DJ, Reid G, et al. Probiotics and prebiotics in intestinal health and disease: from biology to the clinic. *Nat Rev Gastroenterol Hepatol*. 2019;16:605-616.

40. Tsai YL, Lin T-L, Chang C-J, et al. Probiotics, prebiotics and amelioration of diseases. *J Biomed Sci*. 2019;26(3).

41. Fisberg M, Machado R. History of yogurt and current patterns of consumption. *Nutr Rev*. 2015;73(suppl 1):4-7.

42. Warburton DER, Bredin SSD. Health benefits of physical activity: a systematic review of current systematic reviews. *Curr Opin Cardiol*. 2017;32(5):541-556

43. McPhee JS, French DP, Jackson D, Nazroo J, Pendleton N, Degens H. Physical activity in older age: perspectives for healthy ageing and frailty. *Biogerontology*. 2016;17(3):567-580.

44. Chilkoti A. As home workouts rise during coronavirus, gyms sweat. *Wall Street Journal*. May 6, 2020. Accessed December 28, 2020. https://www.wsj.com/articles/as-home-workouts-rise -during-coronavirus-gyms-sweat-11588784616

45. Li Z, Dalaker J. CRS Report: Poverty among Americans aged 65 and older. *Congressional Research Service*. 2019. https://fas.org/sgp/crs/misc/R45791.pdf

46. U.S. Department of Agriculture, Economic Research Service. Definitions of food security. Accessed December 28, 2020. https://www.ers.usda.gov/topics/food-nutrition-assistance /food-security-in-the-us/definitions-of-food-security/. Updated September 9, 2020.

47. Coleman-Jensen A, Rabbitt MP, Gregory CA, Singh A. 2020. Household food security in the United States in 2019, ERR-275, U.S. Department of Agriculture, Economic Research Service.

48. Administration on Aging. Budget request for fiscal year 1972 by the Administration on Aging. Federal Register. August 19, 1972;37(162):16848.

49. Carlin JM. Meals on wheels. In: *Oxford Encyclopedia of Food and Drink in America*. New York: Oxford University Press; 2004.

50. Bechill WD, Wolgamot I. Nutrition for the elderly. The program highlights of research and development nutrition projects funded under Title IV of the Older Americans Act of 1965. Washington, DC: U.S. Department of Health, Education, and Welfare, Administration on Aging; 1973.

51. Administration on Aging. Budget request for fiscal year 2003 by the Administration on Aging. Federal Register. 1972;19;37(162):16848.

52. Millen BE, Silliman RA, Cantey-Kiser J, et al. Nutritional risk in an urban homebound older population: The nutrition and healthy aging project. *J Nutr Health Aging*. 2001;5(4):269-277.

53. National Resource Center on Nutrition, Physical Activity & Aging. Florida International University. https://nutrition.fiu .edu/about_staff.asp

54. National Resource Center on Nutrition and Aging (NRCNA). Accessed September 1, 2021. https://acl.gov/news-and-events /announcements/new-grant-opportunity-national-resource -center-nutrition-and-aging

55. Administration for Community Living. Program Evaluations and Reports. Accessed February 6, 2021. https://acl.gov /programs/program-evaluations-and-reports

56. National Resource Center on Nutrition and Aging (NRCNA). Information, Data, and Evaluation. Accessed February 6, 2021. https://acl.gov/senior-nutrition

57. Robertson RE. U.S. General Accounting Office. Food assistance: options for improving nutrition for older Americans. GAO/ RCED-00-238. Washington, DC: U.S. General Accounting Office. 2000:8-9.

58. USDA Food and Nutrition Service. U.S. Depratment of Agriculture. CSFP: Final caseload assignments for the 2020 caseload cycle and administrative grants. Accessed February 6, 2021. https://www.fns.usda.gov/csfp/final-caseload -assignments-2020-caseload-cycle

59. USDA Food and Nutrition Service. U.S. Depratment of Agriculture. Program Data Review. Accessed February 6, 2021. https:// www.fns.usda.gov/pd/overview

60. Bewell Stanford. Self-managing chronic disease. Accessed February 6, 2021. https://bewell.stanford.edu/self-managing -chronic-disease/

61. U.S. General Accounting Office. GAO-20-18, Nutrition assistance programs: agencies could do more to help address the nutritional needs of older adults. Washington, DC: U.S. General Accounting Office; 2019:9.

62. Perrin A, Duggan M. Pew Research Center. Americans' Internet access: 2000-2015- as Internet use nears saturation for some groups, a look at patterns of adoption. Accessed June 26, 2015. http://www.pewinternet.org/2015/06/26/americans-internet -access-2000-2015/

63. Rideout V. e-health and the elderly: how seniors use the Internet for health. Press release. Menlo Park, CA: Kaiser Family Foundation in consultation with Princeton Survey Research Associates (PSRA). Assessed February 6, 2021. https://www .kff.org/wp-content/uploads/2013/01/e-health-and-the-elderly -how-seniors-use-the-internet-for-health-information-key-findings -from-a-national-survey-of-older-americans-survey-report.pdf

CHAPTER 12

Providing Nutrition Services in Community and Public Health Primary Care

Lauren Melnick, MS, RDN, LDN

(We would like to acknowledge the work of Arlene Spark, EdD, RDN, FADA, FACN, in the past editions of Nutrition in Public Health.)

Learning Outcomes

AFTER STUDYING THIS CHAPTER AND REFLECTING ON THE CONTENTS, YOU SHOULD BE ABLE TO:

1. Define primary health care.
2. Outline 2–3 ways in which telehealth has impacted delivery of preventative care, including nutrition.
3. Describe the impact of the Affordable Care Act on preventative care in the United States.
4. Summarize 3–4 ways in which primary care services are financed.
5. Discuss the scope and breadth of nutrition services available in primary care settings, why barriers exist to providing nutrition services in primary health care, and how those barriers may be overcome.
6. Define at least three federally funded programs designed to close gaps in care among vulnerable populations.

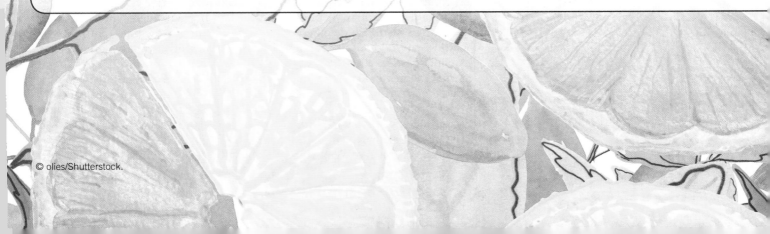

Introduction

Historically, there has been a lack of clarity and consensus around primary care. The confusion may be attributed to the numerous definitions of the word *primary*. Among its many meanings are main, chief, most important, key, prime, principal, crucial, fundamental, core, central, essential, basic, and important as well as first, initial, leading, top, and foremost. If *primary* is understood to be first, initial, or leading in time or order, this results in a relatively narrow concept of primary care as "first contact" or the entry point of healthcare delivery. This narrow definition of primary care connotes only a triage function in which patients are then passed on to a higher level of care. If, on the other hand, *primary* is understood in its sense of chief, principal, or main, *primary care* is understood as central and fundamental to health care. This latter idea supports the multidimensional view of primary care envisioned in the Institute of Medicine's (IOM) report, *Primary Care: America's Health in a New Era*. That *primary care is fundamental to health care* is also the view envisioned in this chapter.[1] The IOM is now called the National Academy of Medicine.

The National Academy of Medicine defines primary care as "the provision of integrated, accessible health care services by clinicians who are accountable for addressing a large majority of personal health needs, developing a sustained partnership with patients, and practicing in the context of family and community."[1] According to this definition, primary care is a function predicated on relationships and collaboration (rather than boundaries between specialties and disciplines). There is emphasis on the clinician's role as the patient's partner and advocate as the patient navigates their way through the healthcare system. The National Academy of Medicine recommends that primary care should be viewed as a central mission of the healthcare system (not as a feeder to tertiary care), and that it should be provided by teams that bring "different kinds of expertise…to bear on the patient's needs through collaborative activity, and…permit the delegation of some tasks by broadening the range of professionals involved in primary care.[1] The vision purported by the National Academy of Medicine includes the idea that primary care should be "patient-centered." Seven criteria have been developed to guide practitioners toward support of a **patient-centered primary care** practice. The concept that patients should have access to primary care that best suits their preferences, needs, and values is one of six domains of quality addressed by the National Academy of Medicine. These criteria will be described in further detail later in the chapter.[2] Primary care is continuing, comprehensive, and preventive personal medical care that, at the intersection of public health, should account for the social, environmental, and community determinants of health that impact one's well-being. The primary care setting has evolved to include all public and/or private outpatient clinics; private practices that offer office-based general medical care; and virtual/telemedicine visits that allow patients with a secure Internet connection to receive care on their computers, tablets, and smart phones. (Although not considered here, primary care settings also include emergency rooms, acute care facilities, chronic care facilities, and addiction treatment facilities.) Typically, primary care practice is defined within the categories of pediatrics, adolescent medicine, general internal medicine, family practice, geriatrics, and obstetrics and gynecology. Providers of primary care include allopathic physicians or medical doctors (MDs) and osteopathic physicians or doctors of osteopathy (DOs). Primary care physicians often work with other healthcare providers, such as physician assistants (PAs), nurse practitioners (NPs), registered nurses (RNs), social workers (MSWs, LMSWs), Registered Dietitian/Nutritionists (RDNs), and

Patient-centered care The provision of healthcare that is respectful of and responsive to individual patient preferences, needs, and values; the patient has a significant role in determining their course of care.

behavioral health practitioners. In fact, there has been a significant push in recent years to provide better coordinated primary care among various allied health practitioners using a multi-disciplinary team approach to practice.

The concept of primary care is so fundamental to community and public health that objectives to address primary care are reflected in several of the *Healthy People 2030* leading health indicators (LHIs). In this most recent iteration of Healthy People, LHIs are categorized by life stages. A majority of indicators are relevant to children and adolescents and adults and older adults.[3]

- Increase the proportion of people who get the flu vaccine every year from 49.2% to 70%.
- Increase control of high blood pressure in adults (18 years and older) from 47.8% of adults with controlled hypertension to 60.8%.
- Reduce the number of diabetes cases diagnosed yearly from 6.5 new cases of diabetes per 1,000 adults aged 18 to 84 years to 5.6 new cases per 1,000 adults.
- Reduce the proportion of children and adolescents with obesity from 17.8% of children and adolescents aged 2 to 19 years to 15.5%.
- Increase the proportion of people with health insurance from 89% of persons under 65 years to 92.1%.
- Increase the proportion of adults who get screened for colorectal cancer from 66.2% of adults aged 50 to 75 years to 74.4%.

Room for Nutrition in Primary Care

Conducted under the aegis of the National Center for Health Statistics, the National Ambulatory Medical Care Survey (NAMCS) is a national survey that provides information about ambulatory medical care services in the United States. Findings are based on a sample of visits to non-federally employed office-based physicians who are primarily engaged in direct patient care. According to the NAMCS, in 2016, an estimated 883.7 million visits were made to physicians' offices in the United States, and 86% of adults and 96% of children had a usual place to receive care. As indicated in **Table 12–1**, only 23% of all office-based physician visits were for the primary reason of preventative care, and this number declined as patients aged. In the context of this survey, preventative care is defined as general medical examinations and routine periodic examinations, including prenatal care, annual physicals, well-child exams, screening, and insurance examinations. Among all office visits, nearly one-half (48%) included an examination or screening that was ordered or provided. Visit rates are highest among females, infants under 1 year of age, and adults 65 years and over.[4]

As evidenced by the information above, most adults are compelled to visit their physician to treat a chronic condition or upon development of a new problem.[4] Children and adolescents (18 years and under) are the most likely population to receive preventative care, which is likely driven by a parent or guardian. Health education and counseling are also more commonly prescribed for children, whereas adults are more frequently provided with diagnostic testing.

In today's healthcare climate, aging Americans are taking a more active role in their health, which translates into increasing numbers of visits to doctors. Among all patients who visited physicians in 2016, middle aged persons (45–64 years) and senior citizens (65 years and older) accounted

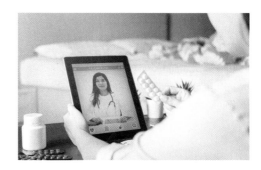

Telemedicine has become a popular way communicate with the primary care physician as well as other health professionals. During the Covid-19 pandemic, telemedicine was used frequently to prevent spreading the virus.

© Asiandelight/Shutterstock.

TABLE 12–1
Reasons for Physician-based Office Visits Among All Age Groups[4]

Percent of All Office Visits	Reason
37	Chronic condition
27	New problem
23	Preventative care
7	Injury
6	Pre- or postsurgical care

Data from Centers for Disease Control and Prevention: Ambulatory Health Care Data. National Ambulatory Medical Care (NAMC) Survey Characteristics of Office-Based Visits, 2016. Accessed December 12, 2020. Available at: https://www.cdc.gov/nchs/products/databriefs/db331.htm

Discussion Prompt

How can community dietitians/nutritionists add to preventative care? Would this save or cost money?

Medicare A federal health insurance program for people who are 65 years or older, certain younger people with disabilities, and people with end-stage renal disease (permanent kidney failure requiring dialysis or a transplant, sometimes called ESRD).

Pandemic Learning Opportunity

Licensure of providers across state lines is another policy that was modified during COVID-19, giving healthcare professionals, including RDNs, the ability to practice in multiple states without meeting strict state-mandated licensure requirement or paying additional fees. It is not expected that HHS will uphold all of these policy changes postpandemic, but there may be some modifications that will allow for easier, seamless provision of these services overall.[7]

for the second and third highest office-based physician visits among all age groups (only infants were higher).[5] Between 2012 and 2050, the number of Americans aged 65 years and older is expected to reach 83.7 million, which is roughly double the current estimate. For this reason, we can expect more physician visits and a greater focus on preventative care. Physicians are also more aggressive in treating chronic disease, which requires more follow-up care.[5]

Nutrition counseling is an appropriate component of treatment for many of the chronic conditions that underlie adult physician visits and promote prescription drug use. According to the National Health and Nutrition Examination Survey (NHANES) from 2016–2017, 45% of adults aged 60–79 years were prescribed lipid-lowering drugs for high cholesterol; followed by antidiabetic agents (23.6%); beta blockers for high blood pressure and heart disease (22.3%); and ACE inhibitors for high blood pressure (21.3%). Adults aged 40–59 years use these drugs less overall, but at a steadily increased rate.[6]

Accessible nutrition therapy intervention as part of preventative care or for the treatment of chronic disease has the potential to decrease both physician office visits and medication use. Email, smart phone/tablets, and two-way conferencing consultations between doctors and their patients have increased significantly as technology and safeguards to protect confidentiality and liability have improved.

Telemedicine/Telenutrition in Primary Care

Telemedicine, the use of virtual, audio, and health information technologies to deliver healthcare, has been gradually adopted by providers, including RDNs, as a means of providing 1:1 or small-group education. Traditionally, it has been viewed as an alternative to in-person care, but not necessarily an ideal modality for those who prefer and or are used to visiting their physician's office. It has also not always been an option for individuals with no or limited Internet access or connectivity.

With the advent of the COVID-19 pandemic in 2020, many of the previous realities about telemedicine shifted and use of this service accelerated at an unprecedented rate. In order to decrease risk of COVID-19 transmission and infection, the U.S. Department of Health and Human Services (HHS) implemented new policy changes around telemedicine to allow for a greater ease and flexibility in delivering services. Some of these changes were related to the platforms and devices in which care is delivered. Previously, there were stringent HIPPA compliance requirements for telemedicine and only certain platforms met this criteria including, but not limited to: Epic MyChart, Doxy, Healthie, Practice Better, and Kalix. As part of COVID-19 precautions, HHS began allowing more commercial applications, such as Apple Facetime, Google Hangouts, Facebook Messenger, Zoom, and Skype, as a means of direct audio and video communication with providers.[7]

Other changes to telemedicine policy due to COVID-19 were related to payers and reimbursement of services. **Medicare** and Medicaid recipients were able to receive the same services covered in person in a virtual manner. Both government and private insurance allowed physicians to see both new and established patients over the phone or through video. Even Federally Qualified Health Centers (FQHCs) and Rural Health Clinics, covered later in this chapter, increased the availability of telehealth services and, in some cases, were able to use phone-only to check on patients without access to applications or Internet.[7]

Nutrition services were no exception to the growth in telehealth. Whereas previous to the pandemic, only approximately 30% of RDNs employed virtual services to their clients,[8] this number is expected to be much higher postpandemic and will likely remain higher long-term. Telenutrition has been embraced by RDNs over the last decade, but more and more nutrition professionals are embracing virtual and audio methods of delivering care for several key reasons outside of the COVID-19 pandemic. One of the foremost reasons is the ability to provide care everywhere. Dietitians who live in rural areas, but who may be specialists in certain niche areas of nutrition, no longer need to worry about traveling to see patients. The same is true for patients who may live in rural or remote areas but are in need of specialized nutrition care. Overall, there is less likelihood of "no shows" for appointments due to weather, work, time constraints, etc., when virtual methods are employed. Bluetooth-compatible devices owned by patients, such as the Apple iPhone, Samsung Smart Phone, or Apple Watch can provide dietitians/nutritionists with helpful monitoring data to inform nutrition care and counseling efforts. Number of steps, physically active minutes, blood pressure, weight, pulse, and blood glucose are examples of key data that can be uploaded or shared from a Bluetooth smart device. Lastly, many of the virtual platforms allow dietitians/nutritionists the ability to speak freely with patients while voice-recognition software captures notes and dialogue from the conversation. This promotes a greater focus on the patient and improved listening as opposed to in-person visits in which charting may need to take place concurrently with counseling.[8]

With any telemedicine initiatives, HHS advises that providers closely evaluate their patients to ensure that virtual or audio options are right for them. Many older adults, adults with disabilities, the under or uninsured, and those with limited English proficiency may not be candidates for telemedicine without the right support mechanisms in place. Telemedicine may save time for the patient in terms of driving and waiting for in-person services, but it can add time to providers who may need to adjust their approach or deal with connectivity issues.[7]

Agency for Healthcare Research and Quality

The Agency for Healthcare Research and Quality (AHRQ) is the lead U.S. federal agency for research on **healthcare quality**, costs, outcomes, and patient safety. It complements the biomedical research mission of its sister agency, the National Institutes of Health (NIH). AHRQ serves as a major source of funding and technical assistance for health services research and research training at leading U.S. universities and other institutions. It is home to research centers that specialize in such major areas of healthcare research as primary care (including preventive services), healthcare organization and delivery systems, and healthcare costs and sources of payment. AHRQ seeks to fulfill their mission of providing safe, quality, accessible, equitable and affordable health care by: a) supporting research that addresses concerns of high public priority, such as the lack of specialists in underserved and rural communities; b) utilizing research to create materials for teaching and training of healthcare systems and professionals; and c) generating measures and data that can be used by primary care providers and policymakers to promote change in the healthcare climate.[9]

The U.S. Preventative Services Task Force (USPSTF) has worked with the AHRQ since 1998 to develop the annual *Guide to Clinical Preventive Services*; individual reports have been released in print and on the AHRQ website as they have been completed.

The current recommendations released between 2014 and 2020 are preventative interventions that have demonstrated effectiveness based on the best available, quality evidence. In evaluating the research, the AHRQ and the USPSTF are tasked with determining the net health benefit (benefit minus

Strategy Tip

Match the appropriate culturally competent dietitian/nutritionist to the client.

Healthcare quality The measured value of providing healthcare services. In healthcare, quality could be related to improved quality of life, effectiveness of treatments, or decreased mortality.

See the AHRQ website at www.ahrq.gov

Visit the USPSTF website at https://uspreventiveservicestaskforce.org/uspstf/

harm) associated with preventative services and assign an "A" or "B" grade to those services that should be discussed with eligible patients and offered as a priority. A variety of clinical preventative services for normal-risk children and adults are recommended (receiving an "A" or "B" rating) by the USPSTF.

The suggested nutrition-related screening and counseling services include[9,10]:

- Abnormal blood glucose and type 2 diabetes mellitus: Screening: Adults aged 40 to 70 years who are overweight or obese
- Breastfeeding primary care interventions: Pregnant women, new mothers, and their children
- Folic acid for the prevention of neural tube defects: Preventive medication: Women who are planning or capable of pregnancy
- Healthy diet and physical activity for cardiovascular risk factors: Behavioral counseling interventions: Adults with cardiovascular disease risk factors
- High blood pressure in adults: Screening: Adults aged 18 years and older
- Obesity in children and adolescents: Screening: Children and adolescents 6 years and older
- Osteoporosis to prevent fractures: Screening: Postmenopausal women younger than 65 years at increased risk of osteoporosis
- Weight loss to prevent obesity-related morbidity and mortality in adults: Behavioral interventions: adults

The USPSTF's entire list can be accessed online at: https://www.uspreventiveservicestaskforce.org/uspstf/recommendation-topics/tools-and-resources-for-better-preventive-care

In order to access and implement these recommendations, the USPSTF has created the Prevention Task Force (formally ePSS) application that is downloadable to smart phones, tablets, and computers. This application is intended for primary care providers who are seeking to identify evidence-based screening, counseling, and preventive medication services that are suitable for patients based on sex, age, and selected behavioral risk factors. USPSTF also has a large library of online resources, including questionnaires, screening tools, and continuing education, for healthcare professionals who are seeking to implement preventative care in their practice.

Since 2014, the Patient Protection and **Affordable Care Act (ACA)**, implemented under the Obama Administration, has ensured that all health plans must cover a set of preventative services at no cost to the insured (as long as the services are provided by a doctor or other provider within your plan's network). The nutrition-related services are outlined below in **Table 12–2**. Other services covered without copayment or coinsurance include: Immunization vaccines, including influenza and HPV; HIV screening (ages 15 to 65 years); statin prevention medication for adults 40 to 75 at high risk; depression screening; and colorectal cancer screening for adults over 50 years. These preventative services are directly related to the "A" and "B" recommendations put forth by the AHRQ and USPSTF. As shown in Table 12–2, several of these no-cost services (within network) are related to nutrition.[11,12]

Affordable Care Act (ACA) The Affordable Care Act refers to two separate pieces of legislation—the Patient Protection and Affordable Care Act (P.L. 111-148) and the Health Care and Education Reconciliation Act of 2010 (P.L. 111-152). Its goal is to provide Americans with better health security by putting in place comprehensive health insurance reforms to expand coverage, hold insurance companies' accountable, lower healthcare costs, guarantee more choice, and enhance the quality of care for all Americans.

Barriers to Providing Nutrition Services in Primary Care and Strategies for Increasing Services

Despite the myriad opportunities to offer the nutrition services that are described in the previous section of this chapter, multiple factors affect the fulfillment of this potential—outside of the patient and their motivation to change behaviors. The physician may be disadvantaged by a lack of confidence and competence in nutrition counseling or just not interested in providing this

TABLE 12-2

Nutrition-Related Free* Preventative Services for Adults, Women, and Children Provided Through the Patient Protection and Affordable Care Act (2014)[12]

Service Provided	Adults (Men and Women)	Women	Children and Adolescents
Alcohol misuse screening and counseling	X		
Anemia screening on a routine basis		X	
Blood pressure screening	X		X (0 months to 17 years)
Breastfeeding comprehensive support and counseling from trained professionals and access to breastfeeding supplies for pregnant and nursing women		X	
Cholesterol screening for adults of certain ages or at higher risk	X		
Diabetes (Type 2) screening for adults 40 to 70 years who are overweight or obese	X	X (for women with a history of gestational diabetes who aren't currently pregnant and who haven't been diagnosed with type 2 diabetes before)	
Dyslipidemia screening			X (all children once between 9 and 11 years; once between 17 and 21 years; and for children at a higher risk of lipid disorders aged 1–17 years)
Diet counseling for those at a high risk of chronic disease	X		
Fluoride chemoprevention supplements; Fluoride Varnish for all infants and children with teeth present			X (for children without fluoride in their water source)
Folic acid supplements for women who may become pregnant		X	
Gestational diabetes screening		X (for women 24 to 48 weeks pregnant and at a high risk for developing gestational diabetes)	
Height, weight, and body mass index (BMI) measurements			X (0 months–17 years)
Hematocrit/hemoglobin screening			X
Iron supplements			X (ages 6–12 months at risk for anemia)
Obesity screening and counseling	X		X
Oral health risk assessment			X (0 months–10 years)
Osteoporosis screening		X (women over 60 years and depending on risk factors)	
Preeclampsia prevention and screening		X	
Phenylketonuria (PKU) Screening			X (newborns)

*Within the plan's network.

Data from Healthcare.gov: *Health Benefits and Coverage: Preventive Health Services*. Accessed December 22, 2020 from: https://www.healthcare.gov/coverage/preventive-care-benefits/

Discussion Prompt

Which is more likely in your community, a lack of RDNs, inadequate third-party reimbursement for their services, or physicians who miss the opportunity to refer patients to RDNS? How can these be remedied?

education. Time constraints coupled with the increased demands of physicians and lack of access to RDNs is another detriment to providing quality service. Finally, there may be inadequate third-party reimbursement for nutrition consultation services, leaving patients with the option of receiving minimal counseling or paying out of pocket for additional services.

Physician Confidence and Skills

Practicing physicians report a lack of confidence and related proficiency in nutrition counseling skills because of inadequate training.[13,14] Despite concerted scientific, educational, and congressional calls to increase nutrition coverage in medicine for more than half a century, most graduating medical students report an inadequate quality and quantity of nutrition training.

Strategies to Improve Confidence and Skills

During the early 1980s through 2000, as the concept of nutrition counseling for weight loss and reduced cardiovascular risk became more popular, there was a significant push to include more nutrition training in U.S. medical school curriculums. Despite early identification of the importance of these concepts as part of traditional university medical education (UME) and graduate medical education (GME), most programs are woefully lacking in time and resources to educate medical students, residents, and fellows. In a compilation of postgraduate program surveys, only about 14% of primary care residents surveyed felt adequately prepared to deliver nutrition counseling to patients.[15] Additionally, despite a vast majority of cardiologists (approximately 70%) agreeing that it is "essential to their role" to include nutrition counseling in their practice, roughly the same percentage of cardiologists said they received minimal to no training on providing effective nutrition counseling.[16] The Accreditation Council for Graduate Medical Education (ACGME), in partnership with the American Heart Association (AHA), has sought to rectify a lack of nutrition science training among cardiology residents and fellows by developing nutrition-specific competencies across six domains: Patient care (assess diet history, diet risk, and refer to an RDN when necessary); medical knowledge (demonstrate basic knowledge of nutrition science, including macro- and micronutrients, and understand how social determinants and lifestyle affect nutrition status); systems-based practice (educate on basics and refer to other specialists, including RDNs, for advanced care); practice-based learning and improvement (continuing to monitor nutrition-related risk factors in patients); interpersonal and communication skills (conveying basic concepts in a concise and understandable manner for all levels of health literacy); and professionalism (displaying empathy when counseling patients and respecting the additional expertise that can be provided by a multispecialty team, including RDNs).[15]

In 1995, the University of North Carolina, Chapel Hill, developed the Nutrition in Medicine (NIM) Project to provide an evidence-based curriculum on core nutrition concepts to medical schools free of charge. Originally provided to schools as a CD-ROM, the NIM curriculum was adapted as an online tool in 2009 as part of the Nutrition Education for Practicing Physicians (NEPP) initiative. Each of the 13 online modules includes information on both preventative and therapeutic aspects of nutrition care, the biochemical basis for nutrition science, and preparation for physicians to answer their patients' most common nutrition-related concerns and questions. As Smartphone and tablet usage has increased, the curriculum has evolved to include three, easily- accessible mobile tools: Pocket notes or one-page, easy-to-access summaries on popular nutrition topics; YouTube Vignettes; and easy-to-access links to Dietary Reference Intakes (DRI) tables.[17] Since its inception, greater than 100 U.S. and international medical schools have accessed NIM in an attempt to enhance existing lectures and curricula.[15]

In general, online programs are viable options for training physicians, as reading and self-directed learning are the primary methods in which physicians receive nutrition training.[17-19] Universities and nonprofit groups offer online training courses that can be completed for Continuing Medical Education (CME) credit. A few examples include: Nutrition Science for Health and Longevity, a 3-hour, self-paced interactive course developed by the Gaples Institute; Introduction to Food and Health—a 2.5-hour online course through Stanford University Center for Continuing Education; and AHA's Healthy Living Continuing Education Series.[15]

Toolkits can also be an effective mechanism for physicians to easily remember and quickly provide key nutrition concepts to patients. One example of an effective toolkit is the product developed by the North Carolina *Eat Smart, Move More* program. The NC toolkit includes pocket reference guides on key clinical nutrition concepts, color-coded BMI charts, resources to use with addressing high blood pressure, and prescription pads that utilize the "5-3-2-1-Almost None" messaging. The 5-3-2-1-Almost None daily concept is in regard to eating fruits and vegetables (five servings or more), three structured meals (breakfast, fewer fast foods, eat at home), 2 hours or fewer of TV or video games, 1 hour or more of moderate to intense physical activity, and limit sugar-sweetened beverages to almost none.[18]

Albert Einstein College of Medicine created other user-friendly tools that make it possible for physicians to quickly determine a patient's diet and exercise habits, as well as provide information to aid in the delivery of effective nutrition counseling. WAVE and REAP are two examples.[19]

The Einstein team developed WAVE and REAP, which are acronyms for tools to help physicians and other healthcare providers conduct nutrition assessments and counseling with their patients in as little as one minute. Weight, Activity, Variety and Excess (WAVE) is designed to encourage provider/patient dialogue about the pros and cons of the patient's status regarding weight, diet, and activity. The Rapid Eating and Activity Assessment for Patients (REAP) is a questionnaire designed to aid providers in performing a quick assessment of diet and physical activity. An accompanying key aids the provider in discussing the patient's answers and provides guidelines for counseling.[19] REAP and WAVE are examples of tools to facilitate nutrition assessment and counseling in the provider office.

Although these tools and similar items developed by insurance companies, professional groups, and the National Initiative for Children's Healthcare Quality (NICHQ) are well received, they are still only used minimally by physicians. Some studies suggest that as low as 30% of all physicians actually use supplemental nutrition resources in practice.[18]

Physician's Time Constraints

The frequency and time spent with nutrition counseling in primary care are not well studied, but a few investigations suggest that the amount of time spent on nutrition depends on the reason for the visit and the patient's age. The question remains: Who receives nutrition counseling and how much time do primary care physicians spend discussing diet? The following research has sought to answer these questions:

- Several studies have found that anywhere from 1 to 8.2 minutes are spent on counseling patients on nutrition, depending on the complexity of the patients' needs. Because of the increased number of preventative measures cited as priorities in the ACA, physicians struggle to prioritize screening recommendations.[18]

- A Canadian study published in 2010 looked at the role of family primary care physicians in managing nutrition-related issues, as well as whether or not current nutrition counseling guidelines are effective in primary care practice. A questionnaire regarding demographic characteristics, attitudes about and perceived barriers to nutrition counseling, training, and current practice was mailed to 757 physicians. Of that number, 451 responded. Although most physicians agreed that 60% of their patients would benefit from nutrition counseling, only 19.1% said that 60% of their patients actually receive counseling. Overall, physicians felt more comfortable addressing general nutrition vs chronic disease. This is due in part to lack of training and time constraints. In fact, lack of time was the number one barrier to providing nutrition counseling reported among those surveyed.[18]

- According to a report published in 2004, when trained medical students observed physician, office, and patient characteristics in 4,344 patient visits in 38 nonmetropolitan primary care physician offices, they found that counseling rates ranged from 0% in some offices to 55% in others. Physicians counseled patients on dietary habits in 25% of visits and exercise in 20% of visits. New patients were counseled 30% more often than established ones. When counseling occurred, physicians (rather than patients) initiated both dietary and exercise counseling 61% of the time. Counseling for dietary habits was associated with counseling for exercise.[20]

- Finally, a 2018 review of survey data related to deficits in nutrition education among physicians found that while 72% of physicians believed that patients understood the nutrition advice being provided to them as part of a physician visit, only 21% of patients actually understood the advice, which was mostly provided in a 3-minute time frame.[16]

Strategies to Reduce Time Constraints

Given the time constraints of a primary care practice and the increased focus on prevention and screening in today's healthcare climate, nutrition counseling needs to be brief and part of an organized office system that is conducive to supporting nutrition services. When necessary, the physician should refer appropriate patients to qualified nutrition professionals (RDNs). The issue remains that RDNs may not be available, particularly in rural environments. In this situation, Telenutrition, as discussed earlier in this chapter, may be a viable solution. Strategies targeting both physicians and the healthcare system may improve the consistency of physician preventive counseling practices.[13]

AHRQ recommends that primary care physicians utilize the "5 As" to deliver nutrition counseling.[9] The 5 As—assess, advise, agree, assist, and arrange—is a mnemonic algorithm that outlines minimal contact interventions that may be provided by clinical staff in primary care settings. Research has demonstrated that although physicians embrace the 5A method, the last two steps, assist and arrange, are not likely to be completed in a busy primary care setting.[17]

The question remains if lengthy interventions are necessarily the best avenue for patients seeking nutrition counseling. Several systematic reviews have shown that behavior change occurs when patients have repeated visits of considerable length; however, research to the contrary has shown that

Strategy Tip

Brainstorm ways that RDNs can reach physicians to prove accessibility for their patients.

small steps, such as those presented by the Eat Less, Move More toolkit, could also be beneficial.[19] The recommendations set forth by USPSTF suggest that counseling and behavior interventions should occur at least twice a month for the first 3 months for all obese patients; however, when considering the other preventative recommendations made by USPSTF, it seems impossible that physicians could spend time on nutrition when they are also being asked to screen for several other issues. Research has shown that if physicians implemented all of the UPSTF recommendations, it would take 7.4 hours per patient.[21]

Time was always be a factor in providing all preventative services; however, the best methods for physicians to confront the constraints associated with nutrition counseling include engaging in further training to provide concise messaging on a few key concepts; referring patients with complex needs to the RDNs, including telenutrition as a viable option; and utilizing shared medical appointments whenever possible and covered by insurance.

Some physicians have an RDN on staff or working as an independent contractor in their offices.

© Lipik Stock Media/Shutterstock.

Compensation and Reimbursement

Traditional **indemnity insurance** is still the most popular form of health insurance, but the nutrition services covered under these plans is still variable. As noted in Table 12–2, the ACA has made possible the addition of several nutrition-related preventative measures for all health plans, including obesity screening and counseling for adults and children who meet specific criteria. This counseling, as noted above, tends to be done quickly or in a SMA format and what is gleaned by the patient in these sessions is uncertain. Medicare Part B recipients are eligible for services related to nutrition management of diabetes, kidney disease and obesity but, just like with the ACA services, certain criteria still need to be met in order for the patient to avoid payment and for the clinician to receive reimbursement.

More in-depth nutrition services are typically paid for out-of-pocket as many third-party payers do not reimburse dietitians for their time. Overall, more dietitians are receiving reimbursement now for MNT and weight-management counseling than they did prior to the ACA, but there is still a lack of uniformity in coverage. Even if a physician can refer their patients to an RDN, the patient may not take advantage of this benefit if they have to pay for the visit. Additionally, the patient may have a low motivation for change, which would further discourage them from using their own dollars for these services. Through their own lack of knowledge or guidance provided by their physician, patients may also not understand the necessity of seeing an RDN.[17] With this said, the Academy of Nutrition and Dietetics, the professional organization for food and nutrition professionals, has created several promotional items and educational toolkits to elevate the perception of the RDN in the eye of the public and to lobby for reimbursement of services.

Systemwide Change Strategies for Reducing the Cost of Medical Care

Population-based medicine and **chronic disease management** are of particular importance to community and public health nutritionists. Population-based medicine addresses the health care of whole populations rather than that of individual patients. It represents a community-based strategy for disease management and health promotion and places each individual patient within the context of the larger community composed of both sick and healthy people. The community may be as small as an individual physician's private medical practice or as comprehensive as a multisite HMO.

Indemnity insurance Also known as "fee-for-service" insurance, indemnity plans allow freedom in choosing healthcare providers, and the insurance company establishes a set dollar amount for the services they will cover.

For more information on how to find a dietitian by geographic area or area of practice, visit: https://www.eatright.org /find-an-expert.

Population-based medicine Assessing the healthcare needs of a specific population (groups of individuals who have one or more personal or environmental traits in common) and making healthcare decisions for the population as a whole rather than for individuals.

Chronic disease management Refers to the oversight of treatments, therapies, and education activities conducted by healthcare professionals to help patients with chronic disease and health conditions live with their illness and maintain motivation to manage their illness.

TABLE 12–3
How the Affordable Care Act Has Impacted Prevention[22]

Year	Preventive Initiative(s)	Other Major Milestones
2010	Providing Free Preventative Care; $15 billion Prevention and Public Health Fund created for health programming; strengthening community health centers; increasing salary for rural healthcare providers.	Prohibition of denying coverage of children based on pre-existing conditions; extending parents' coverage to young adults (up to age 26 years); prohibiting insurance companies from rescinding coverage.
2011	Free preventative care for seniors; increasing access to services at home and in the community.	Improving healthcare quality and efficiency; bringing down healthcare premiums.
2012	Encouraging integrated health systems; understanding and fighting health disparities through increased racial, ethnic, and language data.	Linking payment to quality outcomes (Value-based care).
2013	Improved preventative health coverage through Medicaid.	Open enrollment in the Health Insurance Marketplace begins.
2014	Increasing access to Medicaid.	Prohibiting discrimination due to pre-existing conditions or gender; establishing the Health Insurance Marketplace.
2015	Tax penalty for not having proof of health insurance	Continued above.
2016-2020	Removal of tax penalty for not having proof of health insurance.	Continuation of Health Insurance Marketplace.

HHS.gov. Key features of the Affordable Care Act by year. Accessed December 2, 2015. Available online at: http://www.hhs.gov/healthcare/facts-and-features /key-features-of-aca-by-year/index.html (Years 2015–2020 added by author.)

In population-based medicine, disease groups within a given patient population are identified and new levels of disease monitoring and patient education are used to ensure that best practice is systematically applied across the group, accomplished within the traditional relationship of doctor and patient, but with integral support from nurses, RDNs, pharmacists, health educators, and other members of the healthcare team.

Both population-based medicine and chronic disease management were significantly impacted by the provisions set forth by the ACA. **Table 12–3** demonstrates the extent to which U.S. healthcare was transformed by this new law.[22]

From 2016 to 2020, the Administration made little to no change of preventative health benefits available to Americans.[23] Most changes to the Affordable Care Act made under the Administration were related to operations of the Healthcare Marketplace. For example, the Administration removed the individual mandate or the dollar penalty for not having health insurance that was implemented by the former Administration. In 2017, States were also granted the ability, with federal approval, to ask Medicaid beneficiaries to provide documentation of work or enrollment in school. This action was in opposition to expansion of Medicaid under ACA during the former Administration.[23] As new administrations continue to govern under the ACA, there are sure to be new or revised additions to this legislation that will impact delivery and accessibility of preventative care.

Chronic Disease Management and Self-Management

Disease management is a system of coordinated healthcare interventions and communications for populations with conditions in which patient self-care efforts are significant. Disease management supports the physician or practitioner/patient relationship and plan of care; emphasizes prevention of exacerbations and complications utilizing evidence-based practice guidelines and patient empowerment strategies; and evaluates clinical, humanistic, and economic outcomes on an ongoing basis with the goal of improving overall health. In order to improve health outcomes for the chronically ill, system change interventions that involve primary care and cut across chronic conditions are needed. Chronic disease improvement efforts must create care systems that are designed to meet the needs of patients and their families. The AHRQ and The Robert Wood Johnson Foundation (RJWF), among other organizations, have funded research directed at improving the care of patients with major chronic illnesses. Additionally, valuable experience has been accrued in implementing evidence-based system change ideas in large-scale chronic disease quality improvement programs sponsored by the Bureau of Primary Health Care (BPHC), targeted at funding improvements in health centers and in disease management programs for those with limited access to quality healthcare[23]; the CDC, through their Chronic Disease Prevention and Health Promotion branch; the Administration on Aging (AoA) as part of their Chronic Disease Self-Management Program funding for older adults and adults with disabilities; and The MacColl Center for Healthcare Innovation, formerly a partner in the Improving Chronic Illness Care project (ICIC) that was funded by RWJF and ended in 2011 but resulted in expansion of using the **Chronic Care Model (CCM)** to improve the delivery of preventative healthcare globally.[24,25]

A component of population medicine is chronic disease management (CDM). CDM represents a comprehensive, ongoing, coordinated approach to achieving desired outcomes for a population of patients. These outcomes include improving patients' clinical condition, reducing unnecessary healthcare costs and improving patients' quality of life. To achieve these objectives requires rigorous, protocol-based, clinical management in conjunction with intensive patient education, coaching, and monitoring: In short, a comprehensive system that incorporates the patient, physician, and health plan into one system with one common goal.

Chronic disease management is now a major component of primary health care. The population is aging, and older adults may have several chronic conditions. In addition, with the advent of new technologies, treatments, and medications, some survive for decades with a chronic disease. For several years, the leading causes of death in the United States include the chronic diseases, cardiovascular disease (CVD), and type-2 diabetes. Nutrition is fundamental in the self-management of these conditions. A cost-effective way of delivering nutrition services is through **group** (or cluster) **visits**, also known as **shared medical appointments (SMAs)**.

Group visits or SMAs are a cost-effective means of providing self-care guidance and support to chronically ill patients who need more dietary advice than physicians have the resources (skill and time) to deliver. SMA visits are designed to help patients manage their health, adhere to their physicians' plans of care, and assure that they seek or obtain medical care that they need to reduce their health risks. The term is applied to small groups of patients with similar characteristics rather than individual patient-provider appointments. In this model, the healthcare team (in which the RDN may be included) facilitates an interactive process of care delivery in a periodic group visit program. The group can be conceptualized as an extended doctor's office visit and can be done both in person and virtually. Invitations are extended by the healthcare team to specific patients on the basis of chronic disease history and utilization patterns. Variations of this group format have been used for disease-specific populations, such as

Chronic Care Model (CCM) An organizing framework for improving chronic illness care at both the individual and population levels; typically has six parts self-management support, a well-designed healthcare delivery system, assistance with healthcare decision making, good clinical information (documentation) systems, organized health care, and supportive community stakeholders.

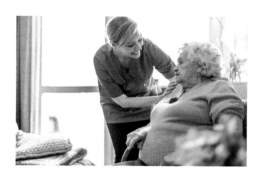

Chronic disease management assists patients in remaining well.

© Pikselstock/Shutterstock.

Group visits or Shared medical appointments (SMAs) An innovative and often cost-effective method in which patients with common needs are brought together in a group setting with one or more healthcare providers to offer education and peer-to-peer support.

Discussion Prompt

What would be the advantage of including a dietitian/nutritionist in an SMA session? Can another healthcare worker replace the RDN? Why or why not?

diabetes, hypertension, dyslipidemia, and weight control. SMA visits offer staff a means to interact with patients that makes efficient use of resources, improves access, and uses group process to help motivate behavior change and improve outcomes. In a 2014 retrospective, 3-year study that looked at the influence of SMAs on patient satisfaction, patients participating in 90-minute SMA sessions were more likely to rate their overall satisfaction of care as "very good" compared with those receiving "usual" (one-on-one appointment) care. SMA participants also found that the care received in the group setting was more accessible and better suited to their needs.[25] At the Cleveland Clinic in Cleveland, OH, SMAs led by RDNs in person and virtually have become hugely popular programming for weight loss and managing nutrition postsolid organ transplant.

Community-based disease self-management programs are another patient-centric alternative to managing chronic disease that is present in both urban and rural areas and is easily accessible to those in the community. Traditionally, community-based disease self-management programs that have the greatest impact tend to have well-defined problem and program objectives; engaged leadership; input from community residents; coordination across stakeholders and settings; integration throughout the organization or community; and a sustainability plan.[26] An example of a successful community-based prevention program is *The Well-Integrated Screening and Evaluation for Women Across the Nation* (WISEWOMAN), funded by CDC. This program provides low-income uninsured women aged 40 to 64 in 21 states and three tribal organizations (per fiscal year 2019 data) with chronic disease risk factor screenings, lifestyle interventions, and referral services. Over the course of a year, WISEWOMAN participants improved their 10-year risk of coronary heart disease by 8.7%, and there were significant reductions in the percentage of participants who smoked and had high blood pressure and high cholesterol.[27]

Chronic diseases have a long course of illness. They rarely resolve spontaneously and generally are not cured by medication. Today, chronic diseases, such as cardiovascular disease (CVD; primarily heart disease and stroke), cancer, and diabetes, are among the most prevalent, costly, and preventable of all health problems. The prolonged course of illness and disability from chronic disease has resulted in extended pain and suffering and decreased quality of life for millions of Americans.

Summary of Health Insurance Plans

With the advent of the ACA, several preventative services that were not previously covered by health insurance plans are now available at no charge to the insured. The nutrition-related services are covered in Table 12–2. It is important to note that annual well-women visits (for women 65 years of age and under), well-baby visits (six visits during the first year), and well-child visits (seven visits between the ages of 1 and 4 years; annual visits for 5–17 years) to primary care physicians/pediatricians are also covered through the ACA.[28]

Indemnity (fee-for-service)

Under fee-for-service or indemnity health coverage, the insured has autonomy to choose doctors, hospitals, and other healthcare providers. The insured can refer himself to any specialist without getting permission, and the insurance company doesn't get to decide whether the visit was necessary. However, most fee-for-service medicine is managed to a certain extent. Fee-for-service plans usually involve more out-of-pocket expenses, often a deductible amount typically of about $100 to $300 a year per covered person or $500 or more per year per family, before the insurance company starts paying. Once the deductible is met, the insurer must pay approximately 80% of the doctor bills, and the policy holder will pay around 20%, which is referred to as coinsurance.[29] The insured may have to pay upfront and then submit the bill for reimbursement, or the provider may bill the insurer directly and the insurance company in turn invoices the individual. Under fee-for-service plans, insurers will usually only pay for reasonable and customary medical expenses, taking into account what other practitioners in the area charge for similar services. If the insured's doctor charges more than what the insurance company considers reasonable and customary, the insured probably has to make up the difference. Fee-for-service plans often include a ceiling for out-of-pocket expenses, after which the insurance company will pay 100% of any costs. Traditional fee-for-service coverage offers flexibility in exchange for higher out-of-pocket expenses. Of all visits made to physicians in 2016, approximately 54% were made by patients who listed private insurance as their primary expected source of payment.[5]

Managed Care

Preferred Provider Organizations

Preferred Provider Organizations (PPOs) are the least-restrictive type of managed care systems. PPOs have made arrangements for lower fees with a network of healthcare providers. PPOs give their policyholders a financial incentive to stay within that network. For example, a visit to an in-network doctor might mean that the insured would pay a $10 to $20 co-pay. If the insured wants to see an out-of-network doctor, they would have to pay the entire bill upfront and then submit the bill to the insurer for an 80% reimbursement. In addition, the insured might have to pay a deductible if they choose to go outside the network or pay the difference between what the in-network and out-of-network doctors charge. With a PPO, the insured can self-refer to a specialist without getting approval and, as long as the specialist is an in-network provider, enjoy the same co-pay. Staying within the network means less money coming out of the insured's pocket. Exclusive Provider Organizations (EPOs) are PPOs that look like **Health Maintenance Organizations** (see below). EPOs raise the financial stakes for staying in the network. The insured is responsible for the entire cost of the visit if they choose a provider outside of the network.[29]

Point-of-Service

A **Point-of-Service (POS)** plan is a less restrictive type of managed care than the PPO. Like PPOs, POS plans have made arrangements for lower fees with a network of healthcare providers and give their policyholders a financial incentive to stay within that network. However, POS plans introduce the gatekeeper or primary care physician (PCP). The insured choose their PCP from among the plan's network of doctors. As with the PPO, the insured can choose to go out of network and still get some kind of coverage. To get a referral to a specialist, one usually goes through the PCP. If the insured chooses to self-refer, he will receive less reimbursement. If the PCP refers the insured to a doctor who is out of the network, the plan should pick up most of the cost. Going outside of the network usually also results in paying a deductible. POS plans may cover additional preventive care services not covered by ACA and may also offer health improvement programs like workshops on nutrition and discounts at health clubs. Rates and coverage vary from state to state.[29]

Preferred Provider Organizations (PPO) A type of health plan that contracts with medical providers, such as hospitals and doctors, to create a network of participating providers. The insured pays less to use providers who belong to the plan's network.

Health Maintenance Organization (HMO) An organization that provides or arranges managed care for health insurance and acts as a liaison to healthcare providers (hospitals, doctors, etc.) on a prepaid basis; these providers have been paid by the HMO and are ensured consistent patients.

Point-of-Service (POS) A managed healthcare insurance plan that offers lower healthcare costs, but limited options.

Health Maintenance Organization

The HMO is the most restrictive type of managed care. Like POSs and PPOs, HMOs have made arrangements for lower fees with a network of healthcare providers and give their policyholders a financial incentive to stay within that network. HMO plans also utilize a gatekeeper PCP. The insured selects a PCP from among the HMO's physician network. HMOs require that the insured sees only doctors within their plan. Visits to a specialist occur only after referral from the insured's PCP. In general, the insured must see only HMO-approved physicians and use HMO-approved facilities, or pay the entire cost of the visit themselves. Like POSs, HMO plans generally cover more preventive care services outside of the ACA and health improvement programs. HMO coverage is a trade-off between premiums paid and plan flexibility. HMOs offer lower premiums but are restrictive when it comes to coverage.[29]

No matter which plan the insurer chooses, the ACA has ensured that every health plan must cover ambulatory patient visits, emergency services, hospitalizations (surgery and overnight stay), laboratory services, and certain prescription drugs, among other vital services.

Government Programs

Medicare

The Health Insurance for the Aged and Disabled Act (title XVIII of the Social Security Act), known as *Medicare*, has made available to nearly every American 65 years of age and older a broad program of health insurance designed to assist with hospital, medical, and other healthcare costs. Medicare is administered by the Centers for Medicare & Medicaid Services (CMS). Formerly, Medicare was administered by the Health Care Financing Administrations (HCFA). With approximately 61 million beneficiaries in 2020 and growing, Medicare is the largest healthcare insurer in the United States. In addition to assisting the elderly, Medicare was also designed to assist persons eligible for Social Security disability payment programs for more than 2 years and individuals with end-stage renal disease (ESRD: permanent kidney failure requiring dialysis or kidney transplant) with payments for medical and healthcare services. All payments ultimately come from the federal Medicare Trust Fund, which is financed by Social Security deductions from employee payrolls. Medicare coverage has two parts: A and B. Part A covers hospital-based inpatient care, skilled nursing facilities (not custodial or long term), home care, and hospice care. Part B covers physician services, outpatient hospital services, durable medical equipment, and other medical services and supplies. There is a monthly premium for individuals who choose to enroll in Part B coverage. Additionally, Medicare prescription drug coverage became available on January 1, 2006.

In order to qualify for nutrition-related services through Medicare Part B, the beneficiary must have diagnosed diabetes, kidney disease, or have had a kidney transplant in the last 36 months. Some of the nutrition-related services available include[30]:

- Intensive Behavioral Therapy for Obesity (Group): As of January 1, 2015, Medicare Part B will cover group obesity counseling, with a group considered 2–10 persons, face-to-face, and 30 minutes in length.
- **Telehealth**: Medicare Part B covers consultations or services that are provided via two-way telecommunications systems by a physician or other healthcare provider, including RDNs.
- **Medical Nutrition Therapy (MNT)** that is ordered by a physician and defined in the legislation as "nutrition diagnostic therapy and counseling services provided by a registered dietitian

Telehealth/Telenutrition The use of telecommunication, virtual health, and health information technologies to provide clinical care when distance is a barrier or when distance is warranted (e.g., illness or infection); may also be more convenient as the healthcare provider and patient can set up a time to communicate that is flexible for both parties.

Medical Nutrition Therapy (MNT) A therapeutic approach to treating medical conditions and their associated symptoms that may involve changes to diet or nutrition support and is typically administered by a registered Dietitian nutritionist (RDN) or a physician.

or nutrition professional for the purpose of managing disease." MNT includes 3 hours of basic coverage, 2 hours in follow-up years, and additional hours as deemed appropriate by the physician when the patient's condition has changed.

- Rural health clinic services and federally qualified health center services.
- Dialysis support (home and facility).
- Diabetes self-management training (DSMT)—a comprehensive. diabetes training program that includes nutrition as one component.

Those who qualify for Medicare do not need to obtain health insurance in the Healthcare Insurance Marketplace, as more preventative benefits are covered under Medicare Part B, including an initial "Welcome to Medicare" wellness visit and subsequent annual wellness visits.

The latest information on Medicare enrollment, benefits covered, and other helpful tools are available at http://www.medicare.gov, the official U.S. government site for Medicare.

Medicaid

Medicaid is the largest source of funding for medical and health-related services for people with limited income. A federally assisted program that became law in 1965, Medicaid is jointly funded by the federal and state governments (including the District of Columbia and U.S. territories) to assist states in providing medical long-term care assistance to people who meet certain eligibility criteria. Medicaid provides assistance with payment of medical care for low-income children (via the Children's Health Insurance Program, or CHIP), pregnant women, individuals with disabilities, and seniors. Each state defines eligibility, benefits, and payment schedules. (For example, in California, the program is known as *Medi-Cal.*) CMS provides Medicaid program guidelines at: https://www.medicaid.gov/index.html.[30]

Primarily, the states define and administer Medicaid programming individually. States are required to cover certain mandatory benefits and can choose to provide other optional benefits. Although nutrition services are not mentioned specifically under the mandatory or optional benefits, there are opportunities for nutrition care through inpatient and outpatient hospital settings, home health services, rural health clinics, and Certified Pediatric and Family Nurse Practitioner services, among other sites.

Medicaid programs expressly cover nutrition services, thanks to the efforts of dietitians practicing or residing in those states. States specify the credentials required for dietetic nutrition practitioners, such as whether they must be state licensed or otherwise certified, the designated setting where the service can be provided, and the number of visits allowed, appropriate code numbers to use, and level of reimbursement.

Medicare + Choice (M+C)

Medicare + Choice is also known as Medicare C and is a health coverage plan that is state licensed, certified by CMS, and offered by private insurance companies or managed care organizations (MCOs), such as HMOs. This plan is a merger of government and managed care plans. They provide at least the same benefits as Medicare Part A and Part B but may offer additional services. Under this plan, MNT for diabetes and nondialysis kidney disease can be offered by dietitians who are have a contract or employment relationship with the private insurance company or HMO. Typically, the elderly enroll in M+C programs to seek protection from costs that Medicare Part B does not cover, namely certain prescription drugs, vision, and hearing care.[31]

Health disparities Refers to the inequalities that occur in the provision of health care and access to health care across different racial, ethnic, and socioeconomic groups. Social Determinants of Health is often used when talking about *health disparities* and refers to the economic and social conditions that influence individual and group differences in health status (e.g., living and working conditions, income, job security, food insecurity, social exclusions/inclusions, race, gender, and disability).

Indian Health Service (IHS) An agency within the Department of Health and Human Services responsible for providing federal health services to American Indians and Alaskan Natives; IHS is the primary federal healthcare provider and health advocate for Indian people, and they seek for these individuals to have optimal health status.

Community-Oriented Primary Care A system of identifying and addressing the health problems of a defined population using the resources of the community and the input of health professionals and community members; the health professionals and community members "treat" the community similarly to how patients are treated individually by physicians.

To become familiar with the IHS agency and its programs, visit its website at: https://www.ihs.gov/

Representative Programs That Deliver Nutrition Services in Primary Care Settings

The Indian Health Service

American Indians and Alaska Natives (AI/AN) born today have a life expectancy that is 5.5 years less (73.0 to 78.5 years, respectively) than the United States. All races, population, and the **health disparities** that exist among these groups are numerous and staggering.[32] The **Indian Health Service (IHS)**, an agency within the DHHS, is responsible for providing federal health services to the AI/AN populations. The provision of health services to members of federally recognized tribes grew out of the special government-to-government relationship between the federal government and Indian tribes. Established in 1787, this relationship is based on Article I, Section 8 of the U.S. Constitution and has been given form and substance through numerous treaties, laws, Supreme Court decisions, and executive orders, namely the Snyder Act of 1921. The IHS is charged with upholding the federal government's obligation to promote healthy AI/AN people, communities, and cultures, and to honor and protect the inherent sovereign rights of tribes. As the principal federal healthcare provider and health advocate for indigenous populations, the goal of the IHS is to assure that comprehensive, culturally acceptable personal and public health services are available and accessible. The IHS provides health services to 2.56 million individuals who belong to more than 574 federally recognized tribes in 37 states, mostly in the western United States and Alaska. For FY 2020, Congress appropriated $6.0 billion, an increase of $1.0 billion over the previous 5 years, to help provide healthcare services to AI/AN.[33] The Affordable Care Act has helped ensure that appropriate funds are available for IHS to deliver quality, accessible care and expand the benefits offered to AI/AN populations through health insurance and Medicaid coverage.[33]

IHS services are provided directly and through tribally contracted and operated health programs at 46 hospitals, 330 clinics, and 133 health stations on or near Indian reservations. Most of the care supported by the IHS is administered through **Community-Oriented Primary Care (COPC)**, an approach to healthcare delivery that undertakes responsibility for the health of a defined population. COPC is practiced by combining epidemiologic study and social interventions with clinical care of individual patients, so that the primary care practice itself becomes a community medicine program. Both the individual patient and the community in which the patient lives are the foci of diagnosis, treatment, and ongoing surveillance.

The IHS employs over 15,000 people, including members of virtually every discipline involved in providing health care, social, and environmental health services. RDNs and others who have health-related degrees have the option of joining the IHS as civil servants or as commissioned officers in the Public Health Service (PHS).[33]

Preventive measures involving environmental, educational, and outreach activities are combined with therapeutic measures into a single national health system. The same is true within the IHS. Within these broad categories are special initiatives in traditional medicine, elder care, women's health, children and adolescents, injury prevention, domestic violence and child abuse, healthcare financing, state health care, sanitation facilities, and oral health. Two examples of preventative efforts through the IHS are its Health Promotion and Disease Prevention (HPDP) program and the IHS Comprehensive School Health Program. HPDP seeks to increase the health of individuals served by the IHS in five primary focus areas: diabetes, nutrition, obesity, physical activity, and tobacco cessation.[34] The IHS Comprehensive School Health Program focuses on increased healthy eating choices and physical activity, as well as

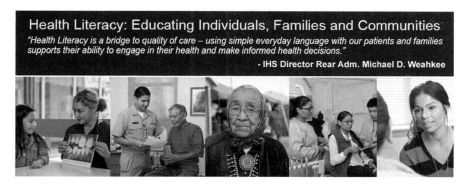

Health Literacy: Educating Individuals, Families and Communities

"Health Literacy is a bridge to quality of care – using simple everyday language with our patients and families supports their ability to engage in their health and make informed health decisions."

- IHS Director Rear Adm. Michael D. Weahkee

Indian Health Service: Diabetes Standard of Care and Practice Resource: Youth and Type 2 Diabetes. Updated 2020. Available online at: https://www.ihs.gov/diabetes/clinician-resources/soc/youth-and -type-2-diabetes

improved mental and oral health, among schools and Head Start program on or near reservations.[35]

Most IHS funds are appropriated for American Indians who live on or near reservations. Congress also authorizes programs that provide some access to care for Indians who live in urban areas rather than on reservations or in Alaska Native villages. The National Council of Urban Indian Health was founded in 1998 to meet the unique healthcare needs of the urban Indian population through education, training, and advocacy. Title V of Public Law 94-437, the *Indian Health Care Improvement Act of 1976*, authorizes the appropriation of funds for urban Indian Health Organizations. Title V funds are but one source of funding for urban Indian health organizations. Urban Indian primary care clinics and outreach programs provide culturally acceptable, accessible, affordable, and accountable health services to an underserved off-reservation urban Indian population. These urban health organizations engage in a variety of activities, ranging from the provision of outreach and referral services to the delivery of comprehensive ambulatory health care.

The IHS's *Patient Education Protocols and Codes (PEPC)* were developed to standardize the provision of health services and documentation of patient education encounters from one health professional to another. Among the nutrition-related topics included in the manual are bariatric surgery, breastfeeding, celiac disease, chronic kidney disease, chronic obstructive pulmonary disease (COPD), eating disorders, electrolyte imbalance, formula feeding, pancreatitis, and nutritional/herbal supplements. For every chronic disease, there is typically a code for the condition, followed by MNT for Medical Nutrition Therapy. One example is cancer (CA): CA-MNT.

Type 2 Diabetes—an Epidemic among American Indian/Alaskan Native Populations

We already know that AI/AN populations are subject to astounding health disparities, and this is reflected in their rate of mortality from both chronic conditions and other causes, such as assault/homicide, intentional self-harm/ suicide, and unintentional injuries. The AI/AN also die at higher rates of chronic liver disease/cirrhosis, diseases of the heart, and chronic lower respiratory disease, among other conditions, compared with all other races.[37]

Type 2 diabetes has been an issue of particular concern in the AI/AN community[38]:

- AI/AN adults have a three times higher likelihood of diagnosed diabetes compared with non-Hispanic whites.

Strategy Tip

Dietitians and nutritionists who belong to the Indian Health Service should be culturally competent. What is meant by culturally competent?

The 21st edition of the IHS's *Patient Education Protocols and Codes* manual is still the most recent and is available online at[36]: https://www.ihs.gov/healthed /index.cfm/patientedprotocols/. Check for future updates.

- AI/AN youth aged 10–19 years have a nine times higher likelihood of diagnosed type 2 diabetes compared with non-Hispanic whites.
- All AI/AN populations have a 2.5 times higher death rate due to diabetes compared with non-Hispanic whites.
- For those AI/AN adults with diabetes, there is a 2.4 times higher incidence rate of diabetes-related kidney failure (ESRD) compared with the general U.S. population.

The Special Diabetes Program for Indians (SDPI) resulted from the identification that type 2 diabetes warranted specific interventions in the AI/AN community. Each year, Congress appropriates $150 million to fulfill the goals of the SDPI. Focused primarily on adults, the SDPI enhanced prevention and treatment services at IHS, Tribal and Urban Indian health settings, allowed the creation of new initiatives to address the epidemic, and improved monitoring of diabetes care and diabetes health-related outcomes.[39] The first year, 2020, since the program's inception in 1997 that the SDPI could report to Congress a lower prevalence of diabetes, mortality from diabetes, and kidney failure related to diabetes; fewer hospitalizations for uncontrolled diabetes; and fewer cases of diabetic eye disease, proving that concerted prevention efforts among vulnerable populations can produce favorable outcomes over time.

Primary prevention efforts by primary healthcare professionals are recommended in two arenas: 1) general community health promotion and health education, and 2) activities in the primary care clinic. Clinically based health promotion activities should not duplicate communitywide health promotion but instead should offer additive benefits. For example, if significant health education is offered at the community level, motivational interviewing and collaborative problem solving can be offered in the clinical setting. Current evidence suggests that modifiable risks for type 2 diabetes mellitus include obesity, which is caused by a lack of physical activity and poor diet. Primary prevention efforts can focus on the prevention of obesity, as is the primary objective of several nonprofit programs targeting improved eating habits and increased physical activity. An example of these efforts is programming through the Partnership for a Healthier America (PHA), a nonprofit entity devoted to transforming the food landscape in pursuit of health equity. Components include: *Veggies Early and Often*, aimed at promoting vegetable consumption at an early age; *Healthy Hunger Relief*, working with food banks to address food insecurity; *FNV (Fruits N Vegetables)* marketing and advertising campaign; and the *Healthier Campus Initiative*, to promote healthy eating and physical activity on college and university campuses.

Preventing obesity in women of childbearing age is another primary prevention goal, because a diabetic pregnancy places the fetus at increased risk of future onset of diabetes. In addition, the mother who has had gestational diabetes is at higher risk for future onset diabetes.

Recognizing the importance of tailoring guidance and initiatives to AI/AN youth, the IHS Division of Diabetes Treatment and Prevention developed best practice guidelines for working with youth type 2 diabetes prevention and treatment. These recommendations are intended for healthcare organizations and communities that serve youth (ages 2–18) who are at risk for or have type 2 diabetes. The best practices can be used by a variety of stakeholders, including primary healthcare teams, educators, community and school workers, and healthcare leaders. **Table 12–4** and **Figure 12–1** highlights some of the key recommendations set forth by the Division.[39]

The IHS Standards of Care for Patients with Type 2 Diabetes was developed and updated by the IHS National Diabetes Program and Area Diabetes Consultants to help provide consistent, quality care to AI/AN patients with

> The PHA program is an expansion of the popular government program, *Let's Move!* created by former first lady, Michelle Obama.[40]

TABLE 12–4
Summary of Evidence-Based Best Practices for AI/AN Youth At-Risk or Living with Type 2 Diabetes*

- Test overweight (BMI >85th percentile) AI/AN youth with any of the following risk factors:
  — Family history of diabetes.
  — Signs of insulin resistance or conditions associated with it (e.g., acanthosis nigricans, PCOS, hypertension, dyslipidemia, small-for-gestational-age (SGA) or large-for-gestational-age (LGA) birth weight).
  — Maternal history of diabetes or gestational diabetes during child's gestation.
- Start testing these higher risk children at age 10 years (or younger if puberty occurs earlier).
- Test at-risk children ≤ every 3 years.
- Glycemic control targets for youth with type 2 diabetes are:
  — A1C < 8% for ages 6 to 12 years
  — A1C < 7.5% for ages 13 to 19 years.
- The only FDA-approved diabetes medications for use in children are metformin and insulin. While other medications are sometimes used in clinical practice, there is less evidence to support their use, and that use would be off-label.

Indian Health Service: Diabetes Standard of Care and Practice Resource: Youth and Type 2 Diabetes. Updated 2020. Available online at: https://www.ihs.gov/diabetes/clinician-resources/soc/youth-and-type-2-diabetes
*Not inclusive of blood pressure and kidney health recommendations.

diabetes. The IHS Diabetes Program supports that those with diabetes should be referred to the RDN for MNT and education or counseling at diagnosis and at least annually. Some people may require more frequent evaluation and counseling.

Health Resources and Services Administration, Bureau of Primary Health Care

The Health Resources and Services Administration (HRSA), an agency of the U.S. DHHS, is the primary federal agency for improving access to healthcare services for people who are uninsured, isolated, or medically vulnerable. HRSA's five bureaus and 11 offices provide leadership and financial support to healthcare providers in every state and U.S. territory. HRSA grantees provide health care to uninsured people; people who are geographically isolated; people living with HIV/AIDS; and pregnant women, mothers, and children. In order to accomplish their strategic goals, HRSA focuses on training health professionals, connecting them to vulnerable populations,

1. Screening for overweight and obesity in all youth.
2. Test for prediabetes and diabetes in all at-risk youth.
3. Use healthy eating and physical activity guidelines for youth.
4. Implement an education and prevention/treatment program for youth who are overweight, obese, have prediabetes, or have diabetes.
5. Engage families in the planning and implementation of the youth and type 2 diabetes prevention and treatment programs.
6. Maintain normal blood glucose in all pregnant women with diabetes.
7. Promote breast-feeding of infants for at least 2 months by all postpartum women.

FIGURE 12–1 Summary of Evidence-Based Best Practices for AI/AN Youth at Risk or Living With Type 2 Diabetes.

Indian Health Service, Division of Diabetes Treatment and Prevention: Indian Health Diabetes Best Practices, Youth and Type 2 Diabetes Prevention and Treatment (2011, addendum 2014). Accessed November 23, 2015. Available online at: http://www.ihs.gov/MedicalPrograms/Diabetes/HomeDocs/Tools/BestPractices/2011_BP_Youth_T2DM_508c.pdf and improving systems of care, including virtual health opportunities and improved Internet bandwidth in rural communities. The HSRA budget projected for FY 2021 is $11.2 billion (Note that federal fiscal year, FY, begins October 1st and ends September 30th.), and this allocation will be used to advance the core goals of this office[41]:

- Improve access to quality health services
- Foster a healthcare workforce able to address current and emerging needs
- Achieve health equity and enhance population health
- Optimize HRSA Operations and strengthen program management

In the following section, the HRSA Bureau of Primary Health Care will be discussed and linked to other healthcare programming intended to alleviate the burden of vulnerable populations.

Bureau of Primary Health Care

Community health centers offer "one-stop shopping" where primary and preventive healthcare visits, lab services, dental and mental health services, and case management are conveniently located, coordinated, and tailored to meet the patient's needs. Ideally, community health center staff and providers are as diverse as the patients they serve; many are bilingual and residents of the community. Since 2000, the number of patients served by community health centers has grown annually from 9.6 million to nearly 30 million in 2020—a 210% increase over 20 years.[41]

Technically known as **Federally Qualified Health Centers (FQHCs)**, community health centers employ nonprofit healthcare providers that serve the communities in which they are located. Almost 1,400 health centers serve as the medical home for patients, and one out of every 12 people living in the United States utilizes one of these centers for primary care in nearly all U.S. states and associated territories (Washington, D.C., Puerto Rico, the Virgin Islands, and the Pacific Basin).[42]

FQHCs were established in the 1960s as part of the federal government's "War on Poverty." In particular, HRSA's primary healthcare programs have their roots in the Migrant Health Act of 1962 and the Economic Opportunity Act of 1964, which established funding for the first community-based clinics. The founders saw quality, personalized medical care as a right of all people and established a policy that no patient would be turned away, regardless of their ability to pay. FQHCs are "by the community, for the community, of the community."[43] Federal law requires that every FQHS have a Board of Directors and that more than half of the Board members must be patients of that center.

Health center patients are among the nation's most vulnerable populations and are people who, even if insured, would nonetheless remain isolated from traditional forms of medical care because of where they live, who they are, the language they speak, and their complex healthcare needs. About half of health center patients reside in rural areas, while the other half tends to live in economically depressed, inner city communities. Health centers serve one in five low-income children. Approximately two-thirds of health center patients have family incomes at or below the U.S. poverty level ($26,300 annual income for a family of four in 2020). Moreover, nearly one in five patients at FQHCs are uninsured and approximately 1.4 million of the 30 million served are considered homeless.[42]

In summary, an FQHC is a community health center that has been designated by the federal government as adhering to regulations pertaining to the scope and quality of health services provided to anyone, regardless of their ability to pay. Similarly, an *FQHC Look Alike* is a health center that has been identified by the Health Resources and Services Administration (HRSA) and

Federally Qualified Health Centers (FQHC) Reimbursement designation significant for several health programs funded (by Bureau of Primary Healthcare and CMS) under the Health Center Consolidation Act (Section 330 of the Public Health Service Act), including: community health centers, Migrant Health Program, Public Housing Primary Care Program, and Healthcare for the Homeless Program. FQHCs provide comprehensive primary care services.

Locations of FQHCs can be found at: http://findahealthcenter.hrsa.gov

certified by the Centers for Medicare and Medicaid Services as meeting the definition of "health center," although it does not receive grant funding from the federal government. These clinics are reimbursed by Medicaid for their services.[42]

There are benefits of being an FQHC, and one of these advantages is increased funding opportunities. The Community Health Center Fund, a 5-year, $11 billion initiative to operate, expand, and construct health centers throughout the nation, was made possible through the ACA. The majority of the funding ($9.5 billion) is reserved for creating new sites in **Medically Underserved Areas** (MUAs) and increasing the number of preventative services related to oral and behavioral health, as well as pharmacies. The remainder of the funding ($1.5 million) is appropriated for construction and renovation projects at existing FQHCs. In 2019, S. 106/H.R. 2328: Community Health Investment, Modernization, and Excellence (CHIME) Act was introduced in the House as a proposal to reauthorize and extend the Community Health Center Fund through FY 2024.[44-46]

Other benefits for FQHCs included: enhanced Medicare and Medicaid reimbursement, medical malpractice coverage through the Federal Tort Claims Act, eligibility to purchase prescription and nonprescription medications for outpatients at reduced cost, access to National Health Service Corps, and eligibility for various other federal grants and programs. Overall, FQHCs in general reduce costs to health systems and reduce the likelihood that patients will need to use expensive care providers, such as emergency departments and inpatient hospital stays.[45]

Each FQHC that receives Public Health Service (PHS) 330 grant funding must meet the requirements of that grant. Community Health Centers must serve a MUA or Medically Underserved Population (MUP). To determine if an area qualifies, search the MUA/MUP database at: http://muafind.hrsa.gov/. If an area does not have the MUA/MUP designation, it can apply for that, as well as for PHS Section 330 grant funding while the designation is being processed. Migrant Health Centers, Health Care for the Homeless, and Public Housing Primary Care Programs do not need to meet the MUA/MUP qualification.[47]

FQHCs offer health care to every member of the family throughout the lifespan. Nutrition is a component of many of the comprehensive support services offered by health centers, including:

- Primary care
- Prenatal care
- Outpatient diabetes self-management training
- MNT for diabetes/renal disease
- Neonatal home visits
- Nutrition assessment and referral
- Blood pressure and cholesterol screening
- Preventative health education
- Well-childcare and screenings
- Expanded virtual health offerings

Other services provided include: dental services, immunizations, social services and case management, family planning, treatment and referrals, pharmacy services, lab testing, 12-step cancer and other health screenings, childbirth flu clinics, transportation, medical interpretation, eye exams, podiatric services, clinical breast exams and mammography referrals, and comprehensive HIV care, including outreach education, prevention, and treatment. As of 2015, the ACA allowed for additional funds targeted to the provision and staffing of mental health services (Integrated Behavioral Health Service Awards) and substance abuse services.[47]

Medically Underserved Areas/Populations Areas or populations designated by the U.S. Health Resources Service Administration (HRSA) as having too few primary care providers, high infant mortality, high poverty, or a high elderly population. Often associated with Health Professional Shortage Areas (HPSAs) or areas/facilities where there are shortages of primary medical care, dental, or mental health providers.

Strategy Tip

Read more about grants and grant writing in Chapter 15.

Patient-Centered Medical Homes A model or philosophy of organizing primary care into a multidisciplinary, team-based approach to allow for better communication and coordination of care; focused on meeting the needs of the patient "right where they are"; significant emphasis on quality and safety.

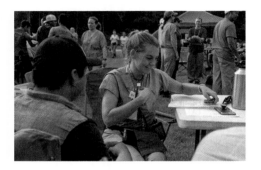

The Migrant Health Program differentiates America from other countries, where the very poor are given healthcare.

Centers for Disease Control and Prevention.

Migrant Health Program Provides support to health centers so that they can provide appropriate and comprehensive preventative and primary health care to migratory and seasonal agriculture workers and their families; focuses on the occupational health and safety needs of this population.

The healthcare delivery model used in the community health center has been described as the *patient-centered medical home* (PCMH). This model seeks to 1) strengthen the provider-patient relationship and 2) replace episodic care based on illness with coordinated care based on prevention. The physician-led PCMH team approach provides for all of the patient's healthcare needs and, when necessary, arranges for referrals to specialists outside of the practice. Across all healthcare avenues, the PCMH became more widely utilized in 2008 when the National Committee for Quality Assurance (NCQA) determined standards for Physician Practice Connections-**Patient-Centered Medical Homes** (PPC-PCMH). Last updated in 2017, these standards also included a recognition system for high-functioning PCMHs.[48] Research on PCMHs has shown that this model improves quality of care, better management of chronic conditions, patient experience, and staff satisfaction while also reducing healthcare costs. More recent guidelines and related funding have focused on improved patient access through virtual visits and after-hours care.[49]

Migrant Health Centers

Since 1962, the Federal **Migrant Health Program (MHP)** has provided grants to community nonprofit organizations for a broad array of medical and support services to migrant and seasonal farm workers and their families.[46] The MHP was originally authorized by the Migrant Health Act, Public Law 87-692, enacted in September 1962 and is currently authorized under section 330(g) of the Public Health Service Act. The vision of the MHP is the universal accessibility to quality and appropriate health care for the nation's migrant and seasonal farm workers (MSFW) and their families. The MHP provides MSFWs and their families' access to comprehensive, culturally competent, primary care services. The MHP supports the delivery of migrant health services including primary and preventive health care, transportation, outreach, dental, pharmaceutical, occupational health and safety, and environmental health. These programs use bilingual and bicultural lay outreach workers and health personnel, as well as culturally sensitive appropriate protocols. They also provide prevention-oriented and pediatric services such as immunizations, well-baby care, and developmental screenings. HRSA FQHCs partner to serve the migrant and seasonal farm worker population of which one million plus workers benefited from health center program care in 2019. Of those recipients, over 75% are living at 100% and below the poverty line.[50]

Public Housing Primary Care Program

According to the U.S. Department of Housing and Urban Development (HUD), there were 10.4 million households living in public housing in 2019, an increase of roughly 8 million since 2015.[51] The individuals residing in public housing are some of our most vulnerable—nearly 68% are seniors, children, or people with disabilities and many credit social security as their primary source of income.

The United States Housing Act of 1937 (P.L. 75-412) created the public housing program. The Act is also known as the Wagner-Steagall Housing Act and the Low-Rent Housing Act. Under the program, the federal government, through the HUD, provides subsidies to local public housing agencies that rent housing to low-income families. Public housing was established to provide decent and safe rental housing for eligible low-income families, the elderly, and persons with disabilities. HUD administers federal aid to local housing agencies that manage the housing for low-income people and also furnishes technical and professional assistance in planning, developing, and managing these developments. Approximately 7 million people live in public housing units.

The **Public Housing Primary Care (PHPC) Program** is a federal grant program created under the Disadvantaged Minority Health Improvement Act of 1990. In 1996, the PHPC Program was reauthorized under the Health Centers Consolidation Act as Section 330(i) of the Public Health Service Act. The PHPC is administered by HRSA, under the same bureau as community health centers. The mission of PHPC is to provide accessible comprehensive primary health care and supportive services in order to improve the overall health and well-being of the public housing community and to eliminate health disparities.

The PHPC Program supports health centers and other health delivery systems in providing services in partnership with other community-based providers of public housing developments or at other locations immediately accessible to residents of public housing. PHPC grantees provide primary healthcare services, including direct medical care, health screening and education, dental, prenatal and perinatal, preventive health, and case management; conduct outreach services to inform residents about health services availability; aid residents in establishing eligibility for assistance under entitlement programs and obtaining government support for health care, mental and oral health, or social services; and train and employ residents of public housing to provide health screenings and health education services.

PHPC health centers have an integrated approach to delivering primary health care, health promotion, and disease prevention. Each PHPC program provides comprehensive primary healthcare services, including internal medicine, pediatrics, OB/GYN care, preventive and restorative dental care, health education, outreach, laboratory services, and case management. Many PHPC health centers also provide behavioral health services, pharmacy, X-ray, optometry, and podiatry, along with nutritional services through the Women, Infants, and Children (WIC) program.[49]

In FY 2018, 106 PHPC grantees were awarded program funds to provide primary healthcare services. HRSA-funded health centers served nearly 2.7 million residents of public housing. The physical and social health of this population is not ideal. Over one-third of those receiving care as a result of a PHPC grant self-reported as being in "poor health," and 71 % were classified as overweight or obese. A majority of these individuals are **Medicaid** recipients and closer to two-thirds live below the federal poverty line. Among primary diagnoses for PHPC patients, the top three were nutrition-related: hypertension, overweight and obesity, and diabetes mellitus, thereby demonstrating the need for nutrition services in this federally sponsored initiative.[50] (https://nchph.org/wp-content/uploads/2019/02/Intro-to-NCHPH-Fact-Sheet.pdf)

Health Care for the Homeless

In the United States, approximately 567,000 people are homeless on any given night. In 2019, almost 400,000 were individuals living without a family and 35,000 were children living unattended. Most of the homeless population lives in one of the following states or U.S. territories: Washington, D.C.; Guam: New York; Hawaii; or California (new reference). The definitions for this population vary, but the U.S. HHS defines **homelessness** as the following:

An individual who lacks housing (regard to whether the individual is a member of the family), including an individual whose primary residence during the night is a supervised public or private facility (e.g.) shelters that provide temporary living accommodations, and individual who is a resident in transitional housing." – Section 330 (h)(4)(A).[52]

Public Housing Primary Care Program Provides residents of public housing with increased access to comprehensive primary healthcare services; services are provided at public housing developments or at other locations immediately accessible to residents.

Medicaid A joint federal and state program that helps low-income individuals or families pay for the costs associated with long-term medical and custodial care, provided they qualify. Medicaid is administered by each state, thus coverage may vary.

Homelessness Condition of people without a regular dwelling; often unable to acquire and maintain regular, safe, secure and adequate housing or lack "fixed, regular, and adequate night-time residence"; may reside during the night in a public or private facility or in transitional housing.

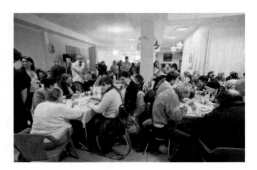

The homeless could benefit from more healthcare.

© Radiokafka/Shutterstock.

Discussion Prompt

What are some barriers to the homeless getting healthcare?

Healthcare for the Homeless Program HRSA grantee program that recognizes the unique needs of homeless persons, focusing on provision of coordinated and comprehensive health care; often includes substance abuse and mental health services.

Homeless people have the same health problems as people with secure housing but get sick with common illnesses much more often than people who are housed. Research has demonstrated that those without homes die an average of 30 years earlier than those in homes.[53,54] First, poor health can lead to homelessness since those who are unable to work because of illness or injury may not have income for housing or to pay their medical bills. Without a home, there is no place to recuperate from an illness or to treat an injury, and health problems tend to get far worse before they get better. Compared with people with housing, the homeless have higher rates of mental illness (approximately one-third of people without homes are mentally ill), current or past drug or alcohol addiction (about one-half), and communicable diseases such as HIV/AIDS and tuberculosis. Infections of every sort are prominent among homeless people, as is trauma resulting from violence and conditions caused by exposure to the elements. Furthermore, medications to help manage or prevent health issues are often not available, lost, or stolen from others.[54]

The HRSA-funded **Health Care for the Homeless (HCH) Program** is a major source of care for homeless persons in the United States, serving patients who live on the street, in shelters, or in transitional housing. In 2017, these health centers served nearly 1.4 million persons experiencing homelessness across 200 health centers in 50 states. As a result of the COVID-19 pandemic, HCH was also able to facilitate 170 COVID-19 testing sites for homeless individuals across the country and in high-demand areas.[52] Programs that deliver primary health care to people without a permanent domicile must be multidisciplinary, as homeless people often have serious, multiple diagnoses. HCH provides primary health care, including diagnosis and treatment for common illnesses, as well as addiction treatment and mental health services. Services such as access to specialty care, transportation, housing, and medical respite care are also part of HCH's provisions. There are HCH programs in every state, the District of Columbia, and Puerto Rico and nearly all major cities in the United States have at least one HCH program.[55] HCH programs are primarily funded by grants from HRSA but also from state and local governments and donations.

Throughout this chapter, it has already been demonstrated that the ACA has made healthcare to vulnerable populations a priority item. The homeless are no exception. The ACA has changed healthcare delivery for homeless persons and people at-risk of becoming homeless by prioritizing the following items[56]:

- Expanding access to affordable healthcare through the Marketplace and Medicaid (for those at-risk)
- Providing better transition care for those persons leaving the homeless environment, including behavioral health care, rehabilitative services, and tenancy supports
- Better coordination of healthcare services with housing and social services that serve the homeless populations

Providers of health care for the homeless need to establish markers of successful outcomes that are unique to the realities of the homeless existence. Seven client-level outcomes have been posited as goals for federally funded HCH projects. Although related, the client-level outcomes can be measured independently of one another. These are improved health status, improved level of functioning, improved quality of life, involvement in treatment, disease self-management, client choice, and client satisfaction.[57]

Special homeless populations, including youth and veterans, are able to use HCH's services. For youth, parental consent is often required, and obtaining this can be a challenge. Veterans are also able to use the Health

Care for Homeless Veterans Program, administered by the Department of Veterans Affairs (VA).

The National Health Care for the Homeless Council (NHCHC) (http://www.nhchc.org/) provides technical assistance to communities trying to obtain HRSA grants or to organizations without federal support. Federal grants are only a fraction of the amount required to create a well-rounded program. For that reason, the NHCHC offers technical assistance and training all stakeholders, including HRSA grantees, educational institutions, and primary care. By working in conjunction with the HRSA, the NHCHC is the pulse for what is happening in the homeless community and determines areas of focus related to the care of homeless persons. For example, the NHCHC had 10 areas of focus in 2015, and those related to primary care include: access to quality health services; building the skills of community healthcare workers; caring for transgendered and gender-nonconforming individuals; legislative advocacy; rural homelessness, including introduction of mobile health services and Telehealth; prevention and care of traumatic brain injury (TBI) in the homeless community; and medical respite care. Medical respite care is also known as recuperative care and is acute and post-acute medical care for homeless persons who are significantly frail and ill, living on the streets, but not sick enough to be in the hospital.[58]

Lack of access to healthy food or enough food to meet energy needs is one more reason why the homeless are plagued by suboptimal health and wellness. There are some provisions in place, however, to ensure that the homeless receive adequate food and nutrition. For example, the homeless are eligible for Supplemental Nutrition Assistance Program (SNAP) or food stamp benefits, even if they do not have a permanent mailing address. In fact, homeless persons have identical rights under the SNAP/Food Stamp Program as persons who are housed, and they also have some additional rights due to the fact that they are homeless.[33] They can use these benefits at grocery stores, farmer's markets or at shelters or soup kitchens where monetary donations are preferred, but not required. Some restaurants will accept SNAP benefits from the homeless as well. Despite this significant benefit, a majority of homeless persons do not take advantage of SNAP for various reasons, including: lack of transportation, lack of knowledge about the program, mental illness, and lack of documentation (photo ID) are some of the common barriers that prevent homeless people from receiving SNAP/Food Stamps.[59]

Many homeless people rely on shelters and soup kitchens for their food intake. For children, additional sources of food are the National School Lunch Program and the School Breakfast Program, as well as the Summer Food Service Program at community sites (churches, libraries, Boys and Girls' Clubs, etc.). Referral to the appropriate USDA food assistance program is one of the most important services we can provide to individuals and families who are homeless.

Summary

Providing quality, comprehensive, affordable primary care is multifaceted, involving many key healthcare professionals, resources, agencies, and funding. Without these factors in place, it becomes difficult to provide primary care to everyone, particularly those populations that are most vulnerable. Several U.S. government agencies have put laws and initiatives in place to alleviate the barriers associated with obtaining preventative care. Healthy People 2030, the Agency for Healthcare Research and Quality, the U.S. Preventative Services Task Force, the Patient Protection and Affordable Care Act, and the Health Resources Service Administration, among others, have provided evidence-based rationale for prioritizing certain preventative measures. They have also worked collectively to develop best practices, creative programming, and health promotion initiatives to help American adults and children to reach optimal health.

While coverage of preventative services has improved significantly with the advent of the Affordable Care Act (ACA), several barriers to primary care provision still exist. Physicians are bound to marked time constraints and lack of training in all areas of preventative care, including nutrition. Less training and education translate to a lack of confidence on the part of the physician to provide suitable nutrition counseling and education. RDNs are not always available to provide nutrition services and/or their services may not be reimbursed by insurance. Even with the expansion of benefits provided under the ACA for all healthcare plans, plus the medical nutrition therapy benefits outlined for Medicare recipients, it remains that some necessary nutrition care may need to be paid for out-of-pocket by the patient. Chronic disease management would be lacking tremendously without nutrition as part of primary care.

In the case of vulnerable populations, such as the AI/AN population, which suffers from high rates of diabetes, obesity, and heart disease, the poor who rely on public housing and other community-based services, and the homeless, who are already prone to greater health issues because they are without a home, preventing and managing disease is extremely challenging. Even with the resources available to these groups through the U.S. government and nonprofit organizations, the vulnerable still face unique obstacles in the healthcare system.

Given the advances that have been made in primary care, even within the last 10 years, particularly with regard to programming, funding, and technology, especially virtual health modalities accelerated by the COVID-19 pandemic, it makes sense that future years will embrace even more valuable provisions to help all Americans to achieve the health they desire. It will continue to take great collaboration from stakeholders, as well as adequate funding, but the fact remains that primary care is a progressive concept and a timeless priority.

Learning Portfolio

© olies/Shutterstock.

Issues for Discussion

1. In this chapter, it was explained that there has been an accelerated use of tele-health and telenutrition due to the COVID-19 pandemic. Prior to the pandemic, telemedicine was slowly adopted by patients and practitioners alike. Do you think this accelerated use of virtual and audio services will continue and take the place of most in-person interactions? What are the pros of using telehealth? What are some of the cons?

2. Physicians play an important role in nutrition, particularly when an RDN is not available. Considering what was discussed regarding barriers to delivering primary care, do you think the expectations are reasonable for physicians when it comes to providing nutrition-related and other preventative care measures? How do you suggest that physicians best utilize their limited time to confront nutrition issues?

3. Despite major efforts by government agencies and professional organizations, Americans continue to be plagued by chronic disease, including obesity, diabetes, and heart disease. Why do you think Americans still struggle with preventing these diseases? Can screening and education ever be effective in the absence of patient motivation? Furthermore, children are one of the highest utilizers of well-visits and preventative care. How can preventative care in childhood better translate to healthier adults?

4. The Affordable Care Act made huge strides in reforming U.S. healthcare. In your opinion, what else still needs to happen in order to improve our healthcare system?

5. Now that you have learned about community health centers, including popula-tions served, funding, services provided, and location, what do you feel is most key to success in a community health center environment? Is there anything else that community health centers should be doing in order to be more successful, particularly as telemedicine options become more available?

6. Government agencies and nonprofits provide healthcare services to the home-less. Even with these resources, the homeless are subject to other issues that may prevent them from receiving healthcare. Can homeless persons really ever improve their health without confronting the other issues exacerbated by homelessness?

Student Activities

1. Consider a popular nutrition topic that could be impactful in working with patients in a primary care setting. For this topic, develop your own version of the "5-3-2-1-Almost None" messaging or an acronym like WAVE that will help physicians to convey the important points of the topic to patients when time is limited.

2. Visit the Healthcare.gov coverage website: https://www.healthcare.gov/get-coverage/. Click on the link to "See Plans and Prices." Answer the required questions about your healthcare needs. Reflect on the experience of seeking out healthcare coverage online. What surprised you about the options available? Did you feel the site and directions were easy to navigate? Do you think someone who has issues with literacy or someone who has limited computer skills would still be able to use this site without assistance? Why or why not?

3. Examine your own health insurance offerings. What nutrition-related services are available through your health plan? Is there a co-pay involved? What are the limitations?

4. Tour and visit a community health center at a nearby location. How does this facility receive funding? What services are offered? What is the primary demo-graphic makeup of patients at the facility? Is accessibility suitable for those utilizing public transportation? Or, if the site is rural, are options provided

Key Terms

Term	page
Patient-centered care	368
Medicare	370
Healthcare quality	371
Affordable Care Act (ACA)	372
Indemnity insurance	377
Population-based medicine	377
Chronic disease management	377
Chronic Care Model (CCM)	379
Group visits or Shared medical appointments (SMAs)	379
Preferred Provider Organizations (PPO)	381
Health Maintenance Organization (HMO)	381
Point-of-Service (POS)	381
Telehealth/Telenutrition	382
Medical Nutrition Therapy (MNT)	382
Health disparities	384
Indian Health Service (IHS)	384
Community-Oriented Primary Care	384
Federally Qualified Health Centers (FQHC)	388
Medically Underserved Areas/Populations	389
Patient-Centered Medical Homes	390
Migrant Health Program	390
Public Housing Primary Care Program	391
Medicaid	391
Homelessness	391
Healthcare for the Homeless Program	392

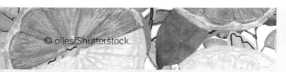
© olles/Shutterstock.

Learning Portfolio

(i.e., telehealth or mobile van) for those who may have issues with getting to the physical location of the health center?

5. Volunteer with meals or food distribution at a local homeless shelter or transitional housing unit and meet with a case manager or healthcare professional. Discuss with the case manager/healthcare professional the issues that homeless persons face in obtaining healthcare. What issues are most prevalent? How are they resolved? What happens when a homeless person's health issues are outside of the shelter or community health center's scope of care?

Case Study 1: Pregnant in Public Housing

Katherine is a 23-year-old female who resides in a public housing complex on the Southside of Chicago, Illinois. Katherine lives with her mother, grandmother, sister, and her sister's two children in a two-bedroom apartment. Currently, Katherine works full-time as a clerk at the local gas station and does some babysitting for the neighborhood kids on the weekends. Her income helps to support the entire family. She is hoping to apply to the local community college for the upcoming fall semester.

Last week, Katherine missed her period and took a pregnancy test to find out that she is expecting. Although this news did not come at a great time as Katherine was separating from the baby's father, she is planning to have the baby and wants to start prenatal care as soon as possible.

Katherine has not been to the doctor's in almost 8 years because she does not have health insurance. Her sister never received care while pregnant with her two children, but Katherine knows that she needs a primary care physician to help her to get healthy for the baby. Already, Katherine is at a greater risk because of her BMI of 30, which is classified as obese, as well as her history of heavy drinking. Katherine vows that she wants to quit drinking, learn to eat a healthy diet, and start taking 15-minute walks each day. Katherine's family cannot afford Internet or smart phones and the nearest library is 15 minutes away; therefore, she does not have the means to look up any information online that might help her to get started on her goals.

On her way home from work, Katherine notices that her neighborhood has a new community health center, and she decides to stop in and make an appointment for the next week.

When Katherine meets with the primary care physician the next week, she receives a test to confirm the pregnancy (she is 6 weeks pregnant) and also has blood drawn for labs. The doctor is concerned, as her fasting blood glucose is 125 mg/dL, which is well over the normal fasting level (70 mg/dl or <). She also has elevated blood pressure. Both of these situations put Katherine at a high risk for complications during pregnancy.

Please answer the following questions based on Katherine's case:

1. Currently, Katherine does not have health coverage; however, because she is low-income, pregnant, and works for a small business that does not provide healthcare coverage, which of the following two insurance options is viable for Katherine, even if a small fee is required?

    a. Medicare Part B or an HMO.

    b. HMOs or private insurance through the healthcare.gov marketplace.

    c. Medicaid or private insurance through the healthcare.gov marketplace.

    d. Medicare + Choice (M+C) or Medicare Part B.

2. The physician working with Katherine refers her to a dietitian at the health center who only works part-time. Coordinating Katherine's schedule with the dietitian's has been very difficult. Which of the following is the BEST option for Katherine so that she can learn more about how to improve her nutrition status during pregnancy?

    a. An online telenutrition session with the RDN.

    b. A shared medical appointment with expectant mothers at the health center, offered four times weekly.

    c. RDN will visit Katherine at her home at Katherine's convenience.

    d. Katherine can miss work to meet with the RDN because it is so important.

3. Katherine learns that the new community health center in her neighborhood was funded by a grant from the government. Which government agency and division likely funded this health center?

    a. Health Resources and Services Administration: Bureau of Primary Health Care.

    b. Centers for Disease Control and Prevention: National Center for Chronic Disease Prevention and Health Promotion.

    c. United States Department of Agriculture: Food and Nutrition Service.

    d. Agency for Healthcare Research and Quality: Center for Quality Improvement and Patient Safety.

4. The Patient Care and Affordable Care Act (ACA) made it possible for adults, women, and children to receive certain nutrition-related preventative services for free. Based on what we know about Katherine's current health status and her health goals, which of the following group of services should Katherine consider receiving FIRST:

    a. Obesity screening and counseling, osteoporosis screening, and cholesterol screening.

    b. Gestational diabetes screening, breastfeeding comprehensive support and counseling, and anemia screening.

    c. Obesity screening and counseling, diabetes (type 2) screening for those with high blood pressure, and alcohol misuse screening and counseling.

    d. Alcohol misuse screening and counseling, cholesterol screening, and gestational diabetes screening.

5. Katherine learns that there may be additional services available to her as part of the Public Housing Primary Care (PHPC) Program. Which of the following statements is MOST accurate in describing the PHCP Program?

    a. PHCP-granted health centers use an integrated model to deliver primary health care, health promotion, and disease prevention, but are not able to help residents with establishing eligibility for assistance.

    b. PHCP grantees provide primary healthcare services, but this does not typically include dental care.

    c. One goal of the PHCP is to provide training and funding for public housing residents who want to become nurses.

    d. The mission of PHCP is to provide accessible, comprehensive healthcare and supportive service of which the Women, Infants, and Children (WIC) program may be one example.

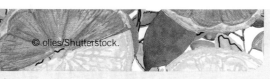

© olies/Shutterstock.

Learning Portfolio

Case Study 2: Health Insurance

Tony is a 40-year-old manager of a popular restaurant and bar in downtown Denver, CO. Due to the success of his business, Tony has very little time for much else outside of work. He is at the restaurant nearly 7 days a week for 10-–12 hours at a time. When Tony is at home, where he lives alone, he mainly catches up on sleep and is thinking about ways to keep his menu and drink offerings innovative. Working for himself, Tony does not have employer-sponsored health insurance, nor does his team of 20 individuals, ranging in age from 18 to 61 years old. Tony has encouraged his team to enroll in the Affordable Care Act so that they are able to have preventative care and coverage in the event of a serious health event. Some of his team has enrolled, but many have not.

For the last 8 years, Tony has enrolled in a plan from the marketplace at healthcare.gov. He is increasingly concerned about his health, particularly after a recent primary care visit that revealed he had high blood pressure (150/100), high LDL cholesterol (175 mg/dL), and elevated fasting glucose (115 mg/dL). This is also the first time that Tony's BMI of 27 has moved him into the overweight category. Given that Tony's father died of a heart attack at 60 years old, he is anxious about how to best take care of himself, especially on limited sleep and with very little time to exercise outside of his day-to-day activity.

1. By utilizing the Affordable Care Act and having regular preventative care, Tony is able to help the CDC meet several of the Healthy People 2030 goals. Which of the following is NOT a HP 2030 goal that Tony is helping to meet through his participation in the ACA?

    a. Increase the proportion of people who get the flu vaccine every year from 49.2% to 70%.

    b. Reduce the number of individuals with side effects from chemotherapy from 75% to 60%.

    c. Increase control of high blood pressure in adults (18 years and older) from 47.8% of adults with controlled hypertension to 60.8%.

    d. Increase the proportion of people with health insurance from 89% of persons under 65 years to 92.1%.

2. At his most recent primary care appointment, Tony's physician suggests that his overall health may benefit from improvements in his diet. Tony thinks that sounds like a great idea and wants to learn more but has no idea where to start. His physician is already 15 minutes late for his next patient. What is the best option for the physician to help Tony?

    a. Provide Tony with a one-page info sheet on the Mediterranean diet as part of his after-visit summary.

    b. Take an extra 15 minutes to explain to Tony a few small steps he can take to improve his diet and offer a follow-up phone call for questions.

    c. Call the nurse back into the exam room to see if she has any nutrition advice for Tony.

    d. Refer Tony to a Registered Dietitian Nutritionist (RDN) who has the ability to see patients in-person or virtually.

3. Tony takes his physician's advice and schedules a telenutrition visit with an RDN. Because of the COVID-19 pandemic and the increase in telemedicine visits, Tony has more options available to him than ever before. Which of the following is true regarding Tony's telenutrition visit, particularly with the new provisions for telemedicine visits implemented as part of the COVID-19 pandemic*?

    a. Tony won't have a co-pay for his telenutrition visit.

    b. Tony will need to follow up with the dietitian after his initial visit.

    c. Tony will be able to use Apple FaceTime for the visit.

    d. Tony will not be able to access his RDN friend in California since he lives in Colorado.

    *Some of these benefits may not be valid currently but were at the time of printing due to the COVID-19 pandemic.

4. It has been 6 weeks since Tony's visit with the RDN, and he is already down 10 pounds and feels full of energy. One of Tony's employees, Barb, comments on his weight loss and asks if Tony will help her enroll in the ACA so that she can get an overall picture of her health and subsequent preventative care. Barb is 61 years old and has a BMI of 29. Which of the following benefits will Barb likely NOT take advantage of as part of her ACA benefits?

    a. Type 2 diabetes screening.

    b. Osteoporosis screening.

    c. None, because the best option for Barb is to enroll in Medicare.

    d. Folic acid supplements.

References

1. Donaldson MS, Yordy KD, Lohr KN, Vanselow NA, eds. Primary care: America's health in a new era. Washington, DC: Institute of Medicine National Academy Press; 1996.

2. Davis K, Schoenbaum SC, Audet AM. A 2020 vision of patient-centered primary care. *J Gen Intern Med*. 2005;20:953-957.

3. U.S. Department of Health and Human Services. Healthy People 2030 Leading Health Indicators. Accessed December 12, 2020. https://health.gov/healthypeople /objectives-and-data/leading-health-indicators

4. Centers for Disease Control and Prevention. National Ambulatory Medical Care (NAMC) Survey Characteristics of Office-Based Visits, 2016. Accessed December 12, 2020. https://www.cdc.gov/nchs/products/databriefs/db331.htm

5. Ortman J, Velkoff VA, Hogan H. An aging nation: the older population in the United States. *Curr Pop Rep*. U.S. Census *Bureau*. 2014;P25-1140.

6. Hales, CM, Servais J, Martin CB, Kohen D. Prescription drug use among adults aged 40–79 in the United States and Canada (NCHS Data Brief No. 347), 2019. Accessed January 5, 2021. https://www.cdc.gov/nchs/products/databriefs/db347.htm

7. U.S. Department of Health and Human Services. Telehealth for patients and providers and policy changes due to the COVID-19 public emergency. Accessed January 21, 2021. https://telehealth.hhs.gov/providers/policy-changes-during-the-covid-19-public -health-emergency/

8. Coughlin K. Telehealth in private practice. *Today's Dietitian*. 2020;22(8):38.

9. U.S. Department of Health and Human Services. Agency for Healthcare Research and Quality: A Profile. 2020. Accessed November 23, 2020. http://www.ahrq.gov/cpi /about/profile/index.html

10. U.S. Preventative Services Task Force. Recommendations topics: See all A and B grade recommendations. Accessed January 5, 2021. http://www.uspreventativetaskforce .org

11. U.S. Preventive Services TaskForce. Prevention TaskForce App: information for professionals. Accessed January 5, 2021. https://www.uspreventiveservicestaskforce.org /apps/

12. Healthcare.gov. Health benefits &coverage: preventative health services. Accessed December 22, 2020. https://www.healthcare.gov/coverage/preventive-care-benefits

13. Eaton CB, McBride PE, Gans KA, Underbakke GL. Teaching nutrition skills to primary care practitioners. *J Nutr*. 2003;133(2):563S-566S.

14. Mihalynuk TV, Scott CS, Coombs JB. Self-reported nutrition proficiency is positively correlated with the perceived quality of nutrition training of family physicians in Washington State. *Am J Clin Nutr*. 2003;77(5):1330-1336.

15. Aspry K, Van Horn L, Carson JAS, et al. Medical nutrition education, training, and competencies to advance guideline-based diet counseling by physicians: a science advisory from the American Heart Association. *Circulation*. 2018;137(23): e821-e841.

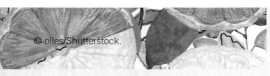

© olies/Shutterstock.

Learning Portfolio

16. Aggarwal M, Devries S, Freeman A, et al. The deficit of nutrition education of physicians. *Am J Med*. 2018;131(4):339-345.

17. University of North Carolina, Chapel Hill. Nutrition education for practicing physicians. Nutrition Medicine. 2014. Accessed December 20, 2021. www.nutritionmedicine.org

18. Wynn K, Trudeau JD, Taunton, K, Gowans M, Scott I. Nutrition in primary care: current practices, attitudes, behaviors. *Can Fam Physician*. 2010;56(e3):e109-e116.

19. Gans KM, Ross E, Barner CW, Wylie-Rosett J, McMurray J, Eaton C. REAP and WAVE: new tools to rapidly assess/discuss nutrition with patients. *J Nutr*. 2003;133(2):556S-562S.

20. Anis NA, Lee RE, Ellerbeck EF, Nazir N, Greiner KA, Ahluwalia JS. Direct observation of physician counseling on dietary habits and exercise: patient, physician, and office correlates. *Prev Med*. 2004;38(2):198-202.

21. Whitlock EP, Orleans CT, Pender N, Allan J. Evaluating primary care behavioral counseling interventions: an evidence-based approach. *Am J Prev Med*. 2002;22(4):267-284.

22. U.S. Department of Health and Human Services: Key features of the Affordable Care Act by Year. 2015. Accessed December 2, 2021. http://www.hhs.gov/healthcare/facts-and-features/key-features-of-aca-by-year/index.html

23. Blumenthal D, Abram MK. The Affordable Care Act at 10 years: what has changed in health care delivery and payment? Accessed September 12, 2021. https://www.commonwealthfund.org/publications/journal-article/2020/feb/aca-at-10-years-changed-health-care-delivery-payment

24. Robert Wood Johnson Foundation. Improving Chronic Illness Care: Our Approach. 2011. Accessed January 3, 2021. http://www.improvingchroniccare.org/index.php?p=About_US&s=6

25. Heyworth, L Rozenblum R, Burgess JF, et al. Influence of shared medical appointments on patient satisfaction: a retrospective, 3-year study. *Ann Fam Med*. 2014;12(4):324-330.

26. Partnership to Fight Chronic Disease. Keeping America Healthy: Essential Elements of Successful Programs. Table 1: Nine Essential Elements of Successful Programs. 2008. Accessed December 15, 2021. http://www.fightchronicdisease.org/sites/default/files/docs/EssentialElements5-28-08.pdf

27. Centers for Disease Control and Prevention. About WISE-WOMAN. 2021. Accessed December 15, 2021. http://www.cdc.gov/wisewoman/

28. U.S. Department of Health and Human Services. Well visits covered by ACA. 2016. Accessed January 3, 2021. http://www.healthfinder.gov

29. Agency for Healthcare Research and Quality. Questions about health insurance: Which type is right for you? 2015. Accessed November 23, 2021. http://archive.ahrq.gov/consumer/insuranceqa/insuranceqa5.htm

30. Centers for Medicare and Medicaid. Benefits covered by Medicare enrollment. 2016. Accessed January 3, 2021. http://www.medicare.gov

31. Academy of Nutrition and Dietetics. How you get paid: Medicare Advantage and Medicare + Choice Plans. Accessed January 3, 2021. www.eatrightpro.org

32. Indian Health Service. Factsheets: disparities. 2019. Accessed December 5, 2020. https://www.ihs.gov/newsroom/factsheets/disparities/#:~:text=American%20Indians%20and%20Alaska%20Natives%20born%20today%20have%20a%20life,to%2078.5%20years%2C%20respectively

33. Indian Health Service. FY 2020 Budget Congressional Justifications. Accessed December 12, 2020. https://www.ihs.gov/aboutihs/annualbudget/

34. Indian Health Service. Health promotion/disease prevention programs. Accessed December 12, 2020. https://www.ihs.gov/hpdp/

35. Indian Health Service. HPDP Programs: School health. 2020. Accessed December 12, 2020. Available online at: https://www.ihs.gov/communityhealth/schoolhealth/

36. Indian Health Service. Patient education protocols and codes: 21st Ed. 2014. Accessed December 5, 2021. https://www.ihs.gov/healthed/index.cfm/patientedprotocols

37. U.S. Department of Health and Human Services, Office of Minority Health. Diabetes and American Indians/Alaskan Natives. Accessed January 15, 2021. https://minorityhealth.hhs.gov/omh/browse.aspx?lvl=4&lvlid=33

38. Indian Health Service. About: Special Diabetes Program for Indians (SDPI). 2015. Accessed December 10, 2021. http://www.ihs.gov/medicalprograms/diabetes

39. Indian Health Service: Diabetes standard of care, clinical practice & educator resources: youth and type 2 diabetes. Accessed January 15, 2021. https://www.ihs.gov/diabetes/clinician-resources/soc/youth-and-type-2-diabetes1/

40. Partnership for a Healthier America. Work & impact: initiatives. Accessed January 20, 2021. https://www.ahealthieramerica.org/initiatives-9

41. Health Resources and Services Administration/Bureaus. About HRSA: organization and bureaus and offices. Accessed January 12, 2021. https://www.ahealthieramerica.org/initiatives-9. https://www.hrsa.gov/about/organization/bureaus/index.html

42. Health Resources and Services Administration, Health Center Program. Impact and growth. Accessed January 12, 2021. https://bphc.hrsa.gov/about/healthcenterprogram/index.html

43. Health Resources and Services Administration. Bureau of Primary Health Care; The Health Center Program. Accessed January 12, 2021. http://bphc.hrsa.gov

44. Health Resources and Services Administration, Health Center Program. Health Center data snapshot: 2020. Accessed January 12, 2021. http://bphc.hrsa.gov

45. Congress.gov. H.R.2328: Reauthorizing and Extending America's Community Health Act (CHIME). Accessed January 12, 2021. https://www.congress.gov/bill/116th-congress/house-bill/2328

46. National Association of Community Health Care Centers. Health care funding worksheet: legislative proposals to extend the community health center fund. Accessed January 12, 2021. https://www.nachc.org/wp-content/uploads/2019/04/Health-Center-Funding-Worksheet_April-2019.pdf

47. Center for Medicare and Medicaid Services. Medicare Learning Network: federally qualified health centers: rural health fact sheet series. 2013. Accessed December 28, 2021. https://www.cms.gov/Outreach-and-Education/Medicare-Learning-Network-MLN/MLNProducts/downloads/fqhcfactsheet.pdf

48. Health Resources and Services Administration. Health center data. 2020. Accessed December 20, 2021. Available online

at: https://data.hrsa.gov/tools/data-reporting/program-data/national

49. National Committee for Quality Assurance (NCQA). About the patient-centered medical home. Accessed December 28, 2020. https://www.ncqa.org/programs/health-care-providers-practices/patient-centered-medical-home-pcmh/

50. U.S. Health Resources and Services Administration. Federally qualified health centers (eligibility). Accessed December 28, 2020. https://www.hrsa.gov/opa/eligibility-and-registration/health-centers/fqhc/index.html

51. U.S. Department of Housing and Urban Development. Humans of HUD: the trials and triumphs of the men and women HUD serves. Accessed January 8, 2021. https://www.hud.gov/humansofhud

52. National Center for Health in Public Housing. Demographic facts: residents living in public housing. Accessed December 28, 2020. https://nchph.org/wp-content/uploads/2019/02/Demographics-Fact-Sheet-2019.pdf

53. National Alliance to End Homelessness. The State of homelessness in America: 2020. Accessed December 22, 2020. https://nchph.org/wp-content/uploads/2019/02/Demographics-Fact-Sheet-2019.pdf

54. National Healthcare for Homeless Council. Policy and advocacy. Medicaid & health care financing. Accessed December 19, 2020. https://nhchc.org/policy-issues/medicaid-health-care-financing/

55. National Healthcare for the Homeless Council. Annual report 2019-2020. Accessed December 19, 2020. http://www.nhchc.org

56. U.S. Interagency Council on Homelessness. The Affordable Care Act's role in preventing and ending homelessness. 2015. Accessed September 12, 2021. https://www.usich.gov/tools-for-action/aca-fact-sheet

57. United States Department of Agriculture (USDA). Are you homeless? SNAP/food stamps and homelessness. 2014. Accessed October 28, 2021. http://www.fns.usda.gov/sites/default/files/Homeless_QA_0.pdf

58. National Healthcare for the Homeless Council. Annual report: July 2, 2014 to June 30, 2015. Accessed January 17, 2021. https://nhchc.org/wp-content/uploads/2019/08/fy16-annual-report-web-final.pdf

59. National Healthcare for the Homeless Council. Supplemental Nutrition Assistance Program (SNAP): health status, homelessness, and hunger: a fact sheet. 2013. Accessed January 17, 2021. http://www.nhchc.org

PART V

Protecting the Public's Nutritional Health

CHAPTER 13

Food Security and Adequate Food Access for the Public

David H. Holben, PhD, RDN, LD, FAND

Learning Outcomes

AFTER STUDYING THIS CHAPTER AND REFLECTING ON THE CONTENTS, YOU SHOULD BE ABLE TO:

1. Define food security, food insecurity, and hunger.
2. Discuss and carry out food security measurement.
3. Interpret food security data from nutrition monitoring and research studies.
4. Understand the consequences of food insecurity and its relationship to selected health issues.
5. Discuss programs that assist the public in securing adequate food.

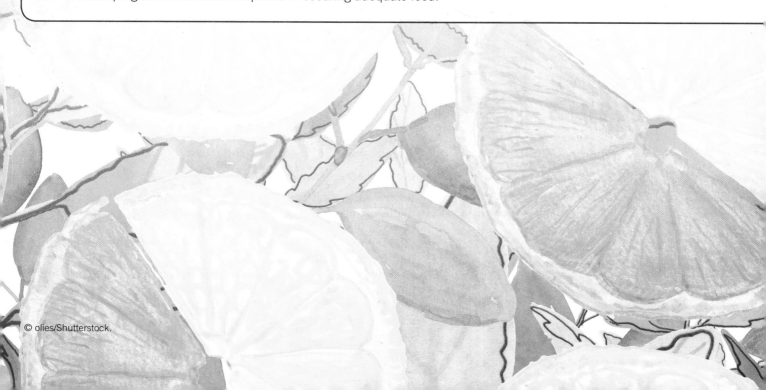

Community food security A situation in which all community residents obtain a safe, culturally acceptable, nutritionally adequate diet through a sustainable food system that maximizes community self-reliance and social justice.[a]

Nutrition security The provision of an environment that encourages and motivates society to make food choices consistent with short- and long-term good health.[d]

Food insecurity Limited or uncertain availability of nutritionally adequate and safe foods or limited or uncertain ability to acquire acceptable foods in socially acceptable ways.[b]

Hunger The uneasy or painful sensation caused by a lack of food. The recurrent and involuntary lack of access to food...[which] may produce malnutrition over time.[b,e]

(Notation: More information on "hunger" and rationale for usage of the terminology, is available.[d])

Food security Access by all people, at all times, to sufficient food for an active and healthy life...[and] includes at a minimum: the ready availability of nutritionally adequate and safe foods, and an assured ability to acquire acceptable foods in socially acceptable ways.[b]

Introduction

Healthy People 2030 establishes data-driven national objectives to improve health and well-being of individuals, organizations, and communities across the United States.[1] Envisioning "A society in which all people can achieve their full potential for health and well-being across the lifespan,"[1] Healthy People 2030[1] has the overarching goals to:

- Attain healthy, thriving lives and well-being free of preventable disease, disability, injury, and premature death
- Eliminate health disparities, achieve health equity, and attain health literacy to improve the health and well-being of all
- Create social, physical, and economic environments that promote attaining the full potential for health and well-being for all
- Promote healthy development, healthy behaviors, and well-being across all life stages
- Engage leadership, key constituents, and the public across multiple sectors to take action and design policies that improve the health and well-being of all

Securing adequate food for the public is paramount to achieving and maintaining health. Yet, **food insecurity** persists at an unacceptable rate in the United States, with the 2019 estimates indicating that 10.5% (13.7 million) of U.S. households were food insecure at some time during 2019.[2]

Food availability is the focus of nutrition and healthy eating in Healthy People 2030. Specifically, the goal is to "improve health by promoting healthy eating and making nutritious foods available." The associated Healthy People 2030[1] objectives are to: 1) Reduce household food insecurity and **hunger** (Nutrition and Weight Status (NWS)-01); and 2) Eliminate very low food security in children (NWS-02).

Food security exists when all people, at all times, have access to sufficient food for an active and healthy life without resorting to emergency food supplies or socially unacceptable ways of obtaining food, including begging, stealing, or scavenging.[3] On the other hand, food insecure families or individuals have limited resources and limited ability to acquire food, which often leads them to resort to socially unacceptable means of food acquisition.[3,4] A possible consequence of food insecurity is hunger, an individual-level physiological condition, due to prolonged, involuntary lack of food.[4,5]

Securing adequate food for the public is paramount. Community and public health nutrition professionals must not only be aware of programs that can assist the public in securing adequate food but also know how to assess:

- Prevalence of food insecurity
- Consequences of food insecurity
- If a particular program designed to improve food security is actually doing so

Therefore, this chapter was designed to:

- Review the definitions of food security, food insecurity, and hunger
- Outline food security measurement strategies
- Summarize the household food security of the United States
- Highlight the consequences of food insecurity and its relationship to selected health issues
- Review how food security measurement can be used for program and client assessment strategies
- Discuss community and public health programs designed to improve food access by the public

Measuring the Food Security Status of the Public

Although food insecurity is broad in scope, its primary dimension is **food insufficiency**, which can be measured along a continuum of successive stages. These stages, as noted by Bickel and others,[6] each have specific characteristics, that is, conditions and experiences related to being unable to fully meet the basic needs of household members followed by the behavioral responses to those conditions and experiences. Community and public health nutrition professionals must be able to understand the federal, state, and local reports related to food security and their implications on public health issues. In addition, they need to be able to develop strategies in order to measure the effectiveness of interventions intended to improve food security.

Household food security status is one outcome measure that provides insight into the public's ability to secure adequate food. The National Nutrition Monitoring and Related Research Act of 1990 (**Table 13–1**) prompted the measurement of household food security status in the United States, which began in 1995. Standardized questionnaires for measuring household food security status and methods for editing and scoring those instruments have been developed.[6,7]

The foundation for measuring the public's food security was laid through work conducted by Radimer and colleagues[8,9] and Wehler and others[10]; their work led to the development of an instrument capable of measuring the food security status of U.S. households. This instrument[6] is called the US Household Food Security Survey Module (**Table 13–2**). Federal estimates of household food security are measured using this instrument as part of the Census Bureau's Current Population Survey (CPS) (https://www.bls.gov/cps/home.htm).[11] The CPS Food Security Supplement and the Spanish Language CPS Food Security Supplement include the Household Food Security Survey Module, as well questions about food expenditures and use of food and

Food insufficiency An inadequate amount of food intake due to a lack of resources.[c]

TABLE 13–1
The National Nutrition Monitoring and Related Research Act of 1990

Facts About This Legislation

- Public Law 101-445
- Enacted October 22, 1990
- Leadership/Responsibility: U.S. Department of Health and Human Services and U.S. Department of Agriculture.
- Reports are filed at least every 5 years on the dietary, nutritional, and health-related status of people in the United States.
- Purposes of the Act
  1. "Make more effective use of Federal and State expenditures for nutrition monitoring and enhance the performance and benefits of current federal nutrition monitoring and related research activities."
  2. "Establish and facilitate the timely implementation of a coordinated National Nutrition Monitoring and Related Program, and thereby provide a scientific basis for the maintenance and improvement of the nutritional status of the people of the United States and the nutritional quality…of food consumed in the United States."
  3. "Establish and implement a comprehensive plan for the National Nutrition Monitoring and Related Research Program to assess, on a continuing basis, the dietary and nutritional status of the people of the United States and the trends with respect to such status, state of the art with respect to nutrition monitoring and related research, future monitoring and related research priorities, and the relevant policy implications."
  4. "Establish and improve the quality of national nutritional health status data related databases and networks, and stimulate research necessary to develop uniform indicators, standards, methodologies, technologies, and procedures for nutrition monitoring."
  5. "Establish a central federal focus for the coordination, management, and direction of federal nutrition monitoring activities."
  6. "Establish mechanisms for addressing the nutrition monitoring needs of federal, state, and local governments, the private sector, scientific and engineering communities, healthcare professionals, and the public in support of the foregoing purposes."
  7. "Provide for the conduct of such scientific research and development as may be necessary or appropriate in support of such purposes."

Office of the Law Revision Counsel. Accessed February 10, 2021. http://uscode.house.gov/browse.xhtml
National Nutrition Monitoring and Related Research Act of 1990. Accessed February 10, 2021. https://www.congress.gov/bill/101st-congress/house-bill/1608
National Nutrition Monitoring and Related Research Act of 1990. Accessed February 10, 2021. https://www.congress.gov/bill/101st-congress/senate-bill/253

TABLE 13–2
US Household Food Security Survey Module

- "(I/We) worried whether (my/our) food would run out before (I/we) got money to buy more." Was that often true, sometimes true, or never true for (you/your household) in the last 12 months?
- "The food that (I/we) bought just didn't last, and (I/we) didn't have money to get more." Was that often, sometimes, or never true for (you/your household) in the last 12 months?
- "(I/We) couldn't afford to eat balanced meals." Was that often, sometimes, or never true for (you/your household) in the last 12 months?
- "(I/We) relied on only a few kinds of low-cost food to feed (my/our) (child/children) because (I was/we were) running out of money to buy food." Was that often, sometimes, or never true for (you/your household) in the last 12 months?
- "(I/We) couldn't feed (my/our) (child/children) a balanced meal, because (I/we) couldn't afford that." Was that often, sometimes, or never true for (you/your household) in the last 12 months?
- "(My/our) (child was/children were) not eating enough because (I/we) just couldn't afford enough food." Was that often, sometimes, or never true for (you/your household) in the last 12 months?
- In the last 12 months, since last (name of current month), did (you/you or other adults in your household) ever cut the size of your meals or skip meals because there wasn't enough money for food? Yes No
- If yes, how often did this happen—almost every month, some months but not every month, or in only 1 or 2 months?
- In the last 12 months, did you ever eat less than you felt you should because there wasn't enough money to buy food? Yes No
- In the last 12 months, were you ever hungry but didn't eat because you couldn't afford enough food? Yes No
- In the last 12 months, did you lose weight because you didn't have enough money for food? Yes No
- In the last 12 months, did (you/you or other adults in your household) ever not eat for a whole day because there wasn't enough money for food? Yes No
- If yes, how often did this happen—almost every month, some months but not every month, or in only 1 or 2 months?
- In the last 12 months, since (current month) of last year, did you ever cut the size of (your child's/any of the children's) meals because there wasn't enough money for food? Yes No
- In the last 12 months, did (CHILD'S NAME/any of the children) ever skip meals because there wasn't enough money for food? Yes No
- If yes, how often did this happen—almost every month, some months but not every month, or in only 1 or 2 months?
- In the last 12 months, (was your child/were the children) ever hungry but you just couldn't afford more food? Yes No
- In the last 12 months, did (your child/any of the children) ever not eat for a whole day because there wasn't enough money for food? Yes No

Note: Questions relating to children are only asked if there are children under 18 in the household. Specific guidelines for using the Core Module, including screening techniques, can be found in the source below.
Bickel G, Nord M, Price C, Hamilton W, Cook J. Guide to measuring household food Security, Revised in 2000. Alexandria, VA: U.S. Department of Agriculture, Food and Nutrition Service; 2000.
Economic Research Service, United States Department of Agriculture. Food security in the United States – survey tools. Accessed February 10, 2021. https://www.ers.usda.gov/topics/food-nutrition-assistance/food-security-in-the-us/survey-tools/

nutrition assistance programs.[12] Several national surveys include a measure of food security.[12] Examples are the:

- Early Childhood Longitudinal Studies[13]
- National Health and Nutrition Examination Survey[14]
- Panel Study of Income Dynamics[15]
- Survey of Program Dynamics[16]

Most recently, in response to the COVID-19 pandemic, the Household Pulse Survey was developed.[12] It is conducted by the Census Bureau and was developed cooperatively by several federal agencies to measure the effects of the pandemic on U.S. households.[12,17] The survey contains questions related to food insufficiency prior to the pandemic, food sufficiency in the last 7 days, reasons for not having enough food, receipt of free food or meals and where it was obtained, food spending (at home; away from home), and confidence of food insufficiency for the next 4 weeks.[12]

Table 13–3 provides a brief summary of some national surveys that include the food security measure. In addition to these, states, academic and private researchers, and public health nutrition professionals use the Household Food Security Survey Module to measure household food security status.

The Food Security Survey Module poses questions to respondents about:

- Anxiety related to food budget or supply and whether the budget is able to meet basic needs

Pandemic Learning Opportunity

Discuss America's national, state, and local response to food insufficiency during the COVID-19 pandemic. What improvement(s) could have been made, if any?

TABLE 13–3
National Surveys That Include Food Security Measurement

Survey	Website	Brief Summary
Current Population Survey	https://www.bls.gov/cps/home.htm	Annual Federal estimates of household food security since 1995.
		"A monthly survey of U.S. households conducted by the U.S. Census Bureau for the Bureau of Labor Statistics. The CPS provides a wide range of information about employment, unemployment, hours of work, earnings, and people not in the labor force."
		Source of Nationally representative data of the noninstitutionalized civilian population used to provide annual U.S. household food security estimates.
Early Childhood Longitudinal Studies (ECLS) Program	https://nces.ed.gov/ecls/	Studies sponsored by the U.S. Department of Education and The National Center for Educational Statistics to track "children's knowledge, skills, and socioemotional development from birth through elementary school."
		"Includes four longitudinal studies that examine child development, school readiness, and early school experiences."
National Health and Nutrition Examination Survey	https://www.cdc.gov/nchs/nhanes/index.htm?CDC_AA_refVal=https%3A%2F%2Fwww.cdc.gov%2Fnchs%2Fnhanes.htm	Managed by the Centers for Disease Control and Prevention's National Center for Health Statistics
		A nationally representative health and nutritional status of the noninstitutionalized civilian population (adults and children).
		Includes interviews and physical examinations.
Panel Study of Income Dynamics	https://psidonline.isr.umich.edu/	Directed by faculty at the University of Michigan.
		Began in 1968 with a nationally representative U.S. sample of more than 18,000 individuals living in 5,000 families.
		"Information on these individuals and their descendants has been collected continuously, including data covering employment, income, wealth, expenditures, health, marriage, childbearing, child development, philanthropy, education, and numerous other topics."
Survey of Program Dynamics	https://www.census.gov/programs-surveys/sipp/about/spd.html	Overseen by the US Census Bureau.
		A nationally representative longitudinal, demographic survey on the economic, household, and social characteristics of the United States.
		Core instrument remained essentially the same over the 1998–2002 period.
		"Core data are collected on employment, income, program participation, health insurance and utilization, child well-being, marital relationships, and parents' depression… [and] topical modules that vary by year.

- Experiences relating to running out of food without being able to obtain more due to financial constraints
- Perceptions of intake adequacy by themselves or other household members
- Food use[6]

This instrument only measures the "sufficiency" dimension of food security and does not measure other aspects of food security, including the nutritional adequacy or safety of diets.[6] Other instruments, therefore, must be used to capture this information in a research project or programmatic evaluation. As seen in Table 13–2, all of the questions in the Household Food Security Survey Module specify financial limitations as the reason for the reported behaviors or conditions and ask about circumstances that occurred within the past 12 months; however, shorter time periods can be utilized.[6] For example, if a public health nutrition intervention (e.g., a community gardening project) was initiated at the beginning of the growing season and concluded at the end of the season, the food security status of participating households could be measured before and after the intervention (e.g., 4–6 months).

TABLE 13–4
Food Security Survey Module Categories of Food Security Status

Food Security	
High food security	No reported indications of food-access problems or limitations.
Marginal food security	One or two reported indications—typically of anxiety over food sufficiency or shortage of food in the house. Little or no indication of changes in diets or food intake.

Food Insecurity	
Low food security	Reports of reduced quality, variety, or desirability of diet. Little or no indication of reduced food intake.
Very low food security	Reports of multiple indications of disrupted eating patterns and reduced food intake.

Economic Research Service, United States Department of Agriculture. *Food security in the United States: definitions of food security.* Accessed February 10, 2021. https://www.ers.usda.gov/topics/food-nutrition-assistance/food-security-in-the-us/definitions-of-food-security.aspx

Responses to the Household Food Security Survey Module questions are tabulated, as summarized by Bickel and colleagues,[6] resulting in a scale that measures the degree of the severity of food insecurity experienced by a household. Based upon the number of positive responses to the questions, a scale score ranging from 0 to 10 is assigned, with larger numbers corresponding to a greater level of food insecurity. Households are categorized into four groupings of household food security status, each representing a range of severity on the food security scale (**Table 13–4**).[6,18]

As summarized by the Economic Research Service of the United States Department of Agriculture,[16] food-secure households can be classified into those with high food security or marginal food security. Households classified as having high food security report no indications of food-access problems or limitations. These households are "fully food secure." While not fully food secure, households classified as having marginal food security have little or no indication of changes in diet or food intake and only report one or two indications of food security, which is typically anxiety over food sufficiency or shortage of food in the house. Essentially, for high or marginally food secure households, there is no or minimal evidence of food insecurity; that is, they are able to secure nutritionally adequate, safe foods in socially acceptable ways.[16]

On the other hand, households that are food insecure can be classified into those with low food security or very low food security. Households with low food security have members who are concerned about the adequacy of the household food supply and management. This may include reduced quality, variety, or desirability of the diet and increased use of unusual coping patterns. However, in this category, little or no reduction in members' food intake is reported. Households at the most severe level, those with very low food security, report multiple indications of disrupted eating patterns and reduced food intake. In fact, some have members who may go one or more entire days with no food due to lack of resources, or food intake may be reduced to an extent that members have repeatedly experienced the physical sensation of hunger. In households with children, typically at the early stages, food reductions are not observed for children. However, at the most severe level, even children have reduced food intake to an extent that physical sensations of hunger have been experienced; however, children are often protected from hunger by other family members.[15] Finally, at the most severe stages of food

Discussion Prompt

Hypothesize areas of your hometown where food insecurity and/or reductions of food intake may be prevalent. What factors are causative in these situations? What are some solutions?

TABLE 13–5
Child-Related Household Food Security Survey Module Questions

- "(I/We) relied on only a few kinds of low-cost food to feed (my/our) (child/children) because (I was/we were) running out of money to buy food." Was that often, sometimes, or never true for (you/your household) in the last 12 months?
- "(I/We) couldn't feed (my/our) (child/children) a balanced meal, because (I/we) couldn't afford that." Was that often, sometimes, or never true for (you/your household) in the last 12 months?
- "(My/our) (child was/children were) not eating enough because (I/we) just couldn't afford enough food." Was that often, sometimes, or never true for (you/your household) in the last 12 months?
- In the last 12 months, since (current month) of last year, did you ever cut the size of (your child's/any of the children's) meals because there wasn't enough money for food? Yes No
- In the last 12 months, did (CHILD'S NAME/any of the children) ever skip meals because there wasn't enough money for food? Yes No
- If yes, how often did this happen—almost every month, some months but not every month, or in only 1 or 2 months?
- In the last 12 months, (was your child/were the children) ever hungry but you just couldn't afford more food? Yes No
- In the last 12 months, did (your child/any of the children) ever not eat for a whole day because there wasn't enough money for food? Yes No

Bickel G, Nord M, Price C, Hamilton W, Cook J. Guide to measuring household food security, revised 2000. Alexandria, VA: U.S. Department of Agriculture, Food and Nutrition Service; 2000.
Economic Research Service, United States Department of Agriculture. Food security in the United States – survey tools. Accessed February 10, 2021. https://www.ers.usda.gov/topics/food-nutrition-assistance/food-security-in-the-us/survey-tools/

insecurity, adults in households with and without children have repeatedly experienced extensive reductions in food intake.[14]

Generally, the Food Security Survey Module takes less than 4 minutes to administer, unless screening is performed, which would decrease the time needed to administer the survey instrument to approximately 2 minutes.[6] Less time is needed because when screening is performed, all questions may not be asked if responses inconsistent with food insecurity are provided for the initial survey questions.

Some public health nutrition professionals may find it difficult to administer the 18-question module for a variety of reasons but are still interested in household food security status as an outcome or factor impacting public health program development and delivery. Therefore, if utilizing the entire Household Food Security Survey Module (all 18 questions) is not possible due to time constraints, an abbreviated six-item subset that is available.[7] This tool also provides food security scale scores for classifying households by level of food security.[6] However, use of this six-item subset does have limitations, since it is less precise, does not measure the most severe levels of food insecurity, and does not ask about children in the household.[7] Consequently, when utilizing this tool in a public health setting, it is important to have a preliminary idea of what levels of food insecurity are likely to exist in the target population before choosing the abbreviated subset.

When the entire Household Food Security Survey Module is used, a subset of the questions can be employed to assess the extent to which children were food insecure in the household.[6,7] **Table 13–5** highlights these questions. A self-administered food security survey tool has also been developed for youth 12 years and older.[7]

Food Security in the United States

The agricultural bounty of the United States has not completely overcome the problem of hunger. In 2019, 89.5% of U.S. households were food secure. However, 10.5% were food insecure at some time during the year,[2] as shown in **Figure 13–1**. Trends in food insecurity and prevalence in the United States are shown in **Figure 13–2**.

Overall, food insecurity was greater among: 1) households with incomes below the official poverty line; 2) households with children, especially

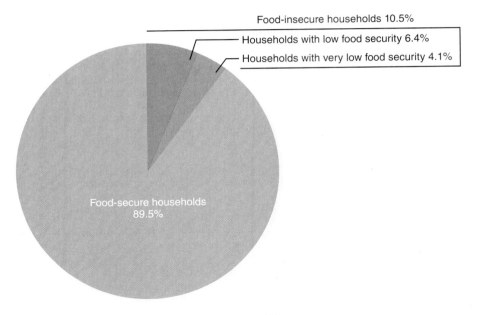

FIGURE 13–1 U.S. Households by Food Security Status, 2019.

Calculated by ERS USDA using data from December 2019 Current Population Survey Food Security Supplement. Key statistics and graphics. Accessed February 15, 2021. Available at http://www.ers .usda.gov/topics/food-nutrition-assistance/food-security-in-the-us/key-statistics-graphics.aspx

those headed by a single woman or man; 3) Black non-Hispanic households; 4) Hispanic households; 5) households located in principal cities; and 6) households located in non-metropolitan (rural) areas.[2]

Although these national estimates paint a picture of the United States as a whole, regions within the United States and particular states may vary with regard to food security status. The prevalence of food security and hunger by state is summarized in **Table 13–6** and **Figure 13–3**.

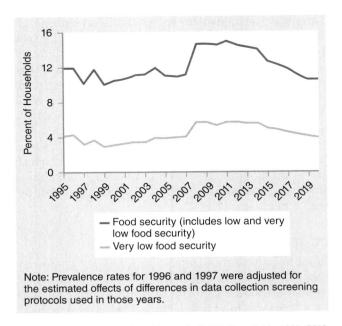

FIGURE 13–2 Trends in the Prevalence of Food Insecurity in U.S. Households, 1995–2019.

Calculated by ERS USDA using data from Current Population Survey Food Security Supplement. Key statistics and graphics. Accessed February 15, 2021. Available at http://www.ers.usda.gov/topics/food -nutrition-assistance/food-security-in-the-us/key-statistics-graphics.aspx

TABLE 13-6
State-level Prevalence of Household-Level Food Insecurity and Very Low Food Security, Average 2017–2019

States	Number of Households Average 2017-19[1] Number	Interviewed Number	Food Insecurity (Low or Very Low Food Security) Prevalence Percent	Margin of Error[2] Percentage Points	Very Low Food Security Prevalence Percent	Margin of Error[2] Percentage Points
U.S.	128,713,000	108,756	11.1	0.19	4.3	0.13
AK	271,000	1,276	10.7	2.34	4.9	1.39
AL	1,985,000	2,009	13.9*	2.31	5.9*	1.33
AR	1,244,000	1,889	13.8*	2.01	5.8*	1.23
AZ	2,761,000	1,851	11.7	1.41	4.2	0.78
CA	14,047,000	8,615	9.9*	0.64	3.6*	0.38
CO	2,403,000	1,152	10.2	1.61	4.3	1.16
CT	1,399,000	983	12.9	2.34	4.5	1.30
DC	327,000	2,265	10.2	1.37	4.0	0.88
DE	375,000	1,130	10.2	1.84	4.2	1.15
FL	9,041,000	4,535	10.9	0.90	4.4	0.58
GA	4,051,000	2,532	10.0	1.51	3.6	0.90
HI	498,000	1,382	8.4*	1.50	3.4*	0.82
IA	1,320,000	1,355	7.9*	1.33	3.6	0.92
ID	653,000	1,862	9.6	1.53	3.4*	0.67
IL	4,996,000	3,068	9.9*	1.17	3.8	0.67
IN	2,741,000	1,742	12.4	1.69	4.1	1.17
KS	1,139,000	1,454	12.5	2.15	5.5	1.30
KY	1,803,000	1,461	13.7*	1.68	4.8	1.20
LA	1,866,000	2,467	15.3*	1.34	7.0*	1.03
MA	2,809,000	2,131	8.4*	1.19	3.2*	0.69
MD	2,367,000	1,323	10.1	1.78	5.0	1.33
ME	563,000	1,127	12.0	2.04	6.2*	1.70
MI	4,111,000	2,458	12.2	1.57	4.7	0.98
MN	2,313,000	1,532	8.3*	1.57	3.4	0.98
MO	2,490,000	1,694	11.7	1.62	4.4	0.97
MS	1,168,000	2,336	15.7*	1.60	6.2*	0.90
MT	458,000	2,214	10.0	1.62	3.9	0.78
NC	4,271,000	2,308	13.1*	1.51	4.9	1.03
ND	324,000	1,687	8.3*	1.20	2.8*	0.78
NE	781,000	1,261	10.8	1.31	4.3	1.11
NH	538,000	1,533	6.6*	1.43	2.6*	0.85
NJ	3,384,000	2,053	7.7*	1.30	3.0*	0.71
NM	846,000	2,106	15.1*	2.45	5.5*	1.11
NV	1,151,000	1,390	12.8	1.85	5.5	1.44
NY	7,838,000	4,208	10.8	1.09	3.9	0.57
OH	4,782,000	3,022	12.6*	1.38	5.4*	0.88
OK	1,516,000	1,606	14.7*	1.84	5.3	1.03
OR	1,709,000	1,751	9.8	1.46	4.3	1.17
PA	5,213,000	2,826	10.2	1.20	4.1	0.68
RI	430,000	1,015	9.1*	1.84	3.1*	1.10
SC	2,129,000	1,674	10.9	2.26	4.0	1.12
SD	357,000	1,341	10.9	1.61	4.7	1.29
TN	2,727,000	2,236	12.5	1.88	5.3	0.95
TX	10,440,000	5,729	13.1*	1.04	4.9*	0.60
UT	1,061,000	1,520	10.7	2.06	3.5	1.64
VA	3,351,000	2,042	9.2*	1.37	3.9	0.88
VT	269,000	1,610	9.6*	1.44	3.2*	0.87
WA	3,013,000	2,134	9.9	1.37	3.5	0.88
WI	2,401,000	1,805	10.1	1.44	3.3*	0.78
WV	749,000	2,400	15.4*	2.26	5.9*	1.20
WY	233,000	1,656	12.2	1.40	5.0	0.89

*Difference from U.S. average was statistically significant with 90-percent confidence (t > 1.645). Standard error of differences assumes that there is no correlation between national and individual State estimates.

[1]Totals exclude households for which food security status is unknown because household respondents did not give a valid response to any of the questions in the food security scale. These exclusions represented about 0.3 percent of all households in 2017, 0.3 percent in 2018, and 0.2 percent in 2019.

[2]Margin of error with 90-percent confidence (1.645 times the standard error of the estimated prevalence rate). Standard errors were estimated using balanced repeated replication (BRR) methods based on replicate weights for the CPS Food Security Supplement.

USDA, Economic Research Service using data from U.S. Department of Commerce, U.S. Census Bureau, 2017, 2018, and 2019 Current Population Survey Food Security Supplements.

Coleman-Jensen, Alisha, Matthew P. Rabbitt, Christian A. Gregory, and Anita Singh. 2020. Household Food Security in the United States in 2019, ERR-275, U.S. Department of Agriculture, Economic Research Service. Accessed September 2020. Retrieved from https://www.ers.usda.gov/webdocs/publications/99282/err-275.pdf?v=1194.6

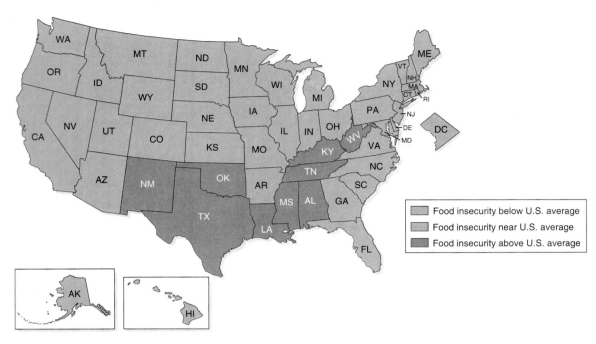

FIGURE 13-3 Prevalence of U.S. Households by State, 2017–2019.

Calculated by ERS using data from Current Population Survey Food Security Supplement. Key statistics and graphics. Accessed February 15, 2021. Available at http://www.ers.usda.gov/topics/food-nutrition-assistance/food-security-in-the-us/key-statistics-graphics.aspx

For 2017–2019, estimated prevalence rates of food insecurity ranged from 6.6% (New Hampshire) to 15.7% (Mississippi).[2] Although a particular state may experience food insecurity below the national average, a community within a state may experience food insecurity exceeding the state and national averages, necessitating the need for programmatic intervention.

Essentially, three factors encompass food security: 1) food availability; 2) food access; and 3) food utilization. In the United States, food insecurity is evident when families have limited resources; lack access to food (due to limited resources, lack of transportation, living in remote areas, or limited access to food stores); depend on food-assistance programs; skip meals; substitute nutritious foods with less-expensive alternatives; and seek assistance from soup kitchens, food pantries, family members, and friends, among others.[19] Food insecurity is strongly related to lacking household resources—poverty, under- and unemployment, and high housing costs.[20,21] Unexpected "energy price shock," such as unexpected increases in vehicle fuel or household energy costs, also contribute to food insecurity.[22]

Coping Strategies Used by the Public to Avoid Food Insecurity

People often use coping strategies to minimize household food security.[2,19] Food management practices used by people with limited resources have been identified by Kempson and colleagues[23] including:

- Strategizing food preparation (e.g., making low-cost dishes; removing mold, insects, and slime from cheese, grain, and meats)
- Rationing the household food supply
- Conserving food
- Inadequately preserving food

- Restricting personal food intake
- Overeating when food is available
- Obtaining food opportunistically
- Cycling monthly eating patterns
- Eating low-cost foods

Supporting some of these ideas, coping strategies used in households with low incomes include many tactics. These tactics included depending upon others (family, friends, community resources), garden fruits and vegetables for home use, hunting or fishing for food, adjusting resources and making trade-offs (securing multiple jobs, not paying medical, utility or other bills or only paying a portion of them in order to have enough money to buy food and other basic needs), adjusting food consumption, decreasing budgets to pay rent and utilities, and obtaining nutrition and shopping knowledge and skills through nutrition education programs.[19,24]

As noted by Coleman-Jensen and others,[2] households with limited resources employ a variety of methods to help meet their food needs, including participating in one or more federal food assistance programs or obtaining food from community emergency food providers to supplement the household food purchased. Coleman-Jensen and others[2] noted, "Households with limited resources use a variety of methods to help meet their food needs. Some participate in federal food and nutrition assistance programs or obtain food from emergency providers in their communities to supplement the food they purchase. Households that turn to Federal and community food and nutrition assistance programs typically do so because they are having difficulty meeting their food needs. The use of such programs by low-income households provides insight into the extent of these households' difficulties in obtaining enough food. The relationship between food security status and the use of food and nutrition assistance programs also provides insight into how low-income households cope with difficulties in acquiring adequate food."

Food and nutrition assistance programs in the United States, that is, the *nutrition safety net*, have been key in helping the U.S. public secure adequate food. In fact, federally funded, including those through USDA Food and Nutrition Service,[25] and community-based programs are vital in helping households make ends meet. Several program summaries follow.

Child and Adult Care Food Program (CACFP)

This program provides "reimbursements for nutritious meals and snacks to eligible children and adults who are enrolled for care at participating childcare centers, daycare homes, and adult daycare centers… and for meals served to children and youth participating in afterschool care programs, children residing in emergency shelters, and adults over the age of 60 or living with a disability and enrolled in daycare facilities."[26] This program is usually administered by the state education agency.

Expanded Food and Nutrition Education Program (EFNEP)

This program uses a holistic nutrition educational approach and is intended to result in individuals and families experiencing improvements in diet quality and physical activity, food resource management, food safety, and food security.[27] Essentially, it helps families with limited incomes acquire knowledge, skills, attitudes, and behavior changes necessary to maintain nutritionally sound diets and enhance personal development, including basic nutrition, food preparation, and resource management skills.

Strategy Tip

As a nutrition professional, be ready to give reasonable ideas for stretching the food dollar. What other ideas can you offer these clients?

More information about CACFP can be found at https://www.fns.usda.gov/cacfp[26]

More information about EFNEP can be found at https://nifa.usda.gov/program/expanded-food-and-nutrition-education-program-efnep

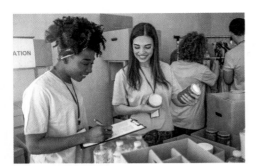

Community food bank.

© Dragana Gordic/Shutterstock.

More information about Feeding America can be found at https://www .feedingamerica.org/[28]

Strategy Tip

Students can volunteer at their local food bank or emergency feeding programs. Which programs are in your town?

More information about USDA Food Distribution can be found at: https://www .usda.gov/topics/food-and-nutrition/food -distribution[29]

More information about SNAP can be found at https://www.fns.usda.gov/snap /supplemental-nutrition-assistance -program[30]

More information about Meals on Wheels America can be found at https://www .mealsonwheelsamerica.org/[31]

Feeding America

This is the largest domestic hunger-relief organization in the United States.[28] They provide food through a network of 200 food banks. Emergency food providers include food pantries, soup kitchens, shelters, and other charitable agencies that provide food to those in need. Annually, it distributes billions of pounds of food to millions of individuals at-risk for or experiencing food insecurity in the 50 states, District of Columbia, and Puerto Rico through community programs, including food pantries, soup kitchens, emergency shelters, after-school programs, and Kids Cafes operated by private nonprofit organizations, government-affiliated agencies, or faith-based agencies affiliated with churches, mosques, synagogues, and other organizations.[28] In 2020, 4 billion pounds of groceries were rescued from going to waste, over 1.8 billion pounds of fresh produce were distributed to families by Feeding America network members, and over 573 million meals were secured for those in need.[28]

Food Distribution Programs

There are several food distribution programs,[29] including:

- Commodity Supplemental Food Program (CSFP)
- Department of Defense (DoD) Fresh Fruit and Vegetable Program
- Food Aid Program
- Food Distribution Disaster Assistance Program
- Food Distribution Program on Indian Reservations (FDPIR)
- Food Purchase Program
- McGovern-Dole International Food for Education and Child Nutrition Program
- National Processing Pilot Program
- Schools/Child Nutrition (CN) USDA Foods Program
- The Emergency Food Assistance Program (TEFAP)
- USDA Foods Processing

Overall, these programs support the nutrition safety net through commodity distribution and other nutrition assistance to families with low incomes, emergency feeding programs, Native American reservations, and older adults.

Supplemental Nutrition Assistance Program (SNAP)

SNAP,[30] historically known as the Food Stamp Program, "provides nutrition benefits to supplement the food budget of needy families so they can purchase healthy food and move toward self-sufficiency." Electronic benefits transfer cards are used to buy eligible food in authorized retail food stores.

Meals on Wheels America

This program[31] supports more than 5,000 community-based programs in the United States. Meals on Wheels empowers programs to "deliver the nutritious meals" and provide "friendly visits and safety checks that enable America's seniors to live nourished lives with independence and dignity."[31] A variety of organizations, including local communities, churches, charitable organizations, and concerned citizens, are examples of participating programs.

National School Lunch and School Breakfast Programs

These programs[32,33] provide nutritionally balanced, low-cost, or free breakfasts and lunches to children enrolled in public and nonprofit private schools and residential childcare institutions. This program is usually administered by the state education agency.

Senior Farmers' Market Nutrition Program (SFMNP)

This program[34] provides older low-income adults with "access to locally grown fruits, vegetables, honey and herbs" with coupons/vouchers that can be used at farmers' markets, roadside stands, and community-supported agriculture programs during the harvest season.

WIC and the WIC Farmers' Market Nutrition Program

Both of these programs[35,36] provide "federal grants to states for supplemental foods, healthcare referrals, and nutrition education eligible pregnant, breast-feeding, nonbreastfeeding postpartum women, and to infants and children up to 5 years of age who are found to be at nutritional risk." Similar to the SFMNP, WIC Farmers Market Nutrition Program provides access to local foods from farmers, farmers' markets, or roadside stands approved by the state to accept the coupons/vouchers.

Summer Food Service Program (SFSP)

This program[37] provides reimbursements to program operators for nutritious breakfasts, lunches, and snacks to ensure that children and teens in areas with lower incomes continue to receive nutritious meals during long school vacations, when they typically would not have access to school meals. Programs vary by area and may be accessed through schools or community organizations. This is a federally funded, state-administered program.

Impact of Food Insecurity on the Public

Food insecurity can have grave consequences on dietary quality, health, and chronic disease risk.[19,38-40] Examples include physical impairments, such as illness and fatigue; psychological suffering, such as feelings of constraint to go against norms and values and stress at home; and sociofamilial disturbances, such as modifications of eating patterns and ritual, disruption of household dynamics, and distortion of the means of food acquisition and management.[38] Holben and Berger-Marshall[19] noted that "Food insecurity is a high priority for public health stakeholders, given its negative impact from public health and economic perspectives.... Across the lifespan, food insecurity often results in disrupted eating patterns that can lead to suboptimal nutritional status..., [contributing] to negative physical and mental [health] outcomes and an increased risk for disease."

Strategies to Assist the Public in Securing Adequate Food

Public health nutrition professionals, registered dietitian nutritionists, nutrition and dietetics technicians, registered nurses, and physicians, along with other healthcare providers and team members, can assist the public in improving food security. This is paramount, since noncompliance with food and nutrition-related suggestions may simply be due to poor access to food rather than a lack of understanding of the regimen. Practical suggestions have been published for incorporating food security principles into practice.[19] During an interview, public health professionals should inquire about issues similar to those assessed in the household food security survey module, including: 1) anxiety related to food budget or supply and whether the budget is able to meet basic needs; 2) experiences relating to running out of food without being able to obtain more due to financial constraints; 3) perceptions of intake adequacy; and 4) food use.[6,7,19]

More information about the National School Lunch and School Breakfast Programs can be found at https://www.fns.usda.gov/nslp[32] and https://www.fns.usda.gov/sbp/school-breakfast-program[33]

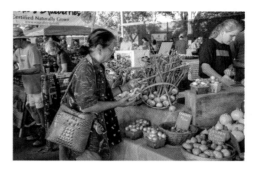

Local Farmer's Market.

© Jen Wolf/Shutterstock.

More information about the Senior Farmers' Market Nutrition Program can be found at https://www.fns.usda.gov/sfmnp/senior-farmers-market-nutrition-program[34]

More information about WIC and the WIC Farmers' Market Nutrition Program can be found at https://www.fns.usda.gov/wic[35] and https://www.fns.usda.gov/fmnp/wic-farmers-market-nutrition-program[36]

Discussion Prompt

Locate some area public schools that offer a Summer Food Service Program. Discuss their contribution to the community and what would occur short-term and long-term without their provisions.

More information about the SFSP can be found at https://www.fns.usda.gov/sfsp/summer-food-service-program[37]

For example, in the context of having inadequate resources, questions could be posed about eating balanced meals, cutting meal size or skipping meals, and experiencing unintentional weight loss. In addition, questions to include should be related to:

- Available resources, including household income, that the individual has for food to implement dietary and nutrition interventions
- Storage facilities for food, including having a refrigerator and/or freezer in the household
- Availability of utilities, including gas, electric, and water, to the household
- Participation in federal and nonfederal food assistance programs in their community, including food pantries, soup kitchens, and community gardens
- How the household acquires food, including gardening practices, hunting for game or fish, and related food safety issues related to dressing fish and game
- Meal planning and purchasing tips related to preserving food resources and reducing food waste.[19]

When working with clients lacking resources, public health nutrition professionals should be prepared to discuss the rationale for federal and nonfederal food assistance programs and their benefits. In addition, being able to assist clients in accessing these programs or referring them to another professional who can assist is vital. In fact, client educational resources with federal and nonfederal programmatic information could be developed and updated periodically.[19,41] To assist clients to preserve scarce resources and reduce food waste, other educational strategies may include an explanation of manufacturers' expiration codes and other information found on packages, such as "use-by" and "sell-by" dates. Food safety education related to food preservation methods, including canning and freezing, and food storage processes should also be included.[19,41]

Summary

Securing adequate food for the public is paramount to achieving and maintaining health. Food security exists when all people, at all times, have access to sufficient food for an active and healthy life without resorting to emergency food supplies or socially unacceptable ways of obtaining food, including begging, stealing, or scavenging.[3] Understanding food security measurement strategies for programmatic evaluation and inclusion in community needs assessments, as well as the consequences of food insecurity and programs designed to assist the public in securing adequate food, is vital for public health professionals. The Economic Research Service of the United States Department of Agriculture is a vital resource for public nutrition professionals to stay abreast of food security-related issues,[4] as is the Food Research and Action Center (FRAC).[42]

More information about FRAC can be found at https://frac.org/[42]

Learning Portfolio

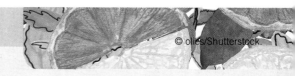
© olies/Shutterstock.

Issues for Discussion

1. You are developing a nutrition intervention that you think will impact the food security status of households in the community. The intervention is planned to be 12 months in length. Develop an assessment/evaluation strategy to assess the impact of the program on household food security status.

2. Individuals in the local community have had trouble securing adequate food for their households, and your agency's public health nutrition team is working with these individuals. During a meeting, you plan to discuss how some of the clients are coping to minimize household food insecurity. Develop a list of strategies that you believe would be generated from such a discussion and the risks associated with those strategies.

3. Select a life stage group—for example, senior adults—and discuss food assistance programs that may be accessed in the community, noting what resources each program provides.

4. Develop an interviewing strategy that will assist you in identifying clients at risk for food insecurity.

Practical Activities

1. Volunteer at a local food pantry, soup kitchen, or free meal program.
2. Interview adults at a senior meal program to learn about their perceptions of the meals and activities offered.
3. Visit a local K–12 school that receives reimbursement for school meals. Observe what is offered, served, and eaten by the children and teens. Also observe what is wasted on the trays.
4. Start a community garden plot or interview a community garden plot gardener or community garden manager to learn about community gardening and its potential role in alleviating food insecurity.
5. For 5–7 days, eat for about $3.00 per day.

Key Terms

	page
Community food security	406
Nutrition security	406
Food insecurity	406
Hunger	406
Food security	406
Food insufficiency	407

Case Study: Food Insecurity

Becky is a 24-year-old mother of two children: Thomas, 2, and Kendall, 7. Becky never finished high school after she had Kendall because she was living with her boyfriend who earned enough money to support the household. A few months ago, her boyfriend left her and now she is left with the burden of all of their household financials and has no job. She has spent almost the last of her savings within the past month. With the little money she has left, she has been buying fast food items off of the "dollar menu" for her and her children for almost every meal of the day. She is worried that she will soon run out of money, but she does not want her children to ever go without food or know that they are in such a tight financial position.

1. What "symptoms" of food insecurity is Becky exhibiting?

2. What program(s) may she and/or her children qualify for?

3. What program may the household qualify for?

4. What community programs would you suggest that Becky seek out?

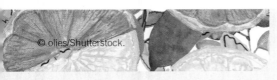
© olies/Shutterstock.

Learning Portfolio

Case Study: Evaluation of Community Program for Families

An agency is developing a community intervention targeted at improving fruit and vegetable intake among families who self-identified as food insecure through a screening questionnaire. The agency would like to measure food security status before and after the intervention, what you recommend to the agency?

1. If the intervention is targeted at households with children and without children?

2. What if respondent burden is a concern?

Resource List

1. USDA Food Security Definitions: https://www.ers.usda.gov/topics/food -nutrition-assistance/food-security-in-the-us/definitions-of-food-security.aspx
2. USDA Food Security Measurement: https://www.ers.usda.gov/topics/food -nutrition-assistance/food-security-in-the-us/measurement.aspx
3. Food Security Survey Tools: https://www.ers.usda.gov/topics/food-nutrition -assistance/food-security-in-the-us/survey-tools/
4. US Food Security Estimates: Coleman-Jenson A, Rabbitt MP, Gregory C, Singh A. Household food security in the United States, 2019 (ERR-275). United States Department of Agriculture, Economic Research Service; 2020.
5. National US Surveys that Include Food Security Measurement: https://www.ers .usda.gov/data-products/food-security-in-the-united-states/documentation .aspx#foodaps
6. USDA Food and Nutrition Assistance Programs: https://www.fns.usda.gov/
7. Healthy People 2030: https://health.gov/healthypeople
8. Feeding America: https://www.feedingamerica.org
9. Food Research and Action Center: https://frac.org/
10. Academy of Nutrition and Dietetics: https://www.eatright.org/

Key Term References

[a]Hamm MW, Bellows AC. Community food security and nutrition educators. *J Nutr Educ Behav.* 2003;35(1):37-43.

[b]Life Science Research Office. Federation of American Societies for Experimental Biology. Core indicator of nutritional state for difficult-to-sample populations. *J Nutr.* 1990;102(suppl 11):1599-1600.

[c]Briefel RR, Woteki CE. Development of food sufficiency questions for the Third National Health and Nutrition Examination Survey. *J Nutr Educ.* 1992;24(1): 24S-28S.

[d]*Food insecurity and hunger in the United States: an assessment of the measure.* Accessed February 10, 2021. http://www.ers.usda.gov/topics/food-nutrition -assistance/food-security-in-the-us/definitions-of-food-security/cnstat-assessment .aspx. Updated on September 9, 2020.

[e]*Nutrition Action themes for the United States: a report in response to the International Conference on Nutrition.* Washington, DC: U.S. Department of Agriculture Center for Nutrition Policy and Promotion; 1996. CNPP-2 Occasional Paper.

References

1. U.S. Department of Health and Human Services. *Healthy People 2030.* Accessed February 10, 2021. https://health.gov/healthypeople

2. Coleman-Jenson A, Rabbitt MP, Gregory C, Singh A. Household food security in the United States, 2019 (ERR-275). United States Department of Agriculture, Economic Research Service; 2020.

3. Economic Research Service, U.S. Department of Agriculture. Food Security in the U.S. – Measurement. Accessed February 10, 2021. Updated on December 18, 2020. https://www.ers.usda.gov/topics/food-nutrition-assistance/food-security-in-the-us/measurement.aspx

4. Economic Research Service, U.S. Department of Agriculture. Food Security in the United States – Definitions of Food Security. Accessed February 10, 2021. Updated on September 9, 2020. https://www.ers.usda.gov/topics/food-nutrition-assistance/food-security-in-the-us/definitions-of-food-security.aspx

5. Economic Research Service, U.S. Department of Agriculture. Food insecurity and hunger in the United States: an assessment of the measure. Accessed February 10, 2021. Updated on September 9, 2020. http://www.ers.usda.gov/topics/food-nutrition-assistance/food-security-in-the-us/definitions-of-food-security/cnstat-assessment.aspx

6. Bickel G, Nord M, Price C, Hamilton W, Cook J. Guide to measuring household food security, revised 2000. Alexandria, VA: U.S. Department of Agriculture, Food and Nutrition Service; 2000.

7. Economic Research Service, U.S. Department of Agriculture. Food Security in the U.S. – Survey Tools. Accessed February 10, 2021. https://www.ers.usda.gov/topics/food-nutrition-assistance/food-security-in-the-us/survey-tools/

8. Radimer KL, Olson CM, Campbell CC. Development of indicators to assess hunger. *J Nutr*. 1990;120(suppl 11):1544-1548.

9. Radimer KL, Olson CM, Greene JC, Campbell CC, Habicht J-P. Understanding hunger and developing indicators to assess it in women and children. *J Nutr Educ*. 1992;24(1):36S-44S.

10. Wehler CA, Scott RI, Anderson JJ. The community childhood hunger identification project: a model of domestic hunger—demonstration project in Seattle, Washington. *J Nutr Educ*. 1992;24(suppl 1):29S-35S.

11. U.S. Bureau of Labor Statistics, U.S. Department of Labor. Labor force statistics from the current Population Survey. Accessed February 11, 2021. https://www.bls.gov/cps/home.htm

12. Economic Research Service, United States Department of Agriculture. Food security in the United States – documentation overview of surveys. Accessed February 15, 2021. https://www.ers.usda.gov/data-products/food-security-in-the-united-states/documentation.aspx#foodaps. Updated on December 18, 2020.

13. National Center for Education Statistics. Early Childhood Longitudinal Studies. Accessed on February 10, 2021. https://nces.ed.gov/ecls/

14. Centers for Disease Control and Prevention. National Center for Health Statistics. National Health and Nutrition Examination Survey. Accessed February 10, 2021. https://www.cdc.gov/nchs/nhanes/index.htm?CDC_AA_refVal=https%3A%2F%2Fwww.cdc.gov%2Fnchs%2Fnhanes.htm

15. Institute for Social Research, University of Michigan. *Panel Study of Income Dynamics*. Accessed February 10, 2021. https://psidonline.isr.umich.edu/

16. United States Census Bureau. Survey of program dynamics. Accessed February 10, 2021. https://www.census.gov/programs-surveys/sipp/about/spd.html

17. United States Census Bureau. Measuring household experiences during the Coronavirus pandemic. Accessed on February 15, 2021. https://www.census.gov/data/experimental-data-products/household-pulse-survey.html

18. Economic Research Service, U.S. Department of Agriculture. Food Security in the U.S.: Definitions of food security. Accessed February 10, 2021. https://www.ers.usda.gov/topics/food-nutrition-assistance/food-security-in-the-us/definitions-of-food-security.aspx

19. Holben DH, Berger Marshall M. Position of the Academy of Nutrition and Dietetics: food insecurity in the United States. *J Acad Nutr Diet*. 2017;117(12):1991-2002.

20. The United States Conference of Mayors. The United States Conference of Majors Hunger and Homelessness Survey: A Status Report on Hunger and Homeless in America's Cities. Accessed February 17, 2021. https://endhomelessness.org/wp-content/uploads/2017/02/US-Conference-of-Mayors-Report-on-Homelessness-and-Hunger_Final.pdf

21. Feeding America. Map the meal gap 2019. Accessed February 17, 2021. https://www.feedingamerica.org/sites/default/files/2019-05/2017-map-the-meal-gap-full.pdf

22. Tuttle CJ, Beatty TKM. The effects of energy price shocks on household food security in low-income households, ERR-233, U.S. Department of Agriculture, Economic Research Service, July 2017.

23. Kempson KM, Keenan DP, Sadani PS, Ridlen S, Rosato NS. Food management practices used by people with limited resources to maintain food sufficiency as reported by nutrition educators. *J Am Diet Assoc*. 2002;102(12):1795-1799.

24. Greder K, Brotherson MJ. Food security and low-income families: research to inform policy and programs. *J Fam Cons Sci*. 2002;94(2):40-47.

25. Food and Nutrition Service, U.S. Department of Agriculture. Food and Nutrition Service – Programs. Accessed February 17, 2021. https://www.fns.usda.gov/

26. Food and Nutrition Service, U.S. Department of Agriculture. Child and adult care food program. Accessed February 17, 2021. https://www.fns.usda.gov/cacfp

27. National Institute of Food and Agriculture, U.S. Department of Agriculture. Expanded food and nutrition education program. Accessed February 17, 2021. https://nifa.usda.gov/program/expanded-food-and-nutrition-education-program-efnep

28. Feeding America. Accessed February 17, 2021. https://www.feedingamerica.org/

29. United States Department of Agriculture. Food distribution. Accessed February 14, 2021. https://www.usda.gov/topics/food-and-nutrition/food-distribution

30. Food and Nutrition Service, U.S. Department of Agriculture. Supplemental nutrition assistance program. Accessed February 17, 2021. https://www.fns.usda.gov/snap/supplemental-nutrition-assistance-program

31. Meals on Wheels America. Accessed February 17, 2021. https://www.mealsonwheelsamerica.org/

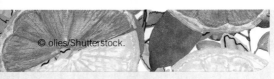
© olies/Shutterstock.

Learning Portfolio

32. Food and Nutrition Service, U.S. Department of Agriculture. National school lunch program. Accessed February 17, 2021. https://www.fns.usda.gov/nslp

33. Food and Nutrition Service, U.S. Department of Agriculture. School breakfast program. Accessed February 17, 2021. https://www.fns.usda.gov/sbp/school-breakfast-program

34. Food and Nutrition Service, U.S. Department of Agriculture. Senior Farmers' Market nutrition program. Accessed February 17, 2021. https://www.fns.usda.gov/sfmnp/senior-farmers-market-nutrition-program

35. Food and Nutrition Service, U.S. Department of Agriculture. Special supplemental nutrition program for Women, Infants and Children (WIC). Accessed February 17, 2021. https://www.fns.usda.gov/wic

36. Food and Nutrition Service, U.S. Department of Agriculture. WIC Farmers' Market Nutrition Program. Accessed February 17, 2021. https://www.fns.usda.gov/fmnp/wic-farmers-market-nutrition-program

37. Food and Nutrition Service, U.S. Department of Agriculture. Summer Food Service program. Accessed February 17, 2021. https://www.fns.usda.gov/sfsp/summer-food-service-program

38. Hamelin A-M, Habicht J-P, Beaudry M. Food insecurity: consequences for the household and broader social implications. *J Nutr*. 1999;129(2):525S-528S.

39. Gundersen C, Ziliak JP. Food insecurity and health outcomes. *Health Aff*. 2015;34(11):1830-1839.

40. Gregory CA, Coleman-Jensen A. Food insecurity, chronic disease, and health among working-age adults, ERR-235, U.S. Department of Agriculture, Economic Research Service, July 2017.

41. Boeing KL, Holben DH. Self-identified food security knowledge and practices of licensed dietitians in Ohio: implications for dietetics and clinical nutrition practice. *Top Clin Nutr*. 2003;18(3):185-191.

42. Food Research & Action Center. Accessed February 17, 2021. https://frac.org/

CHAPTER 14

Safeguarding the Food Supply and Securing the Food Supply

Chloe Giraldi, MS, RDN, LDN

(We would like to acknowledge the work of Rebecca Kahn, MA; Paul N. Taylor, PhD; and Barbara Bruemmer, PhD, RDN, CD; in past editions of Nutrition in Public Health.)

Learning Outcomes

AFTER STUDYING THIS CHAPTER AND REFLECTING ON THE CONTENTS, YOU SHOULD BE ABLE TO:

1. List and describe the roles of federal, state, and local agencies responsible for the safety of the U.S. food supply.

2. List and describe the hazards to food safety.

3. Identify current national food safety issues.

4. Identify organisms that may be disseminated by ingestion and foods most at risk for intentional contamination.

5. Recommend actions that community and public health dietitians/nutritionists can take to promote preparedness for the community and the consumer.

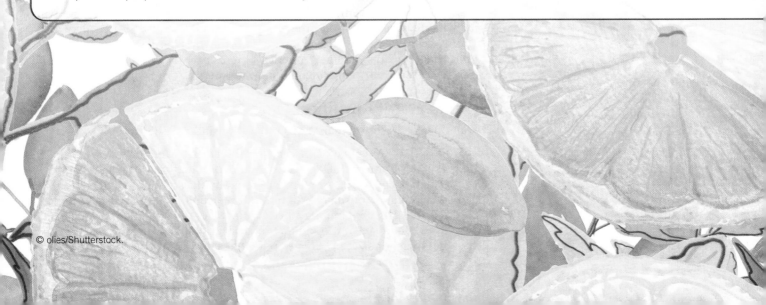

Introduction

America's food supply is among the safest in the world. The federal food safety system was recently strengthened in many areas, with new surveillance systems, better prevention programs, faster outbreak responses, enhanced education programs, more focused and coordinated research initiatives, and better risk assessment activities. According to officials, federal food safety agencies are improving their working relationships with each other.[1]

Despite these efforts, every year, approximately 48 million people contract a foodborne illness, 128,000 are hospitalized, and 3,000 die from foodborne illness.[2] Causative factors include transportation and refrigeration issues, an increasing volume of imported foods, and more people eating more meals away from home. Among those at greatest risk for foodborne illness are children, the elderly, pregnant women, and immunocompromised persons. By 2050, the population of older adults (those over 60 years old) will reach nearly 2.1 billion, and that same age group will also outnumber children and adolescents between the ages of 10 and 24 years old.[3,4]

Americans demand nutritious, wholesome, safe food that is plentiful, varied, and at a reasonable cost. In a rapidly changing world, food producers, processors, vendors, and regulators must constantly adapt to the growing expectations and demands of consumers.

The basic framework of today's federal food safety system was developed early in the 20th century. President Theodore Roosevelt's investigation of Chicago's meat packing industry and Upton Sinclair's exposé of conditions there[5] prompted passage of the Meat Inspection Act of 1906 (concomitant with the Pure Food and Drug Act). Early in this century, terrorist attacks in the United States prompted increased scrutiny of the various food safety regulatory systems and procedures, and passage of anti-bioterrorism legislation.[6] The Department of Homeland Security absorbed some food safety functions by 2003.[7] Against this backdrop, the full range of food safety issues continues to demand vigilance by industry, government, and consumers.

Public health professionals, dietitians/nutritionists, and consumers must not become (or remain) complacent about the safety of the nation's food supply. Significant challenges have not been overcome and new challenges emerge frequently (e.g., globalization of food production, manufacturing, and marketing; geographic centralization and consolidation of food processing; some foodborne pathogens' ability to overcome traditional hurdles such as acidity, temperature, or oxygen, employed against them; new foodborne pathogens evolving or being discovered; and bioterrorism directed at food and water supplies). Old paradigms are increasingly irrelevant; yet, as is human nature, powerful forces resist the changes necessary to keep pace with a dynamic system of food production and supply and to ensure safety at all points in the system. The new paradigm for the 21st century should make this chapter's opening line, "America's food supply is among the safest in the world," obsolete by ensuring global food safety.

Food Safety Defined

Stier defines *food safety* in terms of hazards and risks:

> A safe food may be defined as a product that contains no physical, chemical, or microbial organisms or byproducts of those organisms, which, if consumed by man, will result in illness, injury, or death (an unacceptable consumer health risk). The definition purposely does not use the term contaminants because many of the potential hazards in food … are typically found in or on the food. It is their concentration, numbers, or size that creates potential safety problems.[8]

Hazard expresses a food's capacity to cause harm (i.e., "Any biological, chemical, or physical property that may cause an unacceptable consumer health risk"[8]). The food does not always cause harm; rather, hazard indicates that the food might cause a specified harm. The probability that the specified harm will occur is the hazard's associated "risk."[9]

To evaluate food safety, scientists must first attempt risk assessment (i.e., to "identify hazards related to foods or food components and then estimate the size of the risk that the hazard will occur"[9]). "When conducting a hazard analysis, the [food processor] looks at potential hazards that could realistically cause illness or injury."[8] Risk management involves deciding whether an identified risk is acceptable. "Note that the process outlined…considers all foods to have some degree of risk," that is, "no food is absolutely safe."[9]

Public health and community dietitians/nutritionists must understand food safety issues, using critical thinking to evaluate scientific literature and the press, in order to keep consumers informed in today's environment of "junk science" and pseudoscience. Always a dynamic field, food technologies and food safety regulations are changing at an increasingly rapid rate. Food scientists, environmental health specialists, health educators, and other public health colleagues may be consulted to help educate consumers about food safety issues. These professionals can help consumers sort through the many government and scientific websites that are available. Lists of these websites are maintained by organizations that include The Center for Food Safety[10] (https://center-for-food-safety.uark.edu/), the Simmons College Center for Hygiene and Health in Home and Community (https://www.simmons.edu/academics/research/center-hygiene-and-health),[11] and more than 100 Internet sites in the references to this chapter.

Protecting the Food Supply
Federal Agencies

Several federal agencies, with sometimes overlapping jurisdictions, share responsibility for the safety of the U.S. food supply (**Table 14–1**). The following sections describe the principal federal agencies and their roles.

U.S. Food and Drug Administration

The Department of Health and Human Services' (DHHS) U.S. Food and Drug Administration (FDA) oversees all domestic and imported food (except meat and poultry) sold in interstate commerce, including seafood, shell eggs, bottled water, and wine beverages containing 7% alcohol.[12] The FDA enforces food safety laws governing these foods through inspections; food analysis; safety reviews of food and color additives and animal drugs; monitoring of the safety of food-animal feeds; developing model codes, ordinances, guidelines, and interpretations; working with states to implement such models; establishing good food manufacturing practices (GMP); establishing sanitation and packaging requirements; establishing Hazard Analysis and Critical Control Points (HACCP) programs; collaborating with foreign governments to ensure imported food safety; requesting and monitoring voluntary recalls of unsafe foods; enforcement; research; and industry and consumer food safety education.[12]

Food Safety and Inspection Service

The U.S. Department of Agriculture's (USDA) Food Safety and Inspection Service (FSIS) oversees domestic and imported meat, poultry, and related products (e.g., meat- or poultry-containing stews, pizzas, and other frozen foods), and processed egg products (generally liquid, frozen, and dried pasteurized egg

TABLE 14–1
Federal Agencies with Food Safety Responsibilities

Agency	Unit	Mission	Internet
Department of Agriculture (USDA)	Animal and Plant Health Inspection Service (APHIS)[a] Food Safety and Inspection Service (FSIS) Agricultural Research Service (ARS), National Animal Disease Center (NADC)	Protects and promotes U.S. agricultural health Ensures that the nation's commercial supply of meat, poultry, and egg products is safe, wholesome, and correctly labeled and packaged. Conducts research on animal health and food safety problems	USDA: http://www.usda.gov APHIS: http://www.aphis.usda.gov FSIS: http://www.fsis.usda.gov ARS/NADC: https://www.ars.usda.gov/
Department of Commerce (USDC)	National Oceanic and Atmospheric Administration (NOAA)	Administers National Seafood Inspection Program (NSIP) offering seafood inspection, grading, certification, and other services to the seafood industry (voluntary, fee-for-service)	USDC: http://www.commerce.gov NOAA: http://www.noaa.gov NSIP: https://www.fisheries.noaa.gov /insight/noaas-seafood-inspection-program
Department of Health and Human Services (DHHS)	Centers for Disease Control and Prevention (CDC) Food & Drug Administration (FDA)	Tracks foodborne illness incidents and outbreaks; provides data and information to the other food safety agencies Approves food and drugs for widespread use; its Center for Food Safety and Applied Nutrition (CFSAN) ensures that food is safe, nutritious, and wholesome	DHHS: https://www.hhs.gov/ CDC: http://www.cdc.gov FDA: http://www.fda.gov CFSAN: https://www.fda.gov/about -fda/fda-organization/center-food -safety-and-applied-nutrition-cfsan
Department of Homeland Security (DHS)	Customs & Border Protection (CBP)	Inspects agricultural goods arriving in the United States at ports and borders	DHS: http://www.dhs.gov/dhspublic/ CBP: https://home.treasury.gov/about /history Introducing the new CBP Agriculture Specialist: https://www.cbp.gov/ careers/frontline-careers/as
Department of the Treasury	Bureau of Alcohol, Tobacco, Firearms and Explosives (ATF)	Regulates qualification and operations of distilleries, wineries, breweries, importers, and wholesalers	Treasury: http://www.ustreas.gov ATF: http://www.atf.gov
Federal Trade Commission	Bureau of Consumer Protection (BCP); Division of Advertising Practices (DAP); Division of Consumer Protection (DCP); Division of Enforcement (DE)	Protects consumers against unfair, deceptive, or fraudulent practices; protects consumers from deceptive and unsubstantiated advertising (advertising claims for food, particularly those relating to nutritional or health benefits of foods); conducts law enforcement activities to protect consumers	FTC: http://www.ftc.gov BCP: https://www.ftc.gov/about-ftc /bureaus-offices/bureau-consumer -protection DAP: https://www.ftc.gov/about-ftc /bureaus-offices/bureau-consumer -protection/our-divisions/division-advertising-practices DE: https://www.ftc.gov/about-ftc /bureaus-offices/bureau-consumer -protection/our-divisions/division -enforcement

[a]Some APHIS functions and personnel transferred to the Department of Homeland Security, Customs and Border Protection, on March 1, 2003. Compiled from: https://www.foodsafety.gov/about#:~:text=The%20Food%20Safety%20and%20Inspection,safety%20in%20the%20United%20States, 2019.

products). FSIS enforces food safety laws governing these foods through antemortem and postmortem inspections of food animals, meat, and poultry slaughter and processing plant inspections, monitoring and inspecting processed egg products (together with the USDA Agricultural Marketing Service), food analysis, establishing additive and ingredient standards, inspections of foreign meat and poultry processing plants exporting to the United States, requesting and monitoring unsafe meat/poultry products recalls, meat/poultry safety research, and industry and consumer food safety education.[12]

U.S. Environmental Protection Agency

The Environmental Protection Agency (EPA) regulates pesticides and oversees drinking water quality. Its food safety role for foods made from plants, seafood, meat, and poultry includes regulating toxic substances and wastes to prevent entry into the environment or foods, determining new pesticide safety, setting tolerance levels for pesticide residues in foods, and promoting safe use of pesticides (enforcement of these standards is an FDA function).[12] The EPA also establishes safe drinking water standards and assists states in protecting and monitoring drinking water quality.

Customs and Border Protection

In 2003, the Department of Homeland Security (DHS), Customs and Border Protection (CBP) assumed responsibility for inspecting agricultural goods arriving in the United States. Previously, this was a function of the USDA's Animal and Plant Health Inspection Service (APHIS).[13,14] The transfer "linked and integrated the...scientific mission of agriculture border inspection to the expertise and operational capabilities of the primary CBP mission: to prevent terrorists and terrorist weapons from entering the United States."[13] CBP expects to "play an important role in the Department of Homeland Security's multi-layered approach to protect the food supply from the threats of agroterrorism and bioterrorism,"[13] while also detecting and denying entry to animal and plant pests and diseases that could harm U.S. agriculture.

Centers for Disease Control and Prevention

DHHS's Centers for Disease Control and Prevention (CDC) oversees and directs prevention efforts against foodborne and waterborne infections. Collaborating with other domestic and international agencies, the CDC recently expanded its mission to work toward effective global surveillance and control of foodborne and waterborne pathogens. In the United States, the CDC participates in the National Food Safety Initiative (NFSI) with the FDA, USDA, and other agencies to address food safety problems, and collaborates with the EPA and the drinking water industry to improve drinking water safety.[12,15] The CDC also initiated and participates in addressing emerging infectious diseases and preventing future emergent infectious diseases worldwide.[16]

National Oceanic and Atmospheric Administration

The Department of Commerce, National Oceanic and Atmospheric Administration (NOAA) administers a Seafood Inspection Program offering seafood inspection, grading, and certification; vessel and plant sanitation; label review; laboratory analysis; training; and consultative and information services to the seafood industry on a voluntary fee-for-service basis.[17,18] Processors may use official marks on complying products, indicating that they are federally inspected. (Note: All seafood processors must participate in the FDA's seafood HACCP program,[19,20] under which the FDA inspects the processors annually. FDA provides guidance on fisheries products, hazards, and controls while allowing latitude to industry in implementing their HACCP programs.[21])

Bureau of Consumer Protection

The Federal Trade Commission's (FTC) Division of Advertising Practices, Bureau of Consumer Protection protects consumers from deceptive and unsubstantiated advertising. It enforces laws pertaining to advertising claims for food (particularly those claims relating to nutritional or health benefits of foods), television infomercials (to ensure that format and content are non-deceptive), and general advertising.[22]

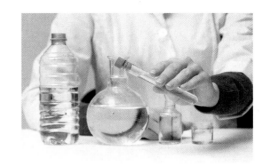

Scientist is analysing and testing a water concept.

© Happy Nati/Shutterstock.

Alcohol and Tobacco Tax and Trade Bureau

The U.S. Department of the Treasury's Alcohol and Tobacco Tax and Trade Bureau (TTB) regulates distilleries, wineries, breweries, and importers and wholesalers in the industry. TTB tests new alcohol products, determines whether products currently marketed pose a health risk to consumers, and ensures that alcohol beverage labels are not misleading.[23]

State and Local Collaboration

State and local governmental agencies oversee all food products within their jurisdictions, in cooperation with federal agencies. Usually, public health departments and state agriculture departments are the delegated authorities, with responsibilities at the state, county, and city level, varying by state. Registered sanitarians, environmental health specialists, and sometimes other classes of employees inspect restaurants, food stores, supermarkets, other retail food establishments, dairy farms, milk-processing plants, grain mills, and food manufacturing plants within local jurisdictions. They also may collaborate with federal agencies to develop and implement food safety standards for foods produced within state borders, and seize unsafe food products made or distributed within their jurisdictions.[12] State food sanitation codes usually meet or exceed model federal standards, and for those states maintaining their own commodity inspection programs (e.g., at least 27 states have state meat inspection programs[24]), the state program must be equivalent to the corresponding federal program and operates under federal oversight.

Community and public health dietitians/nutritionists should know their jurisdiction's regulatory authorities for sanitation and food safety and develop working relationships with them to identify and serve the needs of their communities. Inviting these officials to attend or speak at regional, state, and local dietetic or other association meetings is one way to build networking relationships. Dietitians/nutritionists will find opportunities to assist these officials during natural disasters, in investigating outbreaks of food- and waterborne disease, and during other civil disturbances.[25-27] Hurricane Sandy highlighted the importance of nutrition professionals on emergency preparedness teams. Many people were left without power, safe drinking water, or a way to feed themselves, which was of particular concern for those who were receiving nutrition support through various feeding tubes. Registered dietitians and other nutrition professionals are part of city and regional emergency preparedness plans to protect the public during natural disasters.[28] Civil emergency preparedness and response organizations should include community and public health nutritionists and/or registered dietitians on their teams. (Find out who is on your local team—see the American Civil Defense Association's website at https://tacda.org/contact-us/.[29]) Dietitians/nutritionists are also needed to participate in emergency nutrition and food aid research.[30,31]

Food Safety Laws

Major food safety legislation in the United States began in 1906 with the Pure Food and Drug Act (which created the FDA) and the Meat Inspection Act. **Table 14–2** lists several federal laws with applicability to food safety. Some of these laws are discussed in the following sections.

Federal Meat Inspection Act of 1906

The Federal Meat Inspection Act (amended by the Wholesome Meat Act in 1967) requires continuous inspection (antemortem, during slaughter, and postmortem) by USDA or USDA-sanctioned state meat inspection programs

> ### *Pandemic Learning Opportunity*
> What happened to a large meat-packing plant during the COVID-19 pandemic? How could this have been prevented?

> ### *Pandemic Learning Opportunity*
> How did dietitians assist with the COVID-19 pandemic?

TABLE 14–2
Selected Federal Regulations Important to Food Safety

Year	Legislation	Resource
1906	Pure Food and Drug Act	https://history.house.gov/Historical-Highlights/1901-1950/Pure-Food-and-Drug-Act/
1906	Federal Meat Inspection Act	https://www.fsis.usda.gov/wps/wcm/connect/fsis-content/fsis-questionable-content/celebrating-100-years-of-fmia/overview/ct_index
1967	Wholesome Meat Act	https://www.ncbi.nlm.nih.gov/books/NBK235649/
1968	Wholesome Poultry Products Act	https://www.fsis.usda.gov/wps/wcm/connect/5d43763f-a9aa-459b-94e0-cdf9e3543923/Inspection_and_Grading_What_Are_the_Differences.pdf?MOD=AJPERES
1938	Federal Food, Drug, and Cosmetic Act	https://www.fda.gov/regulatory-information/laws-enforced-fda/federal-food-drug-and-cosmetic-act-fdc-act
1958	Food Additives Amendment	https://www.fda.gov/food/generally-recognized-safe-gras/fdas-approach-gras-provision-history-processes
1960	Color Additives Amendment	https://www.fda.gov/industry/color-additives/color-additives-history
1938	Federal Trade Commission Act (amended for food)	https://www.ftc.gov/enforcement/statutes/federal-trade-commission-act
1957	Federal Poultry Products Inspection Act	https://www.fsis.usda.gov/wps/portal/fsis/topics/rulemaking/poultry-products-inspection-acts
1966	Fair Packaging and Labeling Act	http://www.ftc.gov/os/statutes/fplajump.shtm
1980	Infant Formula Act	https://www.fda.gov/food/guidance-documents-regulatory-information-topic-food-and-dietary-supplements/infant-formula-guidance-documents-regulatory-information
1990	Nutrition Education and Labeling Act	https://www.fda.gov/food/guidance-documents-regulatory-information-topic-food-and-dietary-supplements/labeling-nutrition-guidance-documents-regulatory-information
1990	Organic Foods Production Act	http://www.ams.usda.gov/nop/archive/OFPA.html http://www.ams.usda.gov/AMSv1.0/nop http://www.nal.usda.gov/afsic/pubs/ofp/ofp.shtml Olsson F, Weeda PC. *A Primer on the U.S. Department of Agriculture National Organic Program.* Elmwood Park, NJ: Food Institute. Fishman S. *The Guide to the U.S. Organic Foods Production Act of 1990.* Greenfield, MA: Organic Foods Production Association of North America
1994	Dietary Supplement Health and Education Act	https://ods.od.nih.gov/About/DSHEA_Wording.aspx
1996	Food Quality Protection Act	https://www.epa.gov/laws-regulations/summary-food-quality-protection-act
1996	Safe Drinking Water Act	http://www4.law.cornell.edu/uscode/42/300f.html
2002	Homeland Security Act	http://www.dhs.gov/xlibrary/assets/hr_5005_enr.pdf
2002	Public Health Security and Bioterrorism Preparedness and Response Act	https://www.congress.gov/bill/107th-congress/house-bill/3448
2004	Food Allergen Labeling and Consumer Protection Act	https://www.fda.gov/food/food-allergensgluten-free-guidance-documents-regulatory-information/food-allergen-labeling-and-consumer-protection-act-2004-falcpa
2008	Food, Conservation and Energy Act	https://www.congress.gov/bill/110th-congress/house-bill/2419 https://www.congress.gov/bill/110th-congress/house-bill/2419
2011	Food Safety Modernization Act	www.fda.gov/food/guidance-regulation-food-and-dietary-supplements/food-safety-modernization-act-fsma
2015	Food Safety Modernization Act, Rule on Produce Safety	https://www.fda.gov/food/food-safety-modernization-act-fsma/fsma-final-rule-produce-safety

of all cattle, sheep, swine, goats, and horses at slaughter. Additionally, a federal (or state equivalent) inspector must be present for at least part of every shift while meat products are processed for human or animal consumption. Meat and meat products meeting federal standards are stamped "United States Inspected and Passed by Department of Agriculture" (or state equivalent program). Products bearing the federal mark may be shipped and sold in interstate commerce, whereas products bearing state marks may only be shipped and sold in intrastate commerce. State (and city) meat inspection programs must meet federal standards.[32,33]

Federal Food, Drug, and Cosmetic Act of 1938

The Federal Food, Drug, and Cosmetic Act (FDCA) prohibits entry into interstate commerce of any food that is adulterated: containing poisonous or deleterious substances that may make the food unhealthful; containing filth; decomposed; prepared or handled under unsanitary conditions; from a diseased animal; subjected to radiation except as permitted; having a valuable constituent omitted; having an unauthorized ingredient substitution; having a concealed defect; increased in bulk weight or decreased in strength to deceptively improve appearance; or containing an unapproved or uncertified coloring agent or misbranded (not honestly labeled). The FDA establishes guidance and regulatory requirements under the law, codified in Title 21, Code of Federal Regulations. Although the FDA uses inspections to monitor whether food manufacturers adhere to their legal responsibility of producing safe, wholesome foods, the agency's budget and personnel are insufficient and inspections are infrequent. (The USDA, also lacking funding, and the FDA jointly adopted an industry-operated food safety and inspection system, Hazard Analysis and Critical Control Points.)[32,33]

Food Additives Amendment, 1958

The FDA regulates food additives under the 1958 Food Additives Amendment to the FDCA. The FDA must approve an additive before it can be included in food and requires the additive's manufacturer to prove its safety for the ways it will be used in food. Food additives include substances intentionally added for specific purposes, such as carrageenan (a red seaweed gum used to emulsify, stabilize, or thicken foods)[34] or ozone (as an antimicrobial agent in contact with food),[35] and substances unintentionally added to foods, such as acetone (a component of adhesives) or mineral oil (a lubricant, not to exceed 10 ppm in food).[36]

The Food Additives Amendment provided two exemptions:

1. Those additives in use before 1958, which had been determined by the FDA or USDA to be safe for use in specific foods, were given "prior sanctioned" status.[37] For example, sodium nitrite as a preservative in red meats is prior sanctioned and regulated by the USDA, whereas sodium nitrite when added to fish products is an additive regulated by the FDA.[33]
2. Those additives (such as salt and sugar) whose use in foods is Generally Recognized As Safe (GRAS) by experts,[38-40] based on either an extensive history of common use in food before 1958 or published scientific evidence.[41] Chemicals may be added to or removed from either list as necessary whenever scientific knowledge of the chemical so warrants. The FDA and USDA continuously monitor substances on both lists.[42,43]

Color Additives Amendment, 1960

The Color Additives Amendment to the FDCA brought all colors, natural and synthetic, under federal regulation. The FDA must approve all colors used in foods, drugs, and cosmetics before they can be marketed. Some colors (primarily coal-tar dyes) must be batch-certified (the manufacturer submits samples from each batch produced to the FDA for testing and pays a fee for service); whereas, others (mostly from plant, animal, or mineral sources) are exempt from batch certification.[44,45] Manufacturers and food processors may not use color additives to deceive consumers or to conceal blemishes or inferiorities in food products, and must declare color additives by their common or usual names on labels (e.g., FD&C Yellow 5 or carotene) rather than collectively as "colorings."[46]

The Nutrition Labeling and Education Act of 1990

The Nutrition Labeling and Education Act (NLEA) requires most foods to carry a nutrition label expressing nutrients as a percentage of Daily Values (DVs) for a 2,000-calorie diet rather than the now-outdated Recommended Dietary Allowances (RDAs). The Act also 1) mandates more specific definitions for words such as "free," "light," or "reduced"; 2) restricts the use of the terms "sodium free" and "cholesterol free" to products normally containing sodium and/or cholesterol; 3) defines and regulates health claims, such as calcium helping to prevent osteoporosis; and 4) mandates that the total percentage of juice in juice drinks be declared.[47]

Dietary Supplement Health and Education Act of 1994

The Dietary Supplement Health and Education Act (DSHEA) mandates premarket manufacturer responsibility for dietary supplement safety and requires truthful supplement label information. After supplements reach the market, the FDA monitors supplement safety, including voluntary dietary supplement adverse event reporting; monitors product information (e.g., labeling and claims); and takes action against unsafe supplements. The law does not provide for manufacturer registration, nor does it require manufacturers to seek FDA approval before producing or marketing supplements.[48] The law is controversial because, unlike foods or food additives, which must be proven safe by manufacturers before they are marketed, neither the safety nor the efficacy of supplements needs to be proven by producers.[49] Rather, the FDA must prove that a supplement is unsafe, after marketing, before any action may be taken to remove the product from the market. (For example, it took more than a decade for the FDA to accumulate enough evidence to ban ephedra.[50]) Legislation is pending to address problems with DSHEA and supplement safety.

Food Quality Protection Act of 1996

The Food Quality Protection Act of 1996 (FQPA)[50] amended the FDCA and the Insecticide, Fungicide, and Rodenticide Act (IFRA),[51] changing the way the EPA regulates pesticides (also see the 2003 Pesticide Registration Improvement Act[51]). The zero-tolerance provision of the FDCA's food additives anti-cancer clause (Delaney Clause[33]) was replaced with a new safety standard, "reasonable certainty of no harm resulting from aggregate exposure," to be applied to all pesticides used on foods. With no provision for phasing in the new requirements, the EPA faced enforcing the new regulations while simultaneously learning to evaluate pesticides under the new rules and developing or approving new, scientifically tested methodologies for evaluating aggregate

Discussion Prompt

Describe the differences between the Delaney Act and the more relaxed regulation of dietary supplements. Why does this duality exist?

and cumulative risks.[52-55] Not surprisingly, this led to controversy among the EPA, environmental advocates, and public health organizations.[56,57] In 1993, the EPA was sued by four states and several environmental and public health groups "for allegedly failing to adequately protect children from pesticides used on food…contend[ing] that the EPA set inadequate limits on several organophosphate insecticides."[58]

Public Health Security and Bioterrorism Preparedness and Response Act of 2002

The Bioterrorism Act's Title III specifically addresses food safety, directing:

> …federal agencies, the food industry, consumer and producer groups, scientific organizations, and the States, [to] develop a crisis communications and education strategy with respect to bioterrorist threats to the food supply. Such strategy shall address threat assessments; technologies and procedures for securing food processing and manufacturing facilities and modes of transportation; response and notification procedures; and risk communications to the public.[59]

Title II covers security strategy, food adulteration, detention, registration, records maintenance, prior notice, and marking.[60] Bioterrorism and food is covered at length in Chapter 18.

Food Allergen Labeling and Consumer Protection Act, 2004

The Food Allergen Labeling and Consumer Protection Act (FALCP, effective 2006) provides improved food labeling information to consumers who suffer from food allergies. FALCP requires food labels to identify the presence of any of eight major food allergens: milk, eggs, fish, crustaceans, peanuts, tree nuts, wheat, and soybeans. Concomitant with expanding the number of allergens to be identified, the new requirements represent improvements over present labeling standards:

> …if a product contains the milk-derived protein casein, the product's label would have to use the term "milk" in addition to the term "casein" so that those with milk allergies would clearly understand the presence of an allergen they need to avoid.[61]

Food, Conservation, and Energy Act of 2008

The Food, Conservation, and Energy Act allows federal agricultural programs to continue through fiscal year 2012. Among the 14 titles comprising the Act, two have direct applications to food safety:

1. Title X, "Horticulture and Organic Agriculture," provisions concern:
   - Pest and disease management
   - Organic agriculture
   - Miscellaneous issues
2. Title XI "Livestock," provisions relate to:
   - Livestock mandatory reporting
   - The country of origin labeling
   - The Agricultural Fair Practices Act of 1967 definitions
   - An annual report
   - Production contracts
   - Regulations

Strategy Tip

Most schools now have a food allergy program where allergic students have been identified and epi-pens are available.

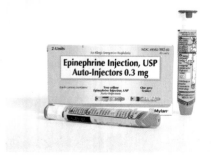

Epi-pens contain epinepherine, a life-saving substance to counteract anaphylaxis from a food allergy. Generic epi-pens can now be obtained, which drastically reduces the cost.

© Amy Kerkemeyer/Shutterstock.

- The sense of Congress regarding pseudorabies eradication program
- The sense of Congress regarding the cattle fever tick eradication program
- The National Sheep Industry Improvement Center
- The trichinae certification program
- Low pathogenic diseases
- Animal protection
- The National Aquatic Animal Health Plan
- The study on bioenergy operations
- The interstate shipment of meat and poultry inspected by federal and state agencies
- For certain small establishments
- Inspection and grading
- Food safety improvement[62,63]

Food Safety Modernization Act of 2011

Prior to the Food Safety Modernization Act (FSMA), the FDA had the authority to respond to threats to the safety of our food supply. This reactionary role meant that the FDA could not interfere in the food processing supply chains freely and could not easily work with state and local regulatory bodies to address potential hazards to the food supply. Furthermore, the FDA did not have, the authority to closely monitor supply chains on imported foods. The FSMA allows the FDA to increase its regulations and hazard prevention policies for food facilities, produce imported food. It also allows the FDA to issue food recalls when food companies fail to voluntarily issue a recall on unsafe food products.[64] Additionally, the FSMA also protects consumers against food fraud. **Food fraud** describes when foods are intentionally misrepresented in terms of the food itself, the packaging, or otherwise.[65] Overall, awareness of the points within the food supply chain where food fraud could occur can help to prevent it. Protecting food from any intentional points of altering or misrepresentation is known as **food defense**. Facilities, and operators can help to ensure that within their company they are aware of the risk points for where food fraud may occur. The FDA also helps with trainings and outreach for companies to understand where food fraud can occur, as well as helps them respond to situations with intentional food alteration.[66]

In 2020, the FDA announced proposed drafts to the FSMA to detail requirements for additional traceability of specific foods, known as the "Food Traceability Proposed Rule," which is a part of the "Blueprint for the New Era of Food Safety," which will be discussed later in this chapter. If approved, this rule would require additional traceability records on the high-risk foods that are included on the "Food Traceability List."[67] Recent updates to the FSMA align with the increasingly data-driven food safety environment and will help consumers access information on food products, as well as help interventions occur within the supply chain to prevent foodborne illness when unsafe products are detected. Some of the food industry's current risk focuses include allergens, food contact surfaces for ready to eat (RTE) foods, new microbe emergence, heavy metals, drug and chemical residues, and new foods considered to be high risk.[68]

Hazard Analysis and Critical Control Points

The Hazard Analysis and Critical Control Points (HACCP) protocol was developed by the Pillsbury Corporation in 1971 to ensure food safety for astronauts in outer space. Its principles focus on preventing hazards that

Food fraud The act of purposely altering, misrepresenting, mislabeling, substituting, or tampering with any food product at any point along the farm-to-table food supply chain.

Food defense Effort to protect food from acts of intentional adulteration.

Discussion Prompt

How could a registered dietitian assist with unsafe food?

could cause foodborne illness by identifying and correcting hazards before they develop, following foods from raw materials to finished products.[69,70] HACCP consists of seven principles:

1. Identify hazard(s)
2. Identify critical control point(s) (CCPs) for controlling each hazard identified
3. Define limits for each CCP
4. Establish specific procedures for monitoring each CCP
5. Establish a procedure for taking corrective action whenever a CCP's limits have been exceeded
6. Implement procedures to verify that the HACCP program is working as intended
7. Thoroughly document the HACCP program and maintain records of CCP monitoring data. Examples of HACCP plans and flowcharts are easily obtained.[9,71,72]

HACCP programs are used in the seafood industry (since 1995; FDA oversight), meat and poultry processing plants (since 1998; USDA oversight), and the juice industry (since 2001; FDA oversight). Other areas of the food industry, such as food service, also use HACCP programs,[73,74] and the FDA is developing HACCP protocols for use in these segments.[62]

Good Manufacturing Practices

Some regulations published by the FDA are collectively called good manufacturing practices (GMPs), or the Code of GMPs.[75] These specify sanitation, safety, and quality assurance procedures to be followed by food processors.[76] For example, the FDA specifies safe procedures for manufacturing, thermally processing, and packing low-acid canned foods to avoid growth of *Clostridium botulinum* and subsequent toxin formation by the pathogen.[77] The FDA also recognizes that it is impossible to manufacture, process, and package foods that are 100% free of poisonous, deleterious, or aesthetically unpleasant substances, and it has established specific tolerances and rules relating to these substances (e.g., fresh, frozen, and canned clams, mussels, and oysters must not contain .80 µg paralytic shellfish poisoning toxin/100 g meat;[78] ground nutmeg poses no inherent hazard to health if it contains 100 insect fragments and/or #1 rodent hair/10 g.[79]

Hazards to Food Safety

Biologic Hazards

Biologic hazards include bacteria, viruses, parasites, and fungi (**Table 14–3**). Although several previously unknown or lesser-known pathogens have emerged in recent years, *Escherichia Coli* (*E. coli*), Norovirus, Salmonella, *Clostridium perfringens*, *Campylobacter*, and *Staphylococcus aureus* are the most common sources of foodborne illness in the United States, according to 2018 updates.[80]

These microbes cause either infections or intoxications. In *infections*, pathogens are ingested and multiply in the body, causing illness; in *intoxications*, toxins made by pathogens cause illness. Intoxications result from ingesting live pathogens that go on to multiply and produce toxin in the body, or they can occur without ingesting the live pathogens, if the pathogens are allowed to grow on food and produce heat-stable toxins. Food processing then kills the organisms but does not damage the toxin.

TABLE 14–3
Some Biologic Hazards Associated with Food[1,2]

Hazard Type	Organism	Examples of Food Vehicles	Signs & Symptoms
Bacteria	Bacillus cereus Campylobacter jejuni Clostridium botulinum Clostridium perfringens Escherichia coli Listeria monocytogenes Salmonella typhi Salmonella enteriditis Shigella dysenteriae Staphylococcus aureus Streptococcus pyogenes Vibrio cholerae Yersinia enterocolitica	Chicken fried rice[3] Unpasteurized milk and cheese[4] Muktuk (whale meat)[5] Ground turkey and beef casserole[6] Raw milk and raw colostrum[7] Jellied pork cold cuts[8] Milk (food handler) and water[9] Dry dog food (unwashed hands)[10] Sugar snaps (peas)[11] Precooked packaged ham[12] Macaroni and cheese/cook[13] Seafood[14] Pork chitterlings[15]	Abdominal pain, diarrhea, headache, and fever
Viruses	Hepatitis A Rotavirus Noroviruses Swine flu (H1N1) Avian flu (H5N1)	Green onions/foodhandlers[16] Deli sandwiches[17] Oysters, raspberries, and other berries[18] Respiratory transmission[43] Direct contact[44]	Gastroenteritis, diarrhea, abdominal pain, nausea, vomiting, and fever.
Fungi	Alternaria spp. Aspergillus spp. Byssochlamys spp. Fusarium spp. Penicillium spp.	Grain[19] Prob. Kombucha tea[20] Fruits, vegetables[21] Corn; sorghum[22] Chestnuts[23]	Low-grade fever
Parasites Flatworms Protozoans Roundworms	Clonorchis sinensis Diphyllobothrium latum Fasciola hepatica Fasciolopsis buski Paragonimus spp. Taenia spp. Cryptosporidium parvum Cyclospora cayetanensis Entamoeba histolytica Giardia lamblia Sarcocystis spp. Toxoplasma gondii Anisakis simplex Ascaris lumbricoides Pseudoterranova decipiens Trichinella spiralis	Fish (frozen, raw, or salted)[24,25] Fish[26] Watercress[27] Raw aquatic plants; untreated water[28] Raw crayfish[29]undercooked crayfish[30] Fecal/oral[31] Chicken salad[32] Guatemalan raspberries[33] Prob. ice and ice cream[34] Prob. taco ingredients[35] Raw beef and pork[36] Raw and undercooked venison[37] Raw fish[38] Fecal/oral[39] Raw fish[40] Bear, cougar, wild boar meats; pork[41]	Diarrhea, abdominal pain, nausea, vomiting, fever.
Prions	Abnormal prion proteins Bovine spongiform encephalopathy (BSE; aka Mad Cow Disease)	Wild game[42] and infected cows[45]	Neurological degeneration, sometimes overextended periods of time.

[1]This is not a complete list.
[2]Compiled by the author from: For excellent reviews of most of these organisms, see: (a) Hui YH, Pierson MD, Gorham MD, eds. *Foodborne Disease Handbook,* 2nd ed. Vol. 1: Bacterial Pathogens, Vol. 2: Viruses, Parasites, Pathogens, and HACCP, Vol. 3: Plant Toxicants, & Vol. 4: Seafood and Environmental Toxins. New York: Marcel Dekker; 2000. (b) Jay JM. *Modern Food Microbiology,* 6th ed. Gaithersburg, MD: Aspen; 2000. (c) Pommerville JC. *Alcamo's Fundamentals of Microbiology,* 9th ed. Sudbury, MA: Jones and Bartlett Publishers: 2011.
[3]Epidemiologic notes and reports *Bacillus cereus* food poisoning associated with fried rice at two child daycare centers—Virginia, 1993. *MMWR Morb Mortal Wkly Rep.* 1994;43:177.
[4]*Campylobacter jejuni* infection associated with unpasteurized milk and cheese—Kansas, 2007. *MMWR Morb Mortal Wkly Rep.* 2009;57:1377.
[5]Outbreak of botulism type E associated with eating a beached whale—Western Alaska, July 2002. *MMWR Morb Mortal Wkly Rep.* 2003;52:24.
[6]*Clostridium perfringens* infection among inmates at a county jail—Wisconsin, August 2008. *MMWR Morb Mortal Wkly Rep.* 2009;58:138.
[7]*Escherichia coli* 0157:H7 infections in children associated with raw milk and raw colostrum from cows—California, 2006. *MMWR Morb Mortal Wkly Rep.* 2008;57:625.

(continues)

TABLE 14–3
Some Biologic Hazards Associated with Food[1,2]   *(continued)*

Hazard Type	Organism	Examples of Food Vehicles	Signs & Symptoms

[8]Pichler J, Much P, Kasper S, et al. An outbreak of febrile gastroenteritis associated with jellied pork contaminated with *Listeria monocytogenes*. *Wiener Klinische Wochenschrift*. 2009;121:149.

[9]Bhunia R, Hutin Y, Ramakrishnan R, Pal N, Sen T, Murhekar M. A typhoid fever outbreak in a slum of South Dumdum municipality, West Bengal, India, 2007: evidence for foodborne and waterborne transmission. *BMC Public Health*. 2009;9:115.

[10]Multistate outbreak of human *Salmonella* infections caused by contaminated dry dog food—United States, 2006–2007. *MMWR Morb Mortal Wkly Rep*. 2008;57:521.

[11]Löfdahl M, Ivarsson S, Andersson S, Långmark J, Plym-Forshell L. An outbreak of Shigella dysenteriae in Sweden, May-June 2009, with sugar snaps as the suspected source. *Eur Surveill*. 2009;14:19268.

[12]Outbreak of staphylococcal food poisoning associated with precooked ham—Florida, 1997. *MMWR Morb Mortal Wkly Rep*. 1997;46:1189.

[13]Farley TA, Wilson SA, Mahoney F, Kelso KY, Johnson DR, Kaplan EL. Direct inoculation of food as the cause of an outbreak of group a streptococcal pharyngitis. *J Infect Dis*. 1993;167:1232.

[14]Crump JA, Bopp CA, Greene KD, et al. Toxigenic *Vibrio cholerae* serogroup O141-associated cholera-like diarrhea and bloodstream infection in the U.S. *J Infect Dis*. 2003;187:866.

[15]*Yersinia enterocolitica* gastroenteritis among infants exposed to chitterlings—Chicago, Illinois, 2002. *MMWR Morb Mortal Wkly Rep*. 2003;52:956.

[16]Hepatitis A outbreak associated with green onions at a restaurant—Monaca, Pennsylvania, 2003. *MMWR Morb Mortal Wkly Rep*. 2003;52:1155.

[17]Foodborne outbreak of group a rotavirus gastroenteritis among college students—District of Columbia, March–April 2000. *MMWR Morb Mortal Wkly Rep*. 2000;49:1131.

[18]Bresee JS, Widdowson M-A, Monroe SS, Glass RI. Foodborne viral gastroenteritis: challenges and opportunities. *Clin Infect Dis*. 2002;35:748.

[19]Liu GT, Qian YZ, Zhang P, et al. Etiological role of *Alternaria alternata* in human esophageal cancer. *Chinese Med J*. 1992;105:394.

[20]Unexplained severe illness possibly associated with consumption of Kombucha tea—Iowa, 1995. *MMWR Morb Mortal Wkly Rep*.1995;44:892, 899.

[21]Moss MO. Fungi, quality and safety issues in fresh fruits and vegetables. *J Appl Microbiol*. 2008;104:1239.

[22]Bhat RV, Shetty PH, Amruth RP, Sudershan RV. A foodborne disease outbreak due to the consumption of moldy sorghum and maize containing fumonisin mycotoxins. *J Toxicol Clin Toxicol*. 1997;35:249-255.

[23]Overy DP, Seifert KA, Savard ME, Frisvad JC. Spoilage fungi and their mycotoxins in commercially marketed chestnuts. *Int J Food Microbiol*. 2003;88:69.

[24]Fan PC. Viability of metacercariae of Clonorchis sinensis in frozen or salted freshwater fish. *Int J Parasitol*. 1998;28:603.

[25]Choi DW. Clonorchis sinensis: life cycle, intermediate hosts, transmission to man and geographical distribution in Korea. *Arzneimittel-Forschung*. 1984;34:1145.

[26]Arizono N, Yamada M, Nakamura-Uchiyama F, Ohnishi K. Diphyllobothriasis associated with eating raw pacific salmon. *Emerg Infect Dis*. 2009;15:866.

[27]LaPook JD, Magun AM, Nickerson KG, Meltzer JI. Sheep, watercress, and the Internet. *Lancet*. 2000;356:218.

[28]Graczyk TK, Gilman RH, Fried B. Fasciolopsiasis: is it a controllable food-borne disease? *Parasitol Res*. 2001;87:80.

[29]DeFrain M, Hooker R. North American paragonimiasis: case report of a severe clinical infection. *Chest*. 2002;121:1368.

[30]Procop GW, Marty AM, Scheck DN, Mease DR, Maw GM. North American paragonimiasis. A case report. *Acta Cytol*. 2000;44:75.

[31]Locally acquired neurocysticercosis—North Carolina, Massachusetts, and South Carolina, 1989–1991. *MMWR Morb Mortal Wkly Rep*. 1992;41:1.

[32]Foodborne outbreak of diarrheal illness associated with *Cryptosporidium parvum*—Minnesota, 1995. *MMWR Morb Mortal Wkly Rep*. 1995;45:783.

[33]Update: Outbreaks of *Cyclospora cayetanensis* infection—U.S. and Canada, 1996. *MMWR Morb Mortal Wkly Rep*. 1996;45:611.

[34]de Lalla F, Rinaldi E, Santoro D, Nicolin R, Tramarin A. Outbreak of *Entamoeba histolytica* and *Giardia lamblia* infections in travellers returning from the tropics. *Infection*. 1992;20:78.

[35]Epidemiologic notes and reports common-source outbreak of giardiasis—New Mexico. *MMWR Morb Mortal Wkly Rep*. 1989;38:405.

[36]Wilairatana P, Radomyos P, Radomyos B, et al. Intestinal sarcocystosis in Thai laborers. *SE Asian J Trop Med Public Health*. 1996;27:43.

[37]Ross RD, Stec LA, Werner JC, Blumenkranz MS, Glazer L, Williams GA. Presumed acquired ocular toxoplasmosis in deer hunters. *Retina*. 2001;21:226.

[38]Bouree P, Paugam A, Petithory JC. Anisakidosis: report of 25 cases and review of the literature. *Comparative Immunol Microbiol Infect Dis*. 1995;18:75.

[39]Hughes RG, Sharp DS, Hughes MC, et al. Environmental influences on helminthiasis and nutritional status among Pacific schoolchildren. *Int J Environ Health Res*. 2004;14:163.

[40]Adams AM, Murrell KD, Cross JH. Parasites of fish and risks to public health. *Revue Scientifique et Technique*. 1997;16:652.

[41]Trichinellosis surveillance—U.S., 1997–2001. *MMWR Morb Mortal Wkly Rep*. 2002;52(SS06):1.

[42]Fatal degenerative neurologic illnesses in men who participated in wild game feasts—Wisconsin, 2002. *MMWR Morb Mortal Wkly Rep*. 2002;52(7):125.

[43]http://www.cdc.gov/h1n1flu/

[44]http://www.cdc.gov/flu/avian/

[45]http://www.cdc.gov/ncidod/dvrd/prions/index.htm

In 1996, the CDC's Emerging Infections Program's Foodborne Diseases Active Surveillance Network (FoodNet) began collecting data from 10 states for laboratory-diagnosed cases of foodborne illness caused by bacterial pathogens *Campylobacter*, Shiga toxin-producing *Escherichia coli* (STEC) O157, *Listeria*, *Salmonella*, *Shigella*, *Vibrio*, and *Yersinia*, and protozoan parasites *Cryptosporidium* and *Cyclospora cayetanensis*. Although the incidence of infections caused by *Campylobacter*, *Cryptosporidium parvum*, *E. coli O157*,

Salmonella, and *Y. enterocolitica* have varied since 1996, infants and young children continue to suffer a high incidence of infections from several of these nine organisms, and this is a major public health concern.[81] Despite this, in the previous decade significant progress was made in meeting objectives set for the food safety Focus Area of Healthy People 2010, however incidence of foodborne infections data was mixed.[81-83] Moving into Healthy People 2030,[84] the overall goal of reducing foodborne illness continues, alongside objectives to improve safe food handling.

Strategy Tip

Swine Flu: H1N1 Virus

Novel influenza A (H1N1) is a flu virus of swine origin that was first detected in Mexico and in the United States in March and April of 2009. The first novel H1N1 patient in the United States was confirmed by laboratory testing at the CDC on April 15, 2009, and the second was confirmed on April 17, 2009. It was quickly determined that the virus was spreading from person to person. On April 22, 2009, the CDC activated its Emergency Operations Center to better coordinate the public health response. On April 26, 2009, the United States government declared a public health emergency. It is thought that H1N1 flu spreads in the same way that regular seasonal influenza viruses spread; mainly through the coughs and sneezes of people who are sick with the virus.

The CDC has developed a polymerase chain reaction (PCR) diagnostic test kit to detect this novel H1N1 virus and has now distributed test kits to all states in the United States and the District of Columbia and Puerto Rico. The test kits are being shipped internationally as well. This will allow states and other countries to test for this new virus.

The U.S. government is aggressively taking early steps in the process to manufacture a novel H1N1 vaccine, working closely with manufacturing. The CDC has isolated the new H1N1 virus, made a candidate vaccine virus that can be used to create a vaccine, and has provided this virus to industry so they can begin scaling up for production of a vaccine, if necessary. Making a vaccine is a multistep process requiring several months to complete.

Centers for Disease Control and Prevention, *2009 SwineFlu*. Accessed February 24, 2010. Available at http://www .cdc.gov/h1n1flu/

Strategy Tip

Avian Influenza: H5N1 Virus

Avian influenza is an infection caused by avian (bird) influenza (flu) viruses. These influenza viruses occur naturally among birds. Wild birds worldwide carry the viruses in their intestines, but usually do not get sick from them. However, avian influenza is very contagious among birds and can make some domesticated birds, including chickens, ducks, and turkeys, very sick and kill them.

(continues)

Infected birds shed influenza virus in their saliva, nasal secretions, and feces. Susceptible birds become infected when they have contact with contaminated secretions or excretions or with surfaces that are contaminated with secretions or excretions from infected birds. Domesticated birds may become infected with avian influenza virus through direct contact with infected waterfowl or other infected poultry, or through contact with surfaces (such as dirt or cages) or materials (i.e., water or feed) that have been contaminated with the virus.

Infection with avian influenza viruses in domestic poultry causes two main forms of disease that are distinguished by low and high extremes of virulence. The "low pathogenic" form may go undetected and usually causes only mild symptoms (i.e., ruffled feathers and a drop in egg production). However, the highly pathogenic form spreads more rapidly through flocks of poultry. This form may cause disease that affects multiple internal organs and has a mortality rate that can reach 90–100%, often within 48 hours.

There are many different subtypes of type A influenza viruses. These subtypes differ because of changes in certain proteins on the surface of the influenza A virus (hemagglutinin [HA] and neuraminidase [NA] proteins). There are 16 known HA subtypes and nine known NA subtypes of influenza A viruses. Many different combinations of HA and NA proteins are possible. Each combination represents a different subtype. All known subtypes of influenza A viruses can be found in birds.

Usually, "avian influenza virus" refers to influenza A viruses found chiefly in birds, but infections with these viruses can occur in humans. The risk from avian influenza is generally low to most people, because the viruses do not usually infect humans. However, confirmed cases of human infection from several subtypes of avian influenza infection have been reported since 1997. Most cases of avian influenza infection in humans have resulted from contact with infected poultry (e.g., domesticated chicken, ducks, and turkeys) or surfaces contaminated with secretions/excretions from infected birds. The spread of avian influenza viruses from one ill person to another has very rarely been reported, and has been limited, inefficient, and unsustained.

"Human influenza virus" usually refers to those subtypes that spread widely among humans. There are only three known A subtypes of influenza viruses (H1N1, H1N2, and H3N2) currently circulating among humans. It is likely that some genetic parts of current human influenza A viruses came from birds originally. Influenza A viruses are constantly changing, and they might adapt over time to infect and spread among humans.

During an outbreak of avian influenza among poultry, there is a possible risk to people who have contact with infected birds or surfaces that have been contaminated with secretions or excretions from infected birds.

Symptoms of avian influenza in humans have ranged from typical human influenza-like symptoms (e.g., fever, cough, sore throat, and muscle aches) to eye infections, pneumonia, severe respiratory diseases (such as acute respiratory distress), and other severe and life-threatening complications. The symptoms of avian influenza may depend on which virus caused the infection.

Centers for Disease Control and Prevention, *Information on Avian Influenza.* Accessed December 5, 2020. Available at http://www.cdc.gov/flu/avian/

Pandemic Learning Opportunity

Discuss how possible viruses can turn into pandemics. Can it happen again? Why?

Bacteria

Campylobacter jejuni, *Campylobacter jejuni subsp. jejuni*, one of about 14 species of *Campylobacter*,[85] is responsible for most cases of foodborne bacterial infection in the United States.[86] It is found in the intestinal tracts of farm livestock (especially poultry),[85,87] wild birds,[88-90] and rodents,[91,92] and in drinking water[93,94] and unchlorinated water[95,96]; it can also be carried by insects.[97,98] Most cases of campylobacteriosis can be traced to eating undercooked poultry or to other foods contaminated by raw poultry.[99] The next most common route of infection is via unpasteurized milk,[85,99-101] but the largest outbreak, where about 2,000 people were infected, was traced to contaminated water.[85,102] Symptoms include abdominal pain, diarrhea, headache, and fever, and infection rates are higher in immunocompromised individuals (e.g., HIV/AIDS patients, infants, the elderly)[99,103-105] In severe cases of campylobacteriosis, there may be bloody diarrhea.[85,105] Among the sequelae to infection are **Guillain-Barré syndrome**[106,107] and **Reiter syndrome**[108]

Escherichia coli *Escherichia coli* (*E. coli*), a known human pathogen since the 18th century,[109] gained widespread recognition in 1971 after an enteritis outbreak was traced to contaminated imported cheeses.[110] *E. coli* is one of four genera of coliform bacteria used as indicators of food safety (microbiological coliform test), and *E. coli* is often specifically assayed because it is more indicative of fecal contamination than the other three genera.[111] Within the genus *Escherichia* there are some 200 O and 30 H serotypes.[110] *E. coli* O157 inhabit the intestinal tracts of cattle; other *E. coli* are normal inhabitants of human intestinal tracts. When people become ill from *E. coli*, the usual transmission vehicles are raw or undercooked ground beef and other red meats, and occasionally prepared foods such as mashed potatoes and cream pies. Untreated water, raw milk, cheeses, and fish have also been implicated. Shiga toxin-producing *E. coli* (STEC) O157:H7 (a toxin similar to that of *Shigella dysenteriae*) was first recognized in 1982.[112-116] Causing either infection or intoxication, symptoms of illness resemble those of shigellosis, including, for infection, bloody diarrhea and colitis, and for intoxication, severe abdominal pain, nausea, vomiting, diarrhea, and sometimes fever.[117,118] Hemolytic uremic syndrome (HUS) and hemorrhagic colitis are especially severe and are particularly serious for children; several fatalities have occurred in the last 20 years. Although STEC is the organism monitored by the CDC, other strains of *E. coli* cause diarrhea (e.g., enteroaggregative *E. coli*[119]). *E. coli* is among the leading causes of travelers' diarrhea (others include Noroviruses, *Campylobacter jejuni/coli*, and *Giardia lamblia*[111]). To prevent foodborne illness caused by *E. coli* (and other pathogens), dietitians/nutritionists should advise that foods be cooked thoroughly and that a thermometer be used to ensure that proper temperatures are reached. Avoiding cross-contamination, proper handling/reheating of leftovers, and handwashing/personal hygiene are also appropriate control measures against *E. coli*.

Listeria The genus *Listeria* has six recognized species. *Listeria monocytogenes*, the primary pathogen, has 13 serovars.[120] For many years, listeriosis was recognized as an animal disease, but *Listeria*'s association with foodborne illness in humans is a recent phenomenon. The organisms are widespread in nature, in wild and domestic animals and birds, in water and soil, and in vegetation. Found in raw milk, soft cheeses, raw meats, and poultry, it can also contaminate raw soil-grown vegetables such as lettuce. Symptoms of listeriosis include nausea, vomiting, and headache, but the health of the host determines the course and severity of the disease—many healthy people never develop clinical manifestations.[120] However, infants may be congenitally infected, and infected pregnant

Guillain-Barré syndrome An inflammatory disorder of the peripheral nerves that is characterized by the rapid onset of weakness and, often, paralysis of the legs, arms, breathing muscles, and face.

Reiter syndrome A peripheral arthritis lasting longer than 1 month.

Strategy Tip

Animal Prion Diseases

Bovine spongiform encephalopathy (BSE)
Chronic wasting disease (CWD)
Scrapie
Transmissible mink encephalopathy
Feline spongiform encephalopathy
Ungulate spongiform encephalopathy

Centers for Disease Control and Prevention, Prion Diseases. Accessed December 5, 2020. Available at http://www.cdc.gov/prions/index.html

women (often with no or mild symptoms) may spontaneously abort, deliver prematurely, or deliver a stillborn infant.[120] Immunocompromised individuals, such as those with HIV/AIDS, are particularly susceptible, and neoplasms, alcoholism, diabetes (especially type 1), cardiovascular disease, renal transplant, and corticosteroid therapy predispose individuals to clinical listeriosis, characterized by meningitis, meningoencephalitis, or encephalitis.[120] *Listeria* can grow at cold temperatures, so refrigeration is inadequate as a control. Thorough cooking, using pasteurized milk and dairy products, avoiding cross-contamination, handwashing/personal hygiene, and maintaining clean, dry food storage and preparation areas are all effective against *Listeria*.

Salmonella The salmonellae are a large group of bacteria, but there are only two species, *Salmonella enterica* and *S. Bongori*. These species are further classified into four subspecies and one subspecies, respectively, and further into 2,324 serovars—these are commonly treated as separate species.[121] *Salmonella spp.* (*spp.* is defined as all individual species within a genus) are found in animal intestinal tracts, including birds, livestock, humans, reptiles, and some insects. Shed in feces, they may then be spread by insects and other vermin.[121] Animal feeds may serve as routes of infection for livestock,[122] and animal carcasses may be contaminated with gastrointestinal salmonellae during slaughter and processing. People who eat undercooked *Salmonella*-contaminated meats, poultry, or eggs, or drink *Salmonella*-contaminated water develop nausea, vomiting, abdominal pain, diarrhea, headache, and fever. The strains most commonly responsible for human illness are *S. Typhimurium* and *S. Enteritidis*. (The incidence of cases of non-typhoid *Salmonella* infections have increased substantially since about 1950.[123]) *S. enteritidis* infections have been increasing since the 1970s and are often associated with eggs, egg products, or egg-containing foods.[121,124-126] Because *S. enteritidis* may be present in fresh, uncracked shell eggs,[127-129] eating undercooked or raw eggs is ill-advised unless the eggs have been pasteurized in the shell.[130,131]

Strategy Tip

Bovine Spongiform Encephalopathy

Bovine spongiform encephalopathy (BSE) is a progressive neurological disorder of cattle that results from infection by an unusual transmissible agent called a prion. The nature of the transmissible agent is not well understood. Currently, the most accepted theory is that the agent is a modified form of a normal protein known as prion protein. For reasons that are not yet understood, the normal prion protein changes into a pathogenic (harmful) form that then damages the central nervous system of cattle.

Research indicates that the first probable infections of BSE in cows occurred during the 1970s, with two cases of BSE being identified in 1986. BSE possibly originated as a result of feeding cattle meat-and-bone meal that contained BSE-infected products from a spontaneously occurring case of BSE or scrapie-infected sheep products. Scrapie is a prion disease of sheep. There is strong evidence and general agreement that the outbreak was then amplified and spread throughout the United Kingdom cattle industry by feeding rendered, prion-infected, bovine meat-and-bone meal to young calves.

The BSE epidemic in the United Kingdom peaked in January of 1993 at almost 1,000 new cases per week. Through the end of 2007, more than 184,500 cases of BSE had been confirmed in the United Kingdom alone in more than 35,000 herds.

Strong epidemiologic and laboratory evidence exists for a causal association between a new human prion disease called variant Creutzfeldt-Jakob disease (vCJD), which was first reported from the United Kingdom in 1996 and the BSE outbreak in cattle. The interval between the most likely period for the initial extended exposure of the population to potentially BSE-contaminated food

(1984–1986) The onset of initial vCJD cases

(1994–1996) Consistent with known incubation periods for the human forms of prion disease.

Centers for Disease Control and Prevention, Prion Diseases. Accessed December 5, 2020. Available at https://www.cdc.gov/index.html

Shigella The genus *Shigella* has four species: *S. dysenteriae*, *S. flexneri*, *S. boydii*, and *S. sonnei*. Although *S. dysenteriae* causes bacillary dysentery and can be carried in food or water, it is not considered a food-poisoning organism.[121] The other three species cause shigellosis infection, characterized by diarrhea, abdominal pain, fever, and chills. *Shigella* is unique among the bacteria discussed thus far, because there are no known nonhuman reservoirs.[121] Poor personal hygiene, therefore, is usually behind outbreaks, with shellfish, raw produce, chicken, and salads the usual vehicles.[121] People may carry *Shigella* for several weeks, excreting the bacteria in their stool. Flies and other vermin also may transmit the bacteria to foods. Control measures include fastidious handwashing/personal hygiene, rapid cooling of foods, vermin control, and use of safe drinking water.

Vibrio The genus *Vibrio* includes approximately 28 species, five being of public health significance: *V. parahaemolyticus*, *V. vulnificus*, *V. hollisae*, *V. alginolyticus*, and *V. cholerae*.[85] These are marine organisms, so the usual vehicle for foodborne illness is seafood, especially shellfish and dried fish, or other foods cross-contaminated by seafood.[85] *V. parahaemolyticus* is the leading cause of foodborne illness in Japan, and in the United States, it has been responsible for many outbreaks, usually associated with eating raw oysters or clams. *V. vulnificus* causes soft-tissue infections and primary septicemia, particularly affecting immunocompromised individuals and those with liver cirrhosis. The organism consumed via raw oysters is responsible for about 95% of seafood-associated mortality in the United States.[85] *V. hollisae* causes gastroenteritis via shellfish consumption, and *V. alginolyticus* can cause gastroenteritis but is more often implicated in soft-tissue and ear infections among swimmers.[85] *V. cholerae* is well known as the causative agent of cholera. Several foodborne gastroenteritis infections have been recorded in the United States, all in patients who had eaten raw oysters. Other foods implicated in small outbreaks (one to six individuals) were raw seaweed, palm fruit, and coconut milk.[85] Control measures against vibriosis include avoiding raw shellfish and seafood, purchasing shellfish/seafood from approved sources, avoiding cross-contamination, and good handwashing/personal hygiene habits.

Yersinia The genus *Yersinia* includes 11 species, among them the plague-causing *Y. pestis*. *Y. enterocolitica* is the primary organism of importance to food safety.[85] Swine are the usual reservoirs, but *Yersinia* is also associated with milk, seafood, and vegetables.[85] Foodborne yersiniosis manifestations include gastroenteritis, pseudoappendicitis, lymphadenitis, and many others.[85] The gastroenteritis is characterized by abdominal pain and diarrhea, and the illness may progress to a variety of systemic syndromes.[85] Children and the elderly are more susceptible than middle-aged adults.

Viruses

Viruses differ from bacteria in that they require a vector (i.e., virus-contaminated food or hands) in order to enter the body and cause disease. Pathogenic viruses have always been associated with foods, but some such as the Norwalk viruses,[132] newly renamed "Noroviruses,"[133] have been known as food-associated pathogens only since the 1970s.[134-136] Before then, causative agents for most gastroenteritis cases could not be identified. Noroviruses are responsible for most of the cases of acute gastroenteritis in the United States.[137] Norwalk virus is "the prototype strain of genetically and antigenically diverse single stranded RNA (ribonucleic acid) viruses,"[132] formerly known as

Strategy Tip

Coronavirus 19 (COVID-19)

In December of 2019, COVID-19, a new virus causing respiratory illness that is easily spread from person to person via respiratory droplets was thought to be identified in Wuhan, China. The severe acute respiratory syndrome coronavirus 2 (SARS-CoV-2) quickly became classified as a **pandemic** by the WHO on March 11, 2020, as it spread across the world.[144] COVID-19 was the first pandemic known to be caused by a coronavirus. Symptoms of COVID-19 include fever, congestion, fatigue, cough, shortness of breath, loss of taste or smell, nausea, and diarrhea. Illness severity ranges from mild to severe, and has been shown to impact older adults, or those with underlying medical conditions.[144] The virus can be spread both by those displaying symptoms and can also be passed through **asymptomatic** carriers. There is currently no evidence to support that COVID-19 may be transmitted through consumption or handling of food. However, it is possible to contract COVID-19 by touching a surface, or packaging that has the virus, and then touching mucous membranes such as the eyes, or mouth. Practices such as proper handwashing, disinfection of cooking, and food-preparation surfaces, and overall good food safety remain important to preventing foodborne illness during the COVID-19 pandemic.

On March 13, 2020, the pandemic was declared a National Emergency and invoked the Stafford and **National Emergencies Act (NEA)** in order to aid in mobilization of funding for state and local governments. The NEA provides increased flexibility in Medicare, Medicaid, and the Children's Health Insurance Portability Act, in order to improve pandemic response efforts.[145]

The **National Emergency** activation in the United States was not only an effort to free up funding for response efforts but also in attempts to control the spread of the virus throughout the country. The National Emergency Activation also ultimately led to ripple effects throughout many industries, including that of food and beverages. Travel into and outside of the United States was halted in an attempt to slow the spread of disease and to prioritize treatment for those who were ill; however, travel bans caused stress and bottlenecks within the food supply chain, which took time to alleviate. While the United States' food supply chain remained under stress throughout the National Emergency, it is important to consider that in developing countries, the food supply chain was likely much harder hit, due to fewer resources, gaps in labor availability, and less-developed logistics chains.[146]

Pandemic An event in which a disease spreads across several countries and affects a large number of people.

Asymptomatic Presenting no symptoms of disease. In the context of COVID-19, no symptoms of fever, cough, shortness of breath, or body aches.

National Emergencies Act (NEA) Authorizes the President of the United States the ability to declare a National Emergency, which can enable the Secretary of Health and Human Services to waive or modify specific program requirements throughout the duration of a pandemic or emergency.

National Emergency A state of emergency resulting from a danger or threat of danger to a nation from foreign or domestic sources and usually declared to be in existence by governmental authority.

small, round structural viruses. It was first identified as the causative agent for a school outbreak of gastroenteritis in 1968, in Norwalk, Ohio.[137] Norovirus outbreaks have been associated with contaminated water, fruits, raw oysters, and scallops,[137-139] and although they are notorious for their association with acute gastroenteritis outbreaks on cruise ships, they are most frequently linked to restaurants with seated dining.[140,141]

In the United States, food- and waterborne hepatitis A outbreaks are relatively uncommon. However, transmission via the fecal-oral route is possible; food handler carriers of hepatitis A are often identified, and raw or undercooked shellfish may carry the virus, so prevention and control measures (see Vibrio previously) are necessary.[142,143]

Supply-Chain, Food and COVID

During the COVID-19 pandemic, the food supply chain experienced new challenges alongside pressures of increased demand and shortages. Throughout the United States of America, regulations and restrictions pertaining to the safety of citizens, such as quarantines, curfews, travel restrictions, and **social-distancing** models differed state by state, which complicated the typical national architecture of moving food supplies. FEMA's National Business Emergency Operations Center developed a virtual clearing house to assist with communications between private industry and public agencies throughout disaster response.[147] The effort to support improved communication streams was key during the emergency situation of the COVID-19 pandemic to ensure that the public remained informed throughout the rapidly changing physical, economic, and political environments.

It is important to remember that the United States supply chain not only relies on national resources but also relies on international imports for the production and distribution of food goods and the machinery used in those processes. During the COVID-19 pandemic, international trade was significantly impacted due to reduced workforce from illness, transportation restrictions, and limited access to certain countries causing overall logistical barriers.[148] Labor shortages not only impacted the food supply due to reduced productivity but also placed increased risk toward food safety if the virus impacted workers' own health or ability to work.[148] One example of the impact of labor shortages during COVID-19 was in April of 2020 when the overall capacity of some meat facilities decreased by approximately 25%.[148] Food plants were not only impacted in labor-shortages due to illness but were also subject to challenges in social-distancing feasibility of employees overall, since workers often needed to be close together on production lines, increasing risk of infection. Ultimately, some food plants closed, hitting the food supply chain with significant impacts, such as product shortages driving up the price of meat products for consumers, or even having purchase limitations put into place at grocery stores.[148]

COVID-19 Impact on Food Industry-Related Businesses

Throughout the COVID-19 pandemic, the food and beverage industry (manufacturers, restaurants via takeout, and retailers) were considered to be **"essential businesses,"** that were allowed to remain open amid restrictions to keep people safe at home. Even so, these businesses were impacted both logistically, and financially. State and local health departments were responsible for regulations related to the safety and sanitation of businesses in the food industry based on CDC guidance. Regulations could vary in stringency based on the local spread of the COVID-19 virus.

Social distancing Also known as "physical distancing," keeping a safe space between yourself and other people who are not a part of your household by maintaining at least 6 feet apart in both indoor and outdoor areas.

Physical distancing See "social distancing."

Essential businesses Businesses that provide a product or service that is considered necessary for everyday life. Definition varies from state to state in the United States.

Temporary guidelines were developed on a larger scale regarding food safety audits for the handling of food from foreign suppliers. The Foreign Supplier Verification Program, (FSVP) required that foreign food suppliers verify their ability to meet import regulations and safety standards set by the United States. In these guidelines, supplier verification could be used in lieu of onsite audits in order to decrease in-person social contact. Regulations accepted by the FSVP included: hazard analysis, and risk-based preventive controls for human food, hazard analysis, and risk-based preventive controls for food for animals, and foreign supplier verification programs. While information on the virus emerged, the FDA provided guidance for increased flexibility in nutrition labeling, as well as to responses to industry questions throughout the pandemic regarding food safety, food policies, and the supply chain.[149] Another resource available to consumers, producers, medical/health professionals and those in the food industry is the FDA Food and Cosmetics Information Center Inquiry form, which provides inquiry submission capabilities where users can submit inquiries related to coronavirus or the FSMA.[150]

Food Purchasing Habits During the COVID-19 Pandemic

Due to initial news reports of the first cases of the SARS-Cov2 virus surfacing from a seafood, meat, and produce market believed to be in Wuhan, consumer fear was driven in the direction of food markets and transmission through food products driving sales of shelf stable products.[148]

Additionally, with emergency-preparedness, and **self-quarantines** occurring throughout the coronavirus pandemic, bulk-buying, or "panic-buying" ensued. Bulk, or panic-buying is when consumers "over-buy" food or supplies in avoidance of social contact during the pandemic. This behavior, in turn, caused shortages, as well as price-gauging in stores across the United States and impacted availability of goods long term. Bulk purchasing of food was discouraged by local governments and stores in order to allow equitable access to supplies for all; however, the behavior continued. Grocers put purchase limits on scarce items such as cleaning supplies, toilet paper, rice, canned vegetables, meat, eggs, flour, dried pasta, bread products, and yeast in order to stop panic-buying and alleviate strain on the supply chains.

When purchasing food in bulk, one important consideration is how to safely store bulk or prepared foods for long periods of time. The CDC posted guidance on handling and storing foods purchased in bulk, which align with their "clean, separate, cook, and chill" method.[151] Although there have been no known cases of COVID-19 due to the virus transmission via food packaging, food consumption, good food safety, and hand hygiene practices are always important when preparing and cleaning food prior to consumption.

Travel restrictions and **stay-at-home orders** caused in-person dining to diminish, or to even be banned at certain points during the pandemic in order to reduce in-person gatherings and virus spread. These restrictions required restaurants to adapt to changing dining habits in order to stay in business. Some adaptations included a changeover to take-out menus, **contact tracing**, curbside pick-up options, touchless payment methods, socially and physically distanced dining options (such as outdoor tents, dispersed and/or reduced seating capacity, plexiglass barriers), in addition to strict food-safety adherence. ServSafe, a food and beverage training conducted by the National Restaurant Association, offered free COVID-19 related training and food service reopening resources to ensure the safety of establishment guests and staff.[152]

Self-quarantine A method of slowing disease spread by staying at home and away from other people. Activities requiring interaction with others or leaving home are avoided.

Stay-at-home order A movement order set to restrict people from leaving their residences aside from undertaking essential activities in order to limit person-to-person contact and slow the spread of a disease.

Contact tracing Identification of any person who has come into contact with an infected person.

Due to nationwide stay-at-home orders, and the closure of in-person dining, it also became important to highlight practices around receiving food delivery, or meal-kits (frozen, prepared, or fresh). Checking temperatures of food upon receipt of delivery, quickly transferring meals to a refrigerator or freezer, handwashing, and using touchless payment methods are all good practices to reduce the risk of illness from foodborne pathogens.

USDA Actions During the COVID-19 Pandemic

During the COVID-19 pandemic, the USDA vowed to "do right and feed everyone," in several ways such as through assistance programs, relief acts, and private-public partnerships to help increase access to nutritious food in a safe manner.

Some of the actions taken to improve access to safe, nutritious food during the COVID-19 pandemic included:

- The Emergency Food Assistance Program (TEFAP), which provided Americans with more than 227 million pounds of food.[153]
- The Families First Coronavirus Response Act (FFCRA)[154] and Coronavirus Aid, Recovery, and Economic Stimulus packages (CARES) act, which provided an additional $850 million in aid to Americans.[155]
- Pandemic EBT (P-EBT), which was launched in order to help provide meals to families with school-aged children even while the schools were closed. P-EBT also waived requirements regarding the timing of serving meals in school settings. The increased flexibility in child nutrition programming allowed for increased access to nutritious meals for those in need during challenging economic times. At the initiation of the Biden Administration in 2021, the President authorized an increase in P-EBT benefits by 15% in order to provide additional funding to school food programs and food banks.[156]
- Disaster Household Distributions were approved in order to provide food products to individuals in areas where access to foods was not available on a regular basis, which included 16 states, territories, as well as 29 tribes.[157]

During the pandemic, public-private partnerships were built in order to combine resources and increase reach of food distribution services throughout the United States in projects such as "Meals to You," which provided breakfast and lunch meal boxes to families eligible for the National School Lunch Program.[158]

Additional calls to action to address hunger during the coronavirus pandemic were put into place at the start of the Biden Administration in January of 2021; including funding improvements and extensions for the Special Supplemental Nutrition Program for Women, Infants and Children (WIC), increased funding to U.S Territories for nutritional assistance and ways to support restaurants as a valuable part of the food supply and also to help feed hungry families.[156,159]

Although the Trump Administration began some work to increase food benefits during the pandemic so that Americans in need could have increased access to food, benefit increases were not made to those Americans who have very low income, which make up a total of 37% of total SNAP households.[160] Through the work of Executive orders early on during 2021, the gaps in these resources for food security for those Americans with very low income through additional funding was tackled, which in turn may help the economy and work to reduce poverty rates.[160]

Emergency Use Authorization A government authorization to allow unapproved medical products, or medical products that have not been approved for a specific use case, to be utilized in an emergency situation (such as COVID-19), when there are no approved alternative treatments.

Discussion Prompt

How did community and public health officials contribute to helping the American people during the COVID-19 pandemic?

Testing and Emergency Vaccine Use Authorization

Testing for the virus became a regular task that could be completed in order to help understand and mitigate disease spread, as well as to better facilitate disease diagnosis and the appropriate usage of healthcare resources. Two types of testing became available to assess for COVID-19 (diagnostic and antibody tests), which were administered at hospitals, clinics, urgent care settings, schools, and pharmacies.

The FDA issued its first-ever **emergency use authorization (EUA)** for the Pfizer-BioNTech developed COVID-19 vaccine to be distributed in the United States during the coronavirus pandemic. An EUA can allow unapproved medical products, or medical products that have not been approved for a specific-use case, to be utilized in an emergency situation (such as COVID-19), when there are no approved alternative treatments.[161] Vaccine distribution efforts of the COVID-19 pandemic brought hope for many industries. Eventual business reopening and loosening of state and local restrictions would hinge on vaccination efforts to ensure the public's safety.

The COVID-19 pandemic impacted the entire food supply chain, food industry, and altered consumer habits and knowledge around food safety, food, and nutrition overall. It is imperative that moving forward, governments consider preparative actions and financial support to secure the food industry in the event of future national emergencies.

Parasites

Parasites include flatworms, roundworms, tapeworms, protozoans, and other organisms that use the body as a host in order to live and multiply. Some familiar parasites are listed in Table 14–3. These are usually ingested in raw or undercooked foods or water in which the parasites live; for example, *Trichinella spiralis* (roundworm of pork, also found in game, like bear and walrus) causes trichinellosis,[122] and *Giardia lamblia*, a waterborne protozoan, causes giardiasis ("beaver fever").[162] Parasites emerging recently as significant to food safety include Cryptosporidium and Cyclospora, and liver flukes (e.g., *Fasciola hepatica* and *F. gigantica*).[163]

Cryptosporidium parvum, a protozoan found in mammals, reptiles, and birds, causes diarrhea in humans (it is particularly severe in immunocompromised individuals). Abdominal pain, nausea, vomiting, and fever are often reported.[164] Cryptosporidiosis is "acquired by at least one of five known transmission routes: zoonotic, person to person, water, nosocomial, or food."[164] People are infected by ingesting oocysts of the parasite, which are shed in the feces of the host.[164] Major outbreaks of cryptosporidiosis have occurred in Maine (1993, unpasteurized apple cider),[165] Minnesota (1995, chicken salad),[166] New York (1996, unpasteurized apple cider),[167] and Washington (1997, raw green onions).[168]

Cyclospora cayetanensis, a protozoan similar to *Cryptosporidium*, causes symptoms similar to cryptosporidiosis in infected humans. Like cryptosporidiosis, cyclosporiasis is much more serious in immunocompromised individuals.[169] The most notorious foodborne cyclosporiasis outbreak "occurred in 1996 in 20 U.S. states and two Canadian provinces, infecting 1,465 people who had eaten imported Guatemalan raspberries."[164]

Prions

Problems in the British beef industry in the 1980s brought prion diseases under increased scientific scrutiny and public curiosity.[137,170-172] Prions, the etiologic agents of, among others, Creutzfeldt-Jakob disease (CJD) and kuru in humans[173,174] and chronic wasting disease and sheep scrapie in animals, are physiologic cellular glycoproteins. The bovine spongiform encephalopathy (BSE; "mad cow disease") prion (PrPSc) is an infectious variant of a normal copper-binding prion (PrPC) on cell surfaces.[175] BSE is one of several transmissible spongiform encephalopathies (the human form of BSE is variant Creutzfeldt-Jakob disease, vCJD[176]) that are emerging, serious public health concerns.[177,178] Critics of U.S. regulatory policies regarding BSE cite half-hearted efforts to monitor for the disease, lack of research funding, and undue meat industry pressure.[179] After two BSE-infected cows were detected in the United States, one each in 2003 and 2004, public, professional, and Congressional lobbying for changes in regulatory oversight ensued. The FDA and USDA have strengthened safeguards protecting consumers from PrPSc, prohibiting "the use of certain cattle-derived materials in human food (including dietary supplements) and cosmetics."[180-182]

Chemical Hazards

Dietitians and nutritionists understand that foods consist of chemicals, but the public grossly misunderstands the word *chemicals*. Several chemical hazards are associated with foods, some naturally occurring (e.g., aflatoxin, alkaloids, histamine), some indirectly added (e.g., pesticides, compounds that migrate from packaging materials, lubricants from food processing machinery), and others directly added (e.g., colors, preservatives).[9]

Naturally Occurring Toxicants Many foods contain natural toxins that may be harmful when consumed at certain levels, such as aflatoxin and mushroom toxins, whereas others contain toxins that are harmful over time, such as mercury. Mycotoxins, potato glycoalkaloids, shellfish toxins, and methylmercury are illustrative of this group, but there are many others, including oxalic acid, goitrogens, hemagglutinens, and protease inhibitors.

Mycotoxins are mold-produced toxins, many of which are of public health importance. The aflatoxins (*Aspergillus flavus* toxin), highly substituted coumarins, are the most studied.[183] Usually associated with corn, cottonseed, peanuts, and products made from them, aflatoxins are also found in milk, cheese,[184] meats, and other foods. Aflatoxins produce liver cancer in animals.[185] Developing countries in Africa and Asia have the greatest incidence of aflatoxin-related cancers.[186] The FDA specifies limits for aflatoxins in animal feeds and foods for human consumption, currently 20 ppb for food, feeds, Brazil nuts, peanuts, peanut products, and pistachios, and 0.5 ppb for milk.[186,187] At the international level, the Codex Alimentarius Commission[188] recommends maximums of 15 µg/kg of aflatoxin in peanuts for further processing and 0.05 µg/kg of aflatoxin in milk.[189]

Other molds, such as *Aspergillus*, *Alternaria*, *Fusarium*, and *Penicillium*, produce toxins in foods. *Aspergillus spp.* produce ochratoxins, found in corn, nuts, grains, meats, and other foods.[183] These heat-stable toxins are hepatotoxic and nephrotoxic in rats.[183] Alternariol and other *Alternaria*-produced toxins have been found in grains and fruits.[190,191] Fumonisins are *Fusarium*-produced toxins found in corn and other grains. These are associated with high rates of esophageal cancer in Africa and Asia.[192,193] Citrinin and patulin are toxins produced by *Penicillium spp.* Citrinin is found in many foods, including bread, rice, other cereal grains, and country-cured hams, and patulin has been found in bread, sausage, fruits, and juices.[183] The Codex Alimentarius Commission recommends maximums of 50 µg/kg of patulin in apple juice and apple juice as an ingredient in other beverages, and 5 µg/kg ochratoxin A in cereals and cereal products.[189]

Mycotoxins survive food-processing methods,[194] but continuous monitoring for them ensures safety of the foods affected. Although mycotoxins are not formed (or are formed in very small quantities) at refrigerator temperatures (generally, 36°–41°F),[195] consumers should be advised to throw out foods that develop molds. Preformed toxins are not affected by refrigeration, freezing, or cooking. Consumers also should be advised to store foods to minimize mold growth, such as by storing foods dry, in small quantities, and/or under refrigeration.

Alkaloids are found in many food products. Various glycoalkaloids are present in potatoes and potato-products[196-202] and can increase with exposure to light,[203-205] heat,[206,207] and insect damage during the growing season.[208] Toxic effects of glycoalkaloids include abdominal pain, diarrhea, and vomiting at low doses; fever, hypotension, neurological disorders, tachycardia, tachypnea,[209] and death[210] at higher doses. Glycoalkaloid poisoning is uncommon; however, and individual responses to glycoalkaloids vary. For many years, dietitians/nutritionists and other health professionals merely cautioned people to avoid eating the green parts of potatoes. The generally accepted safe limit for potato glycoalkaloids is 200 mg/kg.[211] Recently, as scientists have broadened their understanding of the biochemistry of glycoalkaloids, warnings about chronic vs. acute effects of ingested glycoalkaloids have become more strident.[212] Glycoalkaloids increase risk for some cancers[213]; are teratogenic, embryotoxic, and genotoxic[214,215]; and may interfere with or interact with commonly prescribed pharmaceuticals.[216] With the food industry's interest in developing value-added products from potato peels[217,218] (and in reducing the glycoalkaloid content[219]) and the increasing likelihood that dietitians/nutritionists will encounter clients (such as Bangladeshis[198]) for whom potato leaves and potato peels are acceptable food choices, regular monitoring of the scientific literature pertaining to potato glycoalkaloids is warranted.

Toxins causing amnesic shellfish poisoning (ASP), ciguatera poisoning, and paralytic shellfish poisoning (PSP) are not produced by shellfish or fish. Rather, they are produced by microscopic phytoplankton (diatoms and dinoflagellates) consumed by the shellfish and fish. The diatom *Pseudonitzschia pungens* produces domoic acid, which acts as a glutamic acid antagonist in the human central nervous system,[137] producing sometimes fatal ASP.[220] Several outbreaks have occurred since 1988.[221-224]

Ciguatoxin is produced by the dinoflagellate *Gambierdiscus toxicus*. Humans ingest the toxin in predatory fish, such as barracuda, groupers, and sea bass, which in turn have ingested herbivorous fish in which the toxin is concentrated in organs and muscles. Symptoms of ciguatoxin poisoning are similar to those of PSP (nausea, oral paresthesia, and respiratory paralysis), but the onset of symptoms is somewhat longer (3–6 hours vs. 2 hours for PSP). Long considered an illness of the tropics,[225,226] modern food transportation systems can deliver ciguatoxic fish to locations far removed from their home waters.[227-230]

PSP is caused by ingesting toxins (decarbamoyl saxitoxin, neosaxitoxin, gonyautoxins, and others[231,232]) in bivalve mollusks that have eaten dinoflagellates such as *Gonyaulax catenella* and *G. acatenella* (Pacific Coast), and *G. tamarensis* (Atlantic Coast), among others. The toxins are heat-stable and can cause cardiovascular collapse and respiratory failure.[137] PSP mortality can reach 22%.[233]

The National Shellfish Sanitation Program (NSSP),

> …a voluntary, tripartite program composed of state officials, the shellfish industry, and Federal -agencies…is designed to prevent human illness associated with the consumption of fresh and frozen shellfish (oysters, clams, and mussels) through the establishment of sanitary controls over all phases of the growing, harvesting, shucking, packing, and distribution of fresh and frozen shellfish.[234]

The FDA oversees the NSSP and, together with state agencies, manages the sanitation programs at the state level. Foreign countries (e.g., Canada, Chile, Korea, Mexico, New Zealand) may import shellfish into the United States by agreeing to abide by the provisions of the NSSP as set forth in a Memorandum of Understanding between countries. Public health dietitians/nutritionists should consult the Interstate Certified Shellfish Shippers List (ICSSL),[235] published monthly by the FDA, because under the NSSP, all states require that shellfish be from a certified source, proof of which is dealer listing in the ICSSL.

Metals such as mercury are persistent environmental pollutants and can cause foodborne illness. Foods usually implicated are fish, shellfish, and marine mammals. These animals ingest and accumulate methylmercury from their foods. Mercury enters the environment and food chains from both human activities (coal-fired powerplant emissions, medical and electronics wastes, etc.) and natural processes.[236] Methylmercury is neurotoxic[236] and possibly immunomodulating[237] in humans, usually over time with chronic exposure. The human fetus is particularly susceptible to methylmercury poisoning. The FDA's seafood website (https://www.fda.gov/food/guidance-documents-regulatory-information-topic-food-and-dietary-supplements/seafood-guidance-documents-regulatory-information) has links to population-specific seafood advisories[238,239] and data on mercury levels in commonly consumed fish and shellfish.[240,241] One example is the irreversible neurologic damage from the chemical methylmercury found in fish and shellfish living in polluted waters that may be tempered by nutrition.[242-244] Until more is known, some authorities question current recommendations to eat more fish to improve cardiovascular health.[245]

Directly Added Chemicals

Food Additives Humans have added chemicals to food since before recorded history. Primitive food preservation methods included salting, smoking, and fermentation, all still in use today. Herbs and spices were used to retard spoilage and to mask flavors caused by spoilage. Today, with fewer people cooking meals "from scratch" and with fewer meals eaten in the home, consumers are increasingly leaving decisions about which chemicals are added to foods to the food industry and its government regulators. Dietitians/nutritionists are likely to encounter ignorance of the purposes of food additives in foods consumed by their clients as well as fear of the chemical names listed on ingredient labels. At least this may be true for those who actually read the labels; some dietitians/nutritionists believe that many do not read food labels,[246,247] and among those who do, comprehension is not what it should be.[248,249] Many people are influenced by the popular press and news media, where innuendos, half-truths, and patently false statements compete with sound science on issues surrounding chemical use in foods. The food and chemical industries and government regulatory agencies often exacerbate the confusion by offering platitudes in response to accusations. Steps have been taken to restore public confidence in food safety and in the industries themselves.[250-255] This constant interchange between science and pseudoscience is one of the most daunting obstacles a nutritionist is likely to face. We must regularly evaluate the scientific literature and government policy to better inform clients and to provide guidance in critically evaluating claims made about food additives.

Chemicals are added to foods for many reasons: to increase nutritional quality; to aid in food processing; to increase, decrease, or neutralize certain sensory characteristics of foods; to prolong storage stability; and to inhibit microbial growth. Within broad categories of additives (**Table 14–4**), there are usually several alternatives available to gain the same desired effect. For

Discussion Prompt

In recent years, white tuna and sushi have been found to have higher than expected methylmercury levels. What can be done to prevent this poisoning of our fish supply? What have community and public health nutritionists done to communicate this to the public?

some applications, combinations of additives are applied to meet specific requirements (e.g., a manufacturer may use a blend of acesulfame-K and aspartame to obtain an optimum low-calorie sweetener for hot coffee and tea beverages[256]). Development, testing, and approval of new chemical food additives continues at a rapid pace.

Antioxidants Foods containing fats are subject to oxidative rancidity during storage. To enable foods such as crackers, nuts, and potato chips to be packaged and stored while retaining freshness, antioxidant chemicals such as ascorbic acid (vitamin C), butylated hydroxyanisole (BHA), butylated hydroxytoluene (BHT), sulfur dioxide, and tocopherols (vitamin E), among others, are used, singly or in combinations.[9]

Alternative Sweeteners Sweeteners may be classified as nutritive (or caloric; e.g., sucrose, honey, corn syrups) or non-nutritive (or noncaloric; e.g., acesulfame-K, saccharin). Some nutritive alternative sweeteners are

TABLE 14–4
Examples of Chemical Food Additives[1]

Class	Representative Chemicals	Purposes
Antioxidants	Ascorbic acid (vitamin C) butylated hydroxyanisole, butylated hydroxytoluene, sulfur dioxide, tocopherols (vitamin E)	Retard deterioration, rancidity, discoloration from oxidation; free radical scavengers
Flour bleaching agents, flour maturing agents, starch bleaching agents, starch modifiers	Acetone peroxides, calcium bromate, sodium hypochlorite, adipic anhydride (esterifier), propylene oxide (etherifier)	Enhance whiteness of flour or starch; enhance baking qualities of flour; modify starch functional characteristics to applications desired
Buffers, acids, alkalis	Acetic acid, ammonium hydroxide, citric acid, fumaric acid, malic acid, oxalic acid, sodium carbonate, succinic acid, tartaric acid	Lower or raise pH; buffer pH against change
Colors (exempt from batch certification)[2]	Annatto extract, caramel, carmine, grape skin extract, turmeric	Impart, enhance, or preserve food color or shading
Colors (must be batch certified)[3]	FD&C Blue No. 1, FD&C Green No. 3, Orange B, Citrus Red No. 2, FD&C Yellow No. 5	Impart, enhance, or preserve food color or shading
Flavors, chemical	2-acetyl thiazole, 3-heptanone, benzaldehyde, cresyl acetate, decanal, eugenol, quinine sulfate	Impart or enhance a flavor or flavor "note" in food
Nutritional additives	Amino acids (e.g., dl-leucine), β-carotene, kelp, minerals (e.g., ferrous sulfate), vitamins (e.g., biotin)	Necessary for the body's nutritional and metabolic processes
Preservatives	Benzoic acid, butyl P-hydroxybenzoate, calcium benzoate, calcium disodium EDTA, calcium sorbate, cupric sulfate, heptylparaben	Retard microbial spoilage; block ripening and enzymatic processes; antioxidation
Sequestrants	Calcium acetate, calcium disodium EDTA, citric acid, disodium EDTA, glucono δ-lactone	Combine with polyvalent metal ions to form a soluble metal complex; improve product quality and stability
Stabilizers and thickeners	Carrageenan, carob bean gum, dammar gum, dextrin, edible gelatin, modified starches, tara gum	Increase viscosity of solutions; produce/improve dispersions; impart body, improve consistency, or stabilize emulsions
Surface-active agents: etergents; ispersants; efoaming agents; oaming agents; olubilizing agents; etting agents; hipping agents	TERG-A-ZYME™[4] microcrystalline cellulose decanoic acid	Modify surface properties of liquid food components

Miscellaneous additives: alternative sweeteners; anti-caking agents; anti-sticking agents; clarifying agents; fat replacers[5]; firming agents; growth promoters; lubricants; solvents	acacia 1,3-butylene glycol dioctyl sodium sulfosuccinate calcium polyphosphates aspartame, sucralose, tagatose aluminum silicate castor oil polyvinylpolypyrrolidone dextrins, whey protein, olestra aluminum sulfate calcium lactate (yeast food) mineral oil ethylene dichloride	For specific applications

[1]Not a complete list. For extensive lists, see the *NutritionData Food Additive Identifier*, http://www.nutritiondata.com/food-additives.html; "Food Additives Permitted for Direct Addition to Food for Human Consumption," Code of Federal Regulations, Title 21, Vol. 3, (U.S. Government Printing Office, April 1, 2003), Ch. 1, Part 172; "Secondary Direct Food Additives Permitted in Food for Human Consumption," Code of Federal Regulations, Title 21, Vol. 3, (U.S. Government Printing Office, April 1, 2003), Ch. 1, Part 173; "Indirect Food Additives," Code of Federal Regulations, Title 21, Vol. 3, (U.S. Government Printing Office, April 1, 2003), Ch. 1, Parts 174-178.

[2]See "Summary of color additives approved for use in human food. Part 73, Subpart A: Color additives exempt from batch certification," https://www.fda.gov/industry/color-additive-inventories/summary-color-additives-use-united-states-foods-drugs-cosmetics-and-medical-devices#table1A. Accessed December 12, 2020.

[3]See "Color Additives Approved for Use in Human Food. Part 74, Subpart A: Color additives subject to batch certification," https://www.fda.gov/industry/color-additive-inventories/summary-color-additives-use-united-states-foods-drugs-cosmetics-and-medical-devices#table1B. Accessed December 12, 2020.

[4]TERG-A-ZYME consists of sodium linear alkylaryl sulfonate, phosphates, carbonates, and protease enzyme (*Bacillus licheniformis subtilisin Carlsberg*). See Document #123, "TERG-A-ZYME Technical Bulletin" (White Plains NY: Alconox, https://technotes.alconox.com/wp-content/uploads/2016/03/tech_bulletin_tergazyme_english.pdf. Accessed December 12, 2020).

[5]For a current list of fat replacers, see the Calorie Control Council's website at http://www.caloriecontrol.org/frgloss.html. Accessed December 12, 2020.

so much sweeter than sucrose that they are essentially reduced-calorie sweeteners (e.g., aspartame at 4 kcal/g is approximately 200 times sweeter than sucrose[257] and thus is calorically negligible in foods to which it has been added). Reduced-calorie or noncaloric alternatively sweetened foods are popularly used in weight-reducing diets and weight-maintenance plans to reduce the incidence of dental caries or to manage diabetes. Food scientists and food technologists continue to research and develop alternative sweeteners; the most recently approved sweetener is advantame, a non-nutritive sweetener.[258,259]

Dietitians/nutritionists can help consumers recognize the various sugars (e.g., corn syrup, dextrose, fructose, high fructose corn syrup [HFCS], honey, lactose, sucrose) and alternative sweeteners[260] listed on food labels and can also assist them in choosing foods sweetened with additives that are suited to their individual health profiles, diets, and lifestyles. Dietitians/nutritionists may also be asked about alternative sweeteners that, although legally used abroad, are not approved for additive use in the United States, such as stevia (powdered extract of the plant *Stevia rebaudiana Bertoni*),[261] currently regulated and sold as a food supplement. (Stevia is purported to have antihyperglycemic[262] and antihypertensive properties.[263-265]) Finally, dietitians/nutritionists must thoroughly understand the controversial aspects of some additive sweeteners (e.g., the alleged association of HFCS with the increasing worldwide prevalence of obesity[266]; the purported carcinogenicity of sodium saccharin[267,268]; and the alleged adverse health effects of dietary aspartame[269-274] and sucralose[275-278]) as well as critically evaluate the evidence available in order to make the best possible recommendations to consumers. The Dietary Guidelines for Americans,[279] the Dietary Reference Intakes,[280] and the position statement on sweeteners of the Academy of Nutrition and Dietetics[281] are useful guidelines.

Bleaching agents, maturing agents, starch modifiers, and oxidizing agents such as benzoyl peroxide and chlorine dioxide are used to bleach flour color and to mature flour to improve baking properties. Modified food starches are used to improve the appearance, stability, texture, and quality of food products.[9] Starches may be cross-linked with phosphates or adipates, stabilized by etherification or esterification (acetate- or hydroxypropyl-modified), or thinned by dextrinization or acid hydrolysis.[282]

Buffers, acids, and alkalis buffers (e.g., acetic acid/sodium acetate), acids (e.g., acetic, malic, tartaric acids), and alkalis (e.g., ammonium hydroxide, carbonates) are used in foods to control or adjust pH. They may be from natural sources, fermentation-derived, or chemically synthesized.[9,283]

Colors Natural and synthetic colors are added to foods to enhance visual appeal. Natural colors may be obtained from plant (e.g., beets, grapes, saffron), mineral (e.g., iron oxide, titanium dioxide), and animal (e.g., cochineal extract or carmine from female scale insects, Coccus cacti) sources.[9]

Flavors Flavoring agents constitute the largest group of food additives. Natural flavor substances include spices (e.g., anise, paprika, vanilla), herbs (e.g., basil, parsley, thyme), essential oils (e.g., clove, lime, rose), and plant extracts (e.g., almond, garlic, rosemary). Some natural flavor substances may appear in multiple categories; for example, chervil may be added to foods as a spice, an oil, or an extract, among other designations.[284] Synthetic flavoring agents are also used (e.g., allyl disulfide, isopropyl alcohol, thymol). Flavoring agents may be listed on food labels as "flavorings," "natural flavors," "artificial flavors," and "spices." Monosodium glutamate (MSG), a flavor enhancer, is associated with adverse reaction symptoms (chest pain, edema, facial or oral numbness, headache, perspiration, and cranial or facial pressure such as "Chinese Restaurant Syndrome"[285-291] and MSG-induced asthma[292,293]) in some people but is listed GRAS by the FDA and is reported safe by the Joint Food and Agriculture Organization/World Health Organization (FAO/WHO) Expert Committee on Food Additives,[294] in the absence of conclusive proof that it is harmful. Many health professionals do recognize, however, a subpopulation of MSG-sensitive individuals. Dietitians/nutritionists should be prepared to help these consumers identify MSG-containing foods (MSG may be hidden in general ingredient label statements, such as "hydrolyzed vegetable protein," "natural flavorings," "seasonings") and to suggest alternatives.

Nutritional Additives Vitamins and minerals are added as enrichments and fortifiers to several foods. Although there is no legal distinction between *enrichment* and *fortification* in the United States—the FDA uses the terms interchangeably[295])—enrichment usually signifies replacement of nutrients lost in flour and cereal processing. Enriched flour has had B vitamins and iron added, most breakfast cereals are vitamin and mineral enriched, and polished rice is usually enriched. Fortification also signifies the replacement of lost nutrients, usually in foods other than flour and cereals, as well as the addition of nutrients to commonly used foods to redress deficiency of the nutrient(s) in most diets. Milk thus may be fortified with vitamin D because the diet of children and older adults is often deficient in vitamin D[296]; no-fat and low-fat milks have vitamins A (by law) and D (optional) added because these vitamins are lost when fat is removed; salt may be fortified with iodine to prevent goiter; and cereal and grain products are fortified with folic acid to prevent neural tube defects.[297]

Food fortification is one of the leading research areas in food technology today.[298-300] For example, consumers can buy calcium-fortified and vitamin D–fortified orange juice[301] and vitamin-and-herb-fortified spring water (e.g., Nestlé® Pure Life® Fruity Water). Unfortunately, most people purchase fortified foods with little or no knowledge of bioavailability or potential toxicities of the substances used to fortify the foods.[302,303]

Preservatives (e.g., butylated hydroxyanisole [BHA], butylated hydroxytoluene [BHT], sodium propionate, sulfur dioxide) are used as antimicrobial agents to retard microbial spoilage of foods, as metal chelators to block ripening and enzymatic processes that continue in foods after harvest, and as antioxidants to retard rancidity and browning, allowing consumers to enjoy a variety of foods, from global sources, year-round.[304,305] Dietitians/nutritionists may receive questions from consumers concerning the safety of BHA,[306-309] BHT,[306,307,309] sulfites,[310,311] -nitrites,[312-314] and food irradiation ("cold pasteurization," considered a food additive by the FDA).[315-324] Currently, several classes of foods may be irradiated at doses between 4.5 and 7.0 kGy[325] in the United States, including some fresh fruits and vegetables, spices and seasonings, meats, poultry, and prepackaged foods.

Sequestrants Chelating agents (e.g., EDTA, citric acid) are used to sequester metal ions in foods. Left alone, metals such as iron and copper contribute to off colors and catalyze oxidation reactions in foods.[9]

Stabilizers and Thickeners Processed foods, such as gravies, puddings, and salad dressings, are stabilized and thickened by substances such as carboxymethyl cellulose, gums, and pectin.[9] Foods containing little or no fat, such as low-fat salad dressings, are formulated using stabilizers and thickeners to resemble their full-fat counterparts.

Surface-Active Agents Emulsifiers, defoaming agents, and detergents are all active at molecular surfaces. Emulsifiers (e.g., lecithin, mono- and diglycerides, and fatty acids) are used to keep food mixtures, such as oil in water and water in oil, stable.[9]

Miscellaneous Additives Many other additives (e.g., anti-caking and anti-sticking agents, clarifying agents, firming agents, growth promoters, lubricants, solvents) are used for very specific applications.[9] Macrocomponents, such as fat replacers, are added to foods to replace some or all of a food component. Substances such as bean pastes, fruit pastes, or microparticulate whey protein concentrates (e.g., Simplesse®) and emulsifiers may be used to replace some or all of the fat in baked goods.[326,327]

Agricultural Chemicals Agricultural chemicals include antibiotics, growth hormones, herbicides, fertilizers, fungicides, insecticides, and rodenticides, all of which may enter the food supply. Antibiotics at subtherapeutic doses are used to promote animal growth (in the United States) and to prevent disease. Evidence that antibiotic-resistant strains of bacteria develop in food animals and might be passed on to humans, and that consuming antibiotic residues in food might inhibit the efficacy of therapeutic antibiotic use in humans, is controversial.[328,329] Growth hormones, such as recombinant bovine growth hormone (rbGH or BGH) or recombinant bovine somatotropin (rbST or BST), are considered safe when used as directed.[330,331] However, product labeling is controversial, particularly the use of label statements such as "BST-free."[332-335] Herbicides, fertilizers, fungicides, insecticides, and other pesticides are regulated by the EPA. Residues of these chemicals in food[336-339] are under FDA jurisdiction.

Physical Hazards

Physical hazards include extraneous objects or foreign materials in food that may cause illness or injury if consumed. The most common physical hazards found in foods are:

- Metal (from fields, equipment, premises), bullets and BB shot (from animals shot in the field), and hypodermic needles (broken off when treating animals)

Discussion Prompt

What plant fertilizers have been linked to cancer recently in the media? What can we learn from this?

- Jewelry (buttons, earrings, rings, etc.)
- Stones and rocks (from fields, ceilings, walls), wood (from fields, ceilings, walls, boxes, pallets), and insulation (from buildings)
- Glass (from bottles, jars, light fixtures, utensils, equipment)
- Insects, insect parts, and other filth (from fields, premises, entry after processing)
- Bone (from improper processing; also, from fields and premises)
- Plastic (from fields, packaging and packing, employees)
- Personal effects (bandages, pens, pencils, thermometers, etc.)[8]

Less common physical hazards include capsules, crystals (e.g., struvite), paper, pits, scum, shells, and slime.[340] Food processors must identify potential physical hazards and determine procedures to control each hazard; if warranted, control points should be implemented as part of the facility HACCP plan.[341]

Food Safety in the 21st Century

Rapidly digitized systems, new food products, production methods, and increased supply chain demands highlight the need for an increased consideration of efforts to streamline the approach to providing the public with a safe food supply.

Using work completed as part of the FSMA, in 2020, the FDA released "The New Era of Smarter Food Safety Blueprint," a document outlining the approach that the FDA will take to ensure that new technologies, and tools can be leveraged in creating a more traceable, secure food system.[342] The goals of the Blueprint are to improve the response to outbreaks, reduce and prevent foodborne illnesses, and to alert consumers of contamination before food is consumed. Advances in data analytics and technology are key components of stakeholder focus when considering the future of food safety. "The New Era of Smarter Food Safety Blueprint" includes four core elements: technology-enabled traceability, smarter tools and approaches for outbreak prevention response, new business models and retail modernization, and improvements in food safety culture. Food safety and the use of state and federal resources run throughout each of the key elements to consider in the document.[342]

Blockchain and the Food System

One unique concept for the use of new technologies in the food system includes the use of blockchain for food safety data and traceability efforts. Data from each "block" or participant in the network or chain is converted into something called a "hash," a unique fixed type of code that specific data is converted into.[343] As data such as food temperature, humidity, method and location of processing, fertilizer type, storage conditions, etc., cross each participant in the network, the hash will integrate into the next "block" or participant in the chain, thus ensuring that across each pass of information, food data are not lost or tampered with. Use of **blockchain** in the food system may help to expedite the process of food recalls, improve regulatory compliance, increase food supply chain efficiency, and decrease food fraud occurrences by preventing tampering of information across the different network members of the food supply chain.[343] With the technological advances made, more preventive tools will become a part of food safety and supply chain processes globally, increasing efficiency and accuracy of data. However, with these advances comes the need for additional proactive consideration around cybersecurity risks and any threats that could be made to these advanced systems.

Blockchain Digital distributed ledger maintained by a network of multiple computing machines that stores data in the form of blocks that are secured and unable to be changed. It passes information through stages in a process in a fully automated environment. In the context of the food supply, blockchain can be used for transparency throughout the supply chain to store digital records of information to improve food safety and reduce food fraud.

Industrial Internet of Things (IIoT) and Food Safety

Through the use of big data, the food supply chain processes can be improved in order to prevent food fraud occurrences, foodborne illnesses, recalls, and more. The Internet of Things, and Industrial Internet of Things, play a role in food safety from several perspectives. The IIoT can help to improve traceability of foods, increasing transparency in the movement of food goods throughout the supply chain.[344] Use of radio frequency identification chips (RFIDs), can help ensure appropriate storage environments and proper food handling as products are in route to the end consumer.[344] Data from RFID chips can help manufacturers determine if a product needs to be pulled prematurely due to contamination, improper holding, or other information collected by the device in order to ensure a safe deliverable food product. Collaboration among industry operations, such as with manufacturers, government agencies, and researchers, can enhance the ability to provide the safest food, in the most economical way possible. Finally, remote access and automation of the information and transport of foods are improved through the use of **Industrial Internet of Things IIoT**, which allows for the ability to remove unsafe or contaminated products from the supply chain, decrease handling times, and reduce food waste overall.[344]

The following are among many of the food safety issues that will continue to occupy our nation in the 21st century:

Safety of bioengineered foods. Genetically engineered food crops and animals are controversial.[345-347] Whereas most scientists agree that bioengineered foods are safe,[348,349] some make persuasive opposing arguments,[350,351] and consumers hold strong views at either extreme.[351-355] There are also those who question labeling foods with respect to the consumers' right to know what they are buying.[356]

The United States is the world's largest producer of Genetically Modified Organisms (GMOs). Most of the soybeans, cotton, and corn grown in the United States have been modified to resist insects or tolerate herbicides or weed killers, making them GMO crops.[357] GMO production and consumer labeling is a controversial topic; some believe that GMOs are harming the overall diversity of crops we are growing, which in turn harms the soil and overall food supply.[358] Others believe GMOs are necessary to feed the growing world population. GMO crops have expanded the food supply through engineering that allows crops to resist weeds, insects, microorganisms, rodents, and extreme weather.[359] Many people believe that foods produced using GMOs should be labeled as such so consumers can make informed, educated choices.[358,360]

GMOs are currently regulated on the federal level through various agencies, depending on the type of product. Genetically modified plants are regulated by the U.S. Department of Agriculture's Animal and Plant Health Inspection Service Plant Protection Act. GMOs in food and drugs are regulated through the FDA and GMOs in pesticides are regulated through the Environmental Protection Agency.[360] Some states are working toward more stringent GMO regulations and labeling laws so consumers can be aware of foods that are produced using any GMOs. This requires collaboration between states as food rarely remains within state borders. Currently, local authorities have been able to pass legislation banning the cultivation of GMO crops within their boundaries; these include Marin and

Industrial Internet of Things (IIoT) The use of smart sensors, instruments, and analytics to enhance industrial, or mechanical processes.

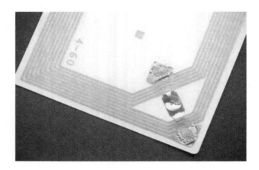

Radio frequency identification chips (RFIDs) can track food storage.

© Bkindler/E+/Getty Images.

Terrorism The unlawful use of force or violence against persons or property to intimidate or coerce a government, the civilian population, or any segment thereof, in furtherance of political or social objectives.

Response Those activities and programs designed to address the immediate and short-term effects of the onset of an emergency or disaster.

Mendocino counties in California and Kauai and Hawaii counties in Hawaii.[360] The FDA does require GMO products to be labeled or named differently when the new product poses a threat to public safety by changing in a way that may obviously cause harm, such as the addition of an allergen.[358,360] Many nongovernmental groups across the US are working to address GMO regulations and labeling. In 2018, the Agricultural Marketing Service of the USDA established the National Bioengineered Food Disclosure Standard, which requires that food manufacturers and importers disclose bioengineered foods and ingredients via labeling.[361]

Agroterrorism and Bioterrorism

For centuries, humans have targeted agricultural crops and employed biological agents in adversarial confrontations with each other,[362] but for most of the 20th century, these methods were thought unlikely to be employed. In the 1990s, government and public health professionals began to assess vulnerabilities and to prepare countermeasures against acts of warfare or **terrorism** directed against the agricultural, food, and water systems of the national infrastructure.[363-365] The CDC identified many biological and chemical agents that could be used for these purposes.[366,367] The effects of several of these, such as mercury, could be insidious, whereas others, such as Salmonella, would make it difficult to distinguish disease outbreaks due to bioterrorism from those due to mundane incidents.

In 1984, a bioterrorist act was perpetrated by a religious cult attempting to gain political control of Wasco County, Oregon. More than 700 people were sickened after *Salmonella* was sprinkled over salad bars in 10 restaurants. What was most frightening about this incident was that it went unrecognized as bioterrorism until disgruntled members of the cult told their stories.[368,369]

Public health dietitians/nutritionists will most likely be involved with bioterrorism directed at food and water systems. A consensus is forming that preventing and detecting these incidents will require more than the usual precautions taken by government and the food and water industries, and that improvements made or contemplated by these entities will be inadequate. Rather, the focus should be on improving surveillance systems with the aim of detecting outbreaks early enough to intervene.[370-372] Consumers are an integral part of this plan but currently do not seek medical care for gastrointestinal illnesses.[372] This is one area where dietitians/nutritionists can help. Public health dietitians/nutritionists are routinely involved in educating consumers and should actively seek ways to expand their roles to encompass antibioterrorism. (As noted earlier, dietitians/nutritionists should be involved in investigating and monitoring outbreaks of foodborne disease and in emergency preparedness planning and **response**.)[373,374]

Food as a Target

Food is not only vulnerable because of the physical need for survival but also because of the complex layers of societal involvement. As illustrated in **Figure 14–1**, both individual and societal factors may be profoundly impacted by an attack on the food supply. The individual components are both physical and psychological; societal components can be economic and political.

Physical

The physical consequences start with our dependence on food for survival. Although this simple statement appears as a *prima fascia* tenet, so obvious that it should not need acknowledgment, it is our assumption that food is

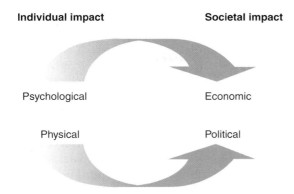

Individual impact   **Societal impact**

Psychological   Economic

Physical   Political

FIGURE 14–1 Potential Consequences of a Major Food Bioterrorism Event.

always available that contributes to our vulnerability. Our population does not regard food insufficiency as a risk that all may face; however, it is certainly recognized as a vulnerability of select groups, such as the homeless and poor. But the concept that a food shortage could occur is generally not considered a threat. The lack of food in the short term could cause physical discomfort, could be associated with mild malnutrition, or in an extreme situation could threaten life. Certain segments of the population could be more vulnerable to shortages, such as groups that may be isolated and unable to obtain emergency supplies, or those who, by their physical limitations, may have fewer reserves or increased needs, such as pregnant women, infants, small children, and older adults.

Another potential physical consequence is the destruction or contamination of food that has been exposed to a biological weapon. This could potentially remove needed food supplies from circulation and cause disruption in the transportation and distribution of replacement food supplies to the public, retail outlets, restaurants, and institutional feeding sites.

Psychological

The terrorist attacks on the United States in 2001, where millions of people experienced anxiety and distress, demonstrated the widespread psychological impact of terrorist events. Individuals would understandably respond to attacks on the food supply in a similar fashion, but the degree of psychological harm may be very difficult to assess and control. Factors that may influence the magnitude of emotional response include the weapon (severity of the attack, type of weapon used, and duration of the attack or multiple attacks), emergency communication (perceived accuracy and timeliness of information, level of detail on individual victims, extent and duration of media coverage), perception of personal risk (uncertainty regarding personal defense strategies), and the coexistence of deprivation or discomfort. Factors that may contribute to public alarm and panic include: rumors and misinformation that establish public mistrust, the appearance of favoritism for some individuals over others, a perception that there is a small chance of escape, requests for isolation, declarations of quarantine, social disruption, and civil discord and violence.[375] The psychological response to an attack on food would certainly be magnified for individuals who have inadequate food, suffer from hunger pains, or would be responsible for others, such as hungry children. Also, the majority of Americans are not accustomed to eating spoiled food, which might be a necessity in the situation of a shortage.

The National Academy of Sciences (NAS) has published a report, *Preparing for the Psychological Consequences of Terrorism: A Public Health*

Recovery As defined here, it includes all types of emergency actions dedicated to the continued protection of the public or to promoting the resumption of normal activities in the affected area.

Strategy,[376] that describes three spheres of psychological consequence: distress response, psychiatric illness, and behavioral change. The authors note that the level of psychological response to terrorism may include "insomnia, fear, anxiety, vulnerability, anger, increased alcohol consumption or smoking; and, a minority will develop psychiatric illnesses, such as posttraumatic stress disorder or depression." Several elements related to food and psychological distress should be considered in public health preparedness. During an attack, availability of basic supplies, including food, is the responsibility of the public health infrastructure. The first of the 10 recommendations from the NAS report is the "Provision of basic resources including food, shelter, communication, transportation, information, guidance, and medical services." During a **recovery** phase, we must recognize that attitudes toward a food or a food group may be altered as a psychological response, particularly if a food has been the vehicle to deliver a terrorist weapon. Such responses may result in short-term or long-term maladaptive behaviors, such as food aversions. Research in this area of behavioral change would not only help us to assure the return to psychological health but may also help us avoid severe economic and/or nutritional consequences of long-term shifts in consumption patterns.

The final element to consider regarding psychological consequences is the amount of damage that potentially may result from small, sporadic terrorist attacks on food, where the main target is psychological health itself. Although few individuals were actually exposed to the anthrax bacterium in 2001, the uncertainty of the exposure and resulting perception created additional "victims" of this attack.

Economic

An attack on our food supply has the potential to cause tremendous economic damage both for domestic consumption and for our export markets and balance of trade. As described by Chalk,[377] an agroterrorism attack would generate costs on three levels:

1. *Direct losses:* From containment measures and the destruction of disease-ridden livestock
2. *Indirect multiplier effects:* From compensation costs paid to farmers
3. *International costs:* From protective trade embargoes imposed by major external trading partners

Following the events of September of 2001, the food industry experienced:

> …a dramatic decline in some travel-dependent sectors of food service, a temporary slowdown in new grocery product introductions, impacts on transportation in small segments of the industry and increased security costs.[378]

Increased economic costs are continuing for agriculture and industry as preparedness plans are developed, implemented, evaluated, and revised. The consequences to our economy are difficult to estimate but could potentially be profound with an agent delivered at a central distribution point with widespread contamination. Even random attacks on the food supply could have major economic impacts if consumers alter eating patterns, shopping habits, and food storage inventory. Also, a stigma with economic consequences may be associated with an industry or a food product. In 1993, after the outbreak of *E. coli,* O157:H7 was traced to Jack in the Box® restaurants in the Pacific Northwest, the parent company, Foodmakers, saw its stock value drop by 30%.[379]

Treatment costs following an outbreak also may be substantial. Trevejo and others reported that the median cost of hospitalization of patients with salmonellosis from 1990 to 1999 ranged from $160,000 to $3.2 million dollars.[380]

Political

How would these factors then impact the political situation? The outbreak of bovine spongiform encephalopathy (BSE; also known as "mad cow disease") led to a loss of confidence in the political system and political destabilization in Great Britain. Much of this fallout was due to communication missteps where the public was given assurances of safety that later proved to be unsubstantiated.[381] Certainly, the election in Spain in the winter of 2004 was influenced by the March 11 train bombings in Madrid. In the United States, the events of September of 2001 and subsequent activities unmistakably influenced the political arena.

Public Health Preparedness for Food Biosecurity

In the face of these consequences of an attack on the food supply, federal agencies, state and local public health jurisdictions, emergency responders, academic institutions, researchers, and community groups have taken specific steps to safeguard the food supply and upgrade the public health infrastructure to lessen risk. The Centers for Disease Control and Prevention (CDC) uses a paradigm for preparedness that includes planning, surveillance, detection, and response. The Department of Health and Human Services also highlights the element of awareness in preparedness efforts.[382] Each of these components has unique challenges with regard to food biosecurity. The issue of awareness is particularly appropriate regarding food security. Although the events of September 2001 certainly maximized awareness of the potential for terrorist attacks, the risk to the food supply is still obscured by complacency that exists at various levels among institutions and individuals.

The elements of effective planning include the identification of appropriate regulatory agencies, which are then responsible for the assessment of areas of risk; development of preparedness priorities, strategies, and plans to diminish risk; communication; training; and evaluation. Planning activities also depend on interagency cooperation. The FBI has prepared a Concepts of Operations Plan (CONPLAN), which provides overall guidance in response to a potential or actual terrorist threat.[383]

To plan a strong defense system, it is important to assess those elements of our food environment that may be involved in a terrorist attack. There are two main approaches to our defense systems. First, we must recognize that food may be a vehicle to deliver a terrorist weapon; second, other types of terrorist activities may compromise the availability of safe food in adequate amounts. In both situations, we must provide defense but also plan and empower local communities and individuals to be prepared with knowledge, skills, and reserves of necessary water and food. Live agents cannot be detected by the human senses. Therefore, the first indication of a biologic attack is usually the first observed casualty, most often detected by local physicians who then report it to local public health officials.

Potential Agents

Food, as a vehicle for the delivery of a bioterrorist weapon, may be contaminated with either biological or chemical weapons that may be viable through

Pandemic Learning Opportunity

Although COVID-19 did not directly affect our food supply, how did it affect it indirectly? Is this also a form of terrorism?

the gastrointestinal tract. The CDC has created a list of agents that have been assigned to categories based on a number of criteria, including:

> …need for hospitalization, mortality rates for exposed untreated persons, potential for initial dissemination to a large population, potential for continued propagation by person-to-person transmission, potential for overall dissemination, capability for mass production, potential for rapid, large-scale dissemination including most effective route of infection and general environmental stability, source of the agent, i.e., soil, animal/insect, or plant source versus laboratory or clinical sources, and main routes of infection, i.e., respiratory versus gastrointestinal.[384]

This report noted several important aspects of this classification process. First, these agents are not ranked on their likelihood of use but on their potential impact. Second, historically, the presumed target for biological weapons was military personnel and military capability. The **virulence** of these agents would be quite different in young, physically fit individuals in the military service compared with a cross-section of the population with varying levels of immune function and comorbidities.

Ingestion of biological agents may occur by:

- Contaminated food or drinking water (nonaerosols can contaminate food supplies or drinking water over long distances)
- Hand-to-mouth contact after touching contaminated surfaces
- Swallowing mucus that contains particles lodged in the nose and throat[385]

Potential targets include food crops, livestock (using aerosols, sprays, and crop dusters), food processing plants, imported foods and food additives, point of sale (i.e., grocery stores), restaurants, institutional feeding sites, and congregate meals.[385] Because the contaminants may be spread from hand to food, packaging may also be a target. Individual packages, such as milk cartons or other sealed containers, may be penetrated with a syringe.

Table 14–5 provides information on the category A and category B agents that may be viable through the gastrointestinal tract. Of these agents, botulism is certainly one that potentially could lead to substantial loss of life. It is considered the most toxic agent known. Knobler and colleagues stated that, "one hundred grams of botulinum toxin evenly distributed in a food or beverage and ingested, could kill over one million people."[386] However, many of the traditional foodborne agents, such as *Salmonella*, that do not have a high fatality rate may still cause significant morbidity, social disruption, and psychological damage, particularly in vulnerable populations.

Healthcare providers and public health professionals should be familiar with the latency periods and presenting symptoms of these agents to assist in communication for early detection and to provide informed responses to the public if one of these agents be suspected in an attack.

Foods at Risk

Two factors influence the magnitude of the impact of a foodborne bioweapon: 1) the range of distribution of the vehicle (food) and 2) the rate of introduction of the vehicle combined with the rate of clearance. Many of our current foods, including dietary staples, are centrally processed and widely distributed. These foods; therefore, would present a more attractive profile with which to deliver a bioweapon. A National Academy of Sciences (NAS) report has noted that food and water supply networks have a ready-made distribution system for the rapid and widespread introduction of biological and chemical weapons.[400] The rate of introduction of the vehicle

Virulence The relative severity of the disease produced by a pathogen.

TABLE 14–5
CDC Information on Bioterrorism Agents and Diseases[387-390]

Category A	Characteristics of Agent	Dissemination	Incubation Period	Symptoms	Case Fatality Ratio (CFR) or Lethality
Anthrax[387,391] *Bacillus anthracis*	Encapsulated, aerobic, gram-positive, spore-forming, rod-shaped bacterium	Aerosol Cutaneous Ingestion	1–7 days	GI: Nausea, anorexia, vomiting, and fever progressing to severe abdominal pain, hematemesis, and diarrhea that is almost always bloody	Gastrointestinal; has mortality rate of 50–100% despite treatment.
Botulism[392,393] Toxin of *Clostridium botulinum*	Most lethal agent known to man. Spore-forming, rod-shaped organisms that grow in anaerobic environments. The toxin interferes with the presynaptic release of acetylcholine at the neuromuscular junction. Seven types of toxin; A-F are toxic in humans. Victims with respiratory symptoms may require ventilatory support. No person-to-person transmission. No natural occurrence of inhalation botulism.	Ingestion Aerosol	18–36 hours (may range from 6 hours to 10 days, dose dependent)	Acute abdomen picture with rebound tenderness may develop. Initial: Blurred vision, double vision, drooping eyelids, slurred speech, difficulty swallowing, dry mouth, muscle weakness. Later: Descending neurologic impairment. GI: nausea, vomiting, abdominal cramps or abdominal pain, diarrhea.[394]	High mortality, 60% if untreated. Hospitalization rate 80%. Lethal dose 1ng/kg.
Plague[389,395] *Yersinia pestis*	Pneumonic plague refers to respiratory infection. Person-to-person transmission from respiratory droplets.	Aerosols	2–6 days	Swollen and tender lymph gland accompanied by pain.	Untreated bubonic plague. CFR 50%
Smallpox[389] *Variola major*	High transmissibility. Quarantine may be necessary for containment.	Aerosol	10–12 days	Fever, hypotension, rash.	Death occurs in 30% of cases.
Tularemia[396] *Francisella tularensis*	Bacterium found in animals. Highly infectious (10–50 organisms can cause disease). May remain alive for weeks in water.	Aerosol (most likely method for bioterrorism); Ingestion	3–5 days (may range 1–14 days)	Depends on site of exposure. Skin ulcers, swollen and painful lymph glands, sore throat, mouth sores, diarrhea, or pneumonia	CFR for Jellison type A: 5–10%
Viral hemorrhagic[387,389] **fevers**	Causes increased capillary permeability, leucopenia, and thrombocytopenia	Contact Aerosol	4–16 days	Fever, easy bleeding, edema, malaise, headache, vomiting, diarrhea, jaundice, shock, sore throat, rash	Lethality is moderate to high

(continues)

TABLE 14–5
CDC Information on Bioterrorism Agents and Diseases[387-390]

Category B (Those that may be ingested)	Characteristics of Agent	Dissemination	Incubation Period	Symptoms	Case Fatality Ratio (CFR) or Lethality
Brucellosis[397] *Brucella species*	Natural *Brucella* species affect sheep, goats, cattle, deer, elk, pigs, dogs, and several other animals.	Ingestion Aerosol cutaneous through skin wounds	5–60 days	Acute form: Nonspecific flu-like symptoms Undulant form: Undulant fevers, arthritis, and epididymo-orchitis in males. Chronic form: Chronic-fatigue syndrome, depression, and arthritis. Nausea, abdominal cramps, watery diarrhea.	CFR: 5%. Hospitalization rate: 55%
Epsilon toxin of *Clostridium Perfringens*[394]	An anaerobic, gram-positive, spore-forming rod commonly found in the intestines of humans and domestic and feral animals [FDA]. The toxins bind to enterocytes and form protein complexes that alter cell permeability [Smedley].*	Ingestion	8–16 hours	Nausea, abdominal cramps, watery diarrhea.	CFR: 0.005% Hospitalization rate: 0.3%

Food Safety Threats	Characteristics of Agent	Dissemination	Incubation Period	Symptoms	Case Fatality Ratio (CFR) or Lethality
Salmonella species	Generally resolves in 5–7 days and does not usually require hospitalization. Victim may require rehydration. Estimated cases per year in the United States: 400,000; mortality: 600. Person-to-person contact likely with fecal-oral transmission. Good hygiene and sanitation essential.	Ingestion	12–72 hours	Diarrhea, fever, abdominal cramps. 3–8 days with a median of 3–4 days.	Nontyphoidal. CFR: 0.8%. Hospitalization rate: 22%. Typhoid. CFR: 0.4%. Hospitalization rate: 75%. Severe bloody diarrhea and abdominal cramps.
Escherichia coli 0:157:H7[398]	Gram-negative rod-shaped bacterium. Estimated cases per year in the United States: 73,000; mortality: 61. Person-to-person contact likely with fecal-oral transmission. Good hygiene and sanitation essential. Children under 5 and the elderly are at risk of the complication of hemolytic uremia syndrome.	Ingestion	3–8 days	Severe bloody diarrhea and abdominal cramps.	CFR: 0.83%. Hospitalization rate: 29.5%.

(continued)

Food Safety Threats	Characteristics of Agent	Dissemination	Incubation Period	Symptoms	Case Fatality Ratio (CFR) or Lethality
Dysentery *Shigella*[399]	Estimated cases per year in the United States: 18,000. Person-to-person contact likely with fecal-oral transmission. Good hygiene and sanitation essential.	Ingestion	3 days**	Diarrhea (often bloody), fever, stomach cramps.	CFR: 0.16%. Hospitalization rate: 0.14%.
Cholera[387,389,397-399] *Vibrio cholerae*	The disease is rare in industrialized nations. Person-to-person contact likely with fecal-oral transmission. Good hygiene and sanitation essential.	Aerosol Ingestion	12–72 hours	Sudden onset of profuse, watery diarrhea, cramps, vomiting, headache	CFR: 0.6%. Hospitalization rate: 34%.
Cryptosporidium Parvum[390,394]	Parasitic infection of the intestinal epithelium. Person-to-person contact likely with fecal-oral transmission. Good hygiene and sanitation essential.	Ingestion	7 days (range, 2–28 days)	Watery diarrhea, abdominal cramps, low-grade fever, malaise, fatigue, anorexia, occasionally nausea and vomiting.	CFR: 0.5%. Hospitalization rate: 0.05%
Q Fever[387] *Coxiella burnetiid*	Acute rickettsial disease.	Aerosol Ingestion	14–16 days	Fever, chills, malaise, headache, myaldia, eye pain, hyperaesthesias, pulmonary syndrome, cough, chest pain.	Untreated CFR, 1%.
Ricin toxin[387] From *Ricinus communis* (castor bean)	Causes damage to the liver and bone marrow.	Aerosol Ingestion	1–12 hours	Vomiting, nausea, diarrhea, cramps, bloody nose, fever, pulmonary edema 18–24 hours after inhalation, severe respiratory distress and death in 36–72 hours.	High lethality.
Staphylococcal Enterotoxin B[387]	Causes damage to the gastrointestinal and respiratory systems.	Aerosol Ingestion	1 hour (range may be 3–12 hours)	Sudden onset of fever, chills, headache, nausea, muscle aches, pulmonary syndrome, vomiting, and diarrhea, if ingested.	Fatality, 1%

Agents that may be disseminated through ingestion are shown in bold type. Compiled from:
*Food and Drug Administration. Bad Bug Book. Accessed April 25, 2021. Available at: https://www.fda.gov/food/foodborne-pathogens/bad-bug-book-second-edition
** Jojosky RA, Groseclose SL. Evaluation of reporting timeliness of public health surveillance systems for infectious diseases. *BMC Public Health*. 2004;4(29). Accessed April 24, 2021. Available at: http://www.biomedcentral.com/1471-2458/4/29
Bioterrorism Agents and Disease. Accessed February 4, 2021. Available at: https://emergency.cdc.gov/agent/agentlist-category.asp

Perishable food Food that is not heat-treated, frozen, or otherwise preserved in a manner so as to prevent the quality of the food from being adversely affected if held for longer than 7 days under normal shipping and storage conditions.

into the food supply and the rate of clearance, however, limits the effectiveness of many distribution systems. Foods that have a long shelf life would be less desirable, because the source of contamination may be identified and isolated before the food reaches many of the intended victims. Highly **perishable foods** with a large distribution range would be most vulnerable to contamination. This category includes dairy products, fresh fruits and vegetables, and certain baked goods. These foods are staples for many of the most vulnerable in our population, such as children. The consequences of an attack on these foods would include a high level of publicity and the associated psychological impact, even though the actual human losses may be limited.

Food Biosecurity Triad: Food Systems Security, Public Health Vanguard, and Consumer Engagement

Our efforts to address the risks are focused in three areas, which are described as a triad: 1) the security of the food supply; 2) mobilizing public health and federal agencies as vanguards in preparedness; and 3) the engagement of individual consumers in this process (**Figure 14–2**).

Food System Security

In this first area, actions have been taken to increase the security of the food supply with increased agency funding, expanded regulations, and revised guidelines for food producers and food importers. Title III of the Public Health Security and Bioterrorism Preparedness and Response Act of 2002 contained specific information related to protecting the food supply. The U.S. Food and Drug Administration (FDA), through the Center for Food Safety and Applied Nutrition (CFSAN), has implemented provisions for registration of food facilities and prior notice of imported food, as noted in **Table 14–6**. These actions will assist with communication regarding food that may have been contaminated, as well as serving as a deterrent.

The U.S. Department of Agriculture (USDA), through the Food Safety and Inspection Service (FSIS), also has taken action regarding meat, poultry, and egg products with guidelines for food processors and for the transportation and distribution of these foods. Many of these actions are based on directives from the Public Health Security and Bioterrorism Preparedness and Response Act of 2002. Additional procedures have been added during times

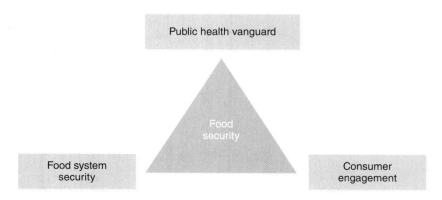

FIGURE 14–2 Triad of Food Security.

TABLE 14–6
Food Biosecurity Triad: Food Systems Security

U.S. Food and Drug Administration (FDA)	
Center for Food Safety and Applied Nutrition *Legislation*: Public Health Security and Bioterrorism Preparedness and Response Act of 2002 Title III: Protecting Safety and Security of Food and Drug Supply *Implementation*: December 12, 2003	Activities related to Bioterrorism Act **Title III, Section 305** • Registration of Food Facilities "Domestic and foreign facilities that manufacture, process, pack or hold food, as defined in the regulation, for human or animal consumption in the US must register with FDA." The purpose is to allow the FDA to: "determine the location and source of a potential bioterrorism incident or an outbreak of food-borne illness and to quickly notify facilities that may be affected." Examples provided by FDA: Included food: • Dietary supplements and dietary ingredients • Infant formulas • Beverages (including alcoholic beverages and bottled water) • Fruits and vegetables • Fish and seafood • Dairy products and shell eggs • Raw agricultural commodities for use as food or components of food • Bakery goods, snack food, and candy (including chewing gum) • Live food animals • Animal feeds and pet food Excluded food: • Food contact substances • Pesticides Facilities that do NOT need to register: • Private residences of individuals • Nonbottled water, such as municipal water systems • Transport vehicles that hold food only in the usual course of their business as carriers • Farms • Restaurants • Nonprofit food facilities [501(c)(3)] • Fishing vessels that harvest and transport fish • Facilities regulated exclusively and throughout the entire facility by the USDA—facilities that handle only meat, poultry, or egg products. For additional information and instructions on registration see https://www.fsis.usda.gov/inspection/establishments/meat-poultry-and-egg-product-inspection-directory#:~:text= FSIS%20is%20responsible%20for%20protecting,poultry%2C%20and%20processed%20 egg%20products. "Act requires that FDA receive prior notice for food imported or offered for import into the U.S. The Act also provides that if an article of food arrives at the port of arrival with inadequate prior notice (i.e., no prior notice, inaccurate prior notice, or untimely prior notice), the food is subject to refusal of admission." https://www.fda.gov/regulatory-information/search-fda-guidance-documents/guidance-industry-prior-notice-imported-food-questions-and-answers-edition-3 **Issued Guidelines:** CFSAN Guidance for Industry: Retail Food Stores and Food Service Establishments: Food Security Preventive Measures Guidance. https://www.fda.gov/regulatory-information/search-fda-guidance-documents/guidance-industry-prior-notice-imported-food-questions-and-answers-edition-3
U.S. Department of Agriculture (USDA)	
Food Safety and Inspection Service (FSIS) Public Health Security and Bioterrorism Preparedness and Response Act of 2002. Responsible for the regulation of meat, poultry, and egg products.	**Actions authorized under the legislation:** • "Enhance the ability of the Service to inspect and ensure the safety and wholesomeness of meat and poultry products. • Improve the capacity of the Service to inspect international products at points of origin and ports of entry.

(continues)

TABLE 14–6
Food Biosecurity Triad: Food Systems Security *(continued)*

U.S. Department of Agriculture (USDA)

• Strengthen the ability of the Service to collaborate with relevant agencies within USDA and other entities within the Federal Government, States and Indian Tribes.
• Otherwise expand the capacity to protect against the threat of bioterrorism."[19]
 	
Issued Guidelines:
FSIS Security Guidelines for Food Processors
Elements include:
  1. Food security plan management: Establish a team with a food security manager; develop and implement a plan; identify potential corrective action and recommendations for recall of adultered products; link to analytical labs; develop a procedure for notification of law enforcement; identify facility entry points; determine local emergency and public health contacts; provide for training, inspections, communication, and response to threats; and liaison with Homeland Security officials.
  2. Checklists for: outside security, general inside security, slaughter and processing security, storage security, shipping and receiving security, water and ice security, mail handling security, and personnel security. See http://www.fsis.usda.gov.
 	
FSIS Safety and Security Guidelines for the Transportation and Distribution of Meat, Poultry, and Egg Products:
Elements include:
  1. Assess vulnerabilities
  2. Emergency operations
  3. Train and test
  4. Screen and educate employees
  5. Secure the facility

Industry Actions	
National Food Processors Association	Includes government agencies, agricultural and food industry organizations. Actions: Food Security Checklist, regarding food plant operations. www.nfpa-food.org Alliance for Food Security
Association of Nutrition and Foodservice Professionals	Articles for Dietary Managers and Food Protection Publications. www.dmaonline.org **https://www.anfponline.org/**

of heightened threat levels (orange or red) to enhance inspection activity; enhance surveillance of transportation, storage, retail sites, and import facilities; conduct random laboratory sampling for threat agents in high-risk commodities; and increase surveillance of human illness.[401] These actions should improve security at sites that could potentially serve as distribution points for an attack. The key to the success of these actions is consistent high standards for compliance and ongoing evaluations. Vigilance in this regard is essential.

Another tool that has been promoted in the food industry is the Hazard Analysis and Critical Control Point (HACCP) approach to food safety. The FSIS has reported a reduction in Salmonella prevalence on raw meat and poultry products with the enforcement of the Pathogen Reduction/HACCP rule.[402] Guidelines for HACCP procedures to diminish the risk of a bioterrorist attack include:

1. Evaluate significant food security hazards and evaluate the likelihood of these risks.
2. Develop and institute preventive or risk control measures to reduce hazards.
3. Determine the points in your operation that are critical for managing a specific risk. These could be locations, processes, functions, or times when your operation is at greatest risk.

4. Develop monitoring procedures for each critical point.
5. Develop a procedure to fix security problems or failures that occur if a critical control has been breached or compromised, similar to a corrective-action program in HACCP.
6. Verify or test your security program periodically.[403]

In November of 2015, the General Accounting Office (GAO) released a report on the Department of Homeland Security's (DHS) Biosurveillance program, BioWatch.[404] The GAO made strong recommendations to correct BioWatch's current capabilities as there have been many false positives; illustrating that the BioWatch system is not yet a foolproof way to survey and protect the public from bioterrorism.[404]

Public Health Vanguard

Progress has been made to create bridge organizations that address interagency coordination, communication, and harmonization activities and to integrate technology into surveillance systems (**Table 14–7**).

The Food Emergency Response Network (FERN; the lead agency of the FDA) coordinates activities among federal, state, regional, and university laboratories to identify bioterrorist agents in food. The FERN Steering Committee has included representatives of numerous federal and local regulatory agencies.[25] Surveillance activities include federal and state sampling programs for domestic and imported food. The agency also examines response and recovery capabilities.

OFSEP was created in 2002 and assumed the function of the Food Biosecurity Action Team (F-BAT).

Strategy Tip

The Department of Homeland Security and the USDA coordinate food security activities through the USDA Homeland Security Council. The Office of Food Security and Emergency Preparedness (OFSEP; the lead agency of FSIS) functions with the FDA and CDC. It is the lead office for emergency preparedness and response; federal/state/industry relations; continuity of operations; scientific expertise in biological, chemical, physical, and radiological terrorism; and security clearance and safeguarding classified information.[2]

While these agencies function to enhance planning, response, and recovery, the function of surveillance is divided among many groups (Table 14–3). The challenge of surveillance of foodborne agents is unique because many of the potential agents (Table 14–1) are common in unintentional foodborne illness. Surveillance thus must distinguish between the background "noise" of seasonal incidents and sentinel events from a bioweapon. The CDC and other agencies have drawn on efforts to enhance food safety to link state and local laboratories with national databases. As noted by Sobel et al.,[405] "The adequacy of response will depend on the capacity of public-health officials to respond to all foodborne disease outbreaks." Technology has greatly enhanced the ability to conduct passive, automated surveillance. **Syndromic surveillance** is an approach that is being tested to examine trends in various syndromic criteria, which may be suggestive of a bioterrorist attack. In theory,

Syndromic surveillance Surveillance activities that enable early detection of epidemics with data analysis for patterns of prodromal illnesses including the use of medications, illness syndromes, or events.

TABLE 14–7
Food Biosecurity Triad: Public Health Vanguard

Agency	Information
Department of Homeland Security Federal Emergency Management Agency (FEMA)	State Homeland Security and Emergency Services. http://www.dhs.gov/dhspublic/ Antiterrorism hazard mitigation information. https://www.fema.gov/pdf/plan/managingemerconseq.pdf NEMB-CAP: National Emergency Management Baseline Capability Assessment Program. A program to assess, analyze, evaluate, and collectively review state capabilities against a national standard. http://www.fema.gov
Department of Health and Human Services (DHHS) Centers for Disease Control and Prevention (CDC) Food and Drug Administration (FDA)	Epi-X: The Epidemic Information Exchange System A secure web-based communication network for public health professionals. http://www.cdc.gov/mmwr/epix/epix.html PHLIS: Public Health Laboratory Information System An electronic reporting system. PHIN: Public Health Information Network. A framework to support communication and data exchange. http://www.cdc.gov/phin/ **CDC Surveillance Systems:** Laboratory Response Network (LRN) to detect links among disease agents during terrorist attacks. https://emergency.cdc.gov/lrn/faq.asp EARS, Early Aberration Reporting System A syndromic surveillance tool. https://knowledgerepository.syndromicsurveillance.org/early-aberration-reporting-system-ears-update-present-and-future FoodNet: Foodborne Diseases Active Surveillance Network A laboratory-based surveillance for foodborne illness. http://www.cdc.gov/foodnet/ NEDSS: National Electronic Disease Surveillance System A component of PHIN. This system promotes standards for data and information systems. https://www.cdc.gov/nndss/about/nedss.html NETSS: National Electronic Telecommunications System for Surveillance A computerized public health system that provides the CDC with weekly data on notifiable diseases. http://www.cdc.gov/epo/dphsi/netss.htm PulseNet National Molecular Subtyping Network for Foodborne Disease Surveillance is a network of public health laboratories that provides an early warning system for foodborne illness. http://www.cdc.gov/pulsenet/ **CDC Response Systems:** HAN: Health Alert Network A system to link local health departments and other organizations for preparedness and response. Other partners for HAN include the National Association of County and City Health Officials (NACCHO) and the Association of State and Territorial Health Officials (ASTHO). https://emergency.cdc.gov/HAN/ CBER, Center for Biologics Evaluation and Research "Responsible for the development of products to diagnose, treat or prevent outbreaks from exposure to the pathogens that have been identified as bioterrorist agents." https://emergency.cdc.gov/agent/agentlist-category.asp eLEXNET: Electronic Laboratory Exchange Network An Internet-based data exchange system for federal, state, and local government food safety laboratories. http://www.mfrpa.org/uploads/1/0/9/7/109760945/jointtues.9am.fda.elexnet_overview_draft[997][1].pdf
U.S. Department of Agriculture (USDA) Food Safety and Inspection Service (FSIS) Multiagency: FDA, CDC, USDA	OFSEP, Office of Food Security and Emergency Preparedness Manages homeland security activities with FDACS. https://www.fdacs.gov/Consumer-Resources/Health-and-Safety/Food-Emergencies-and-Disaster-Preparation FERN, Food Emergency Response Network Coordinates activities among federal, state, regional, and university laboratories to identify bioterrorist agents in food.

this method would provide a more rapid alert system than conventional reporting systems.[406] The CONPLAN highlights specific differences between an attack with weapons of mass destruction and other incidents, noting that the situation may not initially be recognizable until there are multiple casualties, and there may be multiple events with the intent to influence another event's outcome.[383] Thus, time to detection is critical in order for tainted food to be identified and the threat neutralized.

Currently, the quality and safety of food in the United States lies within 16 federal agencies.[407] Due to the fragmentation in responsibility among agencies, the Government Accountability Office reviews current implementation of food safety oversight in order to improve the coordination of efforts, to in turn reduce risk of foodborne illness. In 2018, the U.S. Administration rekindled discussion of creating one singular consolidated food-safety system to be within the USDA.[408,409] The concept of a condensed food-safety authority also came up for discussion under the former U.S. Administration, although the Administration would plan to house this under the Department of Health and Human Services in the FDA, the plan was unsuccessful as it was unable to get past Congress.

During the 2018 U.S. Administration, funding toward the FDA, EPA, and USDA was diverted with the goal of deregulation.[410] The EPA, for example, led the implementation of the "two for one" Executive Order, where for every new regulation issued, two prior regulations would need to be identified for elimination.[411] Programs that were put into place during the former Administration were either eliminated or placed on hold. This would impact the USDA rules for meat inspection at processing plants for pork.[412] Although the plants may see increased efficiency in production time, this came with the increased risk of food contamination due to process.[412] The present U.S. Administration beginning in 2021 will be required to address food safety, the food supply chain, economic impacts of government-run food programming, in addition to considerations on food tariffs placed with foreign countries under the former Administration.[159,160,413]

To combat these challenges, our vanguard of public health agencies must have the resources and structure to respond. However, as noted by a report of the Trust for America's Health, there are many concerns regarding public health preparedness, including insufficient funds; unspent federal aid; agencies unprepared for stockpiling; the exclusion of local agencies, which are unprepared for natural as well as bioterrorist threats; and a workforce crisis.[414]

Consumer Engagement

The third element of the triad is the engagement of individuals/consumers. **Table 14–8** outlines some of the recommendations to consumers to raise awareness and direct action for food reserves and disaster plans in the event of a bioterrorism attack. For example, the Federal Emergency Management Agency (FEMA) has prepared both educational brochures describing personal preparation for emergencies and recommendations for specific items that should be stored in the event of an emergency. This material needs to be reviewed and revised based on simulations and surveys. Recommendations should be founded on the best in evidence-based medicine and practice.

However, should we consider individuals as active or passive partners in preparedness? Government agencies and food industries engage in preparedness activities (e.g., awareness, planning, surveillance, response,

Strategy Tip

Lead agency: For the purposes of the CONPLAN, there are two **lead agencies**: the FBI for crisis management and FEMA for consequence management.

Lead agency The federal department or agency assigned lead responsibility under U.S. law to manage and coordinate the federal response in a specific functional area.

TABLE 14–8
Food Biosecurity Triad: Consumer Engagement

Agency	Activity/Message	Recommendations Regarding Food for Consumers' Preparedness
Department of Homeland Security	• "Preparing makes sense" • "Make a Kit • Make a Plan • Be Informed" Web information: http://www.ready.gov[a]	Make a Kit: Supply Checklists: "Emergency supplies of water, food, and clean air Recommendations include: • Water—One gallon of water per person per day, for drinking and sanitation • Food—At least a 3-day supply of nonperishable food • Can opener for food • Infant formula, if you have an infant"
Federal Emergency Management Agency (FEMA) Shelters	"Toolkit for managing the emergency consequences of terrorist incidents" Guidelines for stocking shelters following a terrorist incident.[b]	Water: Quantity required: • 1–2 gallons per person per day for drinking (infants may need more) • 1–2 gallons per person per day for sanitation needs Possible source: • Bottled water companies • Soft-drink companies • National Guard Food: Quantity required: • Three 800- to 1,000-calorie meals per person per day (prepackaged or hot) • A 4- to 7-day supply should be readily accessible. Possible source: • Red Cross suppliers • Salvation Army suppliers • Local fast-food vendors • Existing supplies in school and church kitchens • Local food growers, farmers, and co-ops
Individuals and families	"Food and Water in an Emergency"[c]	• Short-term (2 weeks) food supply Comments: • "Eat at least one well-balanced meal each day. • Drink enough liquid to enable your body to function properly (2 quarts per day) • Take in enough calories to enable you to do any necessary work • Include vitamin, mineral, and protein supplements in your stockpile to assure adequate nutrition." Other comments and recommendations: • "If activity is reduced, healthy people can survive on half their usual food intake for an extended period and without any food for many days. Food, unlike water, may be rationed safely, except for children and pregnant women."
	"Your Family Disaster Supplies Kit"[d]	Recommendations: • Food: "Include a selection of the following foods in your Disaster Supplies Kit: • Ready-to-eat canned meats, fruits, and vegetables • Canned juices, milk, soup (if powdered, store extra water) • Staples—sugar, salt, pepper • High-energy foods—peanut butter, jelly, crackers, granola bars, trail mix • Vitamins • Foods for infants, elderly persons, or persons on special diets • Comfort/stress foods—cookies, hard candy, sweetened cereals, lollipops, instant coffee, tea bags." Other recommendations: • Practice and maintain your plan. Long-term (greater than 2 weeks)

		Food: "Store large amounts of staples along with a variety of canned and dried foods Stock the following amounts per person per month: • Wheat—20 pounds • Powdered milk (for babies and infants)—20 pounds* • Corn—20 pounds • Iodized salt—1 pound • Soybeans—10 pounds • Vitamin C—15 gms" Supplies: A hand-cranked grain mill to grind the corn and wheat
Department of Health and Human Services (DHHS) FDA Center for Food Safety and Applied Nutrition (CFSAN)	"Food Tampering: An Extra Ounce of Caution"[e]	Recommendations: • Examine food packaging. • Check antitampering devices. • Do not eat food from a package that appears damaged.
U.S. Department of Agriculture (USDA)	"Food Safety and Food Security: What Consumers Need to Know"[f]	Recommendations: • Examine all food product packaging. • Be aware of the normal appearance of food containers. • Contact local health department or law enforcement agency if tampering is suspected and preserve the evidence. "Most of the food safety practices already in place apply equally to intentional contamination." To report unusual characteristics of meat, poultry, and egg products: USDA Meat and Poultry Hotline: 1-888-674-6854

[a]U.S. Department of Homeland Security. *Ready.gov.* Accessed May 13, 2021. Available at http://www.ready.gov

[b]Federal Emergency Management Agency. *Toolkit for Managing the Emergency Consequences of Terrorist Incidents. Appendix A—Biological Weapons.* July 2002. Accessed May 14, 2021. Available at http://www.oregon.gov/OMD/OEM/docs/dom_prep/01-_table_of_contents.pdf

[c]Federal Emergency Management Agency. *Food and Water in an Emergency.* Accessed June 21, 2021. Available at www.fema.gov/pdf/library/f&web.pdf

[d]Federal Emergency Management Agency. *Your Family Disaster Supplies Kit.* Accessed June 21, 2021. Available at www.fdem-mediacenter.org/PDF/Family_Disaster_Supplies.pdf

[e]Center for Food Safety and Applied Nutrition, Food and Drug Administration. *Food Tampering: An Extra Ounce of Caution.* Accessed June 21, 2021. Available at https://www.fda.gov/food/buy-store-serve-safe-food/food-tampering-extra-ounce-caution

[f]Food Safety and Inspection Service, U.S. Department of Agriculture. *Food Safety and Food Security: What Consumers Need to Know.* Accessed May 13, 2021. Available at www.fsis.usda.gov/oa/topics/foodsec_cons.pdf

[g]Food Safety and Security; What Consumers Need to Know. Accessed February 4, 2021. Available at: https://www.fsis.usda.gov/wps/wcm/connect/ebaabfa4-e6a0-4201-9f12-9fd65b46447e/foodsec_cons.pdf?MOD=AJPERES

and recovery), but do individuals? As Figure 14–1 illustrated earlier in this chapter, physical and psychological consequences to the individual are antecedents to economic and political outcomes. So how well prepared are our citizens?

According to the CDC, nearly half of Americans do not have enough food resources, or emergency plans in place in the event of natural disasters, or national emergencies.[415] Additional studies completed on emergency preparedness and food security have shown that although American's are confident that they can survive on food stores and supplies in their homes for about 16 days, more than half of adults surveyed did not have a three-day food supply in their homes,[416] which is the current recommendation from FEMA.[417] During disasters such as the COVID-19 pandemic, food insecurity due to economic downturn further prohibits the consumer with an ability to prepare for long periods in advance. In 2019, the USDA Report on Household Food Insecurity in the United States counted 35 million American's being food insecure, a number that would grow to more than 50 million during the Coronavirus pandemic.[418]

The estimates of the amount of calories that may be necessary to sustain individuals during food shortages varies from the estimates for refugees of 2,100 calories per day[419] to the levels that were available in Biosphere 2, which was 1,780 calories per day.[420] FEMA currently recommends that shelters plan on providing 2,400 to 3,000 calories per person/per day Table 14–4. Certainly, the estimated needs will vary with energy expenditure. Are we prepared to convey messages to individuals to assist them in distinguishing discomfort from true risk?

Our current food culture has substantially lessened the need for food preparation skills and familiarity with raw foods. Yet, the foods recommended by FEMA for long-term food supply (greater than 2 weeks) include the need to grind corn and wheat; food preparation skills are rapidly diminishing in our population. Is the public ready to implement FEMAs recommendations in the event of an emergency, or should public health dietitians/nutritionists advocate for alternatives to meet the current needs of the populations they serve?

We recognize the need for first responders and public health officials to be familiar with response processes, yet consumers do not have specific events to increase food biosecurity awareness. It may be beneficial to have a "vanguard" exercise periodically, such as the last week of June leading up to the Fourth of July. This exercise might serve to raise awareness, build skills, and engage in the preparedness process. Such an exercise may have specific goals, such as:

- Review food and water supplies, including dating and circulating food stocks.
- Stockpile the appropriate amount of water and food for short-term needs.
- Include the preparation of one raw food during the vanguard period.
- Do a food safety check of the home.

These activities could be integrated with other measures to improve preparedness. Families may then be better prepared, both physically and psychologically, for a disruption in food availability that may actually have the most benefit during natural disasters. It would also be an opportunity to raise awareness and support of food banks.

Currently, our citizens are not prepared to make reasonable decisions on food biosecurity. Can these limitations be overcome with central planning and resources? How much physical and psychological damage can be diminished with preparedness, and; therefore, how much can we safeguard against economic and political consequences?

Today, families and households in the United States rely on grocers, convenience stores, food cooperatives, local farms, wholesale clubs, and bulk shops for food purchasing. Food banks, soup kitchens, pantries, and food assistance programming exist to help increase access to safe foods for those in need.

In 2020, during the COVID-19 pandemic emergency economic relief packages were created throughout the crisis in order to help food-insecure Americans. Funding in these packages included $26 billion dollars toward nutrition and agricultural assistance programs, and $400 million dollars to The Emergency Food Assistance Program (TEFAP), the largest food bank supplier.[421] The assistance increased Supplemental Nutrition Assistance Program (SNAP) benefits by 40 percent a month,[422] as well as increased funding to Older Americans, and tribal nutrition assistance programs.

Emergency benefit increases for SNAP provided low-income Americans with additional food purchasing power during the economic crisis of the COVID-19 pandemic.

Additionally, due to the nature of safety in containing the spread of the COVID-19 virus, the economic package also included a budget to the USDA to support the expansion of online payment models for farmer's markets, and mobile payment technology for the EBT system. This allowed consumers to pay at farmer's markets, and small farms via electronic payment or EBT, and also expanded accessibility of online food delivery retailers such as Instacart, Wal-Mart, Amazon, and Aldi for those receiving food-assistance benefits.

Food security is defined as people in a community having safe physical and economic access to food to promote a healthy life. Within this definition are three main components to food security that exist in communities: food access, food availability, and food utilization. Certain demographics are more vulnerable to food insecurity during emergency situations than others, and during a pandemic, the number of those impacted demographics increases exponentially depending on the industries and services that have been affected.

From Awareness to Security

The events of September of 2001 have reshaped our national awareness of food safety related to the potential of a bioterrorism attack. Accomplishments to date have focused on critically vulnerable areas but, given the scope of the challenge, significant risks remain. As previously noted, the FDA has summarized our current situation by concluding that there is a high likelihood of an attack on the food supply.[423] Of additional concern is the potential for engineered bioweapons, which may increase the ability of a virus to kill infected cells, overcome vaccine-induced immunity, increase the agent's ability to survive environmental stress, and increase the potential for dissemination.[424] The technology required to produce such weapons is not obscure, and Smith and others[424] noted that, "The distinction between good biology and its 'dark side' lies only in intent and application."

Public health dietitians/nutritionists possess skills and competencies to support preparedness at all levels, including community interventions and consumer outreach. Consider their didactic and experiential training in food safety, nutritional requirements, nutrition education, and food-service management. Professional associations may play a pivotal role in raising awareness among these individuals who they may serve as responders should a foodborne bioweapon or chemical weapon be suspected or confirmed. Such resources are vital to preserve and sustain food security.

Terms Relevant to Public Health Preparedness

Agroterrorism: The deliberate introduction of a disease agent, either against livestock or into the food chain, for purposes of undermining the socioeconomic stability and/or generating fear.[377]

Biologic toxin: The toxic material of plants, animals, microorganisms, viruses, fungi, or infectious substances of a recombinant molecule, whatever its origin or method of production, including 1) any poisonous substance or biological product engineered as a result of biotechnology produced by a living organism; or 2) any poisonous isomer of biologic products, homolog, or derivative of such a substance.[425]

Carriers: Infected humans who can transmit contagious diseases to other humans.[387]

CDC: Bioterrorism Agents/Diseases

Category A

- Can be easily disseminated or transmitted from person to person
- Result in high-mortality rates and have the potential for major public health impact
- Might cause public panic and social disruption
- Require special action for public health preparedness

Category B

- Are moderately easy to disseminate
- Result in moderate morbidity rates and low mortality rates
- Require specific enhancements of the CDC's diagnostic capacity and enhanced disease surveillance

Category C

- Emerging pathogens that could be engineered for mass dissemination in the future because of availability, ease of production and dissemination, and potential for high morbidity and mortality rates and major health impact.[388]

Consequence management: Includes measures to protect public health and safety; restore essential government services; and provide emergency relief to governments, businesses, and individuals affected by the consequences of terrorism. A consequence management response will be managed by FEMA using structures and resources of the Federal Response Plan (FRP).[383]

Crisis management: Crisis management is predominantly a law enforcement function and includes measures to identify, acquire, and plan the use of resources needed to anticipate, prevent, and/or resolve a threat or act of terrorism.

Debarment: Authorizes the FDA to debar (prohibit from importing food) persons who have been convicted of a felony relating to the importation of any food or who have engaged in a pattern of importing adulterated food that presents a threat of serious adverse health consequences or death to humans or animals.[426]

Disaster field office (DFO): An office established in or near the designated area to support federal and state response and recovery operations. The disaster field office houses the federal coordinating officer (FCO), the emergency response team, and, where possible, the state coordinating officer and support staff.

Emergency operations center (EOC): Site from which civil government officials (municipal, county, state, and federal) exercise direction and control in an emergency.

Emergency public information: Information that is disseminated primarily in anticipation of an emergency or at the actual time of an emergency; in addition to providing information, it frequently directs actions, instructs, and transmits direct orders.

Emergency response team: A team composed of federal program and support personnel, which FEMA activates and deploys into an area affected by a major disaster or emergency.

Emergency support function: A functional area of response activity established to facilitate coordinated federal delivery of assistance required during the response phase to save lives, protect property and health, and maintain public safety.

Evacuation: Organized, phased, and supervised dispersal of civilians from dangerous or potentially dangerous areas, and their reception and care in safe areas.

Federal coordinating officer (FCO): Person appointed by the FEMA director, following a declaration of a major disaster or of an emergency by the president, to coordinate federal assistance.

Federal Response Plan (FRP): Plan designed to address the consequences of any disaster or emergency situation in which there is a need for federal assistance.

First responder: Local police, fire, and emergency medical personnel who first arrive on the scene of an incident and take action to save lives, protect property, and meet basic human needs.

Incubation period: Time between exposure and appearance of symptoms of a disease, syndrome, or illness.

Infectivity: Ease with which a microorganism establishes itself in a host species.

Joint information center (JIC): A center established to coordinate the federal public information activity on scene.

Lead federal agency (LFA): Agency designated by the President to lead and coordinate the overall federal response; it is determined by the type of emergency.

Local government: Any county, city, village, town, district, or political subdivision of any state, Indian tribe or authorized tribal organization, or Alaska Native village or organization, including any rural community or unincorporated town or village or any other public entity.

Mitigate: To cause to become less harsh or hostile; to make less severe or painful.[427]

Public information officer: Official at headquarters or in the field responsible for preparing and coordinating the dissemination of public information in cooperation with other responding federal, state, and local agencies.

Recovery plan: A plan developed by each state, with assistance from the responding federal agencies, to restore the affected area.

Regional director: The director of one of FEMA's 10 regional offices and principal representative for working with other federal regions, state and local governments, and the private sector in that jurisdiction.

Regional operations center (ROC): Temporary operations facility for the coordination of federal response and recovery activities, located at the FEMA regional office.

State coordinating officer: An official designated by the governor of the affected state, upon a declaration of a major disaster or emergency, to coordinate state and local disaster assistance efforts with those of the federal government, and to act in cooperation with the FCO to administer disaster recovery efforts.

Toxicity: Relative severity of the illness or incapacitation produced by a toxin.

Trace backward: Retailers, wholesalers, carriers, and others who have received products from federally inspected meat, poultry, or egg processing establishments should be able to identify the source of the products quickly and efficiently.[428]

Trace forward: Shippers (including operators of federally inspected meat, poultry, and egg-processing establishments) and carriers should have systems in place for quickly and effectively locating products that have been distributed to wholesalers and retailers.[428]

Transmissibility: Ease with which disease is transmitted by victims. Methods may be direct (personal contact), indirect (through material contaminated by the infected person), or secondary (through particles spread by coughing or sneezing).

Vectors: Infected animals or insects that serve as hosts to the organism.

Weaponization for aerosol: As it pertains to the use of anthrax as a bio-terrorist weapon, this generally involves use of a small particle size, a high concentration of spores, treatment to reduce clumping, neutralization of the electrical charge, and use of antimicrobial-resistant strains or genetic modification of the organism to increase virulence or escape vaccine protection.[429]

Weapon of mass destruction (WMD): Any device, material, or substance used in a manner, in a quantity or type, or under circumstances evidencing an intent to cause death or serious injury to persons or significant damage to property.

Summary

Safeguarding the food supply means being aware of the potential dangers to the foods supply, be they naturally occurring biological agents; chemical additives; foreign physical objects that fall into the food supply or intentional hazards from terrorist attacks. Safeguarding the food supply as nutrition professionals also means being part of the safety net wherever possible. As nutrition professionals, we can engage the public in awareness campaigns and participate in local safety drills to ensure public cooperation and safety in the event of a terrorist attack or natural disaster.

Food safety laws and practices exist to protect the public but as nutrition professionals we have an obligation to keep the public informed and hold our nations' suppliers and protective agencies to the high standards set. When current law or practices do not go far enough to keep the food supply and public safe advocacy efforts can eventually bring about change. We have seen this democratic process in action with the recent passing of the Food Safety Modernization Act of 2011, which allows the FDA to act on food threats proactively rather than having to wait until harm is done and merely acting reactively. Furthermore, nutrition professionals can be part of local planning and action committees to ensure the community is safe from any and all threats to the foods supply. This may involve creating collaborative teams of public health departments, colleges and universities training the next generation of public health and medical personnel and current hospitals, and emergency response teams. There are many ways nutrition professionals can engage in maintaining a safe food supply; this chapter offers important aspects of the nutrition professional's toolbox.

Learning Portfolio

© olies/Shutterstock.

Issues for Discussion

1. How can dietitians/nutritionists help consumers understand food safety hazards and risks?
2. How should dietitians/nutritionists approach other health agency staff to offer expertise on food safety issues? How is the nutritionist's perspective likely to differ from other health professionals' perspectives?
3. What possible roles exist for dietitians/nutritionists to identify and combat bioterrorism directed against the food supply system?
4. How can dietitians/nutritionists help to instill a sense of individual responsibility for food safety?
5. How well prepared are our communities to provide food to individuals in the event of an intentional attack on the food supply? In the event of an attack that compromises access to food?
6. In what ways could dietitians/nutritionists improve the delivery of food resources, and/or coordinate food/resource delivery efforts within their communities during quarantines?
7. What priority should food security receive in public health preparedness efforts?
8. What level of investment is appropriate for security of the food supply, and who should provide the funding?
9. What role should nutrition professionals assume for risk assessment, surveillance, planning, response, and recovery in the event of an attack, or in emergency preparedness in general?
10. What are some key issues within the food supply chain that may impact access to foods?

Practical Activities

1. Find out if your school or job offer HACCP training certification programs.
2. Find out where the nearest food safety drills are taking place and participate
3. Ask your schools food service director how they monitor food safety on campus? Do they employ HACCP principles? If so, how?
4. Create food safety sheets for local food pantry guests: safe food storage and cooking instructions for their common foods.
5. Create a top-10 list for students on campus to keep food safe in their dorms, apartments or while they are on the go.
6. Ask about your school's emergency-preparedness plan for food service. What protocols are in place, and how is this information delivered to the student body?
7. Create a top-10 list of shelf-stable foods for students to have on hand in their dorms or apartments in the event of a quarantine, food shortage, or public health emergency.
8. What are some ways that a public health nutritionist can educate the public around food safety in the event of a public health emergency?
9. Do you feel that there were gaps in the COVID-19 pandemic nutrition response? If so, what were the gaps? How could dietitians/nutritionists collaborate to resolve these issues?
10. In what ways can we safeguard the food supply, and prepare a functional supply chain for public health nutrition responses in the future based on what we learned from the COVID-19 pandemic?
11. Create a resource guide to local emergency food assistance programming that is available during emergencies to provide to highly frequented locations such as grocery stores, libraries, community centers, shelters and town halls for distribution.

Key Terms

	page
Food fraud	433
Food defense	433
Guillain-Barré syndrome	439
Reiter syndrome	439
Pandemic	442
Asymptomatic	442
National Emergencies Act (NEA)	442
National Emergency	442
Social distancing	443
Physical distancing	443
Essential businesses	443
Self-quarantine	444
Stay-at-home order	444
Contact tracing	444
Emergency Use Authorization	446
Blockchain	454
Industrial Internet of Things (IIoT)	455
Terrorism	456
Response	456
Recovery	458
Virulence	460
Perishable food	464
Syndromic surveillance	467
Lead agency	469

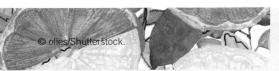
© olies/Shutterstock.

Learning Portfolio

12. Three fundamental considerations when improving food safety in supply chain management include people, processes and technology. Assess these three areas in a common food, or nutrition environment that you have worked in (such as a restaurant, grocer, hospital, etc.). Do you feel that they are progressive in their use of the food supply chain, or are they in need of improvements?

Case Study: Adapting to Pandemic Challenges in an Agricultural Community

During the COVID-19 pandemic food supply, and demand was impacted due to business closures, and movement/travel restrictions. Closures of restaurants, catering, and hotels caused increased demand for supermarkets and forced several adaptations of the food supply chain along the way. In order to support a local agricultural economy, the Whidbey Island Food Cooperative (WIGC) on Whidbey Island, WA, created a multistakeholder cooperative formed of producers (those businesses that grow meat, produce, or ingredients for products), partners (those who buy from producers such as businesses, caterers), and community partners (businesses, individuals, and organizations) in order to connect the local food supply with customers.[430] Available for online ordering with contract free pickup at several locations, the WIGC "Food Hub" provided weekly, seasonal options for produce, dairy, bread, and other ingredients for safe purchase. Additionally, early in the COVID-19 pandemic (April of 2020), several producers within the Food Hub offered weekly "Grocery Bags," which provided staple foods such as milk, eggs, cheese, meat, fish, or vegetarian protein alongside local fruits or vegetables with contact-free payment and pick up options to help community members access foods, when the local grocers were undergoing strain. The WIGC provided a means for individuals to access healthy and safe local foods, for restaurants/caterers to both support community agriculture as well as their own local business economies, and for the agricultural producers to expand their market reach through the community through adaptations and collaboration amongst the local supply chain. What are some ways that a public health nutritionist could work with smaller agricultural communities to further develop cooperative type efforts by expanding into public school systems and local food banks? What are some ways a public health nutritionist could ensure that food safety measures are maintained throughout the cooperative and distribution efforts?

Public health dietitians/nutritionists provide knowledge of the food system, and government food programs. Dietitians/nutritionists help with grant writing for additional funding, provide needs assessments or can liaise conversations between school food service directors and food bank directors in order to help inform about available funding, nutritional requirements needing to be met through programming, and explore ways to connect into the area's agricultural system. In terms of food safety, the public health nutritionist's role includes their experience and knowledge of food service management and the understanding of food safety measures to help cooperative producers ensure food safety throughout the harvesting, preparation, and distribution processes.

Case Study: Potential Bioterrorism Attack

Pitt County, NC, has taken significant measures to prepare their community and health professionals for a potential bioterrorism attack. The Public Health Department held a mock bioterrorism attack in which health officials were tasked with distributing medication to individuals who were potentially exposed to Anthrax. Local Public Health Departments are starting to organize and run these drills across the country.[431] How can public health dietitians/nutritionists help the public prepare?

Online Resources

1. FDA's YouTube channel on Food Safety at home: https://www.youtube.com/user/USDAFoodSafety
2. FDA's video on Food Safety for food consumers: https://www.youtube.com/watch?v=rNwl3ww6wv0
3. The World Health Organization's webpage on GMO foods: http://www.who.int/topics/food_genetically_modified/en/
4. FDA's video on the Food Safety and Modernization Act (FSMA): https://www.youtube.com/watch?v=y_LSrgbXA_w
5. UN Food and Agriculture Organization's fact sheets on biosecurity in the food chain: http://www.fao.org/food/food-safety-quality/publications-tools/food-safety-publications/en/
6. Biosecurity preparedness: Ventura County, California bioterrorism drill: https://www.youtube.com/watch?v=AnUk_VYGtZk

References

1. Schwetz BA. Statement before the Committee on Governmental Affairs, Subcommittee on Oversight of Government Management, Restructuring and the District of Columbia. (October 10, 2001).
2. Centers for Disease Control and Prevention. *Foodborne Germs and Illnesses*, 2020. Accessed October 9, 2020. http://www.cdc.gov/foodsafety/foodborne-germs.html
3. Interagency Forum on Child and Family Statistics. *America's Children: Key National Indicators of Well-Being, 2020.* Accessed October 9, 2020. https://www.childstats.gov/americaschildren/
4. United Nations Department of Economic and Social Affairs. *World Population Ageing.* United Nations Department of Economic and Social Affairs | Population Division; 2015. Accessed November 23, 2020. https://www.un.org/en/development/desa/population/publications/pdf/ageing/WPA2015_Report.pdf
5. Sinclair U. *The Jungle.* New York: Doubleday; 1906. Accessed October 9, 2020. http://www.online-literature.com/upton_sinclair/jungle/
6. Public Health Security and Bioterrorism Preparedness and Response Act of 2002. Accessed July 1, 2021. https://www.govinfo.gov/content/pkg/PLAW-107publ188/pdf/PLAW-107publ188.pdf
7. *Testimony before the Subcommittee on Agriculture, Rural Development, Food and Drug Administration, and Related Agencies Committee on Appropriations*, U.S. House of Representatives. (February 27, 2003). Accessed July 1, 2021. https://appropriations.house.gov/subcommittees/agriculture-rural-development-food-and-drug-administration-and-related-agencies-116th/article/statement
8. Stier RF. The dirty dozen: ways to reduce the 12 biggest foreign materials problems. *FoodSafety Magazine.* 2003;9:44.
9. Potter NN, Hotchkiss JH. *Food Science*, 5th ed. Gaithersburg, MD: Aspen Publishers; 1998:533.
10. University of Arkansas. *Center for Food Safety.* Accessed November 19, 2020. https://center-for-food-safety.uark.edu/
11. Simmons University. *Center for Hygiene and Health in Home and Community.* Accessed November 19, 2020. http://www.simmons.edu/hygieneandhealth
12. U.S. Food & Drug Administration. *FDA Fundamentals.* Accessed October 9, 2020. https://www.fda.gov/about-fda/fda-basics/fda-fundamentals
13. Remarks of Commissioner Robert C. Bonner, Customs and Border Protection National Plant Board Annual Meeting. (August 12, 2003). Accessed July 1, 2021. https://www.govinfo.gov/content/pkg/CHRG-108shrg94810/html/CHRG-108shrg94810.htm.
14. Applebaum RS. Protecting the nation's food supply from bioterrorism. *FoodSafety Magazine.* 2004;10:34;70-71.
15. Centers for Disease Control and Prevention (CDC). *Drinking water.* Accessed October 9, 2020. http://www.cdc.gov/healthywater/drinking/
16. Centers for Disease Control and Prevention. Preventing emerging infectious diseases: a strategy for the 21st century. Overview of the updated CDC plan. *MMWR Morb Mortal Wkly Rep.* 1998;47(15):1.
17. U.S. Department of Commerce, NOAA Fisheries. Seafood Inspection Program. nd. *NOAA Inspection Manual.* Accessed October 9, 2020. https://www.fisheries.noaa.gov/national/seafood-commerce-certification/seafood-inspection-manual
18. Title 50, U.S. Code of Federal Regulations, Part 260-261. Subpart A: Inspection and certification of establishments and fishery products for human consumption. Accessed October 9, 2020. https://www.govinfo.gov/content/pkg/FR-2019-10-15/pdf/2019-22429.pdf
19. U.S. Food & Drug Administration. *FDA's Evaluation of the Seafood HACCP Program for Fiscal Years 2006-2014.* (July 21, 2014). Accessed January 5, 2021. https://www.fda.gov/media/130272/download
20. Foulke J. Seafood safety regulations announced. HHS News, P95-9. 1995. Accessed January 5, 2021. http://www.scienceblog.com/community/older/archives/A/hhs1286.html
21. U.S. Food & Drug Administration. *Fish and Fisheries Products Hazards and Controls Guidance*, 4th ed. 2020. Accessed October 9, 2020. https://www.fda.gov/food/seafood-guidance-documents-regulatory-information/fish-and-fishery-products-hazards-and-controls
22. Federal Trade Commission. *Division of Advertising Practices.* Accessed October 9, 2020. https://www.ftc.gov/about-ftc/bureaus-offices/bureau-consumer-protection/our-divisions/division-advertising-practices
23. Goldammer T. *The Brewer's Handbook. The Complete Book to Brewing Beer*, 2nd ed. Clifton VA: Apex Publishers; 2008:411.
24. United States Department of Agriculture (USDA), Food Safety and Inspection Service (FSIS). States Operating their own MPI programs. (2015). Accessed October 9, 2020. http://www.fsis.usda.gov/wps/portal/fsis/topics/inspection/state-inspection-programs/state-inspection-and-cooperative-agreements/states-operating-their-own-mpi-programs

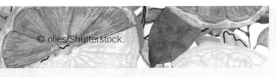

Learning Portfolio

© olies/Shutterstock.

25. Landman J. Food aid in emergencies: a case for wheat? *Proc Nutr Soc.* 1999;58:355-361.

26. Stevens S. Just a matter of time. *Food Manage.* 1990;25(11):116-119, 138.

27. Gemperlein J. When the earth moved. *Food Manage.* 1990;25(1):130-134, 136, 138.

28. Trento L, Allen S. Hurricane Sandy nutrition support during disasters. *Nutr Clin Pract.* 2014;29(5):576-584.

29. The American Civil Defense Association. *Local & State Resources.* 2020. Accessed October 9, 2020. https://tacda.org/contact-us/

30. Marchione TJ. Foods provided through U.S. government emergency food aid programs: policies and customs governing their formulation, selection and distribution. *J Nutr.* 2002;132(7):2104S-2111S. https://doi.org/10.1093/jn/132.7.2104S

31. Reed BA, Habicht J-P, Garza C. Translating nutrition research into action in humanitarian emergencies. *J Nutr.* 2002;132(7):2112S-2116S.

32. HR 875: *Food Safety Modernization Act of 2009.* 2009. Accessed October 9, 2020. http://www.govtrack.us/congress/bill.xpd?bill=h111-875

33. Potter NN, Hotchkiss JH. *Food Science,* 5th ed. Gaithersburg, MD: Aspen; 1998:562.

34. U.S. Food & Drug Administration. Food additives permitted for direct addition to food for human consumption. Code of Federal Regulations (Title 21, Vol. 3, April 1, 2019), Ch. 1, Part 172. *Fed Regist.* 2016;81:22176-22183.

35. Secondary direct food additives permitted in food for human consumption. Code of Federal Regulations (Title 21, Vol. 3, April 1, 2019), Ch. 1, Part 173.

36. Indirect food additives. Code of Federal Regulations (Title 21, Vol. 3, April 1, 2019), Ch. 1, Parts 174-178.

37. Prior-sanctioned food ingredients. Code of Federal Regulations (Title 21, Vol. 3, April 1, 2019), Ch. 1, Part 181.

38. Substances generally recognized as safe. Code of Federal Regulations (Title 21, Vol. 3, April 1, 2019), Ch. 1, Part 182.

39. Direct food substances affirmed as generally recognized as safe. Code of Federal Regulations (Title 21, Vol. 3, April 1, 2019), Ch. 1, Part 184.

40. Indirect food substances affirmed as generally recognized as safe. Code of Federal Regulations (Title 21, Vol. 3, April 1, 2019), Ch. 1, Part 186.

41. Center for Food Safety and Applied Nutrition. Generally Recognized as Safe (GRAS). *U.S. Food and Drug Administration,* 6 Sept. 2019, www.fda.gov/food/food-ingredients-packaging/generally-recognized-safe-gras Accessed November 19, 2020.

42. Rados C. GRAS: time-tested, and trusted, food ingredients. *FDA Consumer.* 2004;38:20.

43. Folkenberg J. A primer on food additives. *FDA Consumer.* 1988;44.

44. Henkel J. From shampoo to cereal. Seeing to the safety of color additives. *FDA Consumer.* 1993.

45. U.S. Food & Drug Administration. (November 2017). *Summary of Color Additives for Use in United States in Foods, Drugs, Cosmetics, and Medical Devices.* Accessed November 19, 2020. http://www.fda.gov/ForIndustry/ColorAdditives/ColorAdditiveInventories/ucm115641.htm

46. United States Department of Agriculture (USDA), FSIS. *Additives in Meat and Poultry Products.* 2015. Accessed November 19, 2020. http://www.fsis.usda.gov/wps/portal/fsis/topics/food-safety-education/get-answers/food-safety-fact-sheets/food-labeling/additives-in-meat-and-poultry-products/additives-in-meat-and-poultry-products

47. U.S. Food & Drug Administration. *How to Understand and Use the Nutrition Facts Label.* 2020. Accessed November 19, 2020. http://www.fda.gov/food/ingredientspackaginglabeling/labelingnutrition/ucm274593.htm

48. Food and Drug Administration. Dietary supplements. 2019. Accessed November 19, 2020. http://www.fda.gov/Food/DietarySupplements/default.htm

49. Hileman B. Reining in dietary supplements. Food additives critics demand changes in the law governing supplement. *Chem Eng News.* 2004;82:21.

50. Food and Drug Administration (FDA). *Food Quality Protection Act of 1996.* (July 28, 2020). Accessed November 19, 2020. https://www.epa.gov/laws-regulations/summary-food-quality-protection-act

51. Environmental Protection Agency (EPA). (2020). *Laws and Regulations.* Accessed November 19, 2020. http://www.epa.gov/pesticides/regulating/laws.htm

52. United States Environmental Protection Agency. *Summary of the Food Quality Protection Act.* Accessed November 19, 2020. http://www.epa.gov/laws-regulations/summary-food-quality-protection-act

53. Tomerlin JR. The US Food Quality Protection Act policy implications of variability and consumer risk. *Food Add Contam.* 2000;17(7):641-648.

54. Sumner D. The Food Quality Protection Act: a public health perspective. *Neurotoxicology.* 2000;21(1-2):183-188.

55. DiFonzo C. Food Quality Protection Act. In: *Pesticide Policy and Michigan Specialty Crops Food Quality Protection Act.* (1997). East Lansing, MI: Michigan State University. Accessed November 19, 2020. http://ipmworld.umn.edu/difonzo-food-quality

56. Measure continues ban on human tests. *Chem Eng News.* 2003;81:21.

57. Wagner JM. Food Quality Protection Act: its impact on the pesticide industry. *Qual Assur.* 1997;5:279.

58. EPA sued over pesticide standards. *Chem Eng News.* 2003;81:25.

59. U.S. Food & Drug Administration. *Public Health Security and Bioterrorism Preparedness and Response Act of 2002 (PL107-188).* Letter from Center Director, 2002. Accessed November 19, 2020. https://www.govinfo.gov/content/pkg/PLAW-107publ188/html/PLAW-107publ188.htm

60. U.S. Food & Drug Administration. *Bioterrorism Act of 2002.* Accessed November 19, 2020. https://www.govinfo.gov/content/pkg/PLAW-107publ188/pdf/PLAW-107publ188.pdf

61. U.S. Food & Drug Administration. FDA commends passage by the House of Representatives of S. 741, a bill providing improved consumer protection and incentives for animal drug development. *FDA News* P04-72. (July 20, 2004). Accessed November 19, 2020. https://www.congress.gov/bill/108th-congress/senate-bill/741/all-info

62. Weber JA. More than a farm bill: food, conservation, and Energy Act of 2008. *Pract Appl Pub Pol News.* 2008;108(9):1432.

63. Congress.gov. *H.R.2419 - Food, Conservation, and Energy Act of 2008*. 2008. Accessed November 19, 2020. https://www.congress.gov/bill/110th-congress/house-bill/2419

64. U.S. Food & Drug Administration (FDA). Background on the Food Safety Modernization Act (FSMA). Accessed November 23, 2020. https://www.fda.gov/food/guidance-regulation-food-and-dietary-supplements/food-safety-modernization-act-fsma

65. Manning L, Soon JM. Food safety, food fraud, and food defense: a fast evolving literature. *J Food Sci*. 2016;81(4):R823-R834. doi: 10.1111/1750-3841.13256

66. Center for Food Safety and Applied Nutrition. Food Defense. U.S. Food and Drug Administration. Published 2019. https://www.fda.gov/food/food-defense

67. U.S. Food & Drug Administration. FSMA proposed rule for food traceability. Published online January 12, 2021. Accessed January 24, 2021. https://www.fda.gov/food/food-safety-modernization-act-fsma/fsma-proposed-rule-food-traceability

68. Pilet J. Industry's resilience with food safety practices will be crucial in 2021. *Food Safety News*. Published January 11, 2021. Accessed January 24, 2021. https://www.foodsafetynews.com/2021/01/industrys-resilience-with-food-safety-practices-will-be-crucial-in-2021/

69. U.S. Food & Drug Administration. *Hazard analysis critical control points (HACCP)*. 2018. Accessed November 19, 2020. http://www.fda.gov/Food/GuidanceRegulation/HACCP/

70. National Restaurant Association. *Applied Foodservice Sanitation: A Certification Coursebook*, 4th ed. Chicago, IL: The Educational Foundation of the National Restaurant Association; 1995:80.

71. U.S. Food & Drug Administration. *Managing food safety: a manual of the voluntary use of HACCP Principles for operators of food service and retail establishments*. 2017. Accessed November 23, 2020. https://www.fda.gov/food/hazard-analysis-critical-control-point-haccp/managing-food-safety-manual-voluntary-use-haccp-principles-operators-food-service-and-retail

72. U.S. Food & Drug Administration. *HACCP Principles & Application Guidelines*. 2017. Accessed November 19, 2020. http://www.fda.gov/Food/GuidanceRegulation/HACCP/ucm2006801.htm

73. Arvanitoyannis IS. *HACCP and ISO 22000: Application to foods of animal origin*. Ames, IO: Wiley-Blackwell; 2009:1-549.

74. Arduser L, Brown DR. *HACCP & sanitation in restaurants and food service operations: A practical guide based on the FDA food code*. Ocala, FL: Atlantic Publishing Group; 2005:1-541.

75. CFR - Code of Federal Regulations, Title 21, Vol. 2, Part 110 (April 1, 2019). *Food and drugs. Current good manufacturing practice in manufacturing, packing, or holding human food*. Accessed November 19, 2020. http://www.accessdata.fda.gov/scripts/cdrh/cfdocs/cfcfr/CFRSearch.cfm?CFRPart=110

76. Gould WA. *Current Good Manufacturing Practices/Food Plant Sanitation*, 2nd ed. Cockeysville, MD: CTI Publications; 1994:Ch. 2.

77. Potter NN, Hotchkiss JS. *Food Science*, 5th ed. Gaithersburg, MD: Aspen; 1998:161.

78. U.S. Food & Drug Administration. *Guidance for Industry: Action Levels for Poisonous or Deleterious Substances in Human Food and Animal Feed*. (2000). Accessed November 19, 2020. https://www.fda.gov/regulatory-information/search-fda-guidance-documents/guidance-industry-action-levels-poisonous-or-deleterious-substances-human-food-and-animal-feed

79. U.S. Food & Drug Administration (FDA). 2018. *Food defect levels handbook*. Levels of natural or unavoidable defects in foods that present no health hazards for humans. Accessed November 19, 2020. http://www.fda.gov/food/guidanceregulation/guidancedocumentsregulatoryinformation/sanitationtransportation/ucm056174.htm

80. Centers for Disease Control and Prevention. Estimates of foodborne illness in the United States | Estimates of Foodborne Illness | CDC. Published February 19, 2019. https://www.cdc.gov/foodborneburden/

81. Vugia D, Cronquist A, Cartter M, et al. Preliminary FoodNet data on the incidence of infection with pathogens transmitted commonly through food - 10 states, 2008. *MMWR Morb Mortal Wkly Rep*. 2009;58(13):333-337.

82. U.S. Department of Health and Human Services. *Healthy People 2010: Understanding and Improving Health*, 2nd ed., Objective 10, Washington, DC: Government Printing Office; November 2000.

83. U.S. Food & Drug Administration, Food Safety Inspection Service, Department of Agriculture. *Food Safety CHAPTER 10*; 2011. Accessed October 24, 2021. https://www.cdc.gov/nchs/data/hpdata2010/hp2010_final_review_focus_area_10.pdf

84. United States Department of Health and Human Services. Foodborne illness—Healthy People 2030 | health.gov. Published 2020. https://health.gov/healthypeople/objectives-and-data/browse-objectives/foodborne-illness

85. Jay JM. *Modern Food Microbiology*, 6th ed. Gaithersburg, MD: Aspen; 2000:560.

86. Tauxe RV. Epidemiology of *Campylobacter jejuni* infections in the United States and other industrialized nations. In: Nachamkin I, Blaser MJ, Tompkins LS, eds. *Campylobacter jejuni: Current Status and Future Trends*. Washington, DC: American Society of Microbiology; 1992:9-19.

87. Blaser MJ. *Campylobacter jejuni* and food. *Food Technol*. 1982;36:89.

88. Moore JE, Gilpin D, Crothers E, Canney A, Kaneko A, Matsuda M. Occurrence of *Campylobacter spp.* and *Cryptosporidium spp.* in seagulls (*Larus* spp.). *Vector Borne Zoon Dis*. 2004;2(2):111-114.

89. Yogasundram K, Shane SM, Harrington KS. Prevalence of *Campylobacter jejuni* in selected domestic and wild birds in Louisiana. *Avian Dis*. 1989;33:664-667.

90. Stelzer W, Mochmann H, Richter U, Dobberkau HJ. A study of *Campylobacter jejuni* and *Campylobacter coli* in a river system. *Zentralblatt für Hygiene und Umweltmedizin*. 1989;189(1):20-28.

91. Pacha RE, Clark GW, Williams EA, Carter AM, Scheffelmaier JJ, Debusschere P. Small rodents and other mammals associated with mountain meadows as reservoirs of *Giardia spp.* and *Campylobacter spp*. *Appl Environ Microbiol*. 1987;53(7):1574-1579.

92. Rosef O, Gondrosen B, Kapperud G, Underdal B. Isolation and characterization of *Campylobacter jejuni* and *Campylobacter coli* from domestic and wild mammals in Norway. *Appl Environ Microbiol*. 1983;46(4):855-859.

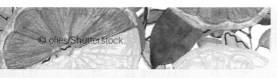

Learning Portfolio

93. Cools I, Uyttendaele M, Caro C, D'Haese E, Nelis HJ, Debevere J. Survival of *Campylobacter jejuni* strains of different origin in drinking water. *J Appl Microbiol.* 2003;94(5):886-892.

94. Moore J, Caldwell P, Millar B. Molecular detection of *Campylobacter spp.* in drinking, recreational and environmental water supplies. *Int J Hygiene Environ Health.* 2001;204(2-3):185-189.

95. Skirrow MB. Epidemiology of *Campylobacter enteritis. Int J Food Microbiol.* 1991;12(1):9-16.

96. Palmer SR, Gully PR, White JM, et al. Water-borne outbreak of *Campylobacter* gastroenteritis. *Lancet.* 1983;321:287-290.

97. Bates C, Hiett KL, Stern NJ. Relationship of *Campylobacter* isolated from poultry and from darkling beetles in New Zealand. *Avian Dis* 2004;48(1):138-147.

98. Gregory E, Barnhart H, Dreesen DW, Stern NJ, Corn JL. Epidemiological study of *Campylobacter spp.* in broilers: source, time of colonization, and prevalence. *Avian Dis.* 1997;41:890-898.

99. Altekruse SF, Stern NJ, Fields PI, Swerdlow DL. *Campylobacter jejuni*—an emerging foodborne pathogen. *Emerg Infect Dis.* 1999;5(1):28-35.

100. Birkhead G, Vogt RL, Heun E, Evelti CM, Patton CM. A multiple-strain outbreak of *Campylobacter enteritis* due to consumption of inadequately pasteurized milk. *J Infect Dis.* 1988;157(5):1095-1097.

101. Hudson PJ, Vogt RL, Brondum J, Patton CM. Isolation of *Campylobacter jejuni* from milk during an outbreak of campylobacteriosis. *J Infect Dis.* 1984;150:789.

102. Vogt RL, Sours HE, Barret T, Feldman RA, Dickinson RJ, Witherell L. *Campylobacter* enteritis associated with contaminated water. *Ann Intern Med.* 1982;96:292.

103. Manfredi R, Nanetti A, Ferri M, Chiodo F. Fatal *Campylobacter jejuni* bacteraemia in patients with AIDS. *J Med Microbiol.* 1999;48:601.

104. Meier PA, Dooley DP, Jorgensen JH, Sanders CC, Huang WM, Patterson JE. Development of quinolone-resistant *Campylobacter* fetus bacteremia in human immunodeficiency virus-infected patients. *J Infect Dis.* 1998;177(4):951-954.

105. Tauxe RV, Pegues DA, Hargrett-Bean N. *Campylobacter* infections: the emerging national pattern. *Am J Public Health.* 1987;77(9):1219-1221.

106. Bereswill S, Kist M. Recent developments in *Campylobacter* pathogenesis. *Curr Opin Infect Dis.* 2003;16(5):487-491.

107. Tsang RS. The relationship of *Campylobacter jejuni* infection and the development of Guillain-Barré syndrome. *Curr Opin Infect Dis.* 2002;15(3):221-228

108. Locht H, Krogfelt KA. Comparison of rheumatological and gastrointestinal symptoms after infection with *Campylobacter jejuni/coli* and enterotoxigenic *Escherichia coli. Ann Rheum Dis.* 2002;61(5):448-452.

109. Neill MA, Tarr PI, Taylor DN, Wolf M. *Escherichia coli.* In: YH Hui, MD Pierson, JR Gorham, eds. *Foodborne Disease Handbook,* 2nd ed., vol. 1: Bacterial pathogens. New York: Marcel Dekker; 2000:196.

110. Jay J M. *Modern Food Microbiology,* 6th ed. Gaithersburg, MD: Aspen; 2000:531.

111. Jay JM. *Modern Food Microbiology,* 6th ed. Gaithersburg, MD: Aspen; 2000:387-406.

112. Besser RE, Griffin PM, Slutsker L. *Escherichia coli* O157:H7 gastroenteritis and the hemolytic uremic syndrome: an emerging infectious disease. *Ann Rev Med.* 1999;50:355-367.

113. Nauschuetz W. Emerging foodborne pathogens: enterohemorrhagic *Escherichia coli. Clin Lab Sci.* 1998;11(5):298-304.

114. Qadri SM, Kayali S. Enterohemorrhagic *Escherichia coli.* A dangerous food-borne pathogen. *Postgrad Med.* 1998;103(2):179-187.

115. Epidemiologic notes and reports isolation of *E. coli* O157:H7 from sporadic cases of hemorrhagic colitis — United States. 1982. *MMWR Morb Mortal Wkly Rep.* 1997;46(30): 700-704.

116. Doyle MP. *Escherichia coli* O157:H7 and its significance in foods. *Int J Food Microbiol.* 1991;12(4):289-301.

117. Griffin PM, Ostroff SM, Tauxe RV, et al. Illnesses associated with *Escherichia coli* O157:H7 infections. A broad clinical spectrum. *Ann Intern Med.* 1988;109(9):705-712.

118. Riley LW, Remis RS, Helgerson SD, et al. Hemorrhagic colitis associated with a rare *Escherichia coli* serotype. *N Engl J Med.* 1983;308:681-685.

119. Nataro JP, Steiner T, Guerrant RL. Enteroaggregative *Escherichia coli. Emerg Infect Dis.* 1998;4(2):251-261.

120. Jay JM. *Modern Food Microbiology,* 6th ed. Gaithersburg, MD: Aspen; 2000:488.

121. Jay JM. *Modern Food Microbiology,* 6th ed. Gaithersburg, MD: Aspen; 2000:511-513.

122. Orriss GD. Animal diseases of public health importance. *Emerg Infect Dis.* 1997;3(4):497-502.

123. Tauxe RV. Emerging foodborne diseases: an evolving public health challenge. *Emerg Infect Dis.* 1997;3(4):425-434.

124. Hogue A, White P, Guard-Petter J, et al. Epidemiology and control of egg-associated *salmonella enteritidis* in the United States of America. *Rev Sci Tech.* 1997;16(2): 542-553.

125. Barnhart HM, Dreesen DW, Bastien R, Pancorbo OC. Prevalence of *Salmonella enteritidis* and other serovars in ovaries of layer hens at time of slaughter. *J Food Prot.* 1991;54(7): 488-491.

126. St. Louis ME, Morse DL, Potter ME, et al. The emergence of grade A eggs as major source of *Salmonella enteritis* infections: new implications for the control of salmonellosis. *JAMA.* 1988;259(14):2103-2107.

127. Guard-Petter J. The chicken, the egg and *Salmonella enteritidis. Environ Microbiol.* 2001;3(7):421-430.

128. Humphrey TJ. Contamination of egg shell and contents with *Salmonella enteritidis*: a review. *Int J Food Microbiol.* 1994;21(1-2):31-40.

129. Perales I, Audicana A. *Salmonella enteritidis* and eggs. *Lancet.* 1988;2(8620):1133.

130. U.S. Department of Agriculture (USDA), Food Safety and Inspection Service. *Shell eggs from farm to table. Fact sheets.* 2019. Accessed November 19, 2020. http://www.fsis.usda .gov/wps/portal/fsis/topics/food-safety-education/get -answers/food-safety-fact-sheets/egg-products-preparation /shell-eggs-from-farm-to-table/CT_Index

131. Mermelstein NH. Pasteurization of shell eggs. *Food Technol.* 2001;55:72.

132. Parashar U, Quiroz ES, Mounts AW, et al. "Norwalk-like viruses": public health consequences and outbreak management. *MMWR Morb Mortal Wkly Rep.* 2001;50(RR-9):1-17.

133. Centers for Disease Control and Prevention (CDC), National Center for Infectious Diseases, Division of Viral and Rickettsial Diseases, Respiratory and Enteric Viruses Branch. *Norovirus: Q&A.* (2019). Accessed November 23, 2020. https://www.cdc.gov/norovirus/

134. U.S. Department of Health and Human Services. Reduce the number of norovirus outbreaks — FSD06 - Healthy People 2030 | health.gov. health.gov. 2019. Accessed November 23, 2020. https://health.gov/healthypeople/objectives-and-data/browse-objectives/foodborne-illness/reduce-number-norovirus-outbreaks-fs-d06

135. Mao Y, Zhu C, Boedeker EC. Foodborne enteric infections. *Curr Opin Gastroenterol.* 2003;19(1):11-22.

136. Lasky T. Foodborne illness—old problem, new relevance. *Epidemiology.* 2002;13(5):593-598.

137. Jay JM. *Modern Food Microbiology*, 6th ed. Gaithersburg, MD: Aspen; 2000:614-615.

138. Norovirus activity—United States, 2006–2007. *MMWR Morb Mortal Wkly Rep.* 2007;56(33):842-846.

139. Acheson D, Bresee JS, Widdowson MA, Monroe SS, Glass RI. Foodborne viral gastroenteritis: challenges and opportunities. *Clin Infect Dis.* 2002;35(6):748-753.

140. Cramer EH, Forney D, Dannenberg AL, et al. Outbreaks of gastroenteritis associated with noroviruses on cruise ships - United States, 2002. *MMWR Morb Mortal Wkly Rep.* 2002;51(49):1112-1115.

141. Centers for Disease Control and Prevention. New report on foodborne disease outbreaks. Published 2019. Accessed October 19, 2019. https://www.cdc.gov/foodsafety/newsletter/new-report-foodborne-disease-outbreaks-9-20-19.html

142. Centers for Disease Control and Prevention. *Viral Hepatitis.* 2020. Accessed November 19, 2020. http://www.cdc.gov/hepatitis/index.htm

143. Archeson D, Fiore AE. Hepatitis A transmitted by food. *Clin Infect Dis.* 2004;38(5):705-715.

144. Centers for Disease Control and Prevention. Coronavirus Disease 2019 (COVID-19). Published September 1, 2020. Accessed August 21, 2020. https://www.cdc.gov/coronavirus/2019-ncov/cdcresponse/about-COVID-19.html

145. National Library of State Legislatures. President Trump Declares State of Emergency for COVID-19. Published March 25, 2020. https://www.ncsl.org/ncsl-in-dc/publications-and-resources/president-trump-declares-state-of-emergency-for-covid-19.aspx

146. OECD. Food Supply Chains and COVID-19: Impacts and Policy Lessons. OECD. Published June 2, 2020. http://www.oecd.org/coronavirus/policy-responses/food-supply-chains-and-covid-19-impacts-and-policy-lessons-71b57aea/

147. Federal Emergency Management Agency. National Business Emergency Operations Center. Homeland Security Digital Library, Published January 1, 1969. Accessed September 3, 2021. https://www.hsdl.org/?abstract&did=723081

148. Aday S, Aday MS. Impacts of COVID-19 on Food Supply Chain. *Food Quality and Safety.* 2020;4(4). doi: 10.1093/fqsafe/fyaa024

149. U.S. Food & Drug Administration. Food Safety and the Coronavirus Disease 2019 (COVID-19). *FDA.* Published online December 3, 2020. Accessed January 18, 2021. https://www.fda.gov/food/food-safety-during-emergencies/food-safety-and-coronavirus-disease-2019-covid-19#foodsupply

150. U.S. Food & Drug Administration. FDA–CFSAN–Outreach and Information Center. Published 2020. Accessed January 18, 2021. https://cfsan.secure.force.com/Inquirypage/

151. Centers for Disease Control and Prevention. Food safety home page. CDC Food Safety. Published 2019. Accessed January 3, 2021. https://www.cdc.gov/foodsafety/

152. National Restaurant Association. Free Courses. ServSafe. Published 2017. Accessed January 18, 2021. https://www.servsafe.com/freecourses

153. U.S. Department of Agriculture, Food and Nutrition Service. FNS Responds to COVID-19 | USDA-FNS. Published 2020. https://www.fns.usda.gov/coronavirus

154. United States Department of Labor. Families First Coronavirus Response Act: Employee Paid Leave Rights | U.S. Department of Labor. Published 2020. https://www.dol.gov/agencies/whd/pandemic/ffcra-employee-paid-leave

155. United States Department of the Treasury. The CARES Act works for all Americans | U.S. Department of the Treasury. Published 2020. https://home.treasury.gov/policy-issues/cares

156. U.S. Department of Agriculture. Biden Administration Expands P-EBT to Benefit Millions of Low-Income and Food Insecure Children During Pandemic. Published January 22, 2021. Accessed January 23, 2021. https://www.usda.gov/media/press-releases/2021/01/22/biden-administration-expands-p-ebt-benefit-millions-low-income-and

157. United States Department of Agriculture. USDA Foods disaster household distribution 2020 | USDA-FNS. Published June 29, 2020. Accessed January 18, 2021. https://www.fns.usda.gov/usda-foods/Disaster-Household-Distribution-2020

158. Meals-to-You. Meals-to-You. Published 2020. Accessed January 10, 2021. https://mealstoyou.org/

159. The White House. Fact Sheet: President Biden's new executive actions deliver economic relief for American families and businesses amid the COVID-19 crises. Published January 22, 2021. Accessed January 30, 2021. https://www.whitehouse.gov/briefing-room/statements-releases/2021/01/22/fact-sheet-president-bidens-new-executive-actions-deliver-economic-relief-for-american-families-and-businesses-amid-the-covid-19-crises/

160. U.S. Department of Agriculture. Biden Administration Expands P-EBT to Benefit Millions of Low-Income and Food Insecure Children During PandemicPublished January 22, 2021. https://www.usda.gov/media/press-releases/2021/01/22/biden-administration-expands-p-ebt-benefit-millions-low-income-and

161. Commissioner of the FDA takes key action in fight against COVID-19 by issuing emergency use authorization for first COVID-19 vaccine. FDA. Published December 14, 2020. Accessed December 29, 2020. https://www.fda.gov/news-events/press-announcements/fda-takes-key-action-fight-against-covid-19-issuing-emergency-use-authorization-first-covid-19#:~:text=Today%2C%20the%20U.S.%20Food%20and

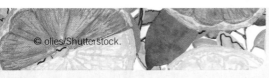
© olies/Shutterstock.

Learning Portfolio

162. Yoder JS, Beach MJ. Giardiasis surveillance—United States, 2003–2005. *MMWR Morb Mortal Wkly Rep: Surv Summ.* 2007;56(SS07):11-18.

163. Slifko TR, Smith HV, Rose JB. Emerging parasite zoonoses associated with water and food. *Int J Parasitol.* 2000;30 (12-13):1379-1393.

164. Jay JM. *Modern Food Microbiology*, 6th ed. Gaithersburg, MD: Aspen; 2000:576-578.

165. Millard PS, Gensheimer KF, Addiss DG, et al. An outbreak of cryptosporidiosis from fresh-pressed apple cider. *JAMA.* 1994;272(20):1592-1596.

166. Centers for Disease Control and Prevention. Foodborne outbreak of diarrheal illness associated with *Cryptosporidium parvum*—Minnesota, 1995. *MMWR Morb Mortal Wkly Rep.* 1996;45(36):783-784.

167. Centers for Disease Control and Prevention. Outbreaks of *Escherichia coli* O157:H7 infection and cryptosporidiosis associated with drinking unpasteurized apple cider—Connecticut and New York, October 1996. *MMWR Morb Mortal Wkly Rep.* 1997;46(1):4-8.

168. Centers for Disease Control and Prevention. Foodborne outbreak of cryptosporidiosis—Spokane, Washington, 1997. *MMWR Morb Mortal Wkly Rep.* 1998;47(27):565-567.

169. Soave R. Cyclospora: an overview. *Clin Infect Dis.* 1996;23(3):429-435.

170. Harris DA, ed. *Mad Cow Disease and Related Spongiform Encephalopathies*. New York: Springer-Verlag: 2004.

171. Yam P. *The Pathological Protein: Mad Cow, Chronic Wasting, and Other Deadly Prion Diseases*. New York: Copernicus Books; 2003:1-284.

172. Brown P, Will RG, Bradley R, Asher DM, Detwiler L. Bovine spongiform encephalopathy and variant Creutzfeldt-Jakob disease: background, evolution, and current concerns. *Emerg Infect Dis.* 2001;7(1):6-16.

173. Pedersen NS, Smith E. Prion diseases: epidemiology in man. *Acta Pathol Microbiol Immunol Scand.* 2002;110(1):14-22.

174. Ironside JW. Prion diseases in man. *J Pathol.* 1998;186(3): 227-234.

175. Kretzschmar HA. Molecular pathogenesis of prion diseases. *Eur Arch Psychiatry Clin Neurosci.* 1999;249(suppl 3):S56-S63.

176. Scott MR, Will R, Ironside J, et al. Compelling transgenetic evidence for transmission of bovine spongiform encephalopathy prions to humans. *Proc Natl Acad Sci USA.* 1999;96(26):15137 -15142.

177. U.S. Food & Drug Administration. *Bovine Spongiform Encephalopathy (BSE) Guidances.* Accessed November 23, 2020. https://www.fda.gov/animal-veterinary/guidance-industry /bovine-spongiform-encephalopathy-bse-guidances.

178. Brown P. The risk of bovine spongiform encephalopathy ("mad cow disease") to human health. *JAMA.* 1997;278(12):1008-1011.

179. Hileman B. Mad cow disease. Regulatory changes stemming from discovery of one diseased cow create new conflicts spawned in part by gaps in scientific understanding. *Chem Eng News.* 2004;82:21.

180. U.S. Department of Agriculture (USDA), FDA. *USDA and HHS Strengthen Safeguards Against Bovine Spongiform Encephalopathy.* 2004. Accessed November 19, 2020. https:// www.fsis.usda.gov/wps/wcm/connect/fsis-archives-content /internet/main/newsroom/meetings/newsletters/constituent -updates/archives/ct_index219

181. U.S. Food & Drug Administration. *Bovine Spongiform Encephalopathy (BSE) and Cosmetics.* 2020. Accessed November 19, 2020. http://www.fda.gov/Cosmetics/ProductsIngredients /PotentialContaminants/ucm136786.htm

182. U.S. Food & Drug Administration. USDA proposes mad cow regulations. *Chem Eng News.* 2004;82:15.

183. Jay JM. *Modern Food Microbiology*, 6th ed. Gaithersburg, MD: Aspen; 2000;595-600.

184. Lie JL, Marth EH. Formation of aflatoxin in cheddar cheese by *Aspergillus flavus* and *Aspergillus parasiticus. J Dairy Sci.* 1967;50(10):1708-1710.

185. Van Rensburg SJ, van der Watt JJ, Purchase IFH, Pereira Coutinho L, Markham R. Primary liver cancer rate and aflatoxin intake in a high cancer area. *S African Med J.* 1974;48(60):2508a.

186. Park DL. Controlling aflatoxin in food and feed. *Food Technol.* 1993;47:92.

187. Labuza TP. Regulation of mycotoxins in food. *J Food Prot.* 1983;46(3):260-265.

188. Food and Agriculture Organization/World Health Organization (FAO/WHO). *FAO/WHO Food Standards.* Codex Alimentarius. Accessed November 23, 2020. http://www.fao .org/fao-who-codexalimentarius/en/

189. Newsome R. Issues in international trade: looking to the Codex Alimentarius Commission. *Food Technol.* 1999;53:26.

190. Stinson EE, Osman SF, Heisler EG, Siciliano J, Bills DD. Mycotoxin production in whole tomatoes, apples, oranges, and lemons. *J Agric Food Chem.* 1981;29:790-792.

191. Stinson EE, Bills DD, Osman SF, Siciliano J, Ceponis MJ, Heisler EG. Mycotoxin production by *Alternaria* species grown on apples, tomatoes, and blueberries. *J Agric Food Chem.* 1980;28:960-963.

192. Marasas WFO, Jaskiewicz K, Venter FS, van Schalkwyk DJ. *Fusarium moniliforme* contamination of maize in oesophageal cancer areas in Transkei. *S African Med J.* 1988;74(3): 110-114.

193. Yoshizawa T, Yamashita A, Luo Y. *Fumonisin* occurrence in corn from high- and low-risk areas for human esophageal cancer in China. *Applied Environ Microbiol.* 1994;60(5):1626-1629.

194. Bennett GA, Richard JL. Influence of processing on Fusarium mycotoxins in contaminated grains. *Food Technol.* 1996;50(5):235-238.

195. Bullerman LB. Mycotoxins and food safety. *Food Technol.* 1986;40(5):59-66.

196. Friedman M, Roitman JN, Kozukue N. Glycoalkaloid and calystegine contents of eight potato cultivars. *J Agric Food Chem.* 2003;51(10):2964-2973.

197. Friedman M, McDonald GM. Glycoalkaloids in fresh and processed potatoes. In: Lee T-C, Kim H-J, eds. *Chemical Markers for Processed and Stored Foods*. Washington, DC: American Chemical Society; 1996:189-205.

198. Phillips BJ, Hughes JA, Phillips JC, Walters DG, Anderson D, Tahourdin CSM. A study of the toxic hazard that might be

associated with the consumption of green potato tops. *Food Chem Toxicol*. 1996;34(5):439-448.

199. Hellenäs KE, Branzell C, Johnsson H, Slanina P. Glycoalkaloid content of early potato varieties. *J Sci Food Agric*. 1995;67(1)125-128.

200. Zhao J, Camire ME, Bushway RJ, Bushway AA. Glycoalkaloid content and in vitro glycoalkaloid solubility of extruded potato peels. *J Agric Food Chem*. 1994;42(11):2570-2573.

201. Friedman M. Composition and safety evaluation of potato berries, potato and tomato seeds, potatoes, and potato alkaloids. *ACS Symposium Series*. (Chapter 35). 1992;484: 429-462.

202. Friedman M, Dao L. Distribution of glycoalkaloids in potato plants and commercial potato products. *J Agric Food Chem*. 1992;40(3):419-423.

203. Edwards EJ, Cobb AH. The effect of prior storage on the potential of potato tubers (*Solanum tuberosum* L) to accumulate glycoalkaloids and chlorophylls during light exposure, including artificial neural network modelling. *J Sci Food Agric*. 1999;79(1):1289-1297.

204. Griffiths DW, Bain H, Dale MFB. Effect of storage temperature on potato (*Solanum tuberosum* L.) tuber glycoalkaloid content and the subsequent accumulation of glycoalkaloids and chlorophyll in response to light exposure. *J Agric Food Chem*. 1998;46(12):5262-5268.

205. Percival G, Dixon GR, Sword A. Glycoalkaloid concentration of potato tubers following exposure to daylight. *J Sci Food Agric*. 1996;71(1):59-63.

206. Coria NA, Sarquis JI, Peñalosa I, Urzúa M. Heat-induced damage in potato (*Solanum tuberosum*) tubers: membrane stability, tissue viability, and accumulation of glycoalkaloids. *J Agric Food Chem*. 1998;46(11):4524-4528.

207. Griffiths DW, Bain H, Dale MFB. The effect of low-temperature storage on the glycoalkaloid content of potato (*Solanum tuberosum*) tubers. *J Sci Food Agric*. 1997;74(3): 301-307.

208. Hlywka JJ, Stephenson GR, Sears MK, Yada RY. Effects of insect damage on glycoalkaloid content in potatoes (*Solanum tuberosum*). *J Agric Food Chem*. 1994;42(11):2545-2550.

209. Rayburn JR, Bantle JA, Friedman M. Role of carbohydrate side chains of potato glycoalkaloids in developmental toxicity. *J Agric Food Chem*. 1994;42(7):1511-1515.

210. Friedman M, McDonald GM, Filadelfi-Keszi MA. Potato glycoalkaloids: chemistry, analysis, safety, and plant physiology. *Crit Rev Plant Sci*. 1997;16(1):55-132.

211. Wood M. New safeguards against glycoalkaloids. *Agric Res*. 1997;45(12):16.

212. Korpan YI, Nazarenko EA, Skryshevskaya IV, Martelet C, Jaffrezic-Renault N, El'skaya AV. Potato glycoalkaloids: true safety or false sense of security? *Trend Biotechnol*. 2004;22(3):147-151.

213. Friedman M, Henika PR, Mackey BE. Effect of feeding solanidine, solasodine, and tomatidine to non-pregnant and pregnant mice. *Food Chem Toxicol*. 2003;41(1):61-71.

214. Smith DB, Roddick JG, Jones JL. Potato glycoalkaloids: some unanswered questions. *Trend Food Sci Technol*. 1996;7(4): 126-131.

215. Nigg HH, Beier RC. Evaluation of food for potential toxicants. In: *Phytochemicals and Health: Proceedings, Tenth Annual Penn State Symposium in Plant Physiology*; 1995 (May 18-20): 192-201.

216. Tanne JH. Foods and drugs alter response to anaesthesia. *BMJ*. 1998;317:1102.

217. Arora A, Camire ME. Performance of potato peels in muffins and cookies. *Food Res Int*. 1994;27(1):15-22.

218. Camire ME, Flint SI. Thermal processing effects on dietary fiber composition and hydration capacity in corn meal, oat meal, and potato peels. *Cereal Chem*. 1991;68(6):645-647.

219. Surjawan I, Dougherty MP, Bushway RJ, Bushway AA, Briggs JL, Camire ME. Sulfur compounds reduce potato toxins during extrusion cooking. *J Agric Food Chem*. 2001;49(6):2835-2838.

220. Teitelbaum JS, Zatorre RJ, Carpenter S, et al. Neurologic sequelae of domoic acid intoxication due to the ingestion of contaminated mussels. *N Engl J Med*. 1990;322:1781-1787.

221. Perl TM, Bédard L, Kotsatsky T, Hockin JC, Todd EC, Remis RS. An outbreak of toxic encephalopathy caused by eating mussels contaminated with domoic acid. *N Engl J Med*. 1990;322:1775-1780.

222. Stewart GR, Zorumski CF, Price MT, Olney JW. Domoic acid: a dementia-inducing excitotoxic food poison with kainic acid receptor specificity. *Exp Neurol*. 1990;110(1):127-138.

223. Zatorre RJ. Memory loss following domoic acid intoxication from ingestion of toxic mussels. *Can Dis Wkly Rep*. 1990;16(suppl 1E):101-104.

224. Iverson F, Truelove J, Nera E, Tryphonas L, Campbell J, Lok E. Domoic acid poisoning and mussel-associated intoxication: preliminary investigations into the response of mice and rats to toxic mussel extract. *Food Chem Toxicol*. 1989;27(6):377-384.

225. Pottier I, Vernoux J-P, Lewis RJ. Ciguatera fish poisoning in the Caribbean islands and Western Atlantic. *Rev Environ Contam Toxicol*. 2001;168:99.

226. Ting JY, Brown AF, Pearn JH. Ciguatera poisoning: an example of a public health challenge. *Austr N Zealand J Public Health*. 1998;22(1):140-142.

227. Pearn J. Neurology of ciguatera. *J Neurol Neurosurg Psychiatry*. 2001;70:4-8.

228. Bruneau A, Mahanty S, al-Azraqui T, MacLean J, Bourque M, Desroches F. Ciguatera fish poisoning linked to the ingestion of barracuda in a Montreal restaurant—Quebec. *Can Commun Dis Rep*. 1997;23(20):153-156.

229. Klemme TM, Lösch RR. Ciguatera-Eine Tückische Fischvergiftung. [Durch Fischimporte ist das Risiko Potentiell auch Hierzulande Gegeben. *Fortschritte der Medizin*.] 1997;115:39. (in German).

230. Sanders WE Jr. Intoxications from the seas: ciguatera, scombroid, and paralytic shellfish poisoning. *Infect Dis Clin N Am*. 1987;1(3):665-676.

231. Lawrence JF, Niedzwiadek B, Menard C. Quantitative determination of paralytic shellfish poisoning toxins in shellfish using prechromatographic oxidation and liquid chromatography with fluorescence detection: collaborative study. *J AOAC Int*. 2005;88(6):1714-1732.

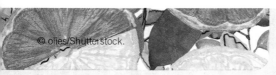

Learning Portfolio

232. Biré R, Krys S, Frémy J-M, Dragacci S. Improved solid-phase extraction procedure in the analysis of paralytic shellfish poisoning toxins by liquid chromatography with fluorescence detection. *J Agric Food Chem.* 2003;51(22):6386-6390.

233. Lehane L. Paralytic shellfish poisoning: a potential public health problem. *Med J Aust.* 2001;175(1):29-31.

234. U.S. Food & Drug Administration, CFSAN. *The National Shellfish Sanitation Program (NSSP).* (2020). Accessed November 19, 2020. http://www.fda.gov/Food/GuidanceRegulation/FederalStateFoodPrograms/ucm2006754.htm

235. U.S. Food & Drug Administration. *Interstate Certified Shellfish Shippers List.* Accessed November 19, 2020. https://www.fda.gov/food/federalstate-food-programs/interstate-certified-shellfish-shippers-list

236. Castoldi AF, Coccini T, Manzo L. Neurotoxic and molecular effects of methylmercury in humans. *Rev Environ Health.* 2003;18(1):19.

237. Sweet LI, Zelikoff JT. Toxicology and immunotoxicology of mercury: a comparative review in fish and humans. *J Toxicol Environ Health. Part B, Crit Rev.* 2001;4(2):161-205.

238. U.S. Food & Drug Administration. *Advice about eating fish: for women who are or might become pregnant, breastfeeding mothers, and young children.* 2020. Accessed November 19, 2020. http://www.fda.gov/Food/FoodborneIllnessContaminants/Metals/ucm393070.htm

239. United States Environmental Protection Agency (EPA). *EPA-FDA Advice about eating fish and shellfish.* 2020. Accessed November 19, 2020. https://www.epa.gov/fish-tech/epa-fda-advice-about-eating-fish-and-shellfish

240. U.S. Food & Drug Administration. *Mercury levels in commercial fish and shellfish (1990-2012).* (2017). Accessed November 19, 2020. http://www.fda.gov/food/foodborneillnesscontaminants/metals/ucm115644.htm

241. U.S. Food & Drug Administration. *Mercury level data in commercial fish (1990–2012).* Mercury concentrations in fish: FDA monitoring program (1990-2004). (2009). Accessed November 19, 2020. https://www.fda.gov/food/metals-and-your-food/mercury-levels-commercial-fish-and-shellfish-1990-2012

242. Clarkson TW, Strain JJ. Nutritional factors may modify the toxic action of methyl mercury in fish-eating populations. *J Nutr.* 2003;133(5, suppl 1):1539S-1543S.

243. Shipp AM, Gentry PR, Lawrence G, et al. Determination of a site-specific reference dose for methylmercury for fish-eating populations. *Toxicol Indust Health.* 2000;16(9-10):335-438.

244. Chapman L, Chan HM. The influence of nutrition on methyl mercury intoxication. *Environ Health Perspec.* 2000;108 (suppl 1):29-56.

245. Chan HM, Egeland GM. Fish consumption, mercury exposure, and heart diseases. *Nutr Rev.* 2004;62(2):68-72.

246. Smith SC, Taylor JG, Stephen AM. Use of food labels and beliefs about diet-disease relationships among university students. *Public Health Nutr.* 2000;3(2):175-182.

247. Elbon SM, Johnson MA, Fischer JG, Searcy CA. Demographic factors, nutrition knowledge, and health-seeking behaviors influence nutrition label reading behaviors among older American adults. *J Nutr Elderly.* 2000;19(3):31-48.

248. Joshi P, Mofidi S, Sicherer SH. Interpretation of commercial food ingredient labels by parents of food-allergic children. *J Allergy Clin Immunol.* 2002;109(6):1019-1021.

249. Levy L, Patterson RE, Kristal AR, Li SS. How well do consumers understand percentage daily value on food labels? *Am J Health Promot.* 2000;14(3):157-160.

250. Verbeke W, Frewer LJ, Scholderer J, De Brabander HF. Why consumers behave as they do with respect to food safety and risk information. *Anal Chim Acta.* 2007;586(1-2):2-7.

251. Henson S, Annou M, Cranfield J, Ryks J. Understanding consumer attitudes toward food technologies in Canada. *Risk Anal.* 2008;28(6):1601-1607.

252. McLellan MR. IFT's strategic plan: changing direction. *Food Technol.* 2002;56:62.

253. Reisch MS. Track us, trust us. American Chemistry Council says will supply the facts to earn the public's trust. *Chem Eng News.* 2004;82:24.

254. Thayer A. ACC convenes amid upheaval. Industry group wrestles with issues of money, resignations, and image. *Chem Eng News.* 2003;81:10.

255. Storck W. ACC tests new ad image program. By stressing "chemistry" not "chemicals," group hopes to change public's view of industry. *Chem Eng News.* 2001;79:13.

256. Pszczola DE. Sweetener 1 sweetener enhances the equation. *Food Technol.* 2003;57(11):48-50.

257. Homler BE. Properties and stability of aspartame. *Food Technol.* 1984;38(7):50-55.

258. Levin GV. Tagatose, the new GRAS sweetener and health product. *J Med Food.* 2002;5(1):23-36.

259. Stankovic, Ph.D. I. *Advantame Chemical and Technical Assessment.* (E Folmer, Ph.D D, ed.); 2013. Accessed December 12, 2020. http://www.fao.org/fileadmin/user_upload/agns/pdf/CTA_Advantame_77.pdf

260. Gilman V. Artificial sweeteners. No-calorie sugar substitutes provide options for enjoying the sweet life. *Chem Eng News.* 2004;82:43.

261. Geuns JM. Stevioside. *Phytochemistry.* 2003;64(5):913-921.

262. Gregersen S, Jeppesen PB, Holst JJ, Hermansen K. Antihyperglycemic effects of stevioside in type 2 diabetic subjects. *Metabolism.* 2004;53(1):73-76.

263. Hsieh M-H, Chan P, Sue Y-M, et al. Efficacy and tolerability of oral stevioside in patients with mild essential hypertension: a two-year, randomized, placebo-controlled study. *Clin Ther.* 2003;25(11):2797-2808.

264. Jeppesen PB, Gregersen S, Rolfsen SE, et al. Antihyperglycemic and blood pressure-reducing effects of stevioside in the diabetic Goto-Kakizaki rat. *Metabolism.* 2003;52(3):372-378.

265. Chan P, Tomlinson B, Chen Y-J, Liu J-C, Hsieh M-H, Cheng JT. A double-blind placebo-controlled study of the effectiveness and tolerability of oral stevioside in human hypertension. *Br J Clin Pharmacol.* 2000;50(3):215-220.

266. Bray GA, Nielsen SJ, Popkin BM. Consumption of high-fructose corn syrup in beverages may play a role in the epidemic of obesity. *Am J Clin Nutr.* 2004;79(4):537-743.

267. Chappel CI. A review and biological risk assessment of sodium saccharin. *Reg Toxicol Pharmacol.* 1992;15(3):253-270.

268. Ellwein LB, Cohen SM. The health risks of saccharin revisited. *Crit Rev Toxicol.* 1990;20(5):311-326.

269. Butchko HH, Stargel WW, Comer CP, et al. Aspartame: review of safety. *Reg Toxicol Pharmacol.* 2002;35(1):S1-S93.

270. Potenza DP, el-Mallakh RS. Aspartame: clinical update. *Connecticut Med.* 1989;53(7):395-400.

271. Yost DA. Clinical safety of aspartame. *Am Fam Physician.* 1989;39(2):201-206.

272. Garriga MM, Metcalfe DD. Aspartame intolerance. *Ann Allergy.* 1988;61(6 pt 2):63-69.

273. Janssen PJ, van der Heijden CA. Aspartame: review of recent experimental and observational data. *Toxicology.* 1988;50(1):1-26.

274. Stegink LD. The aspartame story: a model for the clinical testing of a food additive. *Am J Clin Nutr.* 1987;46(1):204-215.

275. Finn JP, Lord GH. Neurotoxicity studies on sucralose and its hydrolysis products with special reference to histopathologic and ultrastructural changes. *Food Chem Toxicol.* 2000;38 (suppl 2):7-17.

276. Goldsmith LA. Acute and subchronic toxicity of sucralose. *Food Chem Toxicol.* 2000;38(suppl 2):S53-S69.

277. Grice HC, Goldsmith LA. Sucralose–an overview of the toxicity data. *Food Chem Toxicol.* 2000;38(suppl 2):S1-S6.

278. Knight I. The development and applications of sucralose, a new high-intensity sweetener. *Can J Physiol Pharmacol.* 1994;72(4):435.

279. Department of Health and Human Services (DHHS) and USDA. *Dietary Guidelines for Americans*, 8th ed. 2015. Accessed November 19, 2020. http://health.gov/dietaryguidelines/2015/guidelines/

280. United States Department of Agriculture (USDA), National Agricultural Library, Food and Nutrition Information Center. In: *Dietary Guidance*. 2015. Accessed November 23, 2020. National Agricultural Library, Food and Nutrition Information Center.

281. Fitch C, Keim KS. Position of the Academy of Nutrition and Dietetics: Use of nutritive and nonnutritive sweeteners. *Journal Acad Nutr Diet.* 2012;112(5):739-758. doi: 10.1016/j.jand.2012.03.009

282. Tate & Lyle. *Food Starches.* Accessed November 19, 2020. http://www.tateandlyle.com/ingredientsandservices/chooseaningredientorservice/americas/pages/foodstarches.aspx

283. Wittrig B. *Preservative analysis by liquid and gas chromatography.* State College, PA: Restek Corp; 2003. Accessed November 19, 2020. https://www.chromalytic.com.au/pdf2/pres-2003-preserv.pdf

284. Duke J. *Module 19. Botanicals generally recognized as safe.* Accessed November 19, 2020. https://s4.lite.msu.edu/res/msu/botonl/b_online/library/dr-duke/gras.htm

285. Geha RS, Beiser A, Ren C, et al. Review of alleged reaction to monosodium glutamate and outcome of a multicenter double-blind placebo-controlled study. *J Nutr.* 2000;130 (suppl 4):1058S-1062S.

286. Yang WH, Drouin MA, Herbert M, Mao Y, Karsh J. The monosodium glutamate symptom complex: assessment in a double-blind, placebo-controlled, randomized study. *J Allergy Clin Immunol.* 1997;99(6):757-762.

287. Tarasoff L, Kelly MF. Monosodium L-glutamate: a double-blind study and review. *Food Chem Toxicol.* 1993;31(12):1019-1035.

288. Scher W, Scher BM. A possible role for nitric oxide in glutamate (MSG)-induced Chinese restaurant syndrome, glutamate-induced asthma, "hot-dog headache," pugilistic Alzheimer's disease, and other disorders. *Med Hypotheses.* 1992;38(3):185-188.

289. Pulce C, Vial T, Verdier F, Testud F, Nicolas B, Descotes J. The Chinese restaurant syndrome: a reappraisal of monosodium glutamate's causative role. *Adverse Drug React Toxicol Rev.* 1992;11(1):19-39.

290. Sands GH, Newman L, Lipton R. Cough, exertional, and other miscellaneous headaches. *Med Clin N Am.* 1991;75(3):733-747.

291. Scopp AL. MSG and hydrolyzed vegetable protein induced headache: review and case studies. *Headache.* 1991;31(2):107-110.

292. Stevenson DD. Monosodium glutamate and asthma. *J Nutr.* 2000;130(suppl 4):1067S-1073S.

293. Woods RK, Weiner JM, Thein F, Abramson M, Walters EH. The effects of monosodium glutamate in adults with asthma who perceive themselves to be monosodium glutamate–intolerant. *J Allergy Clin Immunol.* 1998;101(6):762-771.

294. Walker R, Lupien JR. The safety evaluation of monosodium glutamate. *J Nutr.* 2000;130(suppl 4):1049S-1052S.

295. Junod SW. *Folic acid fortification: fact and folly.* (2009). Accessed November 19, 2020. https://www.fda.gov/files/about%20fda/published/Folic-Acid-Fortification--Fact-and-Folly.pdf

296. U.S. Food & Drug Administration. PMO 2007: Appendix O. Vitamin fortification of fluid milk products. Grade "A" pasteurized milk ordinance. 2017. Accessed November 19, 2020. https://www.fda.gov/media/114169/download

297. National Institutes of Health Office of Dietary Supplements. *Folate.* 2020. Accessed November 19, 2020. https://ods.od.nih.gov/factsheets/Folate-HealthProfessional/

298. Global trends. (Market trends): Fortified beverages. *Prepared Foods.* 2002;171:9.

299. Health sells!!! Refrigerators, etc. *Business World.* 2002; May 27:38.

300. Fortifying sales: lifestyle choices support demand for fortified foods. *Gourmet Retailer.* 2002;23:42.

301. Food additives permitted for direct addition to food for human consumption; vitamin D3. *Federal Register.* February 27, 2003;68:9000.

302. Penniston KL, Tanumihardjo SA. Vitamin A in dietary supplements and fortified foods: too much of a good thing? *J Am Diet Assoc.* 2003;103(9):1185-1187.

303. Greger JL. Food, supplements, and fortified foods: scientific evaluations in regard to toxicology and nutrient bioavailability. *J Am Diet Assoc.* 1987;87(10):1369-1373.

304. Dalton L. What's that stuff? Food preservatives. *Chem Eng News.* 2002;80:40.

305. Foulke JE. A Fresh Look at Food Preservatives. *FDA Consumer.* (1993; updated 2003). Accessed November 19, 2020. http://www.nettally.com/prusty/formj.htm

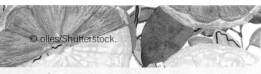
© olies/Shutterstock.

Learning Portfolio

306. Williams GM, Iatropoulos MJ, Whysner J. Safety assessment of butylated hydroxyanisole and butylated hydroxytoluene as antioxidant food additives. *Food Chem Toxicol.* 1999;37(9-10):1027-1038.

307. Whysner J, Williams GM. Butylated hydroxyanisole mechanistic data and risk assessment: conditional species-specific cytotoxicity, enhanced cell proliferation, and tumor promotion. *Pharmacol Ther.* 1996;71(1-2):137-151.

308. Iverson F. Phenolic antioxidants: Health protection branch studies on butylated hydroxyanisole. *Cancer Lett.* 1995;93(1):49-54.

309. Huang M-T, Ferraro T. Phenolic compounds in food and cancer prevention. *ACS Symp Series.* 1992;507:8-34.

310. Lester MR. Sulfite sensitivity: significance in human health. *J Am Coll Nutr.* 1995;14(3):229-232.

311. Lecos C. Reacting to sulfites. *F.D.A. Consumer.* 1995;19(10):17-20.

312. Skovgaard N. Microbiological aspects and technological need: technological needs for nitrates and nitrites. *Food Addit Contam.* 1992;9(5):391-397.

313. Mirvish SS. The significance for human health of nitrate, nitrite and n-nitroso compounds. *NATO ASI Series: Series G: Ecological Sciences.* 1991;30:253.

314. Nitrate, nitrite, and nitroso compounds in foods. *Food Technol.* 1987;41:127.

315. U.S. Food & Drug Administration. *Packaging Materials Listed in 21 CFR 179.45 for Use during Irradiation of Prepackaged Foods.* (2018). Accessed November 19, 2020. https://www.fda.gov/food/irradiation-food-packaging/packaging-materials-listed-21-cfr-17945-use-during-irradiation-prepackaged

316. United States Department of Agriculture (USDA), FSIS. *Irradiation and Food Safety. Answers to Frequently Asked Questions.* (2016). Accessed November 19, 2020. http://www.fsis.usda.gov/wps/portal/fsis/topics/food-safety-education/get-answers/food-safety-fact-sheets/production-and-inspection/irradiation-and-food-safety/irradiation-food-safety-faq

317. Bennett Wood O, Bruhn CM, American Dietetic Association. Position of the American Dietetic Association: food irradiation. *J Am Diet Assoc.* 2000;100(2):246-253.

318. Tritsch GL. Food irradiation. *Nutrition.* 2000;16(7-8):698-701.

319. Pauli GH. *U.S. regulatory requirements for irradiating foods.* (2017). Accessed November 19, 2020. https://www.fda.gov/food/ingredients-additives-gras-packaging-guidance-documents-regulatory-information/regulatory-report-irradiation-food-packaging-materials

320. Farkas J. Irradiation as a method for decontaminating food: a review. *Int J Food Microbiol.* 1998;44(3):189-204.

321. Morehouse KM. Food irradiation: the treatment of foods with ionizing radiation. *Food Test Anal.* 1998;4(3):9.

322. Loaharanu P. Irradiation as a cold pasteurization process of food. *Vet Parasitol.* 1996;64(1-2):71-82.

323. Dodd NJ. Free radicals and food irradiation. *Biochem Soc Symp.* 1995;61:247-258.

324. Lagunas-Solar MC. Radiation processing of foods: an overview of scientific principles and current status. *J Food Protect.* 1995;58(2):186-192.

325. Irradiation in the production, processing and handling of food. *Federal Register.* 1997;62(232):64107.

326. Swanson RB, Munsayac LJ. Acceptability of fruit purees in peanut butter, oatmeal, and chocolate chip reduced-fat cookies. *J Am Diet Assoc.* 1999;99(3):343-345.

327. Pszczola DE. Blends reduce fat in bakery products. *Food Technol.* 1994;48:168.

328. Phillips I, Casewell M, Cox T, et al. Does the use of antibiotics in food animals pose a risk to human health? A critical review of published data. *J Antimicrob Chemother.* 2004;53(1):28-52.

329. Stevens S. "Recent industry poll favors single food safety agency." Milwaukee, WI: Gass Weber Mullins LLC; 2009. Accessed July 1, 2009. http://www.defendingfoodsafety.com/2009/02/articles/food-safety-news/recent-industry-poll-favors-single-food-safety-agency/

330. Center for Science in the Public Interest (CSPI). Congressional leaders call for single food safety agency. CSPI supports effort to modernize food safety laws. 2007. Accessed November 19, 2020. http://cspinet.org/new/200702143.html

331. Committee to Ensure Safe Food from Production to Consumption (Institute of Medicine and National Research Council). *Ensuring Safe Food: From Production to Consumption.* Washington, DC: National Academies Press; 2003:1-206.

332. Bradley T. "Monsanto's victory in Maine rBGH lawsuit a setback for consumers." *Portland Press Herald.* December 30, 2003:10A.

333. Mohl B. "Got growth hormone? Dairies play on fear in marketing milk without the additive." *The Boston Globe.* September 28, 2003:J1. 307.

334. Pray L, Yaktine A. *Managing Food Safety Practices from Farm to Table: Workshop Summary.* Washington, DC: National Academies Press; 2009:Ch. 4.

335. Toops D. A conversation with food safety czar David W.K. Acheson. FoodProcessing.com. 2008. Accessed November 19, 2020. http://www.foodprocessing.com/articles/2008/367.html

336. Hamilton D, Ambrus A, Dieterle R, et al. Pesticide residues in food—acute dietary exposure. *Pest Manag Sci.* 2004;60(4):311-339.

337. Potter TL, Marti L, Belflower S, Truman CC. Multiresidue analysis of cotton defoliant, herbicide, and insecticide residues in water by solid-phase extraction and GC-NPD, GC-MS, and HPLC-diode array detection. *J Agric Food Chem.* 2000;48(9):4103-4108.

338. Cabras P, Angioni A. Pesticide residues in grapes, wine, and their processing products. *J Agric Food Chem.* 2000;48(4):967-973.

339. Mukherjee I, Gopal M. Insecticide residues in baby food, animal feed, and vegetables by gas liquid chromatography. *Bull Environ Contam Toxicol.* 1996;56:381-388.

340. Hyman FN, Klontz KC, Tollefson L. Food and Drug Administration surveillance of the role of foreign objects in foodborne injuries. *Public Health Rep.* 1993;108(1):54-59.

341. University of Nebraska Cooperative Extension. *Physical Hazards.* (2005). Accessed November 19, 2020. http://food.unl.edu/physical-hazards

342. U.S. Food & Drug Administration. New era of smarter food safety. FDA. Published November 6, 2020. Accessed December 29, 2020. https://www.fda.gov/food/new-era-smarter-food-safety

343. Kumar Sharma S, Singh V. Applications of blockchain technology in the food industry. New Food Magazine. Published May 6, 2020. https://www.newfoodmagazine.com/article/110116/blockchain

344. Bouzembrak Y, Klüche M, Gavai A, Marvin HJ. Internet of things in food safety: literature review and a bibliometric analysis. *Trends in Food Science & Technology.* 2019;9454-64. https://doi.org/10.1016/j.tifs.2019.11.002.

345. Polkinghorne JC. Ethical issues in biotechnology. *Trend Biotechnol.* 2000;18(1):8-10.

346. Serageldin I. Biotechnology and food security in the 21st century. *Science.* 1999;285:387.

347. Burke D. Why all the fuss about genetically modified food? Much depends on who benefits. *BMJ.* 1998;316:1845.

348. Kuiper HA, König A, Kleter GA, Hammes WP, Knudsen I. Safety assessment, detection and traceability, and societal aspects of genetically modified foods. European Network on Safety Assessment of Genetically Modified Food Crops (ENTRANSFOOD). Concluding remarks. *Food Chem Toxicol.* 2004;42(7):1195-1202.

349. Perr HA. Children and genetically engineered food: potentials and problems. *J Pediatr Gastroenterol Nutr.* 2002;35(4):475-486.

350. Goldman LR, Koduru S. Chemicals in the environment and developmental toxicity to children: a public health and policy perspective. *Environ Health Persp.* 2000;108(suppl 3):443-448.

351. Käferstein F, Abdussalam M. Food safety in the 21st century. *Bull WHO.* 1999;77(4):347-351.

352. Finucane ML. Mad cows, mad corn and mad communities: the role of socio-cultural factors in the perceived risk of genetically-modified food. *Proc Nutr Soc.* 2002;61:31-37.

353. Hino A. Safety assessment and public concerns for genetically modified food products: the Japanese experience. *Toxicol Pathol.* 2002;30(1):126-128.

354. United States Department of Agriculture (USDA), FSIS and APHIS, and DHHS, FDA. *USDA and HHS Strengthen Safeguards against Bovine Spongiform Encephalopathy.* 2004. Accessed November 19, 2020. https://www.fsis.usda.gov/wps/portal/fsis/topics/food-safety-education/get-answers/food-safety-fact-sheets/production-and-inspection/fsis-further-strengthens-protections-against-bovine-spongiform-encephalopathy-bse/fsis-further-strengthens-protections-against-bse

355. Legname G, Baskakov IV, Nguyen H-O, et al. Synthetic mammalian prions. *Science.* 2004;305(5684):673-676.

356. Consumer protection from an EU regulation on the mandatory labelling of genetically modified food. *Clin Lab.* 2004;50:380.

357. United States Department of Agriculture Economic Research Service (USDA ERS). Adoption of Genetically Engineered Crops in the US, Recent Trends in GE Adoption. (2020). Accessed November 23, 2020. http://www.ers.usda.gov/data-products/adoption-of-genetically-engineered-crops-in-the-us/recent-trends-in-ge-adoption.aspx#.UobvBXL92Dk

358. World Health Organization (WHO). *Food Safety: Frequently asked Questions on Genetically Modified Foods.* (2014). Accessed November 23, 2020. http://www.who.int/foodsafety/areas_work/food-technology/faq-genetically-modified-food/en/

359. Schafer KS, Kegley SE. Persistent toxic chemicals in the US food supply. *J Epidemiol Comm Health.* 2002;56:813-817.

360. Acosta L. *Restrictions on Genetically Modified Organisms: United States.* Library of Congress (2020). Accessed November 23, 2020. http://www.loc.gov/law/help/restrictions-on-gmos/usa.php

361. National Archives. National Bioengineered Food Disclosure Standard. Federal Register. Published December 21, 2018. https://www.federalregister.gov/documents/2018/12/21/2018-27283/national-bioengineered-food-disclosure-standard

362. Jacobs MK. The history of biologic warfare and bioterrorism. *Dermatol Clinics.* 2004;22:231.

363. Martin W. Legal and public policy responses of states to bioterrorism. *Am J Public Health.* 2004;94(7):1093-1096.

364. Hassler KE. *Agricultural Bioterrorism: Why It Is a Concern and What We Must Do.* Carlisle Barracks, PA: U.S. Army War College; 2003:1-44.

365. Pellerin C. The next target of bioterrorism: your food. *Environ Health Perspect.* 2000;108(3):A126-A129.

366. Centers for Disease Control and Prevention (CDC). *Emergency preparedness and response. Bioterrorism agents/diseases.* Accessed November 19, 2020. https://emergency.cdc.gov/agent/agentlist-category.asp

367. Centers for Disease Control and Prevention (CDC). *Emergency Preparedness and Response. Chemical agents.* Accessed November 19, 2020. https://emergency.cdc.gov/agent/agentlistchem.asp

368. Grossman LK. The story of a truly contaminated election. *Columbia Journalism Review.* 2001;39(5):65.

369. Török TJ, Tauxe RV, Wise RP, et al. A large community outbreak of salmonellosis caused by intentional contamination of restaurant salad bars. *JAMA.* 1997;278(5):389-395.

370. Cody MM, Stretch T. Position of the Academy of Nutrition and Dietetics: food and water safety. *J Acad Nutr Dietetics.* 2014;114(11):1819-1829. doi: 10.1016/j.jand.2014.08.023

371. Sobel J, Khan AS, Swerdlow DL. Threat of a biological terrorist attack on the US food supply: the CDC perspective. *Lancet.* 2002;359(9309):874-880.

372. Khan AS, Swerdlow DL, Juranek DD. Precautions against biological and chemical terrorism directed at food and water supplies. *Public Health Rep.* 2001;116(1):3-14.

373. Bruemmer B. Food biosecurity. *J Am Diet Assoc.* 2003;103(6):687-691.

374. Peregrin T. Bioterrorism and food safety: what nutrition professionals need to know to educate the American public. *J Am Diet Assoc.* 2002;102(1):14, 16.

375. Hall MJ, Norwood AE, Ursano RJ, Fullerton CS. The psychological impacts of bioterrorism. *Biosecur Bioterror.* 2003;1(2):139-144.

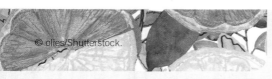

Learning Portfolio

376. Committee on Responding to the Psychological Consequences of Terrorism, National Research Council. *Preparing for the Psychological Consequences of Terrorism: A Public Health Strategy.* Washington, DC: National Academy Press; 2003.

377. Chalk P. *Hitting America's Soft Underbelly: The Potential Threat of Deliberate Biological Attacks Against the U.S. Agricultural and Food Industry.* Santa Monica, CA: RAND Publications; 2004.

378. Neff J. Food industry deals with crisis: from disruptions to previously unimaginable threats, the food industry braces for a new reality post-Sept. 11. *Food Processing.* 2001; Nov 2.

379. Nestle M. *Safe Food: Bacteria, Biotechnology, and Bioterrorism.* Berkeley, CA: University of California Press; 2003.

380. Trevejo RT, Courtney JG, Starr M, Vugia DJ. Epidemiology of salmonellosis in California, 1990–1999: morbidity, mortality, and hospitalization costs. *Am J Epidemiol.* 2003;157(1): 48-57.

381. Center for Food Safety and Applied Nutrition, Food and Drug Administration. *Risk Assessment for Food Terrorism and Other Food Safety Concerns.* October 7, 2003. Accessed November 19, 2020. https://www.federalregister.gov /documents/2003/10/10/03-25850/risk-assessment -for-food-terrorism-and-other-food-safety-concerns-availability

382. Meadows M. The FDA and the fight against terrorism. *FDA Consumer Mag.* 2004: January-February.

383. Federal Bureau of Investigation. *United States Government Interagency Domestic Terrorism Concept of Operations Plan.* 2001. Accessed November 19, 2020. http://fas.org/irp/threat /conplan.html

384. Rotz LD, Khan AS, Lillibridge SR, Ostroff SM, Hughes JM. Public health assessment of potential biological terrorism agents. *CDC Emerging Infect Dis.* 2002;8(2):225-230.

385. Federal Emergency Management Agency. *Managing the Emergency Consequences of Terrorist Incidents.* Accessed November 19, 2020. www.fema.gov/pdf/plan/managing emerconseq.pdf

386. Knobler SL, Mahmoud AAF, Pray LA. *Biological Threats and Terrorism: Assessing the Science and Response Capabilities: Workshop Summary.* Washington, DC: Institute of Medicine, National Academy Press; 2002. Accessed November 19, 2020. https://pubmed.ncbi.nlm.nih.gov/22787686/

387. Federal Emergency Management Agency. *Managing the Emergency Consequences of Terrorist Incidents: Interim Planning Guide for State and Local Governments. Appendix A—Biological Weapons.* July 2002. Accessed November 19, 2020. https:// www.fema.gov/pdf/plan/managingemerconseq.pdf

388. Centers for Disease Control and Prevention. *Emergency Preparedness & Response.* Accessed November 19, 2020. https://emergency.cdc.gov/

389. National Library of Medicine, Specialized Information Services. Biological Warfare. Accessed November 19, 2020. https:// disasterinfo.nlm.nih.gov/biological-agents

390. Mead PS, Slutsker L, Dietz V, et al. Food-related illness and death in the United States. *CDC Emerg Infect Dis.* 2000;5.

391. Centers for Disease Control and Prevention. Anthrax information for healthcare providers. Accessed November 23, 2020. http://www.cdc.gov/anthrax/specificgroups/health-care -providers/index.html

392. Centers for Disease Control and Prevention. Botulism: general information. Accessed November 23, 2020. https://www .cdc.gov/botulism/

393. Centers for Disease Control and Prevention. Anthrax: diagnosis/evaluation (signs and symptoms). Accessed November 23, 2020. http://www.cdc.gov/anthrax/basics/symptoms.html

394. Center for Infectious Disease Research and Policy. Initial Assessment of Food System Biosecurity Threats. Accessed January 6, 2016. http://www.cidrap.umn.edu/cidrap/content /biosecurity/food-biosec/threats/assess.html

395. Centers for Disease Control and Prevention. Frequently asked questions about plague. Accessed November 23, 2020. http:// www.cdc.gov/plague/faq/index.html

396. Centers for Disease Control and Prevention. Tularemia: frequently asked questions about tularemia. Accessed November 23, 2020. https://www.cdc.gov/tularemia/faq/index.html

397. Centers for Disease Control and Prevention. Brucellosis. Accessed November 23, 2020. http://www.cdc.gov /brucellosis/

398. Centers for Disease Control and Prevention. Escherichia Coli O157:H7. Accessed November 23, 2020. http://www.cdc .gov/ecoli/

399. Centers for Disease Control and Prevention. Shigellosis. Accessed November 23, 2020. http://www.cdc.gov/shigella /index.html

400. Committee on Science and Technology for Countering Terrorism, National Research Council. *Making the Nation Safer, the Role of Science and Technology in Countering Terrorism.* Washington, DC: National Academy Press; 2002.

401. Center for Homeland Defense and Security. *Protecting America's Meat, Poultry, and Egg Products: A Report to the Secretary on the Food Security Accomplishments of the Food Safety and Inspection Service.* Accessed November 19, 2020. www.hsdl.org

402. Food Law. Accessed November 19, 2020. https://www .ag.ndsu.edu/foodlaw/overview/introhaccp

403. Centers for Disease Control and Prevention. Salmonellosis. Accessed November 23, 2020. http://www.cdc.gov /salmonella/

404. Government Accounting Office. *Biosurveillance: DHS Should Not Pursue BioWatch Upgrades or Enhancements Until System Capabilities Are Established.* United States Government Accounting Office Report to Congressional Requestors. October 2015. Washington, DC: GAO-16-99.

405. Sobel J, Khan AS, Swerdlow DL. Threat of a biological terrorist attack on the US food supply: the CDC perspective. *Lancet.* 2002;359(9309):874-880.

406. Buehler JW, Berkelman RL, Hartley DM, Peters CJ. Syndromic surveillance and bioterrorism-related epidemics. *Emerging Infect Dis.* 2003;9(10):1197-1204.

407. United States Government Accountability Office. *Food Safety: A National Strategy Is Needed to Address Fragmentation in Federal Oversight. Report to Congressional Requesters.* 2017. Accessed January 4, 2021. https://www.gao.gov/assets /690/682095.pdf

408. Winters DR. Office from 2006-2010. UCLA LAW REVIEW 64 UCLA L. Food law at the outset of the Trump administration. *Rev DisC.* 2017;28. Accessed January 4, 2021.

https://law.ucla.edu/sites/default/files/PDFs/Publications/_RES_PUB_Food%20Law%20at%20the%20Outset%20of%20the%20Trump%20Administration.pdf

409. Flynn D. Trump wants a single federal food safety agency put under USDA. *Food Safety News.* Published June 22, 2018. Accessed January 4, 2021. https://www.foodsafetynews.com/2018/06/president-trump-wants-the-single-federal-food-safety-agency-put-under-usda/

410. Brookings. Tracking deregulation in the Trump era. Published November 12, 2019. Accessed September 3, 2021. https://www.brookings.edu/interactives/tracking-deregulation-in-the-trump-era/

411. United States Environmental Protection Agency. 2019: Year in Review. https://www.epa.gov. Published 2019. https://www.epa.gov/sites/production/files/2020-02/documents/hq_2019_year_in_review.pdf

412. U.S. Department of Agriculture. USDA Announces Proposed Rule to Modernize Swine Inspection. www.usda.gov. Published January 19, 2018. https://www.usda.gov/media/press-releases/2018/01/19/usda-announces-proposed-rule-modernize-swine-inspection

413. Congressional Research Service. *U.S.-EU Trade Agreement Negotiations: Trade in Food and Agricultural Products.* 2020. https://fas.org/sgp/crs/row/R46241.pdf

414. *Trust for America's Health. Ready or Not? Protecting the Public's Health from Disease, Disaster, and Bioterrorism.* 2009. Accessed November 19, 2020. http://healthyamericans.org/report/101/

415. Centers for Disease Control and Prevention. Emergency Kit Preparedness. Published 2020. Accessed January 17, 2021. https://www.cdc.gov/cpr/infographics/00_docs/Emergency-kit-infographic_508.pdf

416. Adelphi University, New York. Poll found Americans are unprepared for disasters. Published October 26, 2012. Accessed January 8, 2021. https://www.adelphi.edu/news/poll-found-americans-are-unprepared-for-disasters/

417. Ready.gov. Build A Kit. Published January 22, 2021. Accessed January 24, 2021. https://www.ready.gov/kit?gclid=Cj0KCQiA3Y-ABhCnARIsAKYDH7vUl6W-Su93n0Bl7riwUhmm8FMwJXaU8E4ODlAUnw-mdM0DdQBquCkaAlEJEALw_wcB#

418. Feeding America. Hunger in America Published 2018. Accessed September 3, 2021. https://www.feedingamerica.org/hunger-in-america

419. United Nations News Service, Relief Web. UN appeals for $10 million to feed refugees in Ethiopia this year. 2004. Accessed November 19, 2020. https://reliefweb.int/report/ethiopia/un-appeals-10-million-feed-refugees-ethiopia-year

420. Walford RL, Harris SB, Gunion MW. The calorically restricted low-fat nutrient-dense diet in Biosphere 2 significantly lowers blood glucose, total leukocyte count, cholesterol, and blood pressure in humans. *Proc Natl Acad Sci.* 1992;89(23):11533-11537.

421. Reiley L. What will the new stimulus package mean for the nearly 50 million food-insecure Americans? *Washington Post.* Accessed September 3, 2021. https://www.washingtonpost.com/business/2020/12/22/coronavirus-stimulus-snap-food-assistance/?wpisrc=nl_sb_smartbrief. Published December 22, 2020.

422. U.S. Department of Agriculture. USDA increases monthly SNAP benefits by 40%. Published April 22, 2020. Accessed September 3, 2021. https://www.usda.gov/media/press-releases/2020/04/22/usda-increases-monthly-snap-benefits-40

423. Federal Registry. *Risk Assessment for Food Terrorism and Other Food Safety Concerns.* 2003. Accessed November 19, 2020. https://www.gpo.gov/fdsys/granule/FR-2003-10-10/03-25850

424. Smith BT, Inglesby TV, O'Toole T. Biodefense R&D: anticipating future threats, establishing a strategic environment. *Biosecur Bioterror.* 2003;1(3):193-202.

425. U.S. Food & Drug Administration. *Chemical and Biological Emergency Response Plan.* Accessed November 19, 2020. http://www.cdc.gov/mmwr/preview/mmwrhtml/rr4904a1.htm

426. U.S. Food & Drug Administration. *The Bioterrorism Act of 2002: Title III. Protecting safety and security of food and drug supply.* Accessed November 19, 2020. https://agr.wa.gov/services/emergency-management/the-bioterrorism-act

427. U.S. Department of Homeland Security. *Ready. Prepare. Plan. Stay Informed.* Accessed November 19, 2020. http://www.ready.gov

428. U.S. Department of Agriculture, Food Safety and Inspection Service. *FSIS Safety and Security Guidelines for the Transportation and Distribution of Meat, Poultry, and Egg Products.* Accessed November 19, 2020. http://www.fsis.usda.gov/oa/topics/transportguide_text_aug.pdf

429. Center for Infectious Disease Research and Policy (CIDRAP) and the Infectious Diseases Society of America. *Anthrax Medical Summary.* Accessed November 19, 2020. http://www.cidrap.umn.edu/infectious-disease-topics/anthrax

430. Whidbey Island Grown Cooperative. About Us. WHIDBEY ISLAND GROWN. Published 2020. Accessed January 9, 2021. https://www.whidbeyislandgrown.com/

431. DiPietro, Gina. *Pitt County Health Department Conducts Mock Bioterrorism Event.* WITN.com. Accessed November 19, 2020. https://wcti12.com/archive/health-dept-training-for-possible-bioterrorism-threat-1

PART VI

Managing Programs

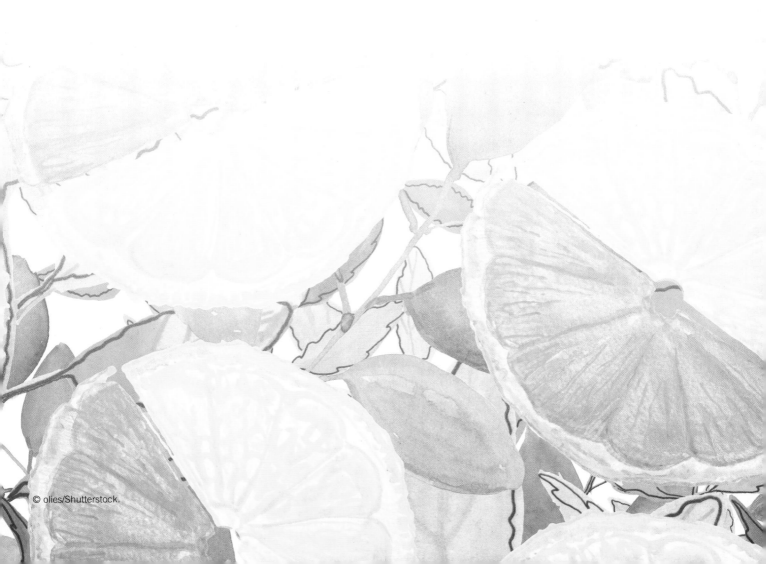

CHAPTER 15

Grant Writing in Community and Public Health Nutrition

Kathleen Cullinen, PhD, RDN

(We would like to acknowledge the work of Elizabeth Barden, PhD, and Katherine Cairns, MPH, MBA, RDN; in past editions of Nutrition in Public Health.)

Learning Outcomes

AFTER STUDYING THIS CHAPTER AND REFLECTING ON THE CONTENTS, YOU SHOULD BE ABLE TO:

1. Discuss the dietitian's/nutritionist's responsibilities in fiscal management.
2. Identify collaborators in fiscal management.
3. Describe the major sources for funding **community** and public health nutrition services.
4. Specify major items in a grant application.
5. List the purposes for which data are needed by nutrition professionals.

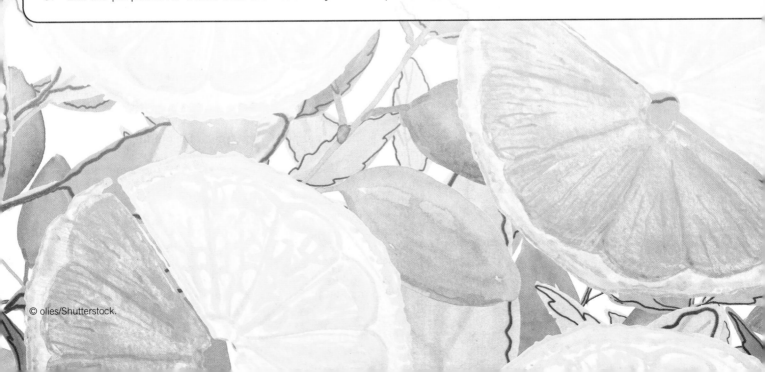

Community A subset of a larger population that is defined on the basis of geographic boundaries, political boundaries, or demographic characteristics.

Introduction: Financing Community and Public Health Nutrition Programs and Services

Providing the community with community and public health nutrition programs that residents need and want requires that the agency allocate dollars to pay personnel salaries, reimburse their travel, buy equipment and supplies, provide for continuing education of nutrition personnel, and purchase other goods needed to deliver services.

The need for accountability and financial transparency are critical for the community and public health manager. Every dietitian/nutritionist who manages a program, service, or project must take responsibility for requesting, justifying, and negotiating a budget and controlling expenditures within the funds that are allocated. Fiscal management means understanding the financing and budgeting process while working closely with the following key people in an organization:

- Department/agency administrator and board members who set the agency's fiscal policy and determine how the agency's budget will be distributed to programs and overhead.
- Finance/fiscal officer or business manager who maintains accounts, controls expenditures, and can provide advice on the organization's written and unwritten fiscal policies and procedures.
- Other program directors who request and manage budgets for programs that should utilize nutrition services. These directors may be convinced to collaborate in funding nutrition services through their internal funding sources or by writing grants for external funding.

As per-capita, inflation-adjusted community and public health spending declines, potentially undermining prevention and weakening responses to health inequalities and new health threats,[1] tighter federal, state, and local government agency budgets require nutritionists to compete for the money they need if they want to turn plans for comprehensive nutrition services into action. Convincing a governmental unit or foundation to invest money and become a stakeholder in nutrition services requires that the value of each proposal be justified with baseline data from different sources, and a work plan for collecting, analyzing, and reporting data to monitor and determine the effectiveness of the services provided. Business planning and compelling answers to the following questions will prepare a nutrition administrator for the competitive public and private funding environment.

- Is there really a community need for the project or service?
- What are the competing options for the available and new money? The plan, budget, service, product, and their evaluation must stand out from the competition.
- Is there a strong and persuasive reason for funding this option over others?
- What support does the competition have for the same funding?
- Does your agency/team have the skills and track record of innovative service and project completion?
- Can cost-effectiveness data be provided for the type of nutrition project or service proposed?
- What stakeholder support and contributions are there for the proposal?
- What additional community support and media attention can be generated prior to, during, and following the funding decisions?

- Are there federal, state, or local requirements/mandates for components of the proposed nutrition project or service?
- What potential does the proposed project or service have to generate income for the agency?
- Are there federal or foundation grants available to establish, maintain, and/or expand the project in the future?
- Is it feasible to implement and maintain the project after external funding ends?

Competitive proposals for spending new or ongoing money must show evidence of support from individuals and organizations in the community who will benefit from the project or service. They can demonstrate their support by paying fees for services; making in-kind contributions of staff, volunteer time, or space in offices or clinics; writing letters of support or collaboration; presenting testimony; lobbying proactively; and donating equipment, materials, or cash contributions.

Interdisciplinary teamwork and networking to increase the number of stakeholders in nutrition programs are discussed in other chapters. Financers prefer to fund a project or service that fits their mission and responds to a demonstrated need that can be met cost effectively. A well-conceived budget for a new project or service details the cost per unit. Projects with high start-up costs should show a reasonable cost per unit after the start-up and within the first six months of operation. Fiscal managers and grant reviewers will ask these questions:

- Will the proposed project or service have a reasonable cost-to-benefit ratio? Funders compare the costs and outcomes of varying types of programming or service delivery options.
- Will the project or service be carried out with the most cost-effective intervention? For example, will reducing anemia in 80% of a **population** group within 6 months of diagnosis be less costly if nutrition counseling is provided by a trained and supervised paraprofessional rather than by a dietitian? Although the outcome may be the same, the costs of different intervention models may vary.

These and additional questions can be used as a checklist in preparing to request the funds needed to initiate the service. Funds for nutrition services may be secured from a variety of sources. The more diversified the funding base, the more stable the program. The more funding sources used to maintain a public health nutrition program, the less dependent the program is on any single source. However, maintaining accountability for too many small funding sources (e.g., $10,000) may be labor intensive or counterproductive.

For grant writing and nutrition program planning and evaluation, all nutrition professionals need to have a basic competence with the acquisition, analysis, and interpretation of diverse types of data from various sources. As with grant writing, this set of skills is particularly important in the current economic climate, where divergent agendas in combination with shrinking resources at times lead to contradictory interpretations of the same data, or at least to differing outlooks on the relative importance of competing priorities. Data are used in many different contexts within nutrition practice. There are at least four dimensions from which data management for nutrition practice can be considered: 1) using data for program planning and conducting needs assessments; 2) using data to assist managerial oversight and to demonstrate the effectiveness of work (program evaluation); 3) using data to monitor a population (nutrition surveillance), define health objectives and

Population All of the inhabitants of a given region (e.g., the U.S. population, or the population of the state of California).

Discussion Prompt

What are some of the health programs in your community that have been funded? What other areas of community health could use funded programs?

Pandemic Learning Opportunities

What did we learn about having extra funding for community food pantries during the COVID-19 pandemic? Were we adequately prepared? Were emergency funds available?

Strategy Tip

Dietitians trained in grant writing can be a great asset to community and public health programs that depend on grant funding for operation.

associated benchmarks (e.g., *Healthy People 2030*[2]), and monitor progress toward meeting those objectives; and 4) collecting and managing new data, and/or accessing existing data sources, to address identified information deficits. This chapter addresses each of these dimensions to give an overview of some of the major issues and processes involved in managing data in a public health nutrition context.

General Revenue

State governments generate funds through state income taxes, sales taxes, various types of business taxes, and taxes on such products as alcoholic beverages and cigarettes. Most recently, taxes on junk food are being explored as an intervention to counter increasing obesity.[3] Several states use lotteries and lawsuit settlement proceeds as revenue for public services. Local government units have the authority to tax property owners for municipal services, such as police and fire departments, schools, recreation, and public health. Tax levies are set annually based on the programs or services needed, the priorities of policymakers, the demands of the taxpayers, and outside interests.

Some local government and many state public health departments derive a portion of their income from general revenue. Public health agencies generally seek a reasonable share of general revenue as a cornerstone of their base income. Usually, there is strong competition for these funds in a health agency because they offer programs some funding stability. However, when governmental entities face increasing economic pressure, the general revenue funds become less stable. If there is no general revenue in the budget for nutrition services, dietitians/nutritionists need to discuss this funding source with agency administrators and business managers to prepare their request for the next budget cycle. Dietitians/nutritionists may need to be persistent and assertive over several years to succeed. Acquiring some funding that is less restrictive to a specific target population provides flexibility to plan more comprehensive, community-responsive programs.

Grants

Federal Grants

A variety of federal funds are used by state, local, and nongovernmental organizations (NGOs) to operate food and nutrition programs. Federal agencies that fund major food/nutrition programs and demonstration projects to over 150 million Americans include:

Request for Proposal (RFP) An invitation to a supplier to bid on supplying products or services that are difficult to describe for a company, or in this example, a public agency.

- The Food and Nutrition Service (FNS) and National Institute of Food and Agriculture (NIFA) of the U.S. Department of Agriculture (USDA) specifically grant funds and innovation grants/contracts
- Centers for Medicare and Medicaid Services (CMS) of the U.S. Department of Health and Human Services (DHHS)
- Centers for Disease Control and Prevention (CDC) of the U.S. Department of Health and Human Services (DHHS)
- Specific health block grant funds from the U.S. Department of Health and Human Services (DHHS)

Personal contacts within each of the major federal or state agencies are useful to obtain advance notice of ***Requests for Proposals*** (RFPs) and special project funding.

State Grants

State departments of health, health and human services, agriculture, and education usually provide some funds for nutrition services. The state funds may support selected statewide and/or local services. In many states, a per capita or pre-established formula is used for allocating state and federal funds to local health agencies. State agencies may have special legislated funding for nutrition programs. State agencies also serve as the conduits for federal funds designated for local program implementation. Specific federal project funds that state that governmental agencies administer through a grants process include:

- Special Supplemental Food Program for Women, Infants and Children (WIC)
- Other supplemental food programs for targeted groups (Farmer's Markets, Senior Food Program, Summer Food Programs, Special Milk Programs, Daycare Programs, School Lunch/Breakfast Programs, Fresh Fruit and Vegetable Program, congregate dining)
- Supplemental Nutrition Assistance Program Education (SNAP-Ed)
- Expanded Food and Nutrition Education Program (EFNEP)
- Nutrition education special projects
- Maternal and child health special projects
- Health promotion special projects
- Chronic disease intervention/reduction special projects
- Targeted agricultural marketing special projects

Each state's grant application procedure has special requirements that need to be determined by consulting the local agency administrator, state agency, or regional/central office nutrition consultants.

Local Grants or Contracts

Local human or social service agencies, home health agencies, area agencies on aging, mental health agencies, developmental disabilities councils, school districts, jails, community colleges, and other governmental units frequently need nutrition services or have special initiatives or ongoing projects that require nutrition expertise. When agencies do not employ a full-time dietitian/ nutritionist on their own staff, they will often contract for these services as the most efficient method for getting the short- or long-term services they need. Those local agencies that need part-time nutrition services frequently maintain lists or files of available contractors and their specialties. It is important to cultivate contacts within the local agencies that can advise on their needs, availability of funding, and interest in developing contracts.

Local voluntary health agencies (e.g., American Heart Association, American Diabetes Association, American Cancer Society, Cystic Fibrosis Association, or March of Dimes chapter or affiliate offices) also may need and contract for nutrition services or offer small competitive project grants. For short-term community projects, funds may be obtained from local businesses, banks, civic organizations, or churches.

Foundation Grants

Millions of dollars of private foundation projects are funded annually for foundation-specific priorities. The Internet and the public library are the most valuable resources for identifying these foundation funders. Foundation and grant information centers maintain information on:

- Names and contact persons for local, state, regional, or national foundations

REQUEST FOR PROPOSAL
SOLICITATION NUMBER: USDA-FS-8-08
AERIAL PHOTOGRAPHY SERVICES
For Arapaho-Roosevelt, NF, CO, White River NF, CO,
Pawnee NGLs & Buffalo NF, WY
Solicitation Issue Date: May 28, 2008
Proposal Due Date: June 27, 2008

U.S. DEPARTMENT OF AGRICULTURE
FARM SERVICE AGENCY
AERIAL PHOTOGRAPHY FIELD OFFICE

NOTICE TO OFFEROR
Any proposal submitted for this RFP must be identified with the following information labeled on the outside of the mailing package:
SOL.NO: USDA-FS-8-08
DUE DATE: 27-JUNE-2008, 4:30 PM
RECEIVING OFFICE: CONTRACTING
Mail To: AERIAL PHOTOGRAPHY FIELD OFFICE
CONTRACTING OFFICER
2222 WEST 2300 SOUTH
SALT LAKE CITY UTAH 84119

NOTICE TO PROSPECTIVE OFFERORS :

OFFERORS ARE CAUTIONED TO NOTE THE FOLLOWING SPECIAL CONTRACT REQUIREMENTS:
Any proposals submitted in response to this solicitation must be presented in two parts, a pricing proposal and a technical proposal. Please limit the size to a maximum of 100 double-sided pages. See Section I. for proposal preparation instructions. (Documentation and samples required in accordance with Attachment A of the contract may be submitted in a separate referenced attachment and will not be counted towards the page limitation).

This solicitation is for direct digital acquisition. (See Section L-3 for Digital Sensor Approval Requirements)

This solicitation includes an option to increase spatial resolution to 30 cm (See Section B-6).

This RFP is subject to the Availability of Funds Clause (FAR 52.232-18). See Section B-1.6, Page 3.

The complete text of any or all clauses referenced herein may be obtained by submitting a request, identifying this solicitation number, to the Contracting Officer, USDA, FSA, Aerial Photography Field Office, 2222 West 2300 South, Salt Lake City, Utah 84119. Complete copies of the FAR in loose-leaf or CFR form may be purchased from the Superintendent of Documents, U.S. Government Printing Office, Washington D.C. 20402.

Requests for Proposals (RFPs) can be found on many governmental websites.

USDA United States Deptartment of Agriculture. https://www.fsa.usda.gov/Internet/FSA_File/usda-fs-8-08_rfp.pdf

Discussion Prompt

Which of these programs utilize dietitians?

- Information on past funding priorities and projects funded
- Dollar amount of awards for foundation projects
- Criteria and format for submitting funding requests
- Timeline for review and award of grant requests

Priorities of foundations may change annually. Putting a new twist on an old idea or need thus may be required for the foundation to consider the proposal. Some foundations prefer that proposals be submitted on behalf of a nongovernmental, nonprofit agency. Dietitians/nutritionists working in a governmental agency who are seeking a foundation grant might collaborate with a nonprofit agency that will submit the proposal and subcontract the nutrition work to the public health agency.

Fee for Services

A fee-for-service adjusted for each target population is a useful method for recovering program costs. A basic market analysis is required to determine the range of fees appropriate to charge the various target populations or program participants. Fees must be based on actual costs, not guesswork. Making a fee-for-service plan more acceptable to clients of a community and public health service is a second task, after calculating actual costs. In presenting a plan to establish fees to administrators, government officials, the public, and coworkers, three alternatives might be offered:

1. **Sliding scale fee-for-service:** The fee is based on the client's ability to pay, with the maximum fee being the actual cost of the service; this can be used for all basic public health services.
2. **Actual cost fee-for-service:** The actual cost of providing a service is calculated and revised annually. It is charged for public health services where there are other private and nonprofit providers of the services within a community. These service charges are not put on a sliding scale because of the potential legal issues of unfair competition by a governmental provider. A public agency will by design have few of these services because of need-based planning.
3. **Cost plus fee-for-service:** This pricing model permits a nonprofit agency to recover the actual cost of a service in addition to a profit, which is then used to subsidize another service within the agency. These "cash cows" may include innovative services or products (healthy cooking demonstrations, diet and fitness classes, customized nutrition services, or educational materials for community organizations), or long-standing, fully capitalized services (laboratory tests).

Third-Party Reimbursement

Third-party reimbursement income is received by billing insurance carriers, such as governmental healthcare programs (Medicaid, Medicare), workers' compensation, health maintenance organizations (HMOs)/managed care organizations (MCOs), and/or other special health insurance pools (catastrophic health, state-sponsored alternative care pools, organized employer groups). Each health carrier has its own billing procedures that the agency's accounting office must determine and continuously keep updated. It is most cost-effective for the agency's accounting department to select the three or four third-party reimbursement sources that cover the majority of the agency's clients and bill these carriers. Clients not covered by those carriers would be treated as fee-for-service clients and advised to collect reimbursement from

---

Strategy Tip

Check www.grantwatch.com for foundation grant opportunities.

Discussion Prompt

Name community and public health programs that are sliding scale, actual cost, and cost-plus fee for service. Does cost choice affect attendance?

their own carrier. Some organizations contract with healthcare reimbursement firms that require an assignment of benefits from all clients and handle all agency billing for a predetermined fee.

With the passage of the Affordable Care Act and the need and demand for population-level disease prevention,[4] emerging opportunities for income generation are developing in the area of third-party reimbursement. Nutrition services are increasingly being reimbursed for preventive services and chronic and acute care interventions. Nutrition and health programs are identifying ways to protect revenue raised from third-party reimbursements to allow a carryover of these funds between fiscal years for program-specific initiatives.

Public Health Department Accreditation

The 2003 *Institute of Medicine* (IOM) report, *The Future of the Public's Health*, called for the establishment of a national Steering Committee to examine the benefits of accrediting governmental public health departments.[5] Launched in 2011, a voluntary national public health department accreditation required a seven-step process in which public health services and systems are charged with producing the evidence needed to address critical uncertainties about how to best organize, finance, and deliver effective public health strategies, including nutrition programs and services, identified by broad cross sections of public health stakeholders.[6] The measurement of health department performance is held against a set of nationally recognized, practice-focused, evidence-based standards with the goal of improving and protecting the health of the public by advancing the quality and performance of tribal, state, local, and territorial public health departments. Many federally funded contractual nutrition services are held to these same standards. Hence, the inclusion of evidence-based nutrition programs or services and sound fiscal and data management practices in grant proposals are more critical than ever for the public health nutritionist seeking competitive federal funding.

Developing Skills in Grant Writing

Although not a typical component of didactic programs in public health nutrition and dietetics, grant-writing skills are valuable assets of nutritionists in public or private practice. In fact, most nutritionists need to become grant writers so that they can obtain outside income to support innovative services, reach new populations, develop and test interventions, and initiate special projects; any or all of these may then turn into long-term, income-producing services. Some grant writing tips are as follows:

- Maintain a grant idea folder in which to file innovative ideas that would require external funding. These can be ideas with a one-paragraph description as contributed by staff members. A community needs assessment (discussed in Chapter 5) will help produce some ideas for needed community programs and services.
- Foster staff development by conducting an internal seed grant program within the section or agency. Allocate a small amount of money each year to this research and development (R&D) fund.
- Find several grant writers and reviewers within the agency with whom to brainstorm ideas and offer advice on writing grant proposals.
- Maintain a large network of project collaborators to work with on grant proposals of mutual interest.
- Identify reliable people and organizations that can be counted on to write letters of support, even on short notice. Some of these

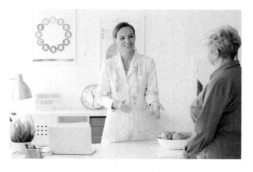

Registered dietitian providing counseling services.

© KatarzynaBialasiewicz/iStock/Getty Images Plus/Getty Images.

individuals/agencies may prefer that the letter of support letter be written for their signature.

- Plan on writing grants that will generate three to four times the dollar amount from the grant as the program is committing.
- Practice writing concisely. If the idea cannot be conveyed in two double-spaced pages, including needs statement, methods, objectives, total funding amount requested, and collaborators, grant writing will be too time-consuming.
- Maintain a file of agency information that can be pulled for grant attachments. Items such as Agency Internal Revenue Tax Exemption 501(c)(3) statements, Indirect Cost Rate Agreement, audited budgets, lists of board members, agency descriptions, federal identification numbers for the agency, and personnel curriculum vitae should be in this file.
- Maintain a file of copies of grants submitted previously.
- Use word processing and spreadsheet software to write the narrative and prepare the budget spreadsheet. This makes it easier to revise the proposal without introducing errors.
- Get on the mailing lists or listservs of every agency and foundation that announces related grant/contract RFPs that can be identified.

Preparing Your Grant Application

Many private foundations have always required a Concept Paper, sometimes referred to as a Letter of Inquiry or a Letter of Intent, to be submitted for review prior to the submission of a full proposal. In recent years, federal and state agencies have also begun to encourage the use of concept papers as a way for applicants to obtain informal feedback on their ideas and projects prior to preparing a proposal. Some of these agencies now require a Concept Paper to be submitted as part of the formal submission process. The purpose of a Concept Paper, from the funding agency's point of view, is to help applicants develop more competitive proposals and to save time by eliminating proposals that are not likely to be funded. The applicant's purpose in developing a Concept Paper is to capture the interest of the funding agency and demonstrate that the idea, project, or program they are proposing is worthy of further consideration via invitation for a complete grant proposal.

Concept Paper

Unless otherwise specified by the funding agency, ideally, your Concept Paper should be limited to three (3) pages (two-page narrative, one-page budget) not including references, with 1" margins and 12-point font. Sections may be single spaced with a double space between sections. The sections of the Concept Paper should be identical to those of the full proposal with the use of section headers to improve the clarity of presentation. Place the name or your organization in the header.

Generally, a Concept Paper describes your idea, the need for your project, how it is to be implemented, and a budget. A Concept Paper is still a funding proposal, so just think of it as a mini funding proposal. Use clear and concise language to best communicate your idea and remember that this is an overview or outline form of your overall project. Avoid vague language and be positive and definite. For example, instead of saying an objective "may be accomplished," indicate that the objective "will be accomplished" by a certain time. Avoid requesting money for "planning" unless that is the purpose of the funding program or a necessary post-award step. Most funding agencies want to fund a project that is beyond early stages of planning. Each section of your narrative for the Concept Paper as well as your full proposal must address the following components:

Project Title

Your project title should be clear and concise and directly reflect the overall content of your proposed project.

Purpose of the Project

This section succinctly describes the purpose, importance, timeliness, and innovation of your project. The relevance and applicability of your project to the sponsor's or funding agency's priorities should also be stated clearly. It concludes with a statement of benefits (or anticipated outcomes) along with a description of who will benefit and how.

Timeframe

Indicate the timeframe (beginning and end) of your project in months and years.

Background and Significance

This section outlines what other public health professionals have published about the general topic and focuses on the gap in knowledge to be filled, the problem to be solved, or the need to be addressed by your proposed project. Supporting statistical data may be included in this section but should be brief. The full proposal requires a more detailed needs assessment described in Chapter 5. Similar to a literature review, this section allows you to state the purpose or need in such a way that your project is the best possible solution to the problem. It provides a statement addressing the significance of the project (showing why the project should be supported) by addressing the unique, unusual, distinctive, innovative, and/or novel aspects of your approach.

Environment and Relevant Experience

List in this section the significant facilities and equipment available for your project, plus information on key personnel and their previous relevant experience. Establish your and/or your agency's credibility. Now convince the funder that you are worthy of their trust—and their money. This may be accomplished by several means. For example, mentioning your and/or your agency's grants track record, naming your agency's board of directors, briefly offering evidence of fiscal stability, or describing ongoing programs. If you are a new organization, or if this is your first project, this can be difficult. You will increase your chances for funding if you partner with relevant experts and/or agencies in your proposed field of study.

Goal(s) and SMART Objectives

The overall goal(s) of your project should be stated succinctly. Objectives must be SMART and should be listed briefly and clearly in a prioritized order. SMART objectives are as follows:

- **S**pecific – target a specific area for improvement
- **M**easurable – quantify or at least suggest an indicator of progress
- **A**ttainable – assuring that an end can be achieved
- **R**elevant – is/are the right objective(s) at the right time for you and/or your agency
- **T**ime-related – specify when the result(s) can be achieved

A goal is an abstract state of being, a condition, an end, or an aspiration while objectives are statements of measurable outcomes that, collectively, will help you measure progress toward your overall goal(s) within the timeframe of your project. Well-written objectives always contain statements that express a quantified result expected within a stated timeframe. For example, a physical activity promotion program at a local hospital could have the following objective: "By June 2023, 45% (up from 20% in January 2021) of County Hospital employees will engage in 150 minutes of moderate-intensity aerobic physical activity (such as brisk walking or tennis) each week."

Sample or Target Population

Briefly describe the sample or who will be participating in your project (e.g., demographics, occupation, geographic location, etc.). In other words, how can you describe the population(s) participating in your project?

Methods or Approach

In this section, you will describe how your project will be conducted and evaluated. It provides an overview of the methodology or approach you will use in your project (sometimes called project activities or work plan). Your methods (or activities) must be appropriate to accomplish your goals and SMART objectives. The methods or activities will need to be congruent with or based on what has been tried in the field in the past. In other words, they must be based on empirical evidence, and they will need to be both reasonable in cost and complexity and accomplishable within your proposed timeframe. In your full proposal, a detailed work plan with timelines, activities, and indicators (i.e., evidence of deliverables including evaluation results that will be reported) is a recommended method for presenting your overall project, and a requirement by some funding agencies. Typically, there are four phases in the post-award period that should be addressed in your work plan: 1) planning; 2) implementation; 3) monitoring and evaluation; and 4) sustainability and/or scaling. In addition to outcome evaluation, process evaluation must be conducted throughout the funding period to ensure *fidelity* in the delivery of the intervention(s) and to make documented project changes as necessary (and with IRB approval when applicable), in order to ensure that the project is on target to meet its overall goals and SMART objectives. A template for a 1-year work plan is provided later in this Chapter.

Budget

Finally, your Concept Paper as well as your full proposal must include your proposed budget. Your proposed budget is used to consider the costs of implementing a successful project. Once your project is clearly outlined, the next question is, "What will your project cost?" Consider all project activities and associated costs (e.g., mailing materials, purchasing supplies, etc.). Only major category totals need to be listed in the budget summary in the Concept Paper. A more detailed budget with expenditures by line item in each major category is required for your full proposal. Cost-sharing contributions, if any, and indirect costs, also known as Facilities and Administrative (F&A) costs, must be itemized. Sample templates for your budget summary for your Concept Paper and an *annotated budget* for your full proposal appear below in **Table 15–1** and **Table 15–2** respectively.

Grant expenditures must be monitored in real-time or at any time point or frequency during the grant award period. The frequency of reporting and/or billing (if a reimbursement grant) will be dependent upon the requirements

TABLE 15–1
Budget Summary for Concept Paper (one-page limit)

Project Title

Project Timeline (MM/DD/YEAR –MM/DD/YEAR)

CATEGORY	AMOUNT
Personnel	
Fringe benefits @48.9%	
Travel	
Equipment	
Supplies	
Consultants	
Contracts (if applicable)	
Other (e.g., Data and Survey Analyses, etc.)	
TOTAL DIRECT COSTS	
Indirect @26%[1]	
Based on $_____ [2]	
TOTAL (DIRECT + INDIRECT)	

[1]There may be a negotiated administrative overhead charge included as a percentage of each budget for overall agency indirect costs.

[2]Indirect cost rates are not based on equipment or contracts (if applicable). Therefore, subtract these costs from your total direct costs before calculating your indirect cost (based on 26% in the template above).

TABLE 15–2
Annotated Budget for Full Proposal

Project Title

Project Timeline (MM/DD/YEAR –MM/DD/YEAR)

CATEGORY	AMOUNT
Personnel	
Full-time (specify FTEs)	
Part-time (specify FTEs)	
Fringe Benefits @48.9%	
Mileage for local travel	
Other travel	
Phone fees: local, long-distance, cell	
Internet and technology allocation	
Postage	
Film/video reproduction	
Printing	
Supplies	
Office	
Food for demonstrations/clients	
Books, other educational materials	
Subscriptions	
Software	
Space, rental allocation	
Equipment rental/allocation[1]	
Copy machines	
Computers	
Telephones	
Video	
Equipment, purchase[2]	
Computer/other hardware	
Other office equipment	
Utilities, actual/allocation	

Staff training and continuing education	
Out-of-town travel	
Lodging	
Registration fees	
Registrations, local	
Memberships	
Other	
Central service charge[3]	
Consultant fees[4]	
Student stipends[5]	
Contingent reserve fund[6]	
TOTAL DIRECT COSTS	
Indirect @26%[7]	
Based on $_____[8]	
TOTAL (DIRECT + INDIRECT)	

[1]Carefully evaluate the rent vs. buy decision on all equipment.

[2]It is important to plan for lifecycle replacement of equipment in each annual budget.

[3]Additional overhead may be charged by the county/city/state to cover the costs of attorneys, accountants, executive directors, and central purchasing that provide service but are outside of the nutrition or health department.

[4]Include fees for graphic consultants, contract professional/technical assistance, external evaluation specialists, and auditor fees for federal funds received. Contract physician fees for grants/third-party reimbursement requirements, especially if third-party reimbursement will cover the costs and result in nutrition reimbursement.

[5]Try to build in student stipends for internships if quality supervision can be provided for the students.

[6]A carryover fund for emergencies, reimbursed initiatives.

[7]There may be a negotiated administrative overhead charge included as a percentage of each budget for overall agency indirect costs.

[8]Indirect cost rates are not based on equipment or contracts (if applicable). Therefore, subtract these costs from your total direct costs before calculating your indirect cost (based on 26% in the template above).

and specifications of the funding agency. A computer spreadsheet is a clear, time-saving tool for preparing the budget summary as well as **annotated budget**. There are many fine financial software or grant management packages available. Most governmental agencies will require their grantees to use their purchased financial software.

Annotated budget A budget with critical or explanatory notes.

Data in Grant Writing for Program Planning and Evaluation

In grant writing, it is essential for nutrition professionals to have a basic competence with the acquisition, analysis, and interpretation of diverse types of data from various sources. Funding is driven by the ability to demonstrate the need for nutrition programming via a needs-assessment, as well as the demonstrated ability to collect, analyze, and interpret data in the design, management, and evaluation of nutrition programming to determine effectiveness.

Data can be defined broadly as information, especially information organized for analysis and decision making.[7] *Data* include, but are not confined to, statistics, which is the branch of mathematics dealing with the collection, analysis, interpretation, and presentation of numerical data.[8] Objective, statistical data (e.g., a community's leading cause of death or per-capita healthcare costs for obesity-related illness) certainly are useful for quantifying and comparing the size of need, degree of achievement toward meeting goals, and costs in relation to accomplishment. However, additional types of data, including subjective information (e.g., a community's perceived needs) are important in accurately characterizing a population and its health service requirements. The definition of what constitutes relevant data to a public health nutrition professional has expanded as the availability of information on all facets of life has become easily accessible. For instance, census data about the presence of a telephone in the household or mobile phone use at first glance may not appear to be relevant nutrition data. However, it is a pertinent factor to know for a nutritionist who is planning a telephone survey in a given neighborhood, where they need to obtain a representative sample of residents, or for a nutritionist who is planning services that include follow-up phone counseling and/or text messaging.

An effective, successful nutrition program is achieved by following a conscientious planning process that justifies its need, inventories available resources and identifies service gaps, identifies relevant goals and SMART objectives, defines tasks and activities to accomplish those goals, and explains how results will be evaluated and disseminated.[9] Data are used during every phase of the grant writing and program planning process to achieve the following outcomes:

- Identify the need for new projects or initiatives
- Recognize the need for changes in program delivery
- Prioritize competing health problems
- Identify the most appropriate at-risk target population
- Define goals and SMART objectives
- Make decisions about allocating limited resources
- Define program performance expectations
- Justify a program's budget
- Develop additional proposals to secure additional funding when necessary

Needs assessment is the portion of the planning process during which a community and its particular health needs are defined. Overall, the needs-assessment phase of the grant writing and program planning process aims to understand the nutrition requirements of the community, prioritize their identified needs, and target resources accordingly and in direct alignment with the specifications of the funding opportunity. Chapter 5 discusses the topic of needs-assessment in detail.

Identifying a specific population with specific health and nutritional status challenges and identifying gaps in existing programs or service delivery is accomplished through close examination of both quantitative and qualitative data. A quantitative assessment includes examination of demographic, socioeconomic, health status, nutritional status, and risk indicators. Data for this assessment come from a review of both regularly published public health reports and scientific research literature that are relevant to the health problem and/or the community. Qualitative methods, such as key informant interviews, focus groups, and informal conversations, derive information from health professionals, community leaders, and community members at-large regarding the community's perceived needs and demands for nutrition-related services. The more subjective information obtained from these sources is necessary to balance the more objective, statistics-driven information that comes from the quantitative assessment; both provide important pieces to the big picture. The needs assessment methodology also includes the compilation of an inventory of existing health and nutrition resources in the community and any major duplication or gaps in available services, as well as program delivery and resource utilization data. A final piece is an assessment by the program planner of the host organization's (usually his or her employer's) mission and willingness to support a proposal for a needs-based nutrition project or program, both financially and institutionally.

Typically, objective quantitative data are used in grant writing and nutrition program planning to address four questions:

1. **What** are the health issues facing a community (problem)?
2. **Where** are the problems (place)?
3. **Who** is at risk (person)?
4. **When** are problems increasing or declining over time (time period)?

Accessing Existing Data Sources

There are many different sources for quantitative, community-level, population-based data on a wide variety of topics. Which types of data and which sources will be used is a matter of strategic choice. Some possible sources include, but are not limited to, population data (e.g., U.S. Census or NHANES), program data (e.g., the WIC program or Head Start), trend data, national objectives (e.g., HP 2030), and cost data. Frequently, national **surveillance** data are also available at the state level, either from the national agency that operates the system or from the state department that submits the data to the national system. All of the online data sources are too numerous to mention. Partners in Information Access for the Public Health Workforce (https://phpartners.org/ph_public/) is a "gateway" to global, national, state, and local public health data tools and statistics from a collaboration of U.S. government agencies, public health organizations and health sciences libraries (https://phpartners.org/ph_public/health_stats), as well as grants and funding opportunities (https://phpartners.org/ph_public/topic/grants). Other sources may be readily located using a web search engine. Many online data sources offer the options of viewing predefined reports or generating custom tables and graphs with data obtained through searches and queries of summary and micro data files. Websites should be visited frequently, because many are constantly in the process of adding new or updated material.

It is important to pay close attention to the data source attribution when using a secondary data source (i.e., data from an agency that is presenting information that its own staff did not collect). For instance, the U.S. Census Bureau is a primary data source because it publishes data collected only by that agency. Community Commons (http://www.communitycommons.org/), on the other hand, utilizes many global, national, state, and local data sources in producing its reports but does not collect its own original data, making it a secondary data source. Failure to note the data's point of origin could result in a program planner collecting data from multiple sources that actually are duplicative rather than complimentary. It is critical to note the time period represented by the data, as well as operational definitions for all measures and technical terms used.

Surveillance The continual, systematic collection of data, as well as its timely interpretation regarding the current and changing condition of a population.

Problem

Planning often begins with an examination of which health and nutrition issues affect a community. An inventory of the leading causes of morbidity and mortality, the prevalence of chronic and infectious diseases, and the leading causes of hospitalization can give a broad overview of the health concerns of the community. These types of data typically are found in regularly published public health reports, such as state or national vital statistics reports and surveillance system reports.

Place

Place describes geographic units, such as the nation, state, county, clinic, region, or neighborhood. Examination of data by place helps to ascertain the geographic extent of the health problem. Maps are an effective way to visually represent differences in health status data by geographic area. Additionally, maps are useful for illustrating disparities in health status among communities that may be segregated in large part on the basis of certain socioeconomic characteristics, such as ethnicity or income. Use of maps to depict the geographic distribution of health problems and suspected factors in the causal pathway can be very effective in attracting the attention of key stakeholders.[10] Maps that include health, social, economic, policy, environmental, and other asset data are relatively easy to construct now that geographic mapping technology is widely available. Community Commons (http://www.communitycommons.org/) offers the ability to make Geographic Information System (GIS) maps and generate indicator reports by accessing more than 10,000 GIS data layers at multiple levels of geography, including state, county, zip code, tract, block group, block, and point levels.

Person

An accurate characterization of *person* is necessary because different groups within a larger population have different health problems and different service requirements. Person may be described in many different ways. The words *population* and *community* are sometimes used interchangeably. Most often, though, population refers to all of the inhabitants of a given region (e.g., the U.S. population, or the population of the state of California). Community, on the other hand, is usually a subset of a larger population that is defined on the basis of geographic boundaries, political boundaries, or demographic characteristics.[11] Another way that communities are defined for planning purposes is on the basis of place of residence, occupation, or other shared personal characteristics; membership in a particular institutional setting; or the clientele of a service-delivery organization. **Table 15–3** presents some examples of different ways a community unit may be conceptualized. For instance, a demographically defined community may be described on the basis of age (e.g., preschoolers or senior citizens), gender, ethnicity, income bracket, occupation, or neighborhood (e.g., residents of Center City, Philadelphia, or San Francisco's Chinatown). More commonly, some combination of factors is used to further aggregate individuals by characteristics that may be associated with some known risk,[12] such as defining a community of teenage mothers who have not graduated from high school and who live in a particular state, or a community of housebound elderly Asian American immigrants living in Chicago. Based on your needs-assessment in the proposal planning process (Chapter 5), a clear, specific definition of the community or target audience that you are proposing your nutrition programming for facilitates program design, intervention, and evaluation.

TABLE 15-3
Different Ways of Defining the Community

Basis of Community	Examples
Geographic (may also be a political unit)	town, city, or state county housing complex school district village or neighborhood zip code area
Setting-based	elementary school community group corporate workplace hospital university church YMCA
Occupational or personal characteristics	physicians, nurses, or dentists immigrants ballet dancers vegans marathon runners
Service delivery-based	patients in a private medical practice patients in a community health center Visiting Nurse Association (VNA) clients Meals on Wheels clients WIC participants

Time Period

It is important to use data to identify changes in health problems over time. This is relevant to establishing whether existing problems have receded or intensified as well as identifying emerging health problems or an increase in disease prevalence among affected groups who were not previously recognized as being at risk. This is often accomplished through the use of trend charts. *Trends* are annual rates reported over a period of time, usually in terms of years. Interpretation of **trends** involves examination of similarities and differences among various parameters. For instance, an investigator may initially examine the pattern of change over time to see whether a problem is increasing or decreasing. More refined analyses may include comparison of one time period to another, a comparison of time series trends in different geographic areas or among different populations, or a comparison of trends among high-risk groups relative to the general population. Often, trend charts concisely present several aspects of data that allow for multiple interpretations. For example, from 1980 to 2014, **Figure 15-1** demonstrates a near doubling of the incidence of diagnosed diabetes in adults aged 65–79 years from 6.9 to 12.1 per 1,000. In adults aged 45–64 years, incidence of diagnosed diabetes showed no consistent change during the 1980s, increased from 1991–2002, and leveled off from 2002–2014. Among adults aged 18–44 years, incidence increased significantly from 1980–2003, showed little change from 2003–2006, then significantly decreased from 2006–2014. The inclusion of additional years of data going forward is necessary to confirm what appears to be a promising trend among persons aged 18—64 years as well as the discouraging upward trend among older adults.

Trends Annual rates reported over a period of time, usually in terms of years.

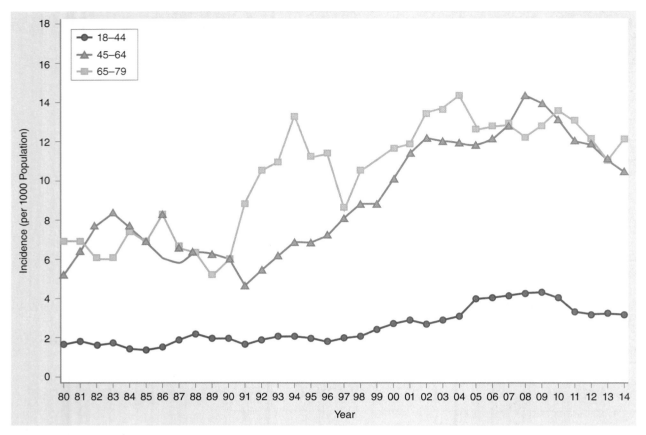

FIGURE 15–1   Incidence of Diagnosed Diabetes per 1,000 Population Aged 18–79 Years, by Age, United States, 1980–2014.

Data from Centers for Disease Control and Prevention (CDC), National Center for Health Statistics, Division of Health Interview Statistics, data from the National Health Interview Survey. Data computed by personnel in the Division of Diabetes Translation, National Center for Chronic Disease Prevention and Health Promotion, CDC. Accessed January 10, 2015. Available at http://www.cdc.gov/diabetes/statistics/incidence/fig3.htm

Data-Driven Program Planning

It is the analysis of the relationship between the parameters of problem, place, person, and time that allows the program planner to draw conclusions about which priority issue should be addressed within which community. Different data elements should be used in combination to more fully characterize the big picture and to help narrow down a target audience for intervention. Data on the leading causes of death in the United States (https://www.cdc.gov /nchs/fastats/leading-causes-of-death.htm) is an example of how important health issues can be identified. That information by itself is not enough for program planning, however, unless the program planner is going to tackle one of the top leading causes of death within the entire U.S. population as the target community! Almost always, the scope of such a project would not be feasible; more commonly, programs are implemented on a much smaller scale. Therefore, it is necessary to narrow the focus. The same data can be ranked by age, gender, race/ethnicity and by geographic location at the state, county, zip code, tract, block group, block, and point-levels (http://www.communitycommons.org/) to help determine the specific priority population(s) or target audience(s) for program planning and funding requests, if the public health nutritionist or the funding agency would like this issue addressed. Reducing the leading cause of death within a target population is an example of a long-term outcome, and the outcome evaluation of the program's effectiveness could not commence for more than 60 years! As a result, many funding agencies may specify a target population and/or require a specific program or intervention that is focused on short- or medium-term outcomes such as increasing fruit and vegetable intake, increasing physical activity, and/or decreasing BMI, as examples, within a specific funding cycle. On the other hand, many grant opportunities, such as those funded by the National Institutes of Health (https://www.nih.gov/), solicit grant proposals with significant and innovative approaches to address need-based outcomes proposed by the nutrition researcher. This is more common in academic institutions than community-based organizations although academic collaboration with community-based organizations to conduct research with populations at high risk for disease is more of a rule than an exception (i.e., community-based participatory research). Federal policy for the protection of human subjects is discussed later in this chapter.

Prioritizing Health Needs

The process of using a range of methods and integrating multiple sources of data to gain a more complete picture of relevant health issues, potential solutions, and effective program evaluation is known as **triangulation**.[13] This technique improves the validity of assessments by reducing biases inherent in the reliance on any single data source or approach.[14] The analysis of health data that is used to derive a list of priority issues for a given community, in order to select a focus of intervention, is based on many sources of information. It is a subjective process to rank the issues based on data collected from the quantitative health assessment, the literature review, and the qualitative sources such as key informant interviews and focus groups. The process is also tempered by the constraints of staff, money, time, community acceptability, and political feasibility; it is because of these factors that resources need to be identified early in the grant planning process, so that realistic and achievable priorities can be established. For example, a publicly funded community health center, with one nutritionist and a limited budget, would likely prioritize local health issues for its program planning differently from would a well-endowed private charitable trust would do, with a charter to focus exclusively on perinatal health. Analysis of published statistics is important, but it is equally important to recognize how things work in the real world. What makes sense theoretically (based on how things look on paper) needs to be balanced with how things work in practice.

For this reason, when preparing a grant proposal and planning a public health nutrition program, it is essential to consider other sources of information than just the results of demographic, socioeconomic, and health risk assessment analyses. It is crucial to speak with key informants to learn their perspectives on where critical needs lie, and on what types of programming might be acceptable to, and be effective with, the chosen target audience. Key informants usually include a combination of the following: subject matter experts, such as local providers (e.g., physicians, nurses, WIC nutritionists, nutrition extension service staff); academics; voluntary health association and professional association spokespeople (e.g., the Academy of Nutrition and Dietetics, the March of Dimes, the American Academy of Pediatrics); community leaders (e.g., elected officials, clergy, venerated elders, school officials); and the constituents themselves, in order to learn what their values and health expectations are. It is important to directly hear the voice of the intended target audience, as their perceived needs and interests may or may not converge with the prioritized needs identified during the quantitative health assessment analysis. To ensure that an audience is receptive, information

Triangulation The process of using a range of methods and integrating multiple sources of data to gain a more complete picture of relevant health issues, potential solutions, and effective program evaluation.

regarding acceptability, appropriateness, and usefulness of planned interventions is a must. Sometimes a community will accept a health program for which there is little community demand (but a quantitatively demonstrated need) when it dovetails with something that is highly desired. For instance, when Supplemental Nutrition Assistance Program Education (SNAP-Ed) was integrated into English as a Second Language (ESL) classes taught at a worksite-training program for recently resettled refugees, a hard-to-reach eligible population was reached. In that way, the target audience received a highly desired product, and the nutritionists were able to convey their education messages simultaneously.[15]

To enhance decision making when prioritizing health needs, objective and subjective data provide the explicit informational criteria upon which the decisions are based. Objective data are often presented using descriptive statistics, such as frequency, mean (a measure of central tendency), and variance and standard deviation (measures of dispersion). These basic statistics can be used to communicate information simply and can be readily computed.[16]

Sample criteria for decision making include the number of persons affected, disease severity, the magnitude of the effects of the problem on quality of life, public perception of the seriousness or changeability of a problem, available resources (including funding, personnel, and redundancy), the political feasibility of intervention, legal mandates, community acceptability, and indicators of organizational support. Criteria should be clearly stated, understood, and agreed upon by those involved in the decision-making process. Assurances should be made that each alternative will be assessed consistently.

Development of grant proposals to secure funds for current or future programming is achieved through a similar examination of data and consideration of priorities and interventions as the process just described. A successful grant proposal (or project proposal) demonstrates health disparities among a particular target audience who are amenable to change through the proposed intervention, so that funders are convinced of the need for action as well as the likelihood that the proposed intervention can meet its stated goals.

Data in Program Management and Evaluation

Evaluation is a core function within program management. The primary purposes of evaluation are to guide program managers and staff members in deciding whether to change or continue a program or specific activities within a program, allow program managers to assess the outcomes of the program on clients' health, and demonstrate to funding sources that their money is being used efficiently and effectively. In the context of program evaluation, data may be used for quality assurance; evaluation of specific initiatives; monitoring of statewide or national data for trends; measurement of progress toward meeting goals and objectives; and assessment of the impact of programs on health outcomes, morbidity, and mortality.[17]

Once a priority health issue and a target community have been selected with interventions appropriate for the target audience and program delivery setting(s), appropriate intervention goals and SMART objectives have been developed (discussed earlier in this chapter); the next phase in the grant-writing process is the development of an evaluation plan. The evaluation process is integrally dependent on quality data that are collected as part of program operations. It is necessary to decide during the planning stage what elements of the program will be evaluated (i.e., how many client visits were scheduled? When were they scheduled? Who did what activities? Were the actual participants members of the expected target audience? At what cost were the activities delivered? What changes occurred among individuals?). This ensures that the appropriate data will be collected during program implementation, provides ongoing management feedback about how the program is being administered, and allows for outcome assessment once the program has ended (or at some regular interval). If evaluation is not considered until after a program has ended, it is unlikely that the required data will be available. For example, consider an 8-week nutrition education lecture series for elderly adults planned at a local community center. Planning to use something as simple as a weekly sign-in sheet would allow the nutritionist to be able to monitor attendance as the course proceeds (which may show whether interest is increasing or decreasing) and demonstrate, at the course's completion, how many persons actually were served. Collecting additional information on the sheet (such as gender or age) would provide additional information about who attended for comparison to the expected target audience's characteristics. If the actual participants differed from the expected target audience (e.g., if the majority of attendees were <65 years old), the evaluation process would have illustrated that the needs of the intended target audience were not being met by the program as currently designed, even if the number of participants met the number expected.

Data collected through the course of program evaluation may also be used for program advocacy. In this instance, the data are used to highlight the need for services and to promote visibility for specific aspects of services and for the program as a whole. In addition, data regarding the number of clients served and achievements in meeting goals and objectives are often used to positively reflect on a program and justify requests for future funding and other types of support.

Nutrition Monitoring and Surveillance

Nutrition monitoring refers to the ongoing description of nutrition conditions in the population, especially among high-risk groups, for the purposes of planning and evaluation.[18] Nutrition monitoring includes ongoing nutrition surveillance systems as well as periodic nutrition surveys. Both are used to monitor trends and patterns among key indicators of nutritional status, with the goals of identifying existing and emerging needs, targeting and developing appropriate nutrition interventions, and determining public policies. *Surveillance* refers to the continuous, systematic collection of data, as well as its timely interpretation regarding the current and changing condition of a population, and the dissemination of those results to those in a position to act on them.[19] The definition of *population* varies according to the specific aims of a given surveillance system; often, nutrition surveillance activities are designed to document the status of nutritionally vulnerable groups, particularly where data are lacking. Then, the data can be used to assess the unmet needs of these groups (e.g., pregnant women, children, the homeless, or the elderly). As previously mentioned, Partners in Information Access for the Public Health Workforce (https://phpartners.org/ph_public/) is a "gateway" to global, national, state, and local public health data tools and statistics, including surveillance data, from a collaboration of U.S. government agencies, public health organizations, and health science libraries (https://phpartners .org/ph_public/health_stats).

Common nutrition-monitoring data elements include nutritional status indicators for pregnant women, infants, children, school-aged children, or elderly adults. These may include food and nutrient consumption data;

knowledge, attitude, and behavior assessments; nutrition program or service utilization, service delivery, and access to care information; and food supply and food access indicators, in order to address issues such as food security and hunger. In the context of evaluation planning in the grant-writing process for nutrition programs, various nutrition surveillance elements may be relevant to define target population characteristics or to demonstrate a health need. In addition, program-specific data can be assessed for monitoring progress toward goals by using surveillance data as a benchmark for comparison.

Protection of Human Subjects

Over the course of the last century, guidelines and regulations have evolved regarding the protection of human subjects in reaction to public and scientific outcry over cases of gross human injustice in human experimentation. And, although typically engaged in program evaluation vs. research, public heath nutritionists must always thoroughly ensure the protection of human subjects or participants in their projects, programming, and in their grant proposals.

The Belmont Report, written in 1979 by the National Commission for the Protection of Human Subjects of Biomedical and Behavioral Research, has heavily influenced the current U.S. system of protection for Human Subjects.[20] In 1981, the Belmont Report, outlining the basic ethical principles in research involving human subjects, drove the revision of the human subjects regulations of the U.S. Department of Health & Human Services and the U.S. Food and Drug Administration to make them as compatible as possible. In 1991, The "Common Rule" or the Federal Policy for the Protection of Human Subjects was published and codified in separate regulations by 15 federal departments and agencies.[21]

Institutional Review Board (IRB) Also known as an independent ethics committee, ethical review board, or research ethics board, an IRB is a committee that has been formally designated to approve, monitor, and review biomedical and behavioral research involving humans.

An **Institutional Review Board (IRB)**, also known as an independent ethics committee, ethical review board, or research ethics board, is a committee that has been formally designated to approve, monitor, and review biomedical and behavioral research involving humans. For all participating academic or community-based organizations, the Common Rule outlines the basic provisions for IRBs, noncoercive or informed consent, and Assurances of Compliance.

In all aspects of public health research or programming, it is critical that researchers and practitioners avoid misrepresentation to human subjects or program participants. Three ethical principles of respect, beneficence, and justice require full and comprehensive disclosure to participants; informed consent; autonomous right of free choice, including the right to terminate participation without penalty; confidentiality; protection of privacy; and equity in participant selection. A public health research project or program should be immediately terminated if, at any point, the data warrant such action. Nutritionists should consult their funding agency for guidance, as well as the academic IRB that they may be proposing to collaborate with to conduct population- or community-based participatory research or programming.

Data Compilation

Data Requirements, Collection, and Management

The recent expansion in data accessibility at the federal, state, and local levels allows nutrition professionals to be more specific in their planning, which increases the likelihood that a true health need will be addressed by nutrition programming and that such efforts will result in a positive change in nutritional status and health for the intended target audience. However, because of the plethora of available data, it is more important than ever to carefully plan for data requirements prior to data retrieval and/or initiation of data collection. Failure to do so can result in a nutritionist becoming mired in data that do not contribute to the primary purpose of the data collection, whether it is for a community profile/needs assessment (Chapter 5), program evaluation, or grant development. Additionally, a nutritionist could end up wasting time and money collecting redundant data that are already available.

The proposed methods or approach that you will employ to achieve your goals and SMART objectives must be included in your grant proposal in the form of a detailed implementation and evaluation plan, also referred to as a work plan. As discussed earlier in this chapter, a detailed work plan with timelines, activities, and indicators (i.e., evidence of deliverables including evaluation results that will be reported) is a recommended method for presenting your overall project, and a requirement by some funding agencies. A template for a work plan to detail the activities, indicators, and timelines for the typical four phases of a project (i.e., planning; implementation; monitoring and evaluation; sustainability and/or scaling) is presented in **Table 15–4** below.

Below are some questions you might ask yourself to ensure that your proposed methods or approach will be able to assess whether or not you will be able to meet your SMART objectives during and after your grant funding cycle.

- Are you employing an evidence-based curriculum or intervention?
- Are the lessons or project activities designed to achieve your SMART objectives?
- How will you ensure that the lessons or project activities will be delivered or implemented with **fidelity** (i.e., delivered as intended)?
- Have you identified valid and reliable evaluation tool(s) or survey(s) to collect short-, medium-, and/or long-term outcomes (e.g., individual knowledge, attitudes, beliefs, behaviors,

Fidelity Assurance that a project or program is implemented or delivered as planned or as designed.

TABLE 15–4
One-Year Work Plan (May 2022–April 2023)

Title of Proposed Project:

Goal(s):

SMART Objective #1:

SMART Objective #2:

Phase of Project	Activities	Indicators	m	j	j	a	s	o	n	d	j	f	m	a
			\multicolumn{12}{} 12-Month Timeframe (Note X for applicable months)											
Planning														
Implementation														
Monitoring and Evaluation														
Sustainability and Scaling														

and/or organizational adoption, implementation and effectiveness of policy, systems, and environmental change)?

• How will the intervention effects be maintained in your target audience and/or target settings over time or after the grant funding has ended?

When available, it is most cost-effective and efficient to use a validated and reliable instrument for evaluating the outcomes of your project. If such an instrument (e.g., survey or questionnaire) is not available, great care must be taken in designing a new instrument to ensure that valid and reliable data may be collected, analyzed, and reported on. For instance, prior to designing a new questionnaire, a program planner should know what problem they are trying to solve, what new information must be acquired to solve it, and who the target population is for the survey. By specifying exactly what one needs to know, the planner can limit the questionnaire to only critical fields and eliminate the collection of potentially interesting but unusable information, thereby reducing the response burden, cost, and processing time. Often, existing monitoring and surveillance systems already may have collected the desired information. If the nutrition program planner does not know what is being searched for, it is necessary to stop and reconsider why a data collection process is being considered in the first place. It is never good practice to collect data on myriad topics and hope that something useful and informative will emerge.

Others who lack those types of skills or who do not have the necessary computer hardware, data collection, and statistical software (and associated technical support) may be better off working from summary statistics in published reports or from third-party summary data sources to report on the outcomes of a funded project. If it is determined that the required data are nonexistent for a given population and a new questionnaire must be implemented, it can be extremely valuable to borrow questions from existing questionnaires. There are at least two advantages to this approach: 1) the data collected locally can be compared with data collected by the original investigators from a larger population (or a population that differs in some other respect, such as income or education); and 2) the existing questionnaire may have been formally validated. The choice of whether to use existing data or to collect new data is also dependent upon the anticipated survey sample size and the method of survey administration (telephone survey, face-to-face interview, web-based survey, mailed survey, etc.)

Final data collection procedural issues to consider include planning for data processing and database management, and deciding when and how results will be presented and disseminated. Although the nutrition program planner may not perform all of these functions, they need to be familiar with them in order to provide managerial oversight. The decision of how results will be presented (particularly with respect to content) can save a lot of time during data analysis by preventing superfluous data analyses or unnecessary formatting of results that are not intended to be used or reported to the funding agency. If results are intended for dissemination via professional forums and refereed journals, as many funding agencies require, perhaps a more polished document with summary results and interpretation highlighted will be prepared.

Prior to Submitting Your Grant Proposal

To help avoid an unsuccessfully funded grant proposal, prior to both preparing and submitting your proposal, consider the following shortcomings that are commonly identified in the external grant review process:

- Diffuse, superficial, or unfocused work plan
- Lack of sufficient detail in methods or approach
- Lack of knowledge of published relevant work
- Unrealistically large amount or scope of work
- Uncertainty concerning future directions
- Lack of specific data in background and significance or needs assessment
- Lack of new or original ideas
- Absence of an acceptable scientific rationale
- Lack of experience in the essential methods or programming
- Outdated methods or programming
- Questionable reasoning in methods or approach
- Poor preparation and presentation

Tips to optimize your chance for funding:

- Have <u>multiple</u> people read your grant application.
- Have a mentor read your application.
- Ask for specific suggestions for improvements.
- Keep readers in mind (avoid acronyms).
- Don't make assumptions—Reviewers will have general knowledge but may be unfamiliar with your specific area of public health nutrition or population. Don't assume reviewers "*will know what you mean.*"
- Read and follow the directions!!!

Characteristics of successful grant proposals include the following:

- Organized and clear writing
- Goals, SMART objectives, methods or approach, and analyses are clearly linked.
- Measures are linked to theory and literature.
- Well-designed tables and figures support and illustrate written points in the proposal.
- Crisp, clear presentation
- Quality formatting (use headings: bold, underline, italicize to make application easy to read).

Summary

An evaluation plan is a critical component of a grant proposal and fiscal and data management are core functions of program management. A nutrition program plan to address a specific health issue is strengthened by data that demonstrate a community's health and nutritional status (based on demographic, socioeconomic, and health and nutritional status data), the community's perceived needs (gathered through qualitative methods), and any major duplication and/or gaps in available community programs or services. The use of data in the needs assessment process assures that resources and activities are directed toward a defined target audience with a prioritized health need.

Accurate, timely information is absolutely critical to decision makers who need to understand a problem's scope as well as its causes and consequences prior to taking action (such as whether to revise a program or initiate something new). Such understanding is achieved through the processes of assessment, analysis, and action. Assessment refers to the detection of the existence of a problem. Analysis is the mechanism by which causes and solutions are identified. Action involves the communication of results to those responsible for initiating action to solve the problem. In addition, related information

> ### *Strategy Tip*
>
> See https://www.grants.gov/web/grants /learn-grants/grants-101.html for more assistance in understanding grants.

is essential to monitoring and evaluating how well (or poorly) their actions have affected the problem.

The utility of nutrition data is far reaching, as it can be used to improve an agency's capacity to assess, analyze, and design resource-relevant actions; improve organizational and public perception and knowledge; increase effective demand for nutrition-relevant information; and ensure adequate resources for action. This is what is meant by "translating data" into public health action.

Undoubtedly, additions will be made to these grant writing tips and they will be shared with other people. Sharing the work and the glory when a new grant comes to the agency is the mark of a true professional. Researching grant funds and writing proposals takes time. Well-written proposals are not always funded. Even experienced grant writers receive rejections. It takes persistence. Funded and unfunded proposals *both* have value and enhance the experience of a grant writer. If a proposal is rejected, ask for a copy of the grant evaluation sheet and try again, and again.

Learning Portfolio

© olies/Shutterstock.

Issues for Discussion

1. What are at least four dimensions from which data management for nutrition practice can be considered?
2. Explain the five characteristics of a SMART objective.
3. What is the role of data in the justification for a proposed intervention among a given target audience?
4. Explain the difference between quantitative and qualitative data and the benefits of each.
5. What are the different ways of defining a community (i.e., on what basis)?
6. What are the characteristics of successful grant proposals?

Practical Activities

1. Identify a significant public health nutrition problem that you would like to address via a funded-grant opportunity.
2. Identify a potential funding source for your proposed project (e.g., https://phpartners.org/ph_public/topic/grants)
3. Develop a three-page Concept Paper composed of no more than a two-page narrative and a one-page budget based on the requirements of the opportunity you have identified.
4. Using the template provided on **Page 517**, develop a 1-year (or year one) work plan for your proposed project.

Key Terms

	page
Community	496
Population	497
Request for Proposal (RFP)	498
Annotated budget	507
Surveillance	509
Trends	511
Triangulation	513
Institutional Review Board (IRB)	516
Fidelity	517

Case Study: Grant Writing Exercise

Using Table 15–4, take the following work plan and decide which months the activities and indicators must be planned within for this mock grant proposal.

Title of Proposed Project: *Farm to Family*

Goal(s): The overall goal of *Farm to Family* is to pilot a direct-to-consumer sales marketing model employing small-scale, direct market farmers and food pantries serving SNAP recipients who purchase new subsidized Community Supported Agriculture (CSA) shares, the increase in which will serve as the primary measure of effectiveness of the pilot.

SMART Objective #1: By April of 2023, participating CSA farmers will report an increase in the number of new SNAP recipient CSA shareholders above the 2021 growing season baseline.

SMART Objective #2: By April of 2023, a convenience sample of pilot SNAP recipients will self-report an improvement in intermediary indicators of fruit and vegetable consumption.

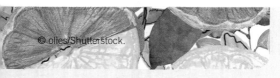
© olies/Shutterstock.

Learning Portfolio

May 2022–April 2023

WORK PLAN

Phase of Pilot	Activities	Indicators	12-Month Timeframe												
			m	j	j	a	s	o	n	d	j	f	m	a
Planning	Participating food pantries complete the USDA FNS authorization process to accept SNAP Electronic Benefit Transfer (EBT) and have readers installed. Participating food pantries install EBT machines at five participating pantries. Print marketing and nutrition education materials. Participating food pantries will distribute marketing materials advertising the reduced-price shares to local SNAP participants (including those accessing emergency food). Farmers in the *Growers Group* are paid to plant an additional 100 CSA half shares on behalf of SNAP recipients accessing participating pantries.	EBT machines installed. Materials printed and distributed. Direct payment made to participating farmers.												
Implementation	SNAP participants will use their SNAP EBT cards to purchase their incentivized half shares at one of five pantries, an authorized EBT retailer. *Growers Group* farmers will deliver CSA half shares on a weekly basis to food pantries for onsite purchase and pickup by pilot SNAP participants. Nutrition education sessions, including cooking demonstrations and taste tests, will be offered at the five participating food pantries on a weekly basis during food distribution hours by nutrition educators funded through the SNAP-Ed Pantry Project who will distribute the self-administered *University of California Fruit and Vegetable Inventory* following the nutrition education sessions. Up to 100 participants per distribution will receive evidence-based nutrition education materials at the point of purchase to reinforce the value and ease of preparation for featured produce, incentivizing current and future consumption.	Purchases of CSA half shares. Logs of CSA half-share distribution and pickup by pilot SNAP participants. Nutrition education sessions, including cooking demonstrations and taste tests, conducted. Surveys completed by *Farm to Family* participants. Evidence-based nutrition education materials distributed.												

Monitoring and Evaluation	A process evaluation will be conducted throughout the funding period to document and assess the process, challenges, and successes throughout **all** four phases of the pilot: 1) planning; 2) implementation; 3) monitoring and evaluation; and 4) sustainability and scaling. Using convenience sampling, the self-administered *University of California Fruit and Vegetable Inventory* will be distributed to pilot SNAP recipients who have purchased at least one CSA half share through *Farm to Family* throughout the implementation months of July of 2022 through December of 2022 during pantry distribution hours and following the provision of nutrition education sessions by SNAP-Ed Nutrition Educators.	Documentation themed by processes, challenges and successes Survey results to assess change in trends over 6-month implementation period in one or more of six constructs related to related to fruit and vegetable consumption: 1) perceived benefits to eating fruit & vegetables; 2) perceived control; 3) self-efficacy; 4) readiness to eat more fruit; 5) readiness to eat more vegetables; and 6) perceived diet quality
Sustainability and Scaling	*Growers Group* farmers adapt their product mix to suit the expressed cultural and dietary preferences of pilot SNAP participants for the 2023 growing season. Meetings will be held on a monthly basis throughout the implementation and postimplementation phase of the pilot with: 1) area foundations to solicit funding incentives in 2023; and 2) communities of faith to discuss subscribing to the 2023 CSA with benevolence dollars (currently devoted to emergency food) or on behalf of congregants paying a subsidizing rate (higher than market value). A statewide presentation and training to SNAP Nutrition Educators will be offered by the Project Lead and Project Evaluator to encourage adoption and scaling as a SNAP-Ed policy, systems, and environmental (PSE) intervention in statewide FY24 SNAP-Ed project proposals.	Farmers product mix tailored to participant preferences. Meetings held and meeting minutes recorded. Funding incentives and/or benevolence dollars allocated with documentation. Presentation and training on *Farm to Family* delivered and evaluated by SNAP Nutrition Educators for feedback on adoption and scaling of pilot. Successfully funded competitive proposals with inclusion of *Farm to Family* as a PSE intervention with integrated direct education and social marketing components.

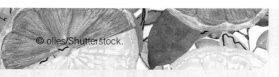
© olies/Shutterstock.

Learning Portfolio

Case Study: Using Data in Grant Writing for Program Planning and Evaluation

Recall that objective quantitative data are used in grant writing and nutrition program planning to address four questions:

1. **What** are the health issues facing a community (problem)?

2. **Where** are the problems (place)?

3. **Who** is at risk (person)?

4. **When** are problems increasing or declining over time (time period)?

For example, let's take a look at the projected impact of the novel coronavirus (COVID-19) on food insecurity in the United States in 2020. Prior to the COVID-19 pandemic, more than 35 million people, including nearly 11 million children, lived in food-insecure households.[1] Although the United States experienced the lowest food insecurity rates in more than 20 years,[2] the pandemic reversed improvements made over the past decade since the Great Recession. In fact, combined data analyses conducted by *Feeding America* at the national, state, county, and congressional district levels, project that the number of people who were food insecure in 2020 is projected to rise to more than 50 million, including 17 million children.[3]

Using *Feeding America*'s website of the projected impacts of COVID-19 on overall food insecurity (https://www.feedingamerica.org/sites /default/files/2021-03/National%20Projections%20Brief_3.9.2021_0.pdf), summarize the projected overall increase in food insecurity rates.

Example: New York City, New York, Nassau County, Congressional District 15

Community Definition	Place of Residence	2018 Overall Food Insecurity Rate	2020 Projected Overall Food Insecurity Rate	Projected Percent Increase in Overall Food Insecurity Rate (2018 to 2020)
State	New York	11.1	16.0	44
County	Nassau	5.3	9.8	83
Congressional District	15	22.3	29.0	30

Similar projections and tabulations may be made for child food insecurity rates using this tool.

To assess the current and future state of local food insecurity, it is critical to understand baseline rates and trends prior to and during the pandemic to develop effective intervention strategies for communities at risk of hunger for grant writing, program planning, and evaluation.

1. Coleman-Jensen A, Rabbitt MP, Gregory CA, Singh A. Household Food Security in the United States in 2019, ERR-275, U.S. Department of Agriculture, Economic Research Service; 2020.

2. Ibid.

3. Feeding America. *The Impact of Coronavirus on Food Insecurity.* Accessed February 9, 2021. Available at https://www.feedingamerica .org/research/coronavirus-hunger-research

Resources

1. **8 Ways to Successfully Navigate NIH Peer Review and Get an R01 Grant** - This 2016 briefing covers the key things that applicants need to know about the submission and review of their R01 NIH grant applications. An R01 grant is a key mechanism by which the National Institutes funds investigator-initiated biomedical research. A Q&A session that follows the presentation answers many common applicant questions. (National Institutes of Health (NIH), HHS). Accessed January 29, 2021. Available at: https://www.youtube.com/watch?v=cW6fzTGCTdw

2. **Applying for Grants to Support Rural Health Projects** - Site provides information on hiring grant-writing consultants, considerations before applying, creating an evaluation plan, and more. (Rural Health Information Hub). Accessed January 29, 2021. Available at: https://www.ruralhealthinfo.org/topics/grantwriting

3. **CDC Grant Funding Profiles** - The CDC Grant Funding Profiles site provides interactive data and summaries of CDC cooperative agreement and grant funding to recipients in U.S. states and territories, and the District of Columbia, starting with fiscal year (FY) 2010. The data are compiled in a format that allows users to view, sort, and analyze funding data by funding opportunity announcement, funding source (CDC funding category and subcategory), geography, and recipient name and type. (Centers for Disease Control and Prevention (CDC), HHS). Accessed January 29, 2021. Available at: https://www.cdc.gov/fundingprofiles/

4. **CDC's Clear Writing Hub** - One of the CDC's goals is to help grantees and partners create environmental health information that the public can understand and trust. CDC has developed this website to help you communicate clearly and effectively to all of the audiences you serve. (National Center for Environmental Health, CDC). Accessed January 29, 2021. Available at: https://www.cdc.gov/nceh/clearwriting/

5. **Debunk the Myths: Grant Application Video Series** - This video explains the grant application process. (Health Resources and Services Administration (HRSA), HHS). Accessed January 29, 2021. Available at: https://www.hrsa.gov/grant-myths/index.html

6. **Grant Writing Basics Blog Series** - A series of blog posts from the Grants.gov team to demystify the federal grant process. (Grants.gov). Accessed January 29, 2021. Available at: https://grantsgovprod.wordpress.com/category/learngrants/grant-writing-basics/

7. **Grants and Proposal Writing-On Demand** - Designed for beginning grant proposal writers, this class presents a general overview of the grant and funding processes as well as the level of detail required in a successful proposal. (National Network of Libraries of Medicine (NN/LM)). Accessed January 29, 2021. Available at: https://nnlm.gov/class/grants-and-proposal-writing-demand/8841

8. **HHS Grant Application Guide** - Use the application instructions found on this page along with the guidance in the funding opportunity announcement to submit grant applications to NIH, the Centers for Disease Control and Prevention, the U.S. Food and Drug Administration, and the Agency for Healthcare Research and Quality. (National Institutes of Health (NIH), HHS). Accessed January 29, 2021. Available at: https://grants.nih.gov/grants/how-to-apply-application-guide.html

9. **How to Apply for a HRSA Grant** - This site is an online technical assistance resource, offering webinars, application and submission guidance, as well as tips for writing successful proposals to HRSA. (Health Resources and Services Administration (HRSA), HHS). Accessed January 29, 2021. Available at: https://www.hrsa.gov/grants/apply-for-a-grant

10. **NIH Data Book** - The NIH Data Book (NDB) provides basic summary statistics on extramural grants and contract awards, grant applications, the organizations that NIH supports, the trainees and fellows supported through NIH programs, and the national biomedical workforce. (National Institutes of Health (NIH), HHS). Accessed January 29, 2021. Available at: https://report.nih.gov/nihdatabook/

11. **NIH Guide for Grants and Contracts** - Link to the NIH Guide for grants and contracts. (National Institutes of Health (NIH), HHS). Accessed January 29, 2021. Available at: https://grants.nih.gov/funding/index.htm

12. **NIH Regional Seminars on Program Funding and Grants Administration** - Semiannual NIH Regional Seminars on Program Funding and Grants. These seminars are intended to help demystify the application and review process, clarify federal regulations and policies, and highlight current areas of special interest or concern. (Office of Extramural Research, NIH). Accessed January 29, 2021. Available at: https://grants.nih.gov/news/contact-in-person/seminars.htm

13. **Proposal Writing** - Training courses, both online and in the classroom at various levels, to learn how to write grant proposals. (Foundation Center). Accessed January 29, 2021. Available at: https://learning.candid.org/topics/proposal-writing/

14. **Proposal Writing Support** - Grant proposal writing tips, tutorials, resources, and classes. (National Network of Libraries of Medicine (NN/LM)). Accessed January 29, 2021. Available at: https://nnlm.gov/funding/support

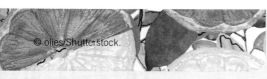
© olies/Shutterstock.

Learning Portfolio

References

1. Himmelstein DU, Woolhandler S. Public Public Health's health's falling falling share share of of US US health spending. *Am J Public Health*. 2016 Jan;106(1):56-57.

2. U.S. Department of Health and Human Services. Office of Disease Prevention and Health Promotion. *Healthy People 2030*. Accessed January 29, 2021. https://health.gov/healthypeople

3. Carter HE, Schofield DJ, Shrestha R, Veerman L. The productivity gains associated with a junk food tax and their impact on cost-effectiveness. *PLoS ONE*. 2019 Jul 22;14(7):e0220209. doi: 10.1371/journal.pone.0220209. PMID: 31329651; PMCID: PMC6645543.

4. Bruening M, Udarbe AZ, Yakes Jimenez E, et al. Stell Crowley P, Fredericks DC, Edwards Hall LA. Academy of Nutrition and Dietetics: standards of practice and standards of professional performance for registered dietitian nutritionists (competent, proficient, and expert) in public health and community nutrition. *J Acad Nutr Diet*. 2015 Oct;115(10):1699-1709.e39.

5. *The future of the public's health in the 21st century*. (2003). Washington, D.C.: National Academies Press; 2003.

6. Consortium from Altarum Institute; Centers for Disease Control and Prevention; Robert Wood Johnson Foundation; National Coordinating Center for Public Health Services and Systems Research. A national research agenda for public health services and systems. *Am J Prev Med*. 2012 May;42(5 suppl 1):S72-S78.

7. *The American Heritage Dictionary of the English Language*, 5th ed. Boston: Houghton Mifflin; 2015.

8. Spicer DA, Kaufman M. Managing data. In: Edelstein S, ed. *Nutrition in Public Health: A Handbook for Developing Programs and Services*, 2nd ed. Sudbury, MA: Jones and Bartlett Publishers; 2006:312-341.

9. Association of State Public Health Nutritionists. *Moving to the Future*. Accessed January 29, 2021. https://movingtothefuture.org/

10. Issel, LM, Wells, R. Health program planning and evaluation. United States: Jones & Bartlett Learning; 2017.

11. Grembowski, D. The practice of health program evaluation. SAGE; 2016.

12. Drummond KE, Murphy-Reyes A. Nutrition research: concepts & applications. United States: Jones & Bartlett Learning; 2017.

13. National Institutes of Health. Health data resources: Common data types in public health research. Accessed January 29, 2021. https://www.nihlibrary.nih.gov/resources/subject-guides/health-data-resources/common-data-types-public-health-research

14. Guest G, Namey E. *Public Health Research Methods*. 55 City Road, London: Sage Publications, Inc.; 2015. doi: 10.4135/9781483398839

15. Gunnell, Sarah, Christensen NK, Jewkes MD, LeBlanc H, Christofferson D. Providing nutrition education to recently resettled refugees: piloting a collaborative model and evaluation methods. *J Immigr Minor Health*. 2015;17(2):482-488.

16. Issel, LM, Wells, R. Health program planning and evaluation. United States: Jones & Bartlett Learning; 2017.

17. Groseclose SL, Buckeridge DL. Public health surveillance systems: recent advances in their use and evaluation. *Annu Rev Public Health*. 2017;38:57-79. doi: 10.1146/annurev-publhealth-031816-044348

18. Kraemer K, Cordaro JB, Fanzo J, et al. What gets measured gets done: how nutrition monitoring, impact evaluation, and surveillance can support program improvement and policy development. In: *Good Nutrition: Perspectives for the 21st Century*. Karger Publishers; 2016:301-311.

19. Celentano Celentano DD, Szklo M. *Gordis Epidemiology*. Netherlands: Elsevier; 2019.

20. U.S. Department of Health and Human Services (DHHS). Office for Human Research Protections. *The Belmont Report: Ethical Principles and Guidelines for the Protection of Human Subjects of Research*. Accessed January 29, 2021. http://www.hhs.gov/ohrp/humansubjects/guidance/belmont.html

21. U.S. Department of Health and Human Services (DHHS). Office for Human Research Protections. *Federal Policy for the Protection of Human Subjects ('Common Rule')*. Accessed January 29, 2021. http://www.hhs.gov/ohrp/humansubjects/commonrule/

CHAPTER 16

Staffing, Managing, and Leading Community and Public Health Nutrition Personnel

Erin Gilfillan, MS, RDN, CDN

Hannah Husby, MS, RDN, CDN

Stephanie Cook, RDN, CSO, LDN

(We would like to acknowledge the work of Esther Okeiyi, PhD, RDN, LDN, and Cynthia Taft Bayerl, MS, RDN, LDN, for their work on past editions of Nutrition in Public Health.)

Learning Outcomes

AFTER STUDYING THIS CHAPTER AND REFLECTING ON THE CONTENTS, YOU SHOULD BE ABLE TO:

1. List at least 10 responsibilities of a public health nutrition director or manager.
2. Describe the six major management functions involved in managing nutrition personnel in the nutrition division of public health.
3. Describe the relationships among the following: job analysis, job description, and job specification.
4. Distinguish between the characteristics of a manager and the characteristics of a leader.
5. Discuss the characteristics of a good performance appraisal.
6. Discuss the importance of public health managers during national and global public health emergencies.

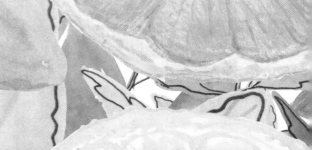

Introduction

There is considerable evidence to show that effective leadership can result in both effective and successful outcomes, especially in healthcare. Sfantou, et al., found that effective leadership is directly correlated with improved healthcare outcomes, regardless of the level of care being provided.[1] It can be inferred that these results also translate to the public health sector. Today's public health nutrition managers recognize the need for a clear understanding and effective application of management principles in day-to-day operations. A manager may feel overwhelmed by the various terms applied in the field of scientific management; therefore, public health nutrition directors or managers need to become familiar with these terms and principles, because no unit in the public health department will provide a greater opportunity for applying these management skills. As early as 1969, Mackenzie posited that the elements managers are faced with are: ideas, things, and people, which remains true even to this day. A manager must think conceptually about issues or matters that need to be resolved, administer to or manage details, and exercise leadership while influencing people so that desired goals can be accomplished.[2] This chapter will examine the role of a manager in the realm of public health nutrition.

The Role of a Public Health Nutrition Director/Manager

A public health manager, also referred to as a director of nutrition services, wears many hats as a leader in their department. The responsibilities of a public health manager or director may include, but are not limited to[3]:

- Providing leadership in all areas of a nutrition division in a public health department.
- Recruiting, orienting, and training dietitians/nutritionists in the nutrition division.
- Supervising dietitians/nutritionists and their work.
- Motivating employees, conducting performance appraisals, and disciplining employees when necessary.
- Maintaining good communication between the nutritionists and staff and between the director and employees.
- Handling concerns and grievances.
- Planning, implementing, and evaluating program and service outcomes.
- Organizing the nutrition division.
- Planning the budget and controlling costs.
- Interacting and working with other divisions in the public health department.
- Representing the health department as an expert in the area of nutrition within and outside of the public health department.
- Promoting morale among the nutritionists and employees.
- Generating income by soliciting grants and writing grant proposals for funding programs and employee positions in the division.
- Networking and collaborating with the community.
- Keeping abreast of laws, changes in the community, community needs, and health needs.

Additionally, the major role of a public health nutrition director or manager can be divided into six areas: planning, staffing, organizing, delegating, leading, and controlling. The director utilizes available resources to accomplish the organizational goals. There are six main resources available to the director, which are known as the "six Ms" of management: manpower, market, machine, method, material, and money. Manpower represents the employees. Market represents the clients and the community that the nutrition division serves. Machines include the equipment used for producing services. Methods represent the processes, policies, procedures, and guidelines stipulated by the division, government, and funding agencies. Materials represent the supplies, software, and training and promotional materials necessary to run the programs. Money represents the financial aspect of the operation. The following sections take a closer look at the major roles of the nutrition director in a public health department.

> Six Ms of management: manpower, market, machine, method, material, and money.

1. **Planning**

   Planning is the establishment of a mission statement, goals, and objectives, and the strategies implemented to accomplish the goals and objectives. A mission statement is the first step in planning; it represents the philosophy or purpose that drives an organization. The division's mission statement must be derived from the overall mission of the public health department and provide an overall direction for the organization. Although goals are stated in general terms, objectives are specific and must be stated in measurable terms related to actions or activities. The following are examples of short-range objectives and goals pertaining to personnel:

   GOALS:

   1. The nutrition division will reduce the employee turnover rate annually.
   2. The nutrition division will help make employees successful.

   OBJECTIVES:

   1. The nutrition division will reduce the employee turnover rate from 50% to 25% by the end of 2025.
   2. The number of employees indicating satisfaction with their productivity will increase 25% by the end of the first year and 50% by the end of the second year.
   3. All employees will participate in at least two professional conferences annually.

   The three types of planning include the strategic plan, the intermediate plan, and the operational plan. The strategic plan involves making decisions about the future, forecasting for the future, and making decisions based on the environment with current and anticipated available resources. A strategic plan serves for 3 to 15 years and should be reviewed regularly. Managers at the top of the organizational structure develop the strategic plan. In strategic planning, performance of the organization is compared with past and future goals utilizing performance measurement systems, such as the SWOT technique (strengths, weaknesses, opportunities, and threats). The strategic plan document serves as a foundation for an intermediate plan, which covers a 1- to 3-year period. Middle-level managers or supervisors may develop an intermediate plan. It is through the intermediate plan that policies are developed. Finally, the operational plan describes a day-to-day action plan. It dictates the plan for a period of 1 year or fewer.

   There are three major levels of managers, each of whom is responsible for a different level of planning. The top managers function at the policy-making level of the organization. They are responsible for broad, comprehensive planning involving strategic planning and long-range goals. The middle-level managers are responsible for developing

Strategy Tip

Use the SWAT technique to bring out successes and failures of the past to reveal new opportunities and identify obstacles.

policies; and first-line managers, at the technical or operational level, are responsible for developing procedures and methods.

The level of managers involved in developing any plan may be based on the size of the organization/unit and the levels of management in that unit. Directors within different nutrition divisions in the public health department may perform different responsibilities, based on the division's size, levels of management, and how the particular organization is structured. For example, the director of nutrition delegates most of the first-line and middle-management functions to the team leaders. The team leaders then plan, orient, train, and provide direct supervision to their designated employees. The nutrition manager or director works with other division managers internally, planning and coordinating efforts relating to the public health department and representing the division by providing expertise in matters relating to nutrition. The nutrition director may contribute ideas regarding how the nutrition division may handle such matters in terms of managing food sanitation and safety. Externally, the manager or director represents the public health department, negotiating for community partnerships, contracts, funding, and projects. In addition, the manager implements nutrition programs and works with other stakeholders, such as government agencies and community services.

A thorough plan is vital for the success of an organization. A well-structured plan prevents many long-term issues for both the director and the division as a whole. Additionally, planning increases effectiveness and efficiency. Effectiveness refers to an operation's ability to accomplish its goals and objectives. Efficiency refers to an operation's ability to achieve maximum results with minimum input. It is important that employees are involved in the planning to ensure everyone remains knowledgeable of what is occurring in the unit. Employees are more likely to follow the plan if they are included as part of the initial planning process.

2. **Staffing**

Managers are responsible for hiring the right people for the positions in their divisions. Once employees are hired, they are introduced to the job and organization during a formal orientation program, and subsequently are given an organized training schedule in preparation for their job. The orientation process may take 3 to 5 days. The amount and length of training are dependent upon each employee's previous training and experience. Over time, the employees are evaluated periodically, typically after the first 90 days on the job and annually by the manager to inform them of how well they are doing. This is referred to as a performance appraisal. A performance appraisal is a formal method of providing constructive feedback to an employee regarding how well or how poorly the employee is performing their job. The objectives are to positively influence, motivate, strengthen, and enhance the employee's work performance. The performance appraisals must be job related. Performance appraisals have many advantages, including:

- Aid employees in defining future goals and provide an objective set of criteria to measure job performance.
- Provide a basis for modifying poor work habits.
- Provide a means of gathering employees' suggestions for improving performance, methods, and morale.
- Serve as a source of documentation in the event of litigation.
- Provide a basis on which to determine promotions and wage increases.

- Provide a means to seek an alternative to termination.
- Help to pinpoint personal weaknesses and strategies to improve them.

Overall, a performance appraisal is an effective motivational tool. The appraisal should not be used as a punishment or as an opportunity for vindictiveness. In addition, it must not be a one-way process, but should be a mutual discussion between the employee and the manager. For the evaluation to be effective, the employee must be informed about the process prior to beginning the job and reminded 2 weeks preceding the actual evaluation. A performance appraisal must be conducted in a private environment. **Table 16–1** provides examples of specific nutrition-related job responsibilities and job competencies that meet set standards of practice. Job competencies are helpful for employees to review periodically prior to performance evaluations to ensure that they are performing to the pre-established standards.

Employees are entitled to know how they are progressing within their jobs as well as the criteria used for progress evaluations. The specified criteria should be discussed with all employees during orientation, training, or in-house meetings with the opportunity for individuals to ask appropriate questions and clarify the objectives being measured. Although there are many evaluation tools available, the Behavioral Anchored Rating Scale (BARS), as documented by Payne-Palacio and Theis, is generally considered one of the most effective resources for employees' performance evaluations.[4] This tool identifies specific behaviors for each performance level in all task and job categories and provides a scale to rate employees. The Management by Objectives (MBO) system is another performance evaluation tool that managers can use. This tool allows both the manager and the employee to collaborate on specific performance objectives and evaluates the employee on how well those objectives are accomplished.

Discipline is ultimately used when all other measures have failed to improve employee performance. Any disciplinary action taken against an employee should be legally defensible. It may be advisable to consult with the legal office of the department before taking disciplinary action. Disciplinary actions should be immediate, consistent, and unbiased. The department rules and regulations must have been communicated to employees prior to any disciplinary action taken in a clear, fair, and reasonable manner, and reviewed regularly.

Disciplinary action should follow specific steps, correlating with the number of prior offenses, scope of the offense, and effect on the department. A manager must be aware of potential grievances of employees, which might lead to one or more offenses. Grievance signs may include indifference toward the job or toward other employees, repeated tardiness and absences, decline in quality of work, and excessive complaints. The first line of action taken by a manager may be to have a face-to-face, private discussion with the employee. The manager may point out changes observed and concerns regarding the employee's progress and future within the department. Mutual discussion can lead to brainstorming strategies for solving the underlying problem. However, if the problem persists, documentation and a formal Grievance Action Form may be completed, which serves as a written warning to the employee. Disciplinary action plans typically include the following steps: mutual discussion, verbal warning, written warning, second written warning, final warning, and termination.

TABLE 16–1

Registered Dietitian Nutritionists' Roles and Responsibilities using the Standards of Practice and Standards of Professional Performance[2,4]

Reproduced from Academy Quality Management Committee. Academy of Nutrition and Dietetics: revised 2017 standards of practice in nutrition care and standards of professional performance for registered dietitian nutritionists. *J Acad Nutr Diet.* 2018;118(1):132-140.e15. doi: 10.1016/j.jand.2017.10.003

Nutrition Roles	Responsibilities and Job Competencies
Clinical practitioner, inpatient or outpatient care	A hospital-based registered dietitian/nutritionist (RDN) in general clinical practice has accepted a new coverage assignment that includes patients with gastrointestinal (GI) disorders. The RDN notes the types of GI disorders and reviews medical nutrition therapy resources and published practice guidelines to identify areas for enhancing knowledge and skills with continuing education and mentoring from a more experienced practitioner. Because the available focus area Scope of Practice (SOP) and Standards of Professional Practice (SOPP) do not specifically address GI disorders, the RDN uses the SOP and SOPP for RDNs as the primary guide for self-evaluation. The RDN recognizes that this self-evaluation and review of GI-related resources will assist with revising their professional development plan to incorporate new competencies, if necessary, and to identify relevant continuing education activities.
Sales representative, national food distributor	An RDN with a management role in hospital foodservice has accepted a sales representative position with a national foodservice distributor. In reviewing resources for the new role, the RDN identifies knowledge and skill areas to strengthen for quality practice. The RDN reviewed the Academy of Nutrition and Dietetics (Academy)/Commission on Dietetic Registration (CDR) Code of Ethics, the Academy's ethics resources, and the SOPP for RDNs to be reminded of areas to consider when in a business practice role. This self-evaluation process identifies knowledge/skill areas for continuing education and mentoring by more experienced RDN colleagues and others with expertise in business and sales. The RDN updates professional development plan to incorporate new practice competencies applicable to the new role in sales.
Quality improvement specialist, multi-hospital system	An RDN with experience as a clinical nutrition manager and as a clinical practitioner in oncology is recruited for an open position in the quality improvement/compliance monitoring department for the hospital system. In evaluating the position description and role expectations, the RDN identifies some knowledge and skill areas for development/enhancement. The RDN uses the SOP and SOPP for RDNs for self-evaluation reflecting on the standards and indicators with the perspective of the quality improvement role. The RDN identifies specific continuing-education activities, updates professional development plan with new essential competencies, and sets a goal to qualify for one of the quality credentials or certifications.
RDN practitioner in a rural Community	An RDN who lives in a rural community works professionally in multiple settings (critical access hospital, clinic at the county health department, and the community's senior meal program) as a part-time employee or contractor. Because of varying professional roles, the RDN uses the SOP and SOPP for RDNs as the guiding self-evaluation resource with each role. This allows the RDN to direct attention to, and reflect on, any new/enhanced knowledge or skills needed for quality and competent practice. Applicable focus area SOP and SOPPs are reviewed as well, to inform this process and to identify any additional resources for investigation (e.g., regulations, practice guidelines, professional organizations, websites, and literature citations). With each role, the RDN evaluates the need for any new essential practice competencies and updates professional development plan as needed.
Telehealth practitioner, nutrition and wellness	An RDN accepts a new position with a national company that provides telehealth wellness information and coaching to enrollees of private insurance providers. The RDN, who has more than 5 years of general clinical practice, including staffing a hospital's wellness center, investigates the requirements for providing telehealth services within the state. The RDN also explores limitations related to licensure and regulations for callers who live in other states. The RDN reviews the SOP and SOPP for RDNs as a self-evaluation tool, accesses the telehealth resources on the Academy's website, and participates in the company's training webinars that incorporate review of policies and procedures to assure legal and competent practice as a licensed practitioner. The RDN updates professional development plan and identifies continuing education opportunities to enhance coaching skills to ultimately qualify for one of the accredited coaching certifications.
RDN, nonpracticing	An RDN takes a leave of absence from the nutrition and dietetics workforce. Because the RDN is maintaining their credential, sustaining professional performance is an expectation. The RDN maintains and establishes networking and professional relationships. The RDN participates in and volunteers for the local and national nutrition and dietetics association. The RDN volunteers within the community to promote healthy lifestyles and responds to public policy calls to action by contacting representatives via social media, correspondence, and personal visits. The RDN obtains continuing professional education units for CDR certification requirement and licensure. The RDN recognizes the need to maintain skills at least at the minimally competent level identified within the SOP in Nutrition Care and SOPP for RDNs.

3. **Delegating**

Workload delegation is an important managerial task, which allows managers to disperse the varying roles within the organization to improve efficiency. Delegating tasks increases employees' sense of self-worth and acts as motivating factors leading to self-driven success. Additionally, delegation enables the manager to gain input from employees, which leads to increased productivity. Employees are delegated to various tasks based on the level of skill and experience. The manager must take full responsibility for each employee's responsibilities within the organization and, therefore, is obligated to oversee the delegated tasks.

A public health manager must coordinate all aspects of the various parts of employees' work to ensure smooth workflow. The public health nutrition director can accomplish this through departmentalization or specialization by functions, clients, geographic areas, number of persons, or time. Some tasks may be delegated to free the director's time to do other tasks. Delegating is essential in distributing workloads. It enriches and enlarges employees' jobs and contributes to employees' improved job knowledge, job motivation, professional development, and job accomplishment.[5] When job responsibilities are delegated, authority must accompany them. The manager must guide the employee to understand the limits of the authority and which decisions and actions can be made without consultation.

4. **Organizing**

In order for the goals and objectives of a nutrition division to be accomplished, the manager must organize the resources in an orderly fashion. Organizing is the act of carefully grouping the organization's resources and activities, including human resources, by type of tasks performed. The organizing process establishes relationships among all functions of management. The organization of the public health nutrition division is based on its mission, goals and objectives, and areas of nutrition services provided to the community. For example, whereas some nutrition divisions in public health departments focus on providing nutrition services to women, infants, and children through the Special Supplemental Nutrition Program for Women, Infants and Children (WIC) program, others focus on preventing and reducing disabilities among individuals or groups, such as the elderly, children, and home-bound individuals. Immunocompromised and lower income individuals, both of whom are at increased nutritional risk, can also utilize nutrition-related services. In all scenarios, the service areas of a public health nutrition division will be easily discernible on the unit's organizational chart. **Figure 16–1** demonstrates an example of an organizational chart for the Center of Food Safety and Applied Nutrition within the department of health and human services.

Strategy Tip

What is the right amount of job duties to delegate to a subordinate employee? How can this go right? How can this go wrong?

The following steps are used in developing an organizational structure:

1. Define organizational goals and objectives.
2. Analyze and classify work to be done.
3. Describe in detail the work or activity in terms of the employees.
4. Organize the employees by tasks and activities and demonstrate their relationship to each other and to management.
5. Clearly delineate staff and line positions. Line positions are in the direct chain of command that is responsible for the achievement

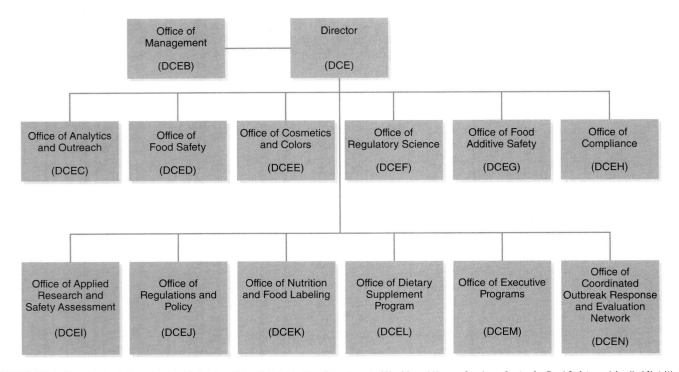

FIGURE 16–1 Organizational Chart for the U.S. Food and Drug Administration, Department of Health and Human Services, Center for Food Safety and Applied Nutrition.

Center for food safety and applied nutrition organization chart. Food and Drug Administration. Published December 16, 2020. Accessed February 21, 2021. https://www.fda.gov/about-fda/fda-organization-charts/center-food-safety-and-applied-nutrition-organization-chart

of organizational goals.[5] Staff positions, in contrast, provide expertise, advice, and support for the line positions. Examples of staff positions are the advisory board, consultants, and secretaries. In an organizational chart, line positions are shown with solid unbroken lines, whereas staff positions are shown with broken lines or dotted lines. The lines depict relationships of communication and control. The Scalar Principle indicates that a clear and unbroken line of authority flows from the bottom position to the top position in the organization.[6]

6. Review and update organizational charts periodically as positions change.

Proper organization of employees requires that managers only oversee a specific number of employees they are capable of managing. This is known as span of control. According to the principle of unity of command, under no circumstance should an employee report to more than one supervisor or manager.

The tools for structuring an organization include job descriptions, job specifications, job breakdowns or analyses, and job design. A job description is an organized list of duties, skills, and responsibilities required in a specific position. A job specification is a written statement of minimum standards that must be met by an applicant for a particular job. It includes duties involved in the job, working conditions specific to the job, and personal qualifications required to carry out the responsibilities successfully. A job analysis or breakdown is written documentation of a study conducted on all aspects of a specific job. It provides information used in developing job descriptions. A job design, developed from job analysis, is used to structure jobs to improve organization efficiency and employee satisfaction. Jobs are divided into manageable units based on employees'

Strategy Tip

What happens when an employee reports to two or more managers?

TABLE 16–2
WIC State Nutrition Coordinator Job Description and Specifications

The State agency ensures that the State Nutrition Coordinator has the following qualifications:

1. One or more of the following skills and experience:
   - Program development skills
   - Counseling skills
   - Community action experience
   - Participant advocacy experience
   - Education background and experience in the development of educational and training resource materials
2. Holds a Masters or Doctoral degree in the field of nutrition from an accredited college or university with emphasis on food and nutrition, community nutrition, public health nutrition, nutrition education, human nutrition, nutrition science, or equivalent *and* has at least 2 years of experience as a nutritionist in education, social service, maternal and child health, public health, nutrition, or dietetics *or*
3. Holds credentials of a Registered Dietitian (R.D.) or is eligible for registration with the Academy of Nutrition and Dietetics' Commission on Dietetic Registration, and if applicable, holds a state license or is certified as a nutritionist/dietitian *and* has a minimum of 2 years of job-related experience *or*
4. Holds a Bachelor degree in the field of nutrition from an accredited college or university and has 3 years of experience as a nutritionist in education, social service, maternal and child health, public health nutrition or dietetics related experience *or*
5. Is qualified as a Senior Public Health Nutritionist under the Department of Health and Human Services guidelines *or*
6. Meets state/Indian health service standards and state personnel qualifications as a public health nutritionist

The state agency ensures that the State Nutrition Coordinator performs the following roles and responsibilities (depending on a state agency's organization, another staff member under the state nutrition coordinator's oversight may perform some of these responsibilities):

1. Develops and evaluates the state's overall WIC nutrition services plan.
2. Provides technical assistance and consultation on nutrition services to state and local agency staff and other health professionals.
3. Provides in-service training and technical assistance for local agency staff involved in providing nutrition education to participants.
4. Keeps current with up-to-date nutrition and breastfeeding information and disseminates this as well as FNS-provided information to other state and local agency staff.
5. Develops state policies, procedures, and/or guidelines that pertain to nutrition services (e.g., nutrition assessment, nutrition education, food package prescriptions, and job descriptions.)
6. Supervises other state nutrition services staff.
7. Participates in the development, management, and implementation of the state nutrition services budget to ensure that it includes required expenditures for nutrition education, including breastfeeding promotion and support.
8. Analyzes and comments on proposed policy or legislation that has potential impact on WIC nutrition services, when necessary.
9. Coordinates nutrition services with other internal WIC Program operations and other nutrition assistance program partners, including both public and private organizations.
10. Provides technical nutrition support in the development and revisions of state management information systems.
11. Evaluates the effectiveness of professional training programs and revises curriculum and materials, as needed.
12. Evaluates progress toward goals and objectives.
13. Identifies or develops appropriate nutrition education resources and materials.

U.S. Department of Agriculture. Qualifications and Roles: State Nutrition Coordinator. Accessed February 23, 2021. Retrieved from https://wicworks.fns.usda.gov /node/qualifications-state-nutrition-coordinator

expertise. **Table 16–2** outlines an example of a nutrition supervisor job description and its specifications.

5. **Leading**

While the terms are often used interchangeably, leadership and management do not mean the same thing. Leadership is the activity of influencing other people's behavior toward the achievement of desired objectives. It involves influencing others without coercion to achieve the organization's goals and objectives. Simply stated, it is getting people to do what you want them to because they want to do it. Management, on the other hand, is the function of running an organization by effectively integrating and coordinating resources in order to achieve desired objectives. Managing a successful nutrition division should incorporate both managerial and leadership qualities.

Leaders share decision making, information, authority, reward, trust, drive, motivation, and vision with their employees. They work well with employees and exhibit respect, concern, and empathy for

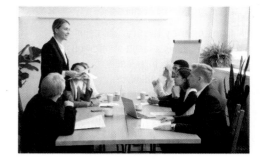

Good leaders communicate with influence, motivation, coordination, and delegation.

© Fizkes/Shutterstock.

Democratic This style is also called participative, because it encourages employee participation in decision making. The manager checks with the employees before making a decision and can act as a coach or problem solver for the group.

Laissez-faire A leadership style also known as the "hands-off" style. The manager provides little or no direction and gives employees as much freedom as possible. All authority or power is given to the employees, and they must determine goals, make decisions, and resolve problems on their own.

Autocratic A leadership style that does not encourage employee input. The manager makes all decisions. Employees are expected to obey management decisions without asking any questions. This type of leadership can be ideal for emergency situations.

McGregor's X and Y theories Different ways in which managers view employees. There are two theories: Theory X and Theory Y.

Theory X Managers believe that workers are motivated by only one thing: money. They are selfish, lazy, and hate work. The manager believes that workers need to be closely controlled and directed.

Theory Y Managers believe that workers are motivated by many different factors apart from money. They enjoy their work. The manager believes that employees will happily take on responsibility and make decisions for the business.

Contingency theory The belief that performance is a result of interaction between two factors: leadership style and situational favorableness.

Maslow's theory The hierarchy of human needs theory. The needs of an individual exist in a logical order (physiological, safety, belonging, esteem, and self-actualization); the basic root needs must be satisfied first.

each individual. They honor differences among employees and integrate those differences within the organization to promote a diverse working environment. Alternatively, a successful manager effectively plans, organizes, and controls productivity, but is less apt to work with employees on a personal level.[7]

One shared characteristic amongst leaders is native intelligence. This means they have the ability to acquire and retain knowledge and respond quickly and productively to a new situation. Leaders have drive, integrity, and self-confidence, and are experts in what they do.[8] Leadership skills are innate and partly learned.[9] Leaders have strong personal mastery that propels them to struggle for change in an organization, seeking out risks, shared dislike, and mundane tasks. They are concerned about the people and strive to help employees achieve personal goals. They derive power from personal relationships and relate with people in intuitive ways. They question established procedures and create new concepts since they are concerned with results.[10] There is a strong correlation between leadership and the ability to relate, influence, motivate, coordinate, delegate, and communicate.[7]

There is no one best style of leadership; rather, style must be adapted to fit the situation. Leaders may use different styles of leadership: **democratic** or participative, **laissez-faire,** or **autocratic,** depending on the employees' responsiveness. The quality and the amount of supervision may determine the success or failure of the organization in accomplishing its goals and its ability to attract government funds to stay afloat.

A. Influencing

The manager and subordinate relationship are critical. **McGregor's X and Y Theories** of leadership differentiate between a leader's attitudes toward employees and its influence on job performance. The **Contingency Theory** of leadership promotes the idea that the type of leadership provided should be contingent on the type of employees and the situation in which the organization exists.[11] Hastings, et al., explained the importance of leader assimilation programs for new leaders entering the organization.[12] Assimilation programs allow for the new leaders to develop a working rapport with employees to encourage a high-performance team. Incorporating assimilation programs into the onboarding process allows employees to preview the new leadership style and provide constructive feedback prior to the full leadership transition.[12]

B. Motivating

Another aspect of leading is creating an environment in which subordinates can be motivated and excited to perform their job well. A leader must understand the concepts of human motivation. To accomplish the goals and objectives of the division, the people who produce the products and services need to be well led and motivated. Interaction between a leader and their subordinates will result in the leader being able to elicit what motivates the employees. There is no one method to create conditions that will motivate employees. Maslow, Herzberg, McClelland, and Vroom all developed theories on how employees are motivated in a work environment.[13-16] An experienced leader may employ Abraham **Maslow's Hierarchy of Needs Theory** by first determining the point of motivational need for each subordinate.[13] **Herzberg's two-factor theory,** which is similar to Maslow's needs theory, identified two major factors, job satisfiers and job dissatisfiers, which can motivate or dissatisfy employees, respectively.[14] Job satisfiers are motivators and include achievement, recognition, responsibility, advancement, the work itself, and potential for growth. The job dissatisfiers are known as maintenance or hygiene factors and must be present for job satisfaction to occur. They include pay, supervision, job security, working conditions, organizational policies, and interpersonal relationships on the job. **McClelland's Motivation Theory** supported Maslow's theory and emphasized that employees are usually at different levels of need, which can be high or low.[15]

An employee will respond positively to motivation if the degree of need is high. **Vroom's Expectancy Theory** stipulates that employees will be motivated if they can link the job performance to the expected reward.[16] For example, if they expect a better reward for better performance, they will be motivated to perform. Motivators can range from an affirmation of work well done, to public recognition of the employee in a meeting, publishing an employee's accomplishments, offering incentives, or rewarding an employee by delegating managerial tasks.[17]

C. Communicating

Effective leadership strongly depends on the ability to communicate with their subordinates. Communication includes being able to transmit ideas and goals, receive messages from internal environments, listen, network, interact with others, and manage both formal and informal organizations. A true leader must resist the temptation of demonstrating favoritism among employees.

The leader represents both the employees and management. The employees look up to the leader as a representative of upper management. The leader, therefore, must be able to: 1) interpret the mission, goals, objectives, and policies of the organization to the employees in a way that garners their cooperation and confidence; 2) motivate and guide employees within each individual role; 3) assist in employees' professional development; 4) listen to and empathize with employees as needed; 5) provide training to individuals and groups; and 6) evaluate employees and implement discipline when necessary.

Leading and directing are synonymous. Directing requires continuous decision making, conveying these decisions to subordinates, and ensuring appropriate actions. It requires coordinating and directing the work of employees to accomplish organizational goals. The director, as a leader, organizes and matches each employee to each specific job based on performance and skills, assists in the orientation and training of employees, listens to and handles grievances, solves problems, and makes decisions in a timely and logical manner. They schedule and conduct employee meetings regularly.

Leaders must also demonstrate effective communication skills to promote inclusion of diverse cultural and ethnic, racial, and gender backgrounds within the organization. A successful leader must demonstrate cultural competency to correct misconceptions, misunderstandings, biases, and stereotyping within and outside of the organization. It is the leader's responsibility to promote cultural dissemination within the workplace to integrate each employee's beliefs, attitudes, and behaviors for the goal of creating a positive workplace culture. Organizations with positive workplace cultures are known to attract driven individuals and enhance overall motivation and job satisfaction.

Herzberg's theory A theory regarding motivation in which employee satisfaction has two factors: hygiene and motivation. Hygiene characteristics are those that are associated with dissatisfaction (i.e., work conditions, pay, and interpersonal relationships), which are contrasted with motivation factors that typically cause satisfaction (i.e., achievement, recognition, and opportunity for growth).

McClelland's theory An individual's motivation and effectiveness in certain job functions are influenced by three needs: achievement, affiliation, and power.

Vroom's theory Assumes that behavior results from conscious choices among alternatives whose purpose is to maximize pleasure and minimize pain. The key elements to this theory are referred to as *expectancy, instrumentality,* and *valence.*

Transformational A leadership style that emphasizes creating relationships among staff. The manager instills confidence and promotes staff respect that results in higher productivity, job satisfaction, and improved communication.

Discussion Prompt

What motivations have you received in the past from employers? Were these motivators successful in enhancing your work?

Leadership communication skills are also essential when diffusing conflicts among employees. A leader cannot ignore conflicts that exist in the workplace or allow them to continue for long periods of time. Conflicts affect team morale, drive, and productivity. The leader must facilitate conflict resolutions by directly influencing behavior change among the individuals involved with the goal of fostering a positive workplace culture.

6. **Controlling**

Controlling is a safeguard used to ensure that resources, quality of services, and client satisfaction are regulated appropriately and adequately. It involves regulating the activities of employees in the division to confirm they meet the established objectives and goals. Control functions require the director to determine which activities need control, such as establishing and communicating standards to employees, measuring performance, and correcting deviations. This includes staffing positions with the correct number of qualified employees, developing and retaining employees, and ensuring quality within programs and services provided to the clients. Additionally, control functions ensure client satisfaction with services provided and guarantee that funding partners are satisfied with the management of their funds. The ability to reallocate personnel or realign the budget when facing financial constraints, while still accomplishing objectives, serves as the main priority for utilizing control measures.

Control functions contribute to a major portion of a manager's responsibility in nutrition and dietetics. Managers must be able to prepare and report financial analyses, control program costs, generate income, detect irregularities in client services or cost overruns, and handle complex projects and programs. The Academy of Nutrition and Dietetics (AND) 2019 Revised Standards of Professional Performance stated that managers or directors in public health are responsible for preparing financial analyses and financial reports, controlling program costs, monitoring program financial performance, documenting program operations, and making decisions regarding capital expenditure.[17,18] The nutrition division usually undergoes periodic review or audits of its accounts. The directors must be able to manage and report the status of the money entrusted into their care.

The community and public health nutrition director must have basic knowledge of accounting, budgeting, interpreting financial documents, and preparing financial reports for all income and expenses generated in the unit. It is important that as the director, they must know how to write for grants, develop the budget for grants, justify the reasons for requesting the amount of money sought after, and manage corresponding programs. Usually, the amount funded is dependent on how well the justification request is written.

Managers and directors must regularly and continuously monitor productivity of their employees. Quality control, quality assurance, continuous quality improvement, and total quality management are all related concepts and can serve as tools for accomplishing this managerial function. Quality control is accomplished by determining if the products or services being provided meet the minimum standards of acceptability. Quality assurance is defined as a process of identifying "problem areas" within a unit and taking action to correct them. The results are monitored over time to see if the problems have been resolved and remain resolved. Quality assurance monitoring may necessitate a development of policies and procedures in patient (client) care protocols, thereby ensuring consistency from practitioner to practitioner. For example, a typical problem may be timeliness in screening to identify high-risk patients. Another example may be inconsistent methods for determining desirable body weight. Quality assurance must be ongoing, using a method such as continuous quality improvement (CQI), which helps identify areas that can be strengthened, and works to improve those areas. When all departments or areas of the organization are studied to determine problem areas and work to correct them, it is referred to as total quality management (TQM).

Within nutrition units in public health departments, quality assurance is a valuable tool. Department may use weekly and monthly meetings as a quality assurance strategy. The team leaders meet weekly with their employees and discuss the week's events and challenges. The team leaders, in turn, meet with the director weekly to share work productivity, issues, and challenges from within individual areas. During the monthly meeting within the division, each of the team leaders presents a progress report to all employees. Controlling, therefore, provides a process for ensuring that established objectives and plans are being accomplished.

Discussion Prompt

Is the dietitian adequately educated in all of these skills to become a nutrition director? Any suggestions to add to the curriculums in most colleges, such that they can take more leadership roles?

The Role of a Public Health Nutrition Director/Manager During Public Health Emergencies

Although relatively uncommon, public health emergencies occur, presenting managers with novel challenges in uncharted territories. In addition to the existing responsibilities of managers, they are required to quickly adapt, regularly assess changing information, efficiently collaborate with other healthcare divisions, and effectively communicate changing needs and policies to others within the organization. Ibrahim, et al., assessed the efficiency of existing response management systems of various countries during the COVID-19 pandemic.[19] During the pandemic, managers were required to reconstruct existing protocols and infrastructure to account for new information collected and the changing needs of the public. The authors analyzed two phases of the COVID-19 pandemic response: Stage 1 consisting of contagion control to minimize spread; Stage 2 consisting of treatment efficacy and active disease tracking. The countries that demonstrated an efficient response management framework and action plan were able to do so partly because of the presence of clear and regular public communication. Conversely, the countries that did not demonstrate an efficient response lacked global collaboration and high-quality data sharing, which may be attributed to the initial lack of guidance from governing bodies. The pandemic altered the existing framework for managers across all healthcare sectors and proved the importance of the role managers play to maintain health security during public health emergencies.

Successful response management during public health emergencies requires continuous needs assessment, identification of existing resources, adequate planning, and timely response with implementation of a thorough plan.[19] Managers are required to analyze other healthcare sectors' responses and compare them with their own organization's response criteria. Public health emergencies are dynamic and require constant reassessment and evaluation of the situation at hand to successfully adapt and ensure that the department and its employees have clear direction. Without emergency response protocol in place, managers are unable to lead a successful organization during an already vulnerable situation, increasing the risk of the organization's foundation to fail, with negative public health repercussions. An organization's public health response capacity is dependent on the ability to manage evolving logistical factors, including supply chain management of resources, continuity planning, and investment in technology to strengthen health security at an organizational level.[20] The Cochrane Library further validated these novel responsibilities of managers during public health emergencies and encouraged continuous monitoring of the emergency situation and impact of interventions taken.[21]

The demand for technology increased significantly during the pandemic, which further impacted managerial roles within public health. Ibrahim, et al., discussed the lack of innovative technology used during early stages of the pandemic's emergency response and the resulting negative effects on contagion control and resource allocation.[19] Another novel responsibility of public health managers is to remain up to date with innovative strategies for obtaining and accessing information and for teaching and communicating with the public. As a result of the COVID-19 pandemic, educators and students were forced to teach and learn remotely. This required the access and knowledge of technology systems, such as Zoom, Microsoft Teams, and Google Classroom to convert existing curriculum from in-person to online. Without adequate leadership, organizations cannot adapt to innovative technologies and, therefore, are faced with the added challenges during crisis management. Mehraeen, et al., discussed the challenges public health managers faced during the COVID-19 pandemic, including those resulting from lack of technology utilization. Policymakers who did not increase technology use placed their organizations at a disadvantage when altering emergency response policies and action plans.[22]

Based on the COVID-19 pandemic response, the Pan American Health Organization (PAHO) developed a set of criteria for public health managers to follow in future emergencies.[23] Importance was placed on maintaining existing emergency plans and resources, while building upon them to account for disaster planning. Public health managers are encouraged to follow four steps when faced with a public health emergency: establish an emergency operations center; continuously assess needs, resources, and response plans; implement the response plan; and prepare for community recovery.[23] Additionally, managers should delegate specific tasks to all employees to ensure every aspect of the emergency response framework is accounted for. This includes having oversight of communications, coordination of information technology, facilitation of first responder and emergency medical activities, and promotion of community-wide health and prevention strategies. Public health nutrition managers should also delegate roles for providing emergency food and food aid, maintaining food safety and security, training of volunteers and public health educators, and short- and long-term relief activities.

Pandemic Learning Opportunity

Describe how your town responded to the COVID-19 pandemic. Do you feel it was handled well? Why or why not? What should have been done differently?

Summary

This chapter discussed how employees in a nutrition division of a public health department are managed. The manager or director must combine management and leadership skills when managing the resources (the six Ms of management) in their unit. The six main functions in directing the activities of the employees must work in tandem to accomplish the goals and objectives of the nutrition division. The manager must create strategies for the success of the organization by continually assessing the competitive environment, and the strengths and areas of improvement for the organization, while looking for opportunities, along with threats. The manager should aim at building their core skills with regard to flexibility in the face of change. The manager must also work to build the skills of their staff. Every active, progressive organization is dynamic, and as organizations grow, the economic, cultural, and political landscape continues to change. There is always a need for the public health leader to grow, expand their skill sets, and manage ambiguity.

Learning Portfolio

© olies/Shutterstock.

Issues for Discussion

1. Why is it important to have job descriptions? How is having appropriate job descriptions a win-win for both the employee and the manager?
2. Discuss some problems you have experienced at your workplace. How could these have been avoided if a good manager was in place? What disciplinary actions should have occurred?

Practical Activity

1. Create an emergency response action plan using the four steps recommended by the PAHO. How would your plan have been affected had there been a lack of adequate management within your hypothetical organization?

Key Terms   page

Key Terms	page
Democratic	536
Laissez-faire	536
Autocratic	536
McGregor's X and Y theories	536
Theory X	536
Theory Y	536
Contingency theory	536
Maslow's theory	536
Herzberg's theory	537
McClelland's theory	537
Vroom's theory	537
Transformational	537

Case Study: Managing Change: How Can Economic Factors Affect the Roles and Responsibilities of a Public Health Nutrition Manager?

One public health organization, discussed throughout this chapter, recently underwent internal staffing changes. Previous directors either progressed to superior positions or retired. As a result, an external candidate was hired to assume the position of nutrition manager within the public health department. When asked what challenges the new manager faced, it was made known that nothing significant had acutely transpired except for expansion of previous job responsibilities of the management position. This was largely due to economic burden and budget cuts, thus reducing the capacity for full-time employees. In addition to the existing job description for the previous manager's role, the new nutrition manager's responsibilities were expanded to include:

- Assume oversight of the diabetes grant funded by the ABC Foundation and the Centers for Medicare and Medicaid Innovations Award. Activities independently related to this grant involve:
  - Recruitment and hiring of specialized registered dietitians, licensed clinical social workers, social workers holding master's degrees, community health workers, health educators, and communications specialists.
  - Ability to oversee issues related to scope of practice, licensure, and reimbursement capabilities for nonregistered dietitian staff.
  - Ability to lead activities related to clinical study and IRB protocols, contract management, and grant writing.
  - Continuous collaboration with local universities, healthcare systems, local nonprofits, and other associated agencies.
  - Regular monitoring of financial activities related to the grant and documentation of expense reports.
- Expand the size and scope of the SNAP-Ed funded program to include activities related to policy change, health disparities, and environmental impact on nutrition.
- Implement programs to promote wellness and nutrition by working regularly with farmer's markets, media outlets, boards of education, and local businesses.
- Recruit and maintain community volunteers interested in a career within public health, and provide regular mentorship, educational opportunities, and community outreach.

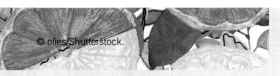
© olles/Shutterstock.

Learning Portfolio

- Hire staff with the skills and competencies necessary to lead community health programs.
- Manage all registered dietitians as well as nonregistered dietitian employees.

Using SWOT management strategy, discuss the strengths, weaknesses, opportunities, and threats associated with the above case. Additionally, discuss how each weakness and threat identified could have been prevented. Discuss the correlation between various economic factors and employee roles within an organization. As a new nutrition manager within a public health department, how might you adapt or respond to the expansion of the previous nutrition manager's job requirements?

Case Study: Job Description

A new WIC Breastfeeding Peer Counselor is being hired. What are some of the titles and subtitles that would be contained in the job description? What would be some of the duties this person must be able to perform?

Resources

1. Bruening M, Udarbe AZ, Yakes Jimenez E, Stell Crowley P, Fredericks DC, Edwards Hall LA. Academy of Nutrition and Dietetics: standards of practice and standards of professional performance for registered dietitian nutritionists (competent, proficient, and expert) in public health and community nutrition. *J Acad Nutr Diet*. 2015;115(10):1699-1709.e39. doi: 10.1016/j .jand.2015.06.374

2. Doley J, Clark K, Roper S. Academy of Nutrition and Dietetics: revised 2019 standards of professional performance for registered dietitian nutritionists (competent, proficient, and expert) in clinical nutrition management. *J Acad Nutr Diet*. 2019;119(9):1545-1560.e32. doi: 10.1016/j.jand.2019.05.013

3. Disaster management in a pandemic: tool 15. Pan American Health Organization. Accessed January 10, 2021. https://www.paho.org/disasters/index.php ?option=com_docman&view=download&category_slug=tools&alias=542 -pandinflu-leadershipduring-tool-15&Itemid=1179&lang=en_Published June 2020

4. Sisk K, Conneally A, Cullinen K. *Guide for developing and enhancing skills in public health and community nutrition*. 3rd ed. Public Health/Community Nutrition Practice Group of the Academy of Nutrition and Dietetics, and the Association of State Public Health Nutritionists; 2018.

5. Workplace health promotion. Centers for Disease Control and Prevention. Published January 10, 2018. Accessed February 21, 2021. https://www.cdc .gov/workplacehealthpromotion/model/assessment/interviews.html

6. Public health nutrition. U.S. Department of Health and Human Services. Accessed February 21, 2021. https://www.ihs.gov/dper/planning/rrm -references/public-health-nutrition/

References

1. Sfantou DF, Laliotis A, Patelarou AE, Sifaki-Pistolla D, Matalliotakis M, Patelarou E. Importance of leadership style towards quality of care measures in healthcare settings: a systematic review. *Healthcare*. 2017;5(4):73. doi: 10.3390/health-care5040073

2. Mackenzie RA. The management process in 3D: a diagram showing the activities, functions, and basic elements of the executive's job. *J Nurs Admin*. 1979;9(11):30-33.

3. Bruening M, Udarbe AZ, Yakes Jimenez E, Stell Crowley P, Fredericks DC, Edwards Hall LA. Academy of Nutrition and Dietetics: standards of practice and standards of professional performance for registered dietitian nutritionists (competent, proficient, and expert) in public health and community nutrition. *J Acad Nutr Diet*. 2015;115(10):1699-1709.e39. doi: 10.1016/j.jand.2015.06.374

4. Payne-Palacio J, Theis M. *Foodservice management: principles and practices*. 13th ed. Pearson; 2015.

5. Riisgaard H, Søndergaard J, Munch M, et al. Work motivation, task delegation and job satisfaction of general practice staff: a cross-sectional study. *Fam Pract*. 2017;34(2):188-193. doi: 10.1093/fampra/cmw142

6. Griffin RW. *Management*. 12th ed. Cengage Learning; 2016.

7. Hudson N, Booth P. *Management practice in dietetics*. 4th ed. Cognella; 2017.

8. George JM, Jones GR. *Understanding and managing organizational behavior*. 6th ed. Pearson; 2011.

9. Boyle MA. *Community nutrition in action: an entrepreneurial approach*. 7th ed. Cengage Learning; 2017.

10. Tamel ME, Reynolds H. *Executive leadership*. Prentice Hall; 1981.

11. McGregor D. *The human side of enterprise*. McGraw Hill; 1985.

12. Hastings NB, Centore LS, Gansky SA, et al. A novel approach for effective integration of new faculty leadership. *J Healthc Leadersh*. 2017;10:1-9. doi: 10.2147/JHL.S150493

13. Maslow AH. A theory of human motivation. *Psychol Rev*. 1943;50(4):370-396.

14. Herzberg F. *Work and nature of man*. World Publishing; 1966.

15. McClelland DC. *The achievement society*. Free Press; 1985.

16. Vroom VH. *Work and motivation*. Jossey-Bass; 1994.

17. Doley J, Clark K, Roper S. Academy of Nutrition and Dietetics: revised 2019 standards of professional performance for registered dietitian nutritionists (competent, proficient, and expert) in clinical nutrition management. *J Acad Nutr Diet*. 2019;119(9):1545-1560.e32. doi: 10.1016/j.jand.2019.05.013

18. Rogers D, Griswold K, Sauer KL, et al. Entry-level registered dietitian and dietetic technician, registered practice today: results from the 2020 Commission on Dietetic Registration entry-level dietetics practice audit. *J Acad Nutr Diet*. 2021;121(2):330-378. doi: 10.1016/j.jand.2020.09.027

19. Ibrahim MD, Binofai FAS, Alshamsi RM. Pandemic response management framework based on efficiency of COVID-19 control and treatment. *Future Virol*. 2020;15(12):801-816. doi: 10.2217/fvl-2020-0368

20. Kandel N, Chungong S, Omaar A, Xing J. Health security capacities in the context of COVID-19 outbreak: an analysis of international health regulations annual report data from 182 countries. *Lancet*. 2020;395(10229):1047-1053. doi: 10.1016/S0140-6736(20)30553-5

21. Nussbaumer-Streit B, Mayr V, Dobrescu AI, et al. Quarantine alone or in combination with other public health measures to control COVID-19: a rapid review. Cochrane Database of Systematic Reviews. Published September 14, 2020. Accessed January 10, 2021. https://www.cochranelibrary.com/cdsr/doi/10.1002/14651858.CD013574.pub2/full

22. Mehraeen M, Dadkhah M, Mehraeen AR. Investigating the capabilities of information technologies to support policy-making in COVID-19 crisis management; a systematic review and expert opinions. *Eur J Clin Invest*. 2020;50(11):e13391. doi: 10.1111/eci.13391

23. Disaster management in a pandemic: tool 15. Pan American Health Organization. Published June 2020. Accessed January 10, 2021. https://www.paho.org/disasters/index.php?option=com_docman&view=download&category_slug=tools&alias=542-pandinflu-leadershipduring-tool-15&Itemid=1179&lang=en

CHAPTER 17

Team Nutrition Members in Community and Public Health Nutrition

Megan Lehnerd, PhD

Joycelyn Faraj, PhD, RDN
(We would like to thank the work of Deepa Arora, PhD, in past editions of Nutrition and Public Health.)

Learning Outcomes

AFTER STUDYING THIS CHAPTER AND REFLECTING ON THE CONTENTS, YOU SHOULD BE ABLE TO:

1. Discuss the benefits and challenges of using a team-based approach in the field of community and public health nutrition.

2. Describe the various members who may be on the community and public health nutrition team and the role each can play.

3. Reflect on the importance of educational training and continuous professional development for community and public health nutrition team members.

4. Outline the key factors needed to develop and maintain an effective community and public health nutrition team.

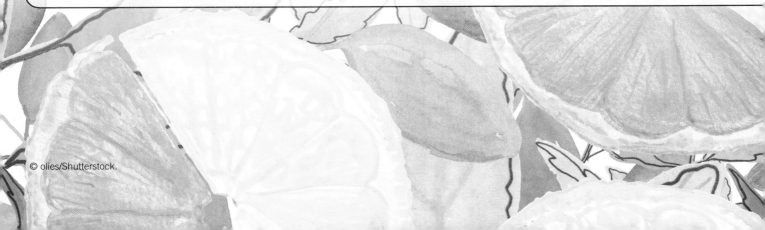

Public health nutrition team A group of key stakeholders working in various sectors who collaborate to support public health nutrition goals and initiatives.

Discussion Prompt

How does the nation's public health policy interface with community nutrition?

Introduction

Community and public health nutrition are a multifaceted approach that applies nutrition and public health principles to design programs, systems, policies, and environments that aim to improve or maintain the optimal health of populations and targeted groups. On one hand, clinical nutrition focuses on individualized medical nutrition therapy, and often addresses a specific set of medical issues. Community nutrition, on the other hand, encompasses individual and interpersonal-level interventions that create changes in knowledge, attitudes, behavior and health outcomes among individuals, families or small, targeted groups within a community setting.[1] Public health nutrition can take advantage of the potential synergy between clinical and community nutrition to strengthen the implementation of population-level public health nutrition initiatives.

Due to its multidimensional approach, the **public health nutrition team** often includes many allied health professionals to help support the public health nutrition initiatives at various levels of the socioecological model. Those trained in community and public health nutrition gain the necessary skills to improve nutritional health and reduce the risk of chronic diseases and obesity by integrating educational and environmental strategies to advance nutrition and physical activity initiatives. Approaches used in public health nutrition include identifying and assessing diet-related health problems among diverse population groups; identifying social, cultural, economic, environmental, and institutional factors that contribute to risk of undernutrition and over nutrition among populations; and creating and monitoring interventions at various levels of the socioecological model. The public health curriculum usually focuses on community nutrition, nutritional epidemiology, food policy, and nutrition research.

Members of the Community and Public Health Nutrition Team

Multilevel interventions are needed to influence the behavioral, environmental, and systemic factors related to maintaining a healthy diet and lifestyle. Therefore, it is essential for the public health nutrition team to involve key stakeholders who work in various sectors. Teams can serve a patient group or a population, and their membership is fluid depending on the needs of the people served. From a socioecological perspective, the public health nutrition team should include members working at the individual, interpersonal, organizational, community, and policy levels. Team functions can include planning, program delivery, program evaluation, and case discussions and conferences. A community or public health nutrition team works together to assess the needs of its target population, identify areas that need emphasis, and design and develop programs to address those needs. Subgroups may form within a team to provide special services. In a team, leadership roles are clearly defined and assigned.

To improve the acceptance and inclusion of suggested dietary modifications, as well as compliance, the desired dietary or health messages must be emphasized repeatedly. Repeated emphasis throughout multiple ecological levels to improve dietary habits and remain healthy will have a greater impact than counseling by a single individual. If the message of managed lives/healthy lives is to be delivered, it thus must entail a combined strong effort by a team of individuals who can shape public health efforts to promote health in communities. It is the responsibility of the community and public health nutrition team to spread the message of nutrition, particularly in areas where the risk for developing preventable chronic disorders like diabetes and heart disease are high.

Individuals and communities must have access to trained/qualified nutrition professionals and other public health and allied health professionals who have received sound training in nutrition. The providers of nutrition information are often registered or licensed **nutritionists** who have fulfilled the requirements and standards established by state and national regulations.

However, there are a variety of other key players involved in public health nutrition interventions who support the provision of total care for the individual and/or community. These individuals can also be important members of the public health nutrition team and may include but are not limited to nutritionists/dietitians, dietetic technicians, health/nutrition educators, foodservice personnel, public health nutrition program directors/ managers, community health workers, physicians, nurses, pharmacists, social workers, psychologists, and physical and occupational therapists, among others.[2] Each of these professionals can contribute their expertise toward the nutritional care of the whole community or to an individual client. The following sections discuss the responsibilities of each member of the public health nutrition team.

Nutritionists/Dietitians and Dietetic Technicians

Nutritionists/dietitians and dietetics technicians play a very important role in providing comprehensive nutrition care. They are an integral part of the professional staff working in hospitals, health clinics, well-baby clinics, nursing homes, schools, childcare centers, and other areas. In hospitals, health clinics, and nursing homes, dietitians assess the nutritional status of patients, provide dietary counseling, prescribe diets, plan menus, and supervise food services. A **registered dietitian nutritionist (RDN)** in a clinical nutrition manager position or director of nutrition and food services may also oversee dining services in healthcare settings. In addition, nutrition and dietetics technicians (NDTR) assist patients in menu selection and record daily dietary intake and data on food acceptance. In schools and childcare centers, dietitians and nutritionists are responsible for planning nutritionally balanced meals for children, providing a variety of foods that meet the Dietary Reference Intakes for different nutrients.

Dietitians/nutritionists with public health and community expertise can become directors, managers, supervisors, consultants, and researchers within a variety of settings from national to state to local levels, such as government agencies, community and professional organizations, nonprofit organizations, and schools.[3] In well-baby community clinics, such as a Special Supplemental Nutrition Program for Women, Infants, and Children (WIC) office, nutritionists and dietitians perform nutrition assessments, counseling, and provide nutrition education, while also collecting data on anthropometrics, nutritional risk, and providing referrals to other health and social services. They can be integral players in the implementation of public health nutrition interventions at an individual and community level.

Another responsibility of the nutritionist or dietitian is to provide updated nutrition information to the other members of the interdisciplinary team. Recent developments related to nutrition in children or adults that focus on normal or therapeutic nutrition, as well as recently published articles from refereed scientific publications or journals, should be shared with the other members of the public health nutrition team. This ensures that all of the team members are on top of new developments in the field.

Strategy Tip

See the qualifications of a registered dietitian posted online at: https://www .eatright.org/food/resources/learn-more -about-rdns

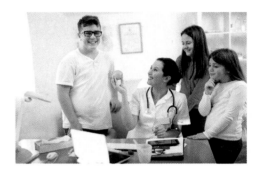

A registered dietitian addressing community team members.

© Jovanmandic/iStock/Getty Images Plus/Getty Images.

Nutritionist The term nutritionist is not a protected term and can be used by individuals who have completed either a bachelor's degree in nutrition, a master's degree in nutrition, or a master's degree in public health with a concentration in nutrition, or even an accelerated program in nutrition.

Strategy Tip

See the qualifications of a Registered Dietetic Technician posted online at: https://www.eatrightpro.org/about-us /what-is-an-rdn-and-dtr/what-is-a -nutrition-and-dietetics-technician -registered

Registered dietitian/nutritionist A food and nutrition expert who has met academic and professional requirements set forth by the Commission on Dietetic Registration to earn the credential of Registered Dietitian/Registered Dietitian Nutritionist.

Nutritionists vs. Dietitians: What is the Difference?

The terms nutritionist and dietitian have certain important differences to be noted. The credentials "registered dietitian nutritionist" (RDN) or "registered dietitian" (RD) are interchangeable and are protected terms, which refer to food and nutrition experts who have met the following criteria[4]:

- **Completed a minimum of a bachelor's degree** at a U.S. regionally accredited university or college and course work accredited or approved by the Accreditation Council for Education in Nutrition and Dietetics (ACEND) of the Academy of Nutrition and Dietetics (as of January 1st, 2024, a master's degree in any field will also be required)
- **Completed an ACEND-accredited supervised practice program** at a healthcare facility, community agency, or a foodservice operation, either as a stand-alone supervised practice or in combination with undergraduate or graduate studies
- **Passed a national examination** administered by the Commission on Dietetic Registration (CDR)
- **Completed continuing professional educational requirements** to maintain registration

In contrast, the term nutritionist is not a protected term, and can be used by individuals who have completed either a bachelor's degree in nutrition, a master's degree in nutrition or a master's degree in public health with a concentration in nutrition. Nutritionists may or may not have necessarily completed the requirements mentioned above to become a registered dietitian.

Another difference between these two positions is that the national credential for RD/RDN is the one accepted in most states. Depending on the type of job, the RD/RDN is sufficient, but some positions will also require a state licensure or certification. Individuals who do not pursue the RD/RDN path may also opt to become a certified nutrition specialist (CNS) or may meet the criteria to be a state-certified/licensed nutritionist based on education, years of experience, and completion of a statewide exam. State licensure criteria vary by state.

Individuals may meet the criteria to be a state Licensed Dietitian Nutritionist (LDN) or Certified Dietitian Nutritionist (CDN) based on education, years of experience, and completion of a statewide exam. State licensure helps protect the consumers against unsafe or inaccurate nutrition counseling or interventions that may lead to poor or dangerous health outcomes.[5]

Within a community or public health setting, such as WIC, both nutritionists and registered dietitians may be able to fulfill the job requirements as they relate to teaching, monitoring, conducting research, and advising the public on how to improve quality of life through healthy eating habits. For many types of jobs in community and public health nutrition, the RD/RDN credential may not be a requirement.

For more information about credentialing, licensing, and educational requirements, please refer to **Table 17–1**.

Within a community or public health setting, such as WIC, both nutritionists and registered dietitians may be able to fulfill the job requirements as they relate to teaching, monitoring, conducting research, and advising the public on how to improve the quality of life through healthy eating habits. For many types of jobs in community and public health nutrition, the RD/RDN credential may not be a requirement.

TABLE 17–1
Credentials and Certifications for Members of the Public Health Nutrition Team

Credential/Certification Name	Website & Description
Registered Dietitian Nutritionist (RDN) or Registered Dietitian (RD)	https://www.eatright.org National credential with specific education, supervised practice, examination, and continuing education requirements.
Certified Nutrition Specialist (CNS)	https://theana.org/certify/CNScandidate State licensure criteria varies by state. For more information about credentialing, licensing, and educational requirements visit the page above by the American Nutrition Association.
Commission on Dietetic Registration State Licensure Licensed or Certified Dietitian Nutritionist (LDN/CDN)	https://www.cdrnet.org/state-licensure State Licensure and certification information for the United States.
Certified Health Education Specialist (CHES) and Master Certified Health Education Specialist (MCHES)	https://www.nchec.org/ National credentials for health educators with education, exam, and continuing education requirements
School Nutrition Specialist (SNS) Credential	https://schoolnutrition.org/certificate-and-credentialing/credentialing-program/ Offering from the School Nutrition Association for school nutrition directors and managers interested in an elevated level of professional development. Includes completion of professional development and an examination of their skills and knowledge of foodservice program management.
School Nutrition Association Certificate Program	https://schoolnutrition.org/certificate-and-credentialing/certificate-program/ Nationwide, tiered certificate program for nutrition directors, managers, and staff seeking to advance their knowledge and skills regarding current issues in the field
Community Health Worker (CHW) Certification	https://www.cthealth.org/wp-content/uploads/2016/02/CHW-Certificaiton-by-State-Final-Final.pdf Specific requirements for certification vary by state but include classroom training on core competencies, work experience, and an evaluation of skills and/or knowledge.
Certified Dietary Manager, Certified Food Protection Professional (CDM, CFPP)	https://www.anfponline.org/become-a-cdm/cdm-cfpp-credential Certification for foodservice professionals in noncommercial settings; requires individuals to pass a nationally recognized CDM credentialing exam and participate in continuing education.

Health and Nutrition Educators

In public health departments, health clinics, and hospitals, **health educators** play a very important role as members of the public health nutrition team. Being education specialists, they design, implement, and assess educational activities that involve all of the other professionals of the public health nutrition team. They can develop and revise the curriculum, select appropriate methods and materials, and also train the staff effectively. Health educators must be able to develop good relationships with the public so that they can identify the needs and problems of the community and then develop programs to address these concerns. The health educator can also market educational campaigns to the target audience.

In the United States, the National Commission for Health Education Credentialing offers two certifications for health education specialists: Certified Health Education Specialist and Master Certified Health Education Specialist.[5] In both cases, individuals need to meet academic eligibility, pass a comprehensive written exam, and satisfy continuing education requirements. The Master Certified Health Education Specialist credential also requires professional experience in the health education field and a more advanced-level commitment to continuing education and professional development.

Pandemic Learning Opportunity

The public health team was able to provide food for the public during the COVID-19 pandemic because of previous design and implementation of this activity.

Health and nutrition educator An education specialist who designs, implements, and assesses health and nutrition educational activities for individuals and communities.

Nutrition educators perform similar tasks as health educators on the community and public health nutrition team, but they focus specifically on supporting individual and community nutrition and healthy food systems. The Society for Nutrition Education and Behavior (SNEB) established a set of evidence-based nutrition educator competencies that outline the knowledge and skills nutrition educators need to develop, implement, and evaluate effective nutrition education.[6] The Nutrition Educator Competencies for Promoting Healthy Individuals, Communities, and Food Systems are divided into 10 themes, under which more specific competencies are outlined below:

1. Basic Food and Nutrition Knowledge
2. Nutrition Across the Lifecycle
3. Food Science
4. Physical Activity
5. Food and Nutrition Policy
6. Agricultural Production and Food Systems
7. Behavior and Education Theory
8. Nutrition Education Program Design, Implementation, and Evaluation
9. Written, Oral, and Social Media Communication
10. Nutrition Education Research Methods

These competencies may be used by educational institutions to develop a curriculum and programs. However, nutrition educators may or may not have formal educational training in nutrition. Therefore, these standards can also be used for individual professional development or for on-the-job training within extension or other programs.

Nutrition educators may work in a variety of settings including schools, WIC offices, hospitals, health centers, Cooperative Extension offices, and other community and public health nutrition programs. As described in Chapter 4, nutrition education is a key component of WIC programs and the Expanded Food and Nutrition Education Program (EFNEP) delivered by state Cooperative Extension offices. One of the strengths of these programs is that they employ paraprofessionals or peer educators to deliver the nutrition education lessons. These **paraprofessionals** are individuals who are native to and/or reside in the community where they work and are better able to tailor the evidence-based nutrition lessons to the community.[7] Paraprofessionals may not always have expertise in nutrition but are skilled teachers, communicators, and community builders who are trained to deliver and evaluate nutrition education programming.[8]

Foodservice Professionals

There are a variety of settings in which foodservice operations provide meals to their community members, including hospitals, postacute care and assisted living facilities, schools and childcare facilities, correctional facilities, colleges and universities, nongovernmental organizations, and corporate cafeterias. **Foodservice professionals** may be RDNs or have a background in nutrition; however, often, a team of individuals with nutrition, culinary and/or management expertise work together to plan and manage the food preparation and ensure food safety.[9]

School nutrition directors, school nutrition managers, and school nutrition assistants or technicians are three key public health nutrition stakeholder groups involved in the provision of nutritious, safe school meals and school-based nutrition education for children and teens.[10] School nutrition directors are those who oversee the district-level operations and day-to-day management

---

Strategy Tip

See the Nutrition Educator Competencies for Promoting Healthy Individuals, Communities, and Food Systems at sneb .org/nutrition-educator-competencies/

Paraprofessional An individual native to and/or residing in the community where they work, making them well suited to tailor nutrition lessons to the community. May also be known as a peer educator.

Foodservice professional An individual with nutrition, culinary, and/ or management expertise who works in one of many foodservice settings to plan and manage food acquisition, preparation, safety, and service.

of the school foodservice program, either on their own or in partnership with other school nutrition professionals. Typically, this position requires higher education in related fields like nutrition, culinary arts, hospitality, and/or business. School nutrition managers oversee the school-level foodservice operations and are typically responsible for menu planning; food procurement, production, and service; food safety/sanitation; recordkeeping; marketing; and personnel management and professional development. School nutrition managers report to the school nutrition director. Finally, school nutrition assistants or technicians are those employees who work in the school cafeteria and directly interface with those eating the meals. They are involved in preparing and serving breakfast and lunch, processing students' transactions at the point of service, and reviewing free/reduced price meal applications. In order to establish nationwide consistency in the training required of school nutrition personnel, the Healthy, Hunger-Free Kids Act of 2010 (HHFKA) required that the United States Department of Agriculture (USDA) establish professional standards for school nutrition professionals and staff. The final rule has been in effect as of July 1, 2015 and applies to all school nutrition professionals who manage and operate National School Lunch and School Breakfast Programs.[11]

In the United States, certification is available for dietary managers who work alongside nutrition professionals to manage foodservice operations. A Certified Dietary Manager, Certified Food Protection Professional (CDM, CFPP) is an expert in noncommercial, foodservice management who must exhibit competence in five key areas: nutrition, foodservice, personnel and communications, sanitation and safety, and business operations. The CDP, CFPP certification requires individuals to pass a nationally recognized CDM Credentialing Exam and participate in continuing education.[12]

Certificate programs and the School Nutrition Specialist (SNS) Credential provide additional opportunities for school nutrition professionals to continue their education and meet the USDA Professional Standards. The School Nutrition Association (SNA) Certificate Program is a nationwide, tiered certificate program for nutrition directors, managers, and staff seeking to advance their knowledge and skills regarding current issues in the field.[13] State-level certificate programs also exist throughout the United States, and many have been accepted by their state department of education as the state-recognized certification for School Nutrition Directors as outlined in the USDA Professional Standards. For example, the Certificate in Excellence in School Nutrition offered by the John C. Stalker Institute of Food and Nutrition at Framingham State University in Massachusetts has been accepted by the Massachusetts Department of Elementary and Secondary Education as the state-recognized certification to be considered when hiring school nutrition directors.[14] The School Nutrition Specialist Credential is an additional offering from the School Nutrition Association for school nutrition directors and managers interested in an elevated level of professional development. School nutrition professionals can earn the SNS Credential through the completion of professional development and through an examination of their skills and knowledge of foodservice program management.[15]

Public Health Nutrition Program Director/Manager

As the leader for the nutrition division of the public health department, the public health nutrition program director or manager is uniquely situated to influence the work of their own team and to impact the broader community. Chapter 16 details the various responsibilities of a nutrition manager

Strategy Tip

See the qualifications of a Certified Dietary Manager and a Certified Food Protection Professional online at: https://www.anfponline.org/become-a-cdm/cdm-cfpp-credential

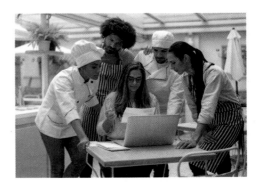

The Certified Food Protection Professional guides the foodservice staff.

© Andresr/E+/Getty Images.

or director, including the role they must play in leading their staff toward accomplishing program and organizational goals. They are also responsible for collaborating with the broader public health nutrition team to advance the health of their community. While Chapter 16 specifically focuses on the role of the manager or director of the nutrition division in a public health department, it should be noted that many of the skills and responsibilities would be the same for any manager of a community nutrition or public health program.

Community Health Worker

Community health worker A public health worker who is a trusted member of the community served, possesses a deeper understanding of said community, and acts as a liaison between health services and the community.

Community health workers are recognized as important members of the public health nutrition team and primary healthcare workforce. A community health worker is defined by the American Public Health Association as a public health worker who is a trusted member of the community served, possesses a deeper understanding of said community, and acts as a liaison between health services and the community.[16] By applying their unique understanding of the experience, language, and culture of the community they serve, community health workers are instrumental in increasing knowledge and self-sufficiency through a range of activities such as outreach, community education, informal counseling, social support, and advocacy. Community health workers have been very effective in high-priority healthcare issues such as managing chronic diseases, improving birth outcomes, maintaining child wellness, and reducing health disparities.[17,18] They facilitate access to public health services while improving the quality and cultural competency of the services delivered. Many community health workers can also provide nutrition education if adequately trained or may perform tasks of a health educator. Community health workers may have a diverse array of background experiences and may come with different job titles, such as health navigators, outreach workers, community health advisors, peer health educators, and peer support specialists, etc.[19]

In the United States, Community Health Worker Certification is available and can be achieved through either work experience or a combination of training and work experience. The specific requirements for certification will vary by state but usually include classroom training on core competencies, work experience, and an evaluation of skills and/or knowledge.[20] The key core competencies for community health workers include:

1. Effective listening and communication skills
2. Cultural responsiveness and the ability to mediate
3. Individual and community assessment
4. Health promotion, including nutrition education to promote healthy lifestyles
5. Advocacy and capacity building
6. Care coordination and systems navigation
7. Crisis identification and problem-solving

The purpose of certification is to create a better understanding and recognition of the value of community health workers, although it is not necessarily a requirement to be able to work as a community health worker.

Strategy Tip

See the criteria needed by each state online to acquire a Community Health Worker Certification at: https://healthcare accessnow.org/community-health-worker -jobtraining/

Consultant

As a part of the public health nutrition team, public health consultants can work with government agencies, nongovernmental agencies, businesses, communities, and healthcare facilities to help improve the overall health of a population. They function as independent experts who provide advice based on careful assessment of guidelines or current operations, policies, and procedures to optimize health-related outcomes.

Different tasks and job duties of a community and public health consultant include, but are not limited to:

1. Conducting professional research and analysis to improve and update strategies to tackle community and public health nutrition challenges
2. Presenting research findings and opinions to government agencies or other entities to develop policies and procedures
3. Reviewing current programs and policies that target community and public health nutrition initiatives and determine areas of improvement
4. Monitoring and evaluating outcomes of community and public health nutrition initiatives

In short, a community and public health nutrition consultant works with various groups to help determine whether efforts can be improved, and what would be the best strategies. In order to do so, an individual would need a recommended skillset and experience that includes strong analytical skills, good writing and communication skills, and a willingness to work in different settings, as it is common for consultants to do field work coupled with administrative work. In addition to experience in the field and the abovementioned skillset, a master's degree in public health or a related field is usually preferred. Certifications from a variety of agencies focusing on public health are also available.

Medical Professionals

Primary Care

Primary Care Providers (PCPs) refer to physicians, nurse practitioners, clinical nurse specialists, or physician assistants who provide preventive care and management of medical conditions. PCPs are a key point of contact with the public and play an important role in shaping the community and public health nutrition message. PCPs obtain anthropometric, clinical, biochemical, and general dietary information from their patients to diagnose disease and assess the health and nutritional status of the patient. Following the diagnosis, they recommend the type and course of treatment in order to control the disease and prevent further health deterioration.

As part of treatment as well as disease prevention and health promotion, PCPs play a role in nutrition education and also make referrals to qualified nutritionists/dietitians for detailed assessment, planning, and patient counseling for behavioral change.

In 1985, the Committee on Nutrition in Medical Education, a branch of the Food and Nutrition Board of the National Research Council, identified the lack of adequate training for medical students in the United States and recommended that nutrition be added to the curriculum as a required course.[21] The National Nutritional Monitoring and Related Research Act was passed in 1990 to ensure that medical students and practicing physicians in the United States have adequate training for medical students and physicians in the discipline of nutrition; however, the curriculum offered at many U.S. medical schools still does not adequately concentrate on this discipline. This is reflected in clinical practice, where physicians provide very limited nutrition education during patient care in the treatment of nutrition-related diseases like diabetes, heart disease, obesity, osteoporosis, and anemia, among others. This underscores the importance of the PCP's connections to others on the public health nutrition team who are better qualified to provide individualized nutrition care.

Discussion Prompt

What are the detailed ramifications of leaving nutrition out of the medical school curriculum? What are the far-reaching consequences?

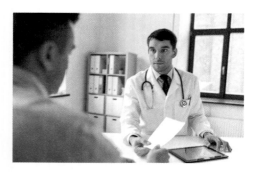

A physician can refer patients to a registered dietitian in the community.

© Syda Productions/Shutterstock.

Discussion Prompt

What are the detailed ramifications of leaving nutrition out of the pharmacy school curriculum? What are the far-reaching consequences?

Discussion Prompt

What are the detailed ramifications of leaving nutrition out of the physical and occupational therapist school curriculum? What are the far-reaching consequences?

Discussion Prompt

What are the detailed ramifications of leaving nutrition out of the dental school curriculum? What are the far-reaching consequences?

PCPs may go beyond primary care to demonstrate competencies in public health sciences, such as epidemiology, biostatistics, and surveillance, planning, implementing and evaluation of programs and policies, leadership, collaboration, advocacy, and communication to improve population health. It is not uncommon for PCPs to pursue a Master of Public Health degree to complement their clinical skills to better address health and wellness from both the perspective of the individual patient as well as in the community and the general population.

Pharmacists

Pharmacists are increasingly responsible for effective, safe, and efficient use of medicines, yet, they are underutilized as public health professionals.[22] Pharmacists work in a variety of settings including hospitals, drug, grocery, and retail stores, and nursing homes, providing ample opportunity in which to support the community and public health nutrition team. Pharmacists are an essential member of clinical nutrition support and healthcare teams. In community settings, pharmacists provide information to the patient on possible interactions between different drugs and food, thus contributing to nutrition education of the public. Pharmacists can be involved in health screenings (e.g., diabetes, cholesterol, osteoporosis), immunizations, pain control, participatory and clinical research, and counseling and health education.[23] They also provide information on self-management of chronic and diet-related conditions such as hypertension and asthma; smoking cessation; alcohol, tobacco, and other drug use prevention; and medication indications and conditions.[23]

Physical and Occupational Therapists

Physical and occupational therapists examine each person and provide individualized care while interacting closely and for an extended period of time with clients in need of therapy to improve their ability to move, reduce or manage pain, restore function, and prevent disability. As it relates to nutrition, patients who have difficulty eating or swallowing need help from these therapists to overcome their handicap to function more efficiently. Therefore, therapists in a clinical setting must work closely with the nutritionist or dietitian to decide which foods will be appropriate for the patient as well as provide the desired nutrition. Subsequently, they interact with the family and the client to train them as to appropriate feeding procedures and regimen. During each session, these therapists could prove invaluable in transferring nutrition-related information to the client.

The work of physical and occupational therapists can have broad public health nutrition implications as well. Physical therapists provide education, behavioral strategies, patient advocacy, and identification of resources to help support tobacco-free living, preventing drug abuse and excessive alcohol use, healthy eating, and active living.[24]

Dentists and Dental Hygienists

Promoting oral hygiene and preventing the development of cavities and tooth-related disorders is the function of the dentist. Dentists and dental hygienists, in their interaction with the client, discourage the use of high-sugar food items and encourage the use of nutritive foods. In other words, these professionals also contribute significantly to improving the nutritional status of their clients on an individual level.

On a population level, the American Dental Association (ADA) recognized the specialty of Dental Public Health in 1950 and has supported this specialty's mission to prevent and control disease and promote dental health through organized community efforts, highlighting the regular assessment to determine need, development of community-based prevention and treatment programs, and ongoing surveillance of populations.[25]

Veterinarians

The American Public Health Association recognized the need for veterinarians in public health services, in every health department and health clinic.[26] The Association recommended that schools of public health and applied public health programs provide facilities for continuing education and recruitment outreach to veterinarians. Furthermore, the veterinary profession has a recognized specialty for practitioners of public health and preventive medicine. The American College of Veterinary Preventive Medicine (ACVPM) certifies core competencies of epidemiology, infectious disease, environmental health, food safety, and public policy. Therefore, veterinarians can serve as essential public health workers in state health departments, play an important role in promoting food safety, especially pathogen control, and in the surveillance of foodborne diseases.[26]

Social Workers

Social workers are dedicated to improving human well-being using ecological, clinical, and biopsychosocial approaches to work at multiple levels of society, ranging from individuals and families to neighborhoods, organizations, and government.[27] In a healthcare setting, social workers help those patients who are in need of placement services. They are able to assess the physical, emotional, financial, and social stresses encountered by the patient that would prevent them from following the recommended medical and dietary advice after discharge while providing guidance to help patients face these challenges and find workable solutions. At the community level, social workers play a crucial role in the Department of Transitional Assistance, assisting and empowering low-income individuals and families to meet their basic needs, improve their quality of life, and achieve long-term economic self-sufficiency. Assisting with applications for programs like the Supplemental Nutrition Assistance Program (SNAP) and health insurance is an essential function of social workers on the public health nutrition team.

Although most social workers practice in direct patient care roles, such as counseling, health education, crisis intervention, and care managers, social workers can also make a difference at a population level by getting involved in health administration, prevention and health promotion, research, advocacy, and policy.[27] To better integrate public health concepts into social work, the Master of Social Work-Master of Public Health (MSW-MPH) program was created to build on the synergy between these two fields. The MSW-MPH focuses on the practice of all core public health services, from community mobilization and health promotion to program evaluation and surveillance.

Psychologists

The traditional role of the psychologist is to counsel clients on their mental health condition and suggest a course of treatment. In healthcare settings, psychologists carry out clinical interviews and behavioral assessments and focus on direct patient counseling by employing behavior change techniques such as self-monitoring and goal-setting to foster emotional and physical well-being. They can also participate in interventions with individuals or groups, such as in programs to help people manage eating disorders, reduce stress, quit smoking, and avoid sedentary behaviors.[28] Health psychology is a specific branch of psychology that deals with how patients handle illness,

Discussion Prompt

What are the detailed ramifications of leaving nutrition out of the social work school curriculum? What are the far-reaching consequences?

and how to most effectively help patients control pain, change health habits, and adhere to medical advice. In order to tackle broader public health nutrition issues, health psychologists can provide support and training for others on the public health nutrition team, like health- and social-care workers, to enhance their skills regarding behavior change techniques and counseling.[29] Psychologists may also be involved in community and public health nutrition research, studying the causes and prevention of diet-related conditions and exploring why certain groups do not seek care when they need it. In this manner, psychologists can participate in wider-reaching population level initiatives by designing, monitoring, and evaluating sustainable, cost-effective interventions that can help inform policy development.

While a bachelor's degree is the foundation for a career in psychology, most careers in health psychology require a doctoral degree. A master's degree would be adequate for research assistant or behavior specialist positions, typically working under the supervision of a licensed psychologist.[28] Those who earn a doctoral degree can work independently and supervise research or clinical teams, including those working in areas of weight management and obesity prevention, pain management, and physical activity promotion.[28]

Researcher/Academic

Public health nutrition researchers play a crucial role in generating scholarship that can inform, influence, and shape initiatives to improve population health. Professionals contributing to public health nutrition research come from a variety of educational backgrounds and training including public health, nutrition, medicine, nursing, social work, allied health professionals, engineering, environmental sciences, biology, and microbiology, among others. Research and academia tend to be closely related, as those working in systems of higher education generally have an important role in knowledge generation. Academic researchers conduct basic and applied research in disciplines pertinent to public health nutrition, educate and train the future generation of public health nutrition workers, and engage in community, public, and professional service. Furthermore, academic institutions often collaborate with public health, governmental, and nongovernmental agencies and carry out community-based research. It is through these collaborations that many students are able to participate in service, learning to gain experience in the field, while allowing researchers to create joint, community-driven research efforts that can guide policy creation and ultimately translate initiatives into action.

Policymakers

As outlined in Chapter 3, local, state, and federal policymakers play an essential role in the creation, funding, implementation, and evaluation of community and public health nutrition programs.[30] This means that they can have substantial influence on the nutrition and health of the public and should be considered an important part of the nutrition team. Through advocacy efforts, collaborations between policymakers and others on the community and public health nutrition team can lead to the development of more evidence-based policies and regulations that better meet the needs of the public at the local, state, and federal levels.

The Public

Public health nutrition should not be limited to only experts who advise the public on what to do and what not to do. There are not enough public health professionals available to interact with the public. The onus of improving the

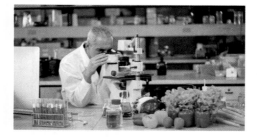

A registered dietitian can be found performing nutrition research for community and public health.

© Witthaya Prasongsin/Moment/Getty Images.

diet and health of communities also lies with the public itself. More active participation is required of the public.[31] Each individual must recognize their own responsibility toward maintaining good health and advocating for changes that support the health of their community. Each individual must consider their own actions to understand what needs to be changed to improve nutritional status and maintain good health.

It would be ideal if each trained professional could associate with a community-based organization long enough to train some of their members. The responsibility thereafter could be taken up by these members to train others in the organization. The organization could then expand its educational activities to other organizations. A chain reaction would follow whereby one individual would educate another until the whole community was informed. "Each one, educate one." Such could be the motto of all community organizations to achieve good nutrition and health for all.

Education Programs

As the demand for trained professionals in the field of public health nutrition has increased, universities worldwide are offering more programs and certificates to help meet this need. Furthermore, free resources for training and continuing education have become widely available through governmental and educational institutions alike.

Bachelor's or Master's in Public Health

A public health major is a degree path that prepares students to understand and advocate for individual and community health and well-being through the development of critical thinking and analysis skills necessary to confront issues such as foodborne diseases, drug overdoses, the obesity epidemic, and health promotion. A Master's degree in Public Health (MPH) is an option for those interested in health and health care on a broader scale than provider-to-patient care and pairs well with other degree options. Both public health degree pathways will prepare individuals to work with specific populations and communities to improve their health through awareness, education, policy, and research. An MPH will provide students with a more advanced understanding of the core disciplines of public health (biostatistics, epidemiology, environmental health, health policy and administration, and social and behavioral sciences).[32] Many advanced clinical degrees also offer a dual-degree option with an integrated MPH, such as Medicine, Dentistry, Masters in Nursing, Social Work, Public Administration, or Nutrition.

Nutrition Education for Public Health Nutrition Team Members

If the members of the public health nutrition team have a responsibility to provide advice that impacts dietary choices, it is important for them to have adequate training in the discipline of nutrition. Registered dietitians and nutritionists will have such training, as discussed above. In order to maintain their professional status, registered and licensed dietitians must take a certain number of **continuing education** credit hours every 5 years to update their skills and knowledge. The Academy of Nutrition and Dietetics holds registered dietitians to high standards to assure they are reliable and trustworthy sources of nutrition information.

Other professionals involved in the public health nutrition team may also pursue nutrition education to strengthen efforts to fight nutrition-related epidemics. Despite recommendations put forth by the 1990 National

Continuing education Additional formal learning to refresh knowledge, skills, and current practices in a particular field.

Nutritional Monitoring and Related Research Act to ensure that medical students and practicing physicians in the United States have adequate training in the field of nutrition and how it relates to human health,[21] the curriculum offered at many U.S. medical schools still does not adequately concentrate on this discipline. Therefore, the Nutrition Academic Award program was developed in 1997 by the National Heart, Lung and Blood Institute to improve nutrition-related knowledge and skills among medical school students, residents, fellows, faculty, and practicing physicians.[33] This initiative is intended to improve the application of nutrition principles in patient care and clinical practice. It should reinforce the existing efforts to improve the qualifications and training of physicians in the science of nutrition. In addition to training medical students, some recipients of the Nutrition Academic Award provide training to students from other health professional schools, such as dental programs, dietetic programs, nursing schools, pharmacy schools, physician assistant programs, public health programs, exercise physiology programs, physical education programs, and health ecology programs.

Professional Societies and Continuing Education

In addition to satisfactory training in the principles of nutrition, many dietitians and nutritionists seek membership in relevant professional societies, such as the Academy of Nutrition and Dietetics, American Society for Clinical Nutrition, Society for Nutrition Education and Behavior, and Institute of Food Technologists. These professional societies are groups of other similarly trained individuals who want to stay informed of recent advances in the field of food and nutrition. Specific to public health nutrition, the American Public Health Association (APHA) offers membership to a multidisciplinary group focused on local, national, and global food and nutrition issues that works to influence policies, programs, research, and education related to public health nutrition.[34] Furthermore, the Association of State Public Health Nutritionists and the Academy of Nutrition and Dietetics offers resources for continuing education and training to support the professional development of public health nutrition leaders.[35] **Table 17–2** and **17–3** lists many of the professional societies for public health nutrition-related resources and memberships.

Strategy Tip

What would be the career benefits to belonging to some of these memberships?

TABLE 17–2
Professional Societies for Public Health Nutrition-Related Resources and Memberships

Professional Society	Website and Society's Mission
Association of State Public Health Nutritionists (ASPHN)	https://asphn.org/ The Association of State Public Health Nutritionists is a professional organization for public health nutritionists whose mission it is to strengthen nutrition policy, programs, and environments for all people through development of public health nutrition leaders and collective action of members nationwide.
Society for Nutrition Education and Behavior (SNEB)	https://www.sneb.org/ The Society for Nutrition Education and Behavior is dedicated to promoting effective nutrition education and healthy behaviors through research, policy, and practice and has a mission to advance food and nutrition education research, practice, and policy that promote equity and support public and planetary health.
Institute of Food Technologists (IFT)	http://www.ift.org The Institute of Food Technologists was founded in 1939, and its mission is to advance the science of food and its applications across the global food system.
School Nutrition Association (SNA)	https://schoolnutrition.org/ The School Nutrition Association is a national organization of school nutrition professionals committed to advancing the quality of school meal programs through education and advocacy.

TABLE 17–3
Free Governmental Resources for Nutrition Education

Governmental Programs	Website and Description
Team Nutrition Initiative	http://www.fns.usda.gov/tn/ Team Nutrition Initiative, professional development for school food service personnel.
Supplemental Nutrition Assistance Program Education (SNAP-Ed)	https://snaped.fns.usda.gov/ Grant program for all U.S. states and territories that provides nutrition education resources and supports the delivery of nutrition messages through social marketing and policy, system, and environmental change.
Dietary Guidelines for Americans 2020-2025 (DGA)	https://www.dietaryguidelines.gov/ The DGA are renewed every 5 years and provide advice on what to eat and drink to build a healthy diet that can promote healthy growth and development, help prevent diet-related chronic disease, and meet nutrient needs.
Expanded Food and Nutrition Education Program (EFNEP)	https://nifa.usda.gov/program/about-efnep EFNEP uses community outreach to provide nutrition education for low-income populations through land-grant universities.
Food Safety	https://www.foodsafety.gov/ Food safety resources for all ages and recalls.
Academy of Nutrition and Dietetics (AND)	http://www.eatright.org The Academy of Nutrition and Dietetics is the world's largest organization of food and nutrition professionals; founded in 1917, its mission is to accelerate improvements in global health and well-being through food and nutrition.
American Society for Nutrition (ASN)	http://www.nutrition.org/ The American Society for Nutrition is a professional society whose mission is to advance the science, education, and practice of nutrition with a focus on areas of nutrition science-based information and practice, education and professional development, science policy, and advocacy.
American Public Health Association (APHA)	https://www.apha.org/ The American Public Health Association is a professional organization for public health professionals founded in 1872, whose mission it is to improve the health of the public and achieve equity in health status. APHA offers a Food and Nutrition section dedicated to local, national, and global food and nutrition issues.

Teamwork
Developing an Effective Public Health Team

A team consists of a group of individuals working together to achieve a shared goal.[2] In an ideal team, members function synergistically, leading to increased efficiency and productivity. The emphasis is seldom placed on individual team members; rather, the team as a total entity is always paramount. To achieve the shared goal, team members are involved in activities that are interdependent instead of independent. With different individuals contributing their skills and knowledge to the team, each member of the team learns about the important role and position of different professional contributors on the team. They learn to respect each other's expertise and also appreciate how all of the disciplines come together to address a common goal. In the public health arena, teamwork is crucial because the efforts of a great diversity of team members contributes tremendously toward improving the health and nutritional status of the individual, family, or community. As discussed earlier, such integrated efforts are necessary to address the physical, emotional, social, economic, cultural, and personal issues linked to the individual, family, or community. Not only can these professionals address the problem from different perspectives but they also can reinforce the messages of health and nutrition to bridge the gap between knowledge and practice. Teamwork thus can prove to be an economical way of addressing the health and nutrition needs of an individual, family, or community.

Strategies and Characteristics of a Properly Functioning and Effective Team

For a team to function in the most productive and efficient manner, its members have to be focused on the objectives, share leadership roles, and be accountable for their actions. Some defining features of a successful team are the following[36,37]:

- *Zero in on the objectives:* Any team should, at the onset, be aware of the goals to be achieved. Each member of the team should be very clear about the goals and objectives of the project. Additionally, the team members should be in agreement regarding the specific outcomes and parameters to be used to assess whether the goals have been adequately reached.

- *Accentuate a participatory style:* In a team as diverse as a public health nutrition team, different ideas are bound to arise because members originate from different disciplines. Members must be encouraged to listen and acknowledge alternate points of view in order to obtain a view of the "big picture." As team members begin to respect each other, recognize each other's contributions, and trust each other, they can address the health issue more appropriately. While some members look at the broader picture, others look at small details; while some address the physical aspect, others deal with emotional issues; while others stress the economic aspect, some will focus on social influences. This is perhaps one of the best ways of finding solutions together.

- *Increase the sense of belonging and connectedness:* The work of any team is considerably enhanced if the members have a strong sense of connection with other team members and with the objectives of the team. All members of the team should have a sense of belonging and a strong desire to meet the defined goals and objectives.

- *Organize the team:* The specific responsibilities for the team should be mutually agreed upon by all team members. Because a public health nutrition team is inherently multifaceted, as are the problems it intends to address, clear leadership roles should be defined for different team activities. Team members should be identified by discipline, knowledge, skills, specialization, experience, and interests.

- *Promote team responsibility:* Given the interdependent nature of any team, members of the team must be encouraged to take responsibility for completing individual duties in a timely manner. When necessary, team members also should assist one another to collectively achieve the objectives of the team.

- *Encourage equal influence:* The team must be built on the premise that the viewpoints and contributions of all members are of equal value, and; therefore, all members must be willing to yield influence on all issues facing the team. Each member of the team must recognize and respect the contributions made by the other members of the team. Members must pay close attention to the suggestions made by others and then collectively arrive at one decision.

- *Establish a timeline for the work to be done and commit to allotting time to do the work:* After the activities necessary to achieve the desired goals and objectives are planned and explained to all the members of the team, every member must then assume responsibility for the activities and make the necessary time commitment to work toward them.

- *Define measurable outcomes and work products:* As per the commitment of each team member, at the end of the time period designated for the activity, tangible work products should be visible. Each person on the team must show their contribution toward attaining the planned goals and objectives of the team. The resources available to the team must be shared equally by all of the members; there should be no competition or turf guarding. Team members come from different disciplines, so there should be complete understanding among all of the members about the role and responsibilities of each member. Cooperation with each other along with administrative support will allow the team to function efficiently and effectively.

- *Discuss and resolve all problems together:* As each member of the team undertakes activities to move in the planned direction, some problems and challenges may arise. For smooth resolution of all such problems, the team members must communicate on a regular basis to discuss and formulate solutions. All challenges thus must be faced by the team collectively and solutions finalized with mutual consent.

Cultural Considerations for the Public Health Nutrition Team

By providing nutrition programs to communities at risk of developing nutrition-linked chronic diseases, public health nutrition workers hope to provide information, skills, and reinforcements in order to encourage people to introduce modifications into their dietary patterns to protect or improve their health. Providing nutrition education not only involves dispensing knowledge and information but also supplying ways and means to change attitudes and behavior. The challenge is for people to retain and follow the recommended changes in dietary practices. It is just not enough to design programs and deliver information to the public in a one-time interaction.[38] To bring about any significant change in the lifestyle of individuals or communities and impact health in a positive manner, the process of imparting knowledge and encouraging changes has to be continued over a period of time. The approach has to be slow, but consistent. To produce a strong desire to change and an intense motivation to incorporate changes into their dietary patterns, people need more than just knowledge transfer, information availability, and attitude change. Skills and adequate resources must be available to support the motivated individual. Social support and rewards for the behavioral change are necessary if the changes are to be incorporated and sustained over time. Public health nutrition professionals must, therefore, train individuals, families, employers, community leaders, and influential people in the community to provide support for recommended changes in their dietary habits.

A major barrier faced by nutrition educators is the lack of linguistically and culturally appropriate services.[39] There is a lack of translated materials in different languages for audiences who speak English as a second language. This problem is further compounded by the fact that the number of bilingual providers and trained interpreters are limited. The public health team must be cognizant of this issue and have appropriate training and structures in place to provide linguistically and culturally responsive programming to meet the needs of their community. Another consideration that the public health nutrition team must keep in mind is that dietary habits are linked to culture. Health promotion programs that emphasize nutrition will have to be designed specifically, or be "custom-made," for the target communities, keeping in mind their dietary food habits, regional food choices and selection, food preferences, and cultural practices. Any recommendation that is not culturally appropriate will not be easily acceptable to the public. In a policy adopted in 2001, the American Public Health Association advocated that federal agencies use resources that are culturally sensitive and linguistically relevant, along with translators.[40] The association also encouraged healthcare providers to collaborate with federal agencies to provide culturally and linguistically appropriate services.

The public health team also must recognize the need to remove cultural barriers that impede the progress of healthy change in communities. Along with outreach programs for health promotion and nutrition education, additional programs must address the problem of cultural and social barriers to change.

It is also important to keep in mind that if nutrition education and health-promotion programs are to be successful, they should be imparted not only at the level of the individual but also at the level of the community. Public health professionals in community health centers and community-based organizations can reach communities that are otherwise disenfranchised. They can target their programs toward specific populations so the message can be delivered more effectively and be better retained and implemented. Community-based organizations are important because many of them arise out of personal experiences and thus better understand the pulse of the community.[41]

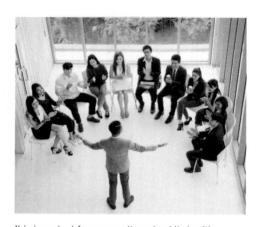

It is important for community and public health nutrition team members to be culturally competent.

© CMYK/Shutterstock.

Chapter Summary

This chapter discusses the importance of a multidimensional, team-based approach to designing, implementing, and evaluating public health nutrition initiatives. It outlines the various stakeholders who may collaborate to provide nutrition education and programming for the community, including public health professionals like nutritionists/dietitians, dietetic technicians, health/nutrition educators, foodservice personnel, public health nutrition program directors/managers, community health workers, physicians, nurses, pharmacists, social workers, psychologists, and physical and occupational therapists. Notably, forming a team of professionals from diverse backgrounds is essential to support communities in creating long-term change, and those team members must be dedicated to continued education and professional development. This chapter describes the educational training and certifications available to prepare those on the public health nutrition team, some of whom are required to hold the positions or titles described. Public health nutrition team members are encouraged to take advantage of the educational opportunities offered by professional societies, government agencies, and others, and examples of professional societies and continuing education opportunities are outlined in this chapter. Finally, strategies are discussed for developing and supporting a properly functioning and effective public health nutrition team. Specific cultural considerations are suggested so that members will be best able to adapt to the community's changing needs and incorporate advances in nutrition and public health into their programming.

Learning Portfolio

© olies/Shutterstock.

Issues for Discussion

1. Why is taking a team-based approach to public health nutrition a more effective strategy than individuals working on their own?
2. Who is responsible for providing nutrition guidance and education within the public health nutrition team? When would the services of a registered dietitian/licensed nutritionist be required?
3. What level of training in the field of nutrition is considered to be "adequate" for medical school students and allied health professionals?
4. What measures can be taken to reduce the challenges faced by the public health nutrition team?
5. What are some ways that the public health nutrition team could work together to make their programming more culturally responsive to their community?

Practical Activities

1. Research a public health or community nutrition program in your community. Using the social ecological model, see if you can map out all of the types of stakeholders who are involved in the public health nutrition team for that organization or program. You may need to explore the website for the program to get the information you need.
2. Do an online search for jobs in the field of public health nutrition. Which types of positions did you find? Choose three positions and create a table that outlines the position name, the educational requirements, the job experience requirements, and the additional qualities that are desired in a candidate. Then compare and contrast what you find about the three positions. How does what you find compare to what you learned in this chapter?
3. Visit the website of the Academy of Nutrition and Dietetics, the Society for Nutrition Education and Behavior, or any of the other professional societies mentioned in this chapter (Table 17–2). Explore the webinar and training opportunities for members of these professional societies. What types of opportunities do they have available? Then, visit the membership section to learn about the cost and benefits of membership. Do they have student memberships available?

Key Terms

	page
Public health nutrition team	546
Nutritionist	547
Registered dietitian/nutritionist	547
Health and nutrition educator	549
Paraprofessional	550
Foodservice professional	550
Community health worker	552
Continuing education	557

Case Study: Assembling a Team

You are the director of your state's department of health and human services, and you are proposing to tackle the opioid epidemic through increased funding to state-run halfway homes and recovery centers. Part of the multipronged approach includes providing workshops to staff on ways to reduce stress, enhance physical activity, impart nutrition education groups, and improve the nutritional offerings at these centers.

Consider the following questions:

1. Who would you want to include in your team to plan and deliver the program? List all potential members and their roles.
2. How would you determine which approach to take as it relates to nutrition and physical activity programs that can be implemented? Where would you find reliable, evidence-based information and educational resources on healthy dietary practices and physical activity?
3. If you wanted team members to gain nutrition training, how would you do this?
4. Would you want to provide a one-time workshop or ongoing education to staff members? Defend your answer.

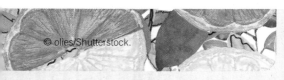
© olies/Shutterstock.

Learning Portfolio

Case Study: Nutrition Education Program

Tiny Tots, a childcare center in Georgia, provides daycare for 0–3 year olds and also offers state-funded pre-K curriculum to 4-year-old children of different races including Caucasians, African Americans, Asians, and Hispanics. The Director has observed that almost 50% of the children attending this childcare center are either overweight or obese. She would like to plan a nutrition education program to address the needs of the population she is serving.

1. Who should be involved in the planning of the nutrition education program for the childcare center?

2. What principles must be kept in mind while planning the nutrition education campaign?

3. How will you ensure the involvement of children in this campaign?

4. How much involvement of parents should be considered?

5. What resources can be used to build a standards-based nutrition education curriculum?

References

1. Academy of Nutrition and Dietetics. Public Health and Community. Accessed January 25, 2021. https://www.eatrightpro.org/practice/practice-resources/public-health-and-community

2. Kaufman. *Leveraging nutrition education through the public health team.* Aspen Publications; 1990.

3. Andersen D, Baird S, Bates T, et al. Academy of Nutrition and Dietetics: revised 2017 scope of practice for the registered dietitian nutritionist. *J Acad Nutr Diet.* 2018;118(1):141-165. doi: 10.1016/j.jand.2017.10.002

4. Academy of Nutrition and Dietetics. What is a registered dietitian nutritionist.? Accessed January 25, 2021. https://www.eatrightpro.org/about-us/what-is-an-rdn-and-dtr/what-is-a-registered-dietitian-nutritionist

5. National Commission for Health Education Credentialing. Health Education Specialist Certification - CHES®, MCHES® | NCHEC. Accessed January 25, 2021. https://www.nchec.org/

6. Society for Nutrition Education and Behavior (SNEB). *Nutrition educator competencies.* Accessed January 25, 2021. https://www.sneb.org/nutrition-educator-competencies

7. Expanded food and nutrition education program (EFNEP) Paraprofessional Supervision. Crucial components for program success. Published online February 2017. Accessed January 25, 2021. https://nifa.usda.gov/sites/default/files/resource/EFNEP-Supervision-White-Paper-2.15.17.pdf

8. National Institute of Food and Agriculture. United States Department of Agriculture. Core Competencies - EFNEP & SNAP-Ed. Accessed January 25, 2021. https://nifa.usda.gov/resource/core-competencies-efnep-snap-ed

9. Academy of Nutrition and Dietetics. Foodservice. Accessed January 25, 2021. https://www.eatrightpro.org/practice/practice-resources/foodservice

10. School Nutrition Association. Qualifications & Job Opportunities. Accessed January 25, 2021. https://schoolnutrition.org/school-meals/careers/qualifications-and-job-opportunities/

11. United States Department of Agriculture. Professional standards for all school nutrition program employees - FNS-486. Published online May 2015. Accessed January 25, 2021. https://fns-prod.azureedge.net/sites/default/files/cn/profstandards_flyer.pdf

12. Association of Nutrition & Foodservice Professionals (ANFP) - CDM, CFPP Credential. Accessed January 25, 2021. https://www.anfponline.org/become-a-cdm/cdm-cfpp-credential

13. School Nutrition Association. Certificate program. Accessed January 25, 2021. https://schoolnutrition.org/certificate-and-credentialing/certificate-program/

14. Framingham State University. Undergraduate certificate in excellence in school nutrition. Accessed January 25, 2021. https://www.framingham.edu/academics/continuing-education/undergraduate-certificates/undergraduate-certificate-in-excellence-in-school-nutrition

15. School Nutrition Association. SNS Credentialing. Accessed January 25, 2021. https://schoolnutrition.org/certificate-and-credentialing/credentialing-program/

16. American Public Health Association. Community health workers. Accessed January 25, 2021. https://www.apha.org/apha-communities/member-sections/community-health-workers

17. Ingram M, Sabo S, Rothers J, Wennerstrom A, de Zapien JG. Community health workers and community advocacy: addressing health disparities. *J Community Health*. 2008;33(6):417-424. doi: 10.1007/s10900-008-9111-y

18. Balcázar HG, de Heer H, Rosenthal L, et al. A *promotores de salud* intervention to reduce cardiovascular disease risk in a high-risk Hispanic border population, 2005-2008. *Prev Chronic Dis*. 2010;7(2):A28.

19. MA Association of Community Health Workers. Who are community health workers? Accessed January 25, 2021. https://machw.org/

20. Carey M, London K, Russell K. Community health worker certification requirements by state. *Conn Health Found*. Published online February 2016:10.

21. Pearson TA, Stone EJ, Grundy SM, et al. Translation of nutritional sciences into medical education: the Nutrition Academic Award Program. *Am J Clin Nutr*. 2001;74(2):164-170. doi: 10.1093/ajcn/74.2.164

22. Mossialos E, Courtin E, Naci H, et al. From "retailers" to health care providers: Transforming the role of community pharmacists in chronic disease management. *Health Policy*. 2015;119(5):628-639. doi: 10.1016/j.healthpol.2015.02.007

23. American Public Health Association. The role of the pharmacist in public health. Accessed January 25, 2021. https://www.apha.org/policies-and-advocacy/public-health-policy-statements/policy-database/2014/07/07/13/05/the-role-of-the-pharmacist-in-public-health

24. Health Priorities For Populations And Individuals | APTA. Accessed January 25, 2021. https://www.apta.org/apta-and-you/leadership-and-governance/policies/health-priorities-populations-individuals

25. Robinson LA. Private sector response to improving oral health care access. *Dent Clin North Am*. 2009;53(3):523-535. doi: 10.1016/j.cden.2009.03.016

26. American Public Health Association. Recognizing the role of veterinarians in the public health workforce. Accessed January 25, 2021. https://www.apha.org/policies-and-advocacy/public-health-policy-statements/policy-database/2014/07/15/13/30/recognizing-the-role-of-veterinarians-in-the-public-health-workforce

27. Ruth BJ, Marshall JW. A history of social work in public health. *Am J Public Health*. 2017;107(S3):S236-S242. doi: 10.2105/AJPH.2017.304005

28. American Psychological Association. Pursuing a career in health psychology. Accessed January 26, 2021. https://www.apa.org/action/science/health/education-training

29. Lawrence W, Barker M. Improving the health of the public: what is the role of health psychologists? *J Health Psychol*. 2016;21(2):135-137. doi: 10.1177/1359105314528013

30. Mozaffarian D, Angell SY, Lang T, Rivera JA. Role of government policy in nutrition—barriers to and opportunities for healthier eating. *BMJ*. 2018;361:k2426. doi: 10.1136/bmj.k2426

31. Avery B. Who does the work of public health? *Am J Public Health*. 2002;92(4):570-575.

32. Find and compare public health degrees. Accessed January 26, 2021. https://www.publichealthdegrees.org

33. Hark LA, Eaton CB. Nutrition curriculum guide for training physicians. 65.

34. American Public Health Association. Food and Nutrition. Accessed January 26, 2021. https://www.apha.org/apha-communities/member-sections/food-and-nutrition

35. ASPHN: Association of State Public Health Nutritionists. Accessed January 26, 2021. https://asphn.org/

36. Franklin CM, Bernhardt JM, Lopez RP, Long-Middleton ER, Davis S. Interprofessional teamwork and collaboration between community health workers and healthcare teams: an integrative review. *Health Serv Res Manag Epidemiol*. 2015;2. doi: 10.1177/2333392815573312

37. UC Berkeley. Steps to Building an Effective Team | People & Culture. Accessed January 28, 2021. https://hr.berkeley.edu/hr-network/central-guide-managing-hr/managing-hr/interaction/team-building/steps

38. Breckon D, Harvey J. Current perspectives of practice and professional preparation. In: *Community Health Education—Settings, Roles and Skills for the 21st Century*. Aspen Publication; 1998.

39. National Academy of Medicine. Language, interpretation, and translation: a clarification and reference checklist in service of health literacy and cultural respect. Accessed January 26, 2021. https://nam.edu/language-interpretation-and-translation-a-clarification-and-reference-checklist-in-service-of-health-literacy-and-cultural-respect/

40. American Public Health Association. Support for culturally and linguistically appropriate services in health and mental health care. Accessed January 26, 2021. https://www.apha.org/policies-and-advocacy/public-health-policy-statements/policy-database/2014/07/15/15/31/support-for-culturally-and-linguistically-appropriate-services-in-health-and-mental-health-care

41. Chillag K, Bartholow K, Cordeiro J, et al. Factors affecting the delivery of HIV/AIDS prevention programs by community-based organizations. *AIDS Educ Prev Off Publ Int Soc AIDS Educ*. 2002;14(3 suppl A):27-37. doi: 10.1521/aeap.14.4.27.23886

PART VII

Surviving in a Competitive World

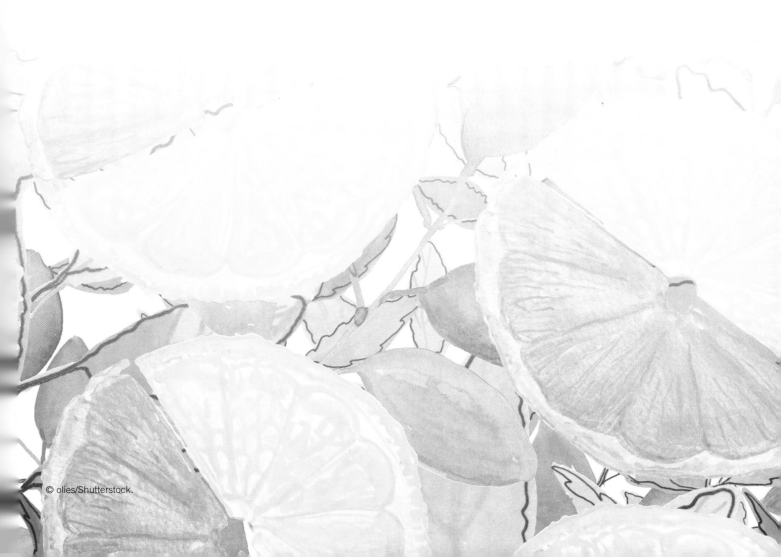

CHAPTER 18

Networking for Nutrition and Earning Administrative Support

Farrell Frankel, MS, RDN

(We acknowledge the work of Sharon Gallagher, Med, RDN, LDN; Patti S. Landers, PhD, RDN/ LDN; and Jeannette Beasley, PhD, MPH, RDN in the past editions of Nutrition in Public Health.)

Learning Outcomes

AFTER STUDYING THIS CHAPTER AND REFLECTING ON THE CONTENTS, YOU SHOULD BE ABLE TO:

1. Discuss the difference between networks, alliances, and coalitions.

2. Give examples of nutrition issues that might be addressed by networks or coalitions.

3. Describe the responsibilities of a lead agency and steering committee in maintaining a nutrition coalition.

4. Review environmental factors that influence the administration's priorities.

5. Describe components of the strategic plan that help to provide insight into administrative goals and objectives.

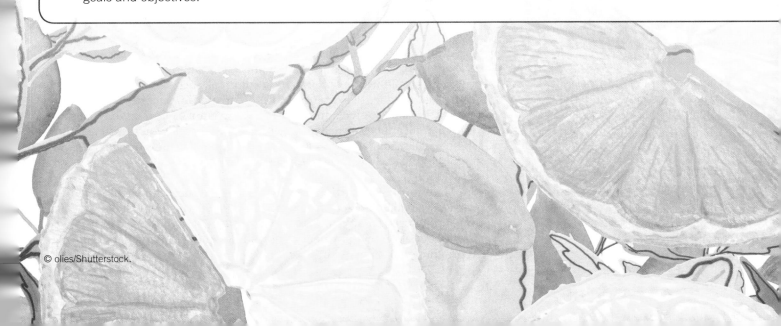

Introduction

For a program to ultimately be successful, it takes assessment, planning, and evaluation, as discussed in previous chapters. To increase the odds of success, it is important to pay attention to factors that can lay the foundation for support. One of those factors is networking. Think of your network of contacts as a professional family. Networks are important, both personally and professionally. One objective of this chapter is to explore how relationships are constructed and nourished. These interactions can also benefit you personally. They are vital to promoting nutrition and making better health available to the individuals and families whom we seek to reach and serve. Later in the chapter, you will find tips about how to improve your own networking skills.

Another important factor to ensure success of a program is earning the support of the administration within your agency. This begins with understanding both external and internal forces influencing agency priorities. By remaining current with the agency's focus, the nutrition department can adapt the plan to meet the changing needs of the agency and survive in the current healthcare environment.

Networks, Alliances, Coalitions, and Consortiums

Call it a clan, call it a network, call it a tribe, call it a family. Whatever you call it, whoever you are, you need one.[1]

Nutrition experts interact with one another at varying levels of the organization. There are many terms used to describe these groups. They are often called networks, alliances, associations, coalitions, consortiums, leagues, or **federations**. Here we discuss a few of these terms that are representative of them all.

In the most informal sense, a **network** is a group of people who form relationships to share ideas, information, and resources. **Alliances** are often semi-official and loosely organized. In alliances, instead of people acting as individuals, the members tend to be made up of representatives from different organizations with similar goals. **Coalitions** are the most structured type of group, and are more formal in nature. Built for a specific purpose, coalitions are often formed to address a particular problem or need in the community. **Consortiums** are similar; they are large groups of organizations, formed to undertake enterprises beyond the resources of any one member.

Networks

We all have methods of communication that can be used as networking tools to connect us with like-minded individuals. Some methods are more structured in nature, such as attending district, state, or national meetings as a means of keeping up with new information and maintaining continuing education requirements. Other methods are more informal, such as **social networking**. In the last decade, the explosion of **social media**, such as **Instagram™**, **TikTok™**, **Facebook™**, and **Twitter™** has launched an entirely new way of communicating and networking, especially among younger generations. These social media platforms led the way for more business-oriented networking platforms such as **LinkedIn™**, which is primarily used for professional networking.

Many professional organizations offer Internet **listservs**, which also provide valuable contacts and a way to interact with individuals who have similar interests. These types of informal networks can be an excellent way of finding out about employment opportunities and gathering data to be used in program planning and evaluation.

Federation An organization that is made by loosely joining together smaller organizations.

Network A group of people who form relationships to share ideas, information, and resources.

Alliance A merging of efforts or interests from representatives of different organizations with similar goals.

Coalition A formal, structured group that forms for a specific purpose or cause.

Consortium Large groups of organizations, formed to undertake enterprises beyond the resources of any one member.

Social Networking The use of dedicated websites and applications to interact with other users, or to find people with similar interests to oneself.

Social Media Websites and applications that enable users to create and share content or to participate in social networking.

Instagram™ A social media platform where users create videos, post pictures, and interact with other users by commenting, liking, reposting, or linking other users' stories and pictures.

TikTok™ A social networking platform in which users create short video content and can interact with other users.

Facebook™ An online social networking service.

Twitter™ An online social networking service that enables users to send and read short messages called "tweets"

LinkedIn™ An online professional networking service.

Listserv An application that distributes messages to subscribers on an electronic mailing list.

Specific websites can be used as a community for nutrition students and dietitians. An example might be the state's dietetic association website. There may be a message board on which students exchange information about class work, explore different academic programs, and discuss internships. A career center part of the website may provide information about writing resumes and offer examples of which questions to expect at a job interview. It can even tell prospective employees how to negotiate for a better salary. Employers may pay to place listings on the site. Job seekers may sometimes post their resumes for free and view a list of open positions and their locations. A speaker's network may be available, where an organization needing a speaker can view people's credentials. Or, members can enroll in a referral network, if it exists, where others wanting nutrition services can find contact information.[2]

At a higher level, nutrition networking efforts can be encouraged or even mandated by funding agencies. The Food and Nutrition Service (FNS) of the United States Department of Agriculture (USDA) provides matching funds for states and communities to provide education to those who receive Supplemental Nutrition Assistance Program (SNAP) benefits (formerly known as Food Stamps). The goal is to increase the likelihood that all SNAP recipients will make healthy food choices and engage in active lifestyles consistent with the Dietary Guidelines for Americans and MyPlate. Because of the tremendous growth in expenditures for SNAP Education (SNAP-Ed), from $661,000 in 1992 to over $343 million in 2008 and $441 million in 2020,[3] networking has become very important and is being mandated by the USDA to avoid duplication of services.

The following provides an example of how the USDA promotes networking: If a **Cooperative Extension Service** or community agency writes a SNAP-Ed plan that includes breastfeeding education, the group must document that it is collaborating with WIC (the Special Supplemental Nutrition Program for Women, Infants and Children). Why? Both SNAP and WIC are USDA programs and many women participate in both. USDA wants to be sure that the information each woman receives is consistent. Because the WIC program has primary responsibility for breastfeeding education, it takes the lead.[4]

Cooperative Extension Service A research-based program that provides outreach services and education to consumers.

Alliances

According to the *Merriam-Webster Dictionary*, "An alliance is the state of being allied: a bond or connection between families, states, parties, or individuals."[5]

Alliances and coalitions may be composed of multiple organizations. For example, The National Alliance for Nutrition and Activity (NANA) is made up of more than 500 national, state, and local organizations. It was established to advocate for policies and programs that promote healthy eating and physical activity.[6] The NANA coalition led the successful effort to pass the Healthy, Hunger-Free Kids Act in 2010, legislation that authorized funding and set policy for the national school lunch program.

Local groups also form alliances to meet a community need. The Metropolitan Area Neighborhood Nutrition Alliance (MANNA) is a group of over 1,000 volunteers and a small paid staff who provide over 60,000 home-delivered, medically appropriate meals per month to people with life-threatening illnesses.[7] Alliances such as MANNA can significantly increase the impact on the community compared with the efforts of a single group or program.

Consortia and Coalitions

As defined by the *Merriam-Webster Dictionary*, "A consortium is a group formed to undertake an enterprise beyond the resources of any one member, while a coalition is defined as a temporary alliance of distinct parties, persons, or states for joint action."[5] Coalition building is considered a formal process in which public and private agencies, communities, businesses, and volunteers unite as partners to combine resources and work together toward a common goal.

An example of a consortium at the national level is the U.S. Department of Health and Human Services' Healthy People. Since 1979, the initiative has promoted partnerships designed to enable diverse groups to work together to improve health. There are partners from all sectors. Federal agencies serve as coordinators. All state and territorial health departments and a multitude of national membership organizations, including the Academy of Nutrition and Dietetics, the American Public Health Association, and the Institute of Food Technologists, belong to the Healthy People Consortium.[8] The plan is updated every 10 years as the U.S. Department of Health and Human Services (DHHS) leverages scientific insights and lessons learned from the past decade, along with new knowledge of current data, trends, and innovations. Healthy People 2030 reflects assessments of major risks to health and wellness, changing public health priorities, and emerging issues related to our nation's health preparedness and prevention. The main objectives of Healthy People 2030 focus on health conditions, health behaviors, settings and systems, and social determinants of health.[8]

By engaging in networks, alliances, coalitions, and consortia, nutritionists can design interventions and services that are more likely to meet community needs and priorities. In order to effectively network, the nutritionist must have community-leader contacts, so it is important to dedicate time to community and professional service. At the heart of an effective network are successful relationships that lead to productive partnerships. Some benefits of networking include:

- Expanding understanding about an issue
- Generating innovative approaches
- Overcoming political, cultural, and bureaucratic barriers
- Reducing duplication of effort
- Bringing together complementary resources
- Sharing risks and limiting liability

Discussion Prompt

Students can discuss groups to which they have belonged that have assisted them in networking.

Collaborating with Others for Nutrition Networks

When forming a nutrition network, alliance, or coalition, the first step is to bring individuals together to explore an issue and clearly identify their purpose or define a problem. It is vital to come to a consensus about purpose and problem.

After you have assembled a group of potential partners, one of the most important features of this stage is relationship building. Each person must feel that they have had an opportunity to give a perspective and that others in the group have heard them. This may take several meetings and a significant amount of time.

After a problem or general purpose has been identified, it is helpful if each member of the group tells how their organization is related to the problem. As illustrated in **Figure 18–1**, you may want to use a RACK analysis to inventory partners. This acronym stands for *Resources, Access, Constraints, and Knowledge.*

Consider the example problem of hunger in a community. The following RACK analysis gives examples of resources, access, constraints, and knowledge that can be provided by members of a community nutrition network. These represent inputs that community agencies make toward the problem or purpose of the network or coalition.

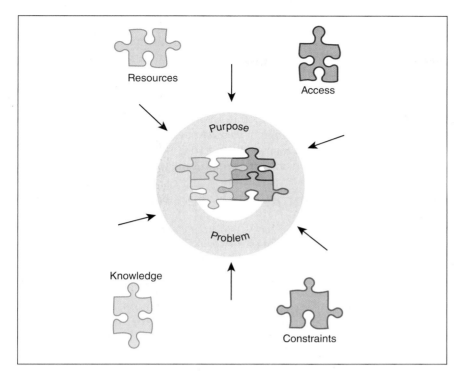

FIGURE 18–1 Elements of a RACK.

Developed by Patti Landers, PhD, RD/LD.

Resources

A primary resource would be food or funds to buy food. Which agencies would you want to enlist who could help with this resource? Examples would include emergency food assistance pantries, a regional food bank, area food markets and food processors, and the local agencies that are responsible for administering the Food Stamp program and other food distribution programs such as WIC.

Other resources, such as space, furniture, telephones, office equipment, and supplies, would also be needed. The next issue is: Who could provide personnel to take applications from hungry people and send them to the right agencies? This may be solved in the "access" category.

Access

Who has access to people who do not have enough food? Partners who can help in this area may include schools, places of worship, healthcare facilities, childcare centers, and social service agencies. Even if we know who needs the food; however, constraints may prevent distribution.

Constraints

Most partners in a network will have constraints of one kind or another. For example, a regional food bank may have plenty of food but be unable to distribute it directly to hungry people. Local food pantries can perform that role. Other constraints may be cultural or political barriers to service. For example, a community agency may be able to provide office space and telephones but may have no funds to hire personnel who speak languages other than English.

Knowledge

A university may have expertise in research and how to evaluate a program but may lack access to data for analyses. Social service or cooperative extension agencies may employ nutritionists or paraprofessionals who are trained as nutrition education aides to provide instruction about dietary quality, food safety, and food resource management; however, they may not be able to teach hungry people who are not enrolled in their programs.

Any coalition should engage in frequent evaluation. New problems may be identified and a RACK analysis may prove helpful in identifying which new partner agencies or business the coalition should seek to involve.

Developing a Community-based Nutrition Network

The Community Tool Box[9] provides over 6,000 Internet pages of practical skill-building information on over 250 different topics, including how to build partnerships and coalitions. In his book, *Quick Tips: Principles for Coalition Success*,[9] Tom Wolff of AHEC/Community Partners states that a shared mission and goal is vital to a successful coalition. Members must be able to set aside their own self-interest in favor of what will benefit the target audience. Wolff also emphasizes that the coalition membership must be diverse and should include representatives from business, government, and the clergy as well as members of neighborhood groups, young people, and the disenfranchised.

When forming a nutrition coalition, it is essential to identify a lead agency. This organization should be willing and able to commit personnel and financial resources as well as have some experience in coalition building. If an agency, rather than an individual, is committed to lead the group, the project will continue even if a personnel vacancy occurs and the individual who was serving as contact person leaves.

Because coalitions are formal and structured, it is important that members write a mission statement, goals, and objectives. Bylaws should be put in place too. Most coalitions have a steering committee. This subgroup may also be called the executive or coordinating committee. Typically, the steering committee includes the coalition chairperson and a representative from the lead agency. The chair or facilitator is often, but not always, from the lead agency and conducts coalition meetings.[10] Some groups prefer to rotate the position. Although someone must chair the group, leadership should be shared as much as possible, and everyone should feel that they have input into decisions through a clear, democratic process. To aid in good communication, the coalition should have regular meetings. The chair or secretary should send out minutes to all members.

Successful coalitions have clear short-term and long-term goals. The members plan often, focus efforts, and measure results. They engage in ongoing evaluation at all stages of their work. The coalition should have an annual meeting that includes all of the members. The chair or steering committee should publish and distribute a yearly report. **Table 18–1** lists examples of potential issues and partners who might come together in a nutrition coalition.

Professional Networking

Professional organizations provide a support and networking system for public health nutritionists. The Academy of Nutrition and Dietetics (AND) is the nation's largest organization of food and nutrition professionals and serves the public by promoting optimal nutrition, health, and well-being.[11]

Strategy Tip

See Community Tool Box: Available at http://ctb.ku.edu.

Discussion Prompt

To start a nutrition club on campus, which members should be included? Go back to Chapter 3 for some considerations.

TABLE 18–1
Food and Nutrition Potential Partners

Organization or Agency	Website
U.S. Department of Health and Human Services (DHHS)	https://www.hhs.gov/
Centers for Disease Control and Prevention	http://www.cdc.gov
Federal Interagency Forum on Child and Family Statistics	http://www.Childstats.gov
National Consumer Protection (a group of 17 federal and private agencies)	http://consumer.gov/ncpw/
U.S. Department of Health and Human Services (DHHS)	http://www.dhhs.gov
U.S. Food and Drug Administration	http://www.fda.gov
President's Council on Physical Fitness and Sports (DHHS)	http://www.fitness.gov
Federal Food Safety Information	http://www.FoodSafety.gov
Grants.gov (a group of seven federal agencies sponsor this online grant search and application site)	http://www.grants.gov
Office of Disease Prevention and Health Promotion (DHHS)	http://www.health.gov
U.S. Department of Health and Human Services (DHHS)	http://www.healthfinder.gov

AND has state, district, and student affiliate groups that provide for excellent peer networking through meetings and the annual Food & Nutrition Conference & Expo. AND members can also choose to participate in the Nationwide Nutrition Network. At the AND website (http://www.eatright.org), consumers, doctors and other healthcare professionals, restaurant owners and managers, and food manufacturers and distributors can enter a zip code to find local dietetics professionals for individual consultations, program development, workshops and seminars, and special projects. AND holds an annual Public Policy Workshop in Washington, D.C., where dietitians network and focus on how they can become involved with members of Congress to impact legislative issues key to the profession and to the nutritional health of Americans. AND dietetic practice groups (DPGs) also provide opportunities for networking with others. Of particular interest to public health nutritionists are the following DPGs: Public Health/Community Nutrition, School Nutrition Services, Hunger and Environmental Nutrition, Nutrition Education for the Public, Gerontological Nutritionists, Nutrition Educators of Health Professionals, Pediatric Nutrition, Weight Management, Women's Health and Reproductive Nutrition, Nutrition Entrepreneurs, and Sports Cardiovascular and Wellness.

The American Public Health Association (APHA) is the oldest and largest organization of public health professionals in the world. APHA has been influencing policies and setting priorities in public health for over 125 years. Throughout its history, it has been at the forefront of numerous efforts to prevent disease and promote health.[12] The APHA Food and Nutrition section contributes to long-range planning in food, nutrition, and health policy, which may affect the nutritional well-being of the public. Priorities of the section include promotion of public health nutrition policy, elimination of racial and ethnic health disparities, education and training for public health workers, and increasing and strengthening membership. An advantage of membership in APHA is the opportunity to not only interact with nutrition professionals but also with the wider public health community, including physicians, nurses, and health educators.

The Society for Nutrition Education (SNE) is an international organization of nutrition education professionals who are dedicated to promoting healthful, sustainable food choices and who share a vision of healthy people in healthy communities.[13] Members conduct research in education, behavior, and communication; develop and disseminate innovative nutrition education strategies; and communicate information on food, nutrition, and health issues to students, professionals, policymakers, and the public. SNE members share ideas and resources through the *Journal of Nutrition Education and Behavior*, a newsletter, an annual conference, and a members-only Email listserv. Divisions offer networking opportunities for members with similar interests and expertise.[13] Groups of special interest may include the Public Health Nutrition and the Social Marketing Networks divisions.

Networking Tips

Developing a strong network requires planning and deliberate action. First, list your personal and professional goals and the contacts you need to make in order to achieve them. The book titled, The *WetFeet Insider Guide to Networking*[14] suggests that your existing and potential contacts are composed of your inner circle, your expanded network, and the network you never knew you had. People who know you well are in your inner circle; these are your family, friends, and current and former colleagues. Your expanded network includes acquaintances with whom you've had brief contact, other members of professional groups, or Email correspondents. The network you never knew you had includes "friends, relatives, and colleagues, relatives, and colleagues or friends."[14]

Here are some tips that will help you develop your personal network:

- Cultivate a wide circle of friends and acquaintances in many different venues.
- Stock a good supply of business cards and carry them with you at all times. Every time you meet someone you believe might be a good contact, take out one of your cards. Make sure your cards include a phone number, your Email address, links to your website or blog (if you have one), and social media handles. Write a personal note on the back before you give it to them. This will let the person know about your interests and make them more likely to keep up with your contact information. They will usually offer you one of their business cards in return. Immediately write a reminder to yourself on the back. Just a phrase like "childhood obesity poster in Atlanta" will help you to remember them. Then, when you contact that person later, they will be impressed that you know who they are and what they did.
- Have an electronic calendar with you and keep it current. If you hear of professional education or networking opportunities, you can add them to your schedule right away.
- Keep an updated resume template on file at all times. You will want to customize it for each specific situation. For example, your resume needs different emphasis areas, depending on the type of position you are seeking. If applying for a job as a clinical dietitian, you would highlight education and work in hospital settings. If you are looking for a position in a nonprofit agency, you would stress your training and experience in collaborating with other people. Listing volunteer activities that show your community

involvement would be important. Demonstrating skill with grant writing would be especially impressive.

- Establish a LinkedIn profile and keep it current. Ask colleagues to endorse you. Continue to seek out LinkedIn connections with relevant individuals.
- Be a member of one or more professional organizations. Always attend local and state meetings. Volunteer to be on committees and help at events. Always do a good job, even with small tasks. Your skills will become known and soon you will be asked to take a leadership role.
- Attend a national conference, at least every other year. If possible, travel with someone in the organization whom you do not know well. Getting out of town and having a block time to network is very important.
- Immediately follow up with contacts you make with a card, brief phone call, or Email message. Send them a request to connect on LinkedIn.
- Prepare in advance for follow-up meetings.
- Work to improve social skills. Good social skills are essential to networking. At meetings or parties, be outgoing, even if it is not natural for you. Do not stand in a corner by yourself. Go up to others who look lonely and strike up a conversation, or join a group and introduce yourself. Do not forget your business cards. Keep them handy, even at social events. You should be ready to electronically send your business information, as well. If social occasions are painful, investigate a public speaking group like Toastmasters where you can improve communication skills.
- Monitor your social media handles, such as Instagram, TikTok, Twitter, and Facebook to ensure that all pictures, comments, and quotes portray you as a professional.
- Follow other people in your field or organizations on social media, such as Instagram, TikTok, Twitter, and Facebook. Engage in meaningful conversations via comments, reposts, likes, and direct messaging.
- Be sincere. Help others and they will help you.
- Always remember to say thank you.

Earning Administrative Support

Networking is often used as a way to establish contacts outside of your primary place of work. But what about making those connections within your organization? Building internal relationships with one's administration is a key to strengthening contacts, especially for a public health nutritionist who is looking for support in establishing nutrition programs.

An important strategy to increase the relevancy of the nutrition division within your organization is to partner with other divisions sharing common goals. Along with developing positive working relationships internally, involvement with the policy board as well as the local media can increase the exposure and value of the nutrition division in the eyes of both the agency administration and the general public.

In networking with the community, gaps in nutrition-related services may be identified and brought to the attention of the administration. If funding is a barrier to developing a new program, identify potential external funding sources and seek administrative support to apply for grant monies.

Discussion Prompt

What are some other websites to keep a job profile?

Pandemic Learning Opportunity

During a pandemic, online networking will be imperative for safety reasons. FaceTime and other visual web-interviews and communications will be necessary. Working from home may become a norm.

The Administration's Perspective

Management and delivery of healthcare services is influenced by economic, political, and social forces. To promote nutrition services within your organization, it is critical to analyze the dynamics operating within your agency. By doing so, you will better understand the influences and motivations of the administration. In Shortell and Kaluzney's *Healthcare Management: Organization Design and Behavior*,[15] the authors identified several key forces impacting healthcare delivery that have implications for management, and for the nutrition department in particular, including the increased focus on evaluation of programs and services, the integration of information technology, the aging of the population, and changing demographics of the United States that are leading to increased cultural diversity.

Understanding the impact of these trends on the healthcare system is important in ensuring that the nutrition division progresses along with the rest of the agency. In this environment of increased accountability, evaluating both the implementation and the effectiveness of existing nutrition programs and services is now routinely expected. Nutrition departments that integrate information technology into daily practices will be more time- and cost-efficient. Reaching out to elderly populations by implementing programs to improve food security for community members who do not have convenient access to grocery stores is an example of addressing the aging of the population. Consider ethnic and cultural diversity by providing nutrition education materials in languages that are highly prevalent in your community and provide culturally sensitive recipes and meal plans. Examples such as these illustrate to the administration that the nutrition division is current with issues critical to improving the community's public health infrastructure.

Healthy People (HP) 2020 and HP 2030 (as discussed in other chapters) provide a framework for understanding national priority areas for health promotion and disease prevention. The objectives in focus areas offer guidelines for focusing program planning within healthcare organizations. Reviewing the *HP 2020/2030* objectives listed in the Nutrition and Overweight focus area, along with focus areas related to nutrition including cancer, chronic kidney disease, and diabetes, can provide the nutrition professional with a better understanding of the healthcare needs of the nation, the government's priorities with respect to funding initiatives, and the administrator's perspective. Furthermore, nutrition-related *HP 2020/2030* objectives can be used to build administrative support for initiatives. For example, one in four adults and one in five adolescents in the United States meet the guidelines for muscle strength training and aerobic activities.[8] HP 2030 sets an objective at increasing and improving the aerobic and muscle strength training of adolescents and adults. Using this information and presenting this to administration can assist in the justification and support for nutrition and physical activity programs within the division.

Understanding the Agency Vision and Strategic Plan

The extent to which each of these environmental factors and *HP 2020/2030* objectives influence the vision, goals, and objectives of individual public health agencies may be better understood by reviewing the organization's planning documents, such as the strategic plan, annual report, and budget. By reviewing the agency's strategic plan, the nutrition professional will better understand the underlying philosophy of the agency as well as the current priorities and perspectives of the administrators. The following are the key components of a strategic plan, along with a description of how they can assist you in identifying areas of interest to the agency administration:

- *Mission statement:* Defines the purpose of the organization and can often provide a better understanding of the underlying philosophy of the agency.
- *Major objectives:* Highlight the priorities of the organization with realistic, measurable, achievable outcomes.
- *Action plan:* Delineates a method for achieving objectives. This section provides an indication of the agency's approach to finding solutions to current issues of interest.
- *Resources needed:* Includes personnel, funds, equipment, and space required to meet objectives. Identify areas where nutrition-related resources could assist in achieving goals and bring these to the attention of the administrator. If funds are being requested, it is ideal to identify them early on in the project planning phase before the budget is developed.
- *Evaluation system:* Delineates the process for assessing the effectiveness of the plan. A description of the evaluation process can provide insight into ways in which the performance of the administration is measured within the organization.

Synergizing with the Strategic Plan

By reviewing the agency's planning documents in concert with the community needs assessment (discussed in Chapter 5), public health nutritionists can evaluate whether their role in the organization is meeting the needs of the public they are serving and is within the framework of the organization's goals. Using components of the community needs-assessment can be an effective tool in garnering support for nutrition services from administrators, funding agencies, and the public alike. The following list describes how elements of the community needs-assessment can be used to directly increase administrative support for nutrition programs:

- *Assessment:* Composed of copious amounts of data related to community demographics, the health and nutrition of community members, perceived needs, and community assets; this section can be reframed for presentation to decision makers to highlight the need for nutrition services in the community. If your assessment included focus-group data regarding the impact of the WIC program on participants, share a direct quote from a participant about ways the program can be improved along with program numbers to support these suggestions. By providing both testimonials from community members and data to support initiatives, you are showing the administration that your department is in touch with the needs of the community.
- *Priorities, goals, and objectives:* Present concise, realistic, measurable objectives to the administrators in order to show that the nutrition department is organized around common goals that are relevant to community needs.
- *Nutrition plan:* Use the nutrition plan to highlight the steps required to achieve the stated objectives. Emphasize the assets of the nutrition department, and also identify gaps along with proposed solutions for addressing barriers to achieving the objectives.
- *Implementation:* Summarize the implementation process to the extent needed to highlight the efficiency, organization, and

teamwork of the nutrition division in working toward common goals.

- *Promotion:* It is important to consider how best to reach and/or influence the key stakeholders. Social media might be used to highlight the proposed program or issue and get others involved quickly and effectively.
- *Evaluation:* As discussed in Chapter 6, evaluating activities of the nutrition division is important for documenting program impact as well as identifying areas for continuous quality improvement.

Prior to preparing evaluation results for presentation to the administration, review the agency's annual report for ideas on how to format results. For example, if the report relies heavily on charts and graphs rather than qualitative data, recognize that the administrator is more familiar with reviewing quantitative data within agency documents. In addition to increasing the likelihood that the administrator will respond favorably to the activities of the nutrition division, results presented in this manner will be more likely to be included in next year's annual report, thereby increasing exposure of the nutrition division's activities to policymakers and budget reviewers.

Partnering to Achieve Shared Goals

Forging partnerships between the nutrition division and groups sharing common goals and objectives provides the opportunity to capitalize on the benefits of combining resources and avoiding the duplication of services. Although the administration's expectations of the nutrition division may seem ambitious given the limited staff and budget allocated to the department, a review of the responsibilities of other divisions within the organization may provide insight into opportunities for working together on initiatives with common goals.

Effective teams focus on the shared purpose of the collaboration by developing goals and priorities required to fulfill the need. In doing so, the process is directed toward a shared commitment, and members identify skills and contributions required for the effort. Fostering positive relations with team members further integrates the nutrition division into the framework of the healthcare organization and provides the potential to increase the overall productivity of the agency.

Relations with the Policy Board

The Board of Health or Board of Directors, often appointed by elected officials, is responsible for approving policies and programs, appointments of personnel, budgets, and legislative initiatives. Special interests of individual board members may influence policy decisions that directly impact the nutrition department.

Representing the nutrition division at board meetings and advocating for nutrition-related programs will increase the likelihood that nutrition services will be viewed as important to improving the public's health, rather than being marginalized as major events shift resources to high priority areas. Therefore, it is important for representatives from the nutrition department to attend meetings and interact with board members in order to remain current with the priorities of the Board.

For example, an outbreak of foodborne illness in the community resulting in hospitalizations and lost productivity provides an opportunity for nutritionists to educate food service workers regarding proper procedures for prevention of further outbreaks. By reaching out to the community when the relevancy of the issue is high, you increase the likelihood that food safety tips

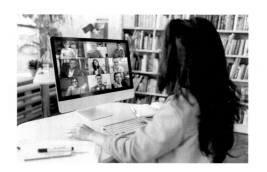

Pandemic Tip: Effective teams work together seamlessly, even online. And will be used after the pandemic.

© Kate Kultsevych/Shutterstock.

Strategy Tip

Remember the discussion about Special interest groups from Chapter 3.

will be translated into behavior change. Furthermore, the education campaign increases exposure of the nutrition department to the community as well as policymakers, and will show the administrator that the nutrition division is responsive to high-priority health issues within the community.

Communications with the Media

Another opportunity for strengthening both administrative and community support for nutrition-related initiatives is to build a good rapport with the local media. There are several ways to build a relationship with the media, including inviting the media to cover events sponsored by the nutrition division, providing copy for nutrition-related topics of interest to the public, and answering questions for nutrition-related news stories. Each of these methods can promote positive public relations between the public and the public health agency.

Before communicating with the media, it is important to contact both the public relations division within your agency and your administrator to be certain you understand the rules and regulations associated with media communications. For example, you may need to obtain approval of press releases from the public relations department prior to dissemination to media outlets.

Preparing and Distributing Press Kits

Press kits are packets of information describing an event or program written in a format conducive to dissemination by media outlets. Press kits can include a press release, pictures, program logos, press passes to the event, an invitation to participate in the program, and/or fact sheets related to program activities and timelines. By announcing programs and events in advance, the publicity could result in increased attendance and lead to a more successful intervention.

To increase the likelihood that your information will be noticed by various local media organizations, including radio, television, and newspaper outlets, ask the public relations department within your agency for strategies that have worked in the past. There may be a particular person at each organization to whom health information press kits should be directed, or a template that facilitates publicizing the event in the format familiar to each specific organization. If your agency doesn't have a public relations department to assist you, contact a colleague who has worked successfully with the organization in the past, or call the organization directly for assistance. More and more marketing is done online and an experienced online marketer may be needed to assist you. More information on marketing your message is in Chapter 26.

Promoting Nutrition Messages Through Media

Nutrition is in the news daily, hitting the headlines with topics ranging from newly released surveillance statistics and epidemiologic evidence associating particular foods with risk for cancer to the latest fad diet book extolling the benefits of a particular dietary regimen. The media seeks credible sources to interpret the implications of research findings on the public's health. Registered dietitians have a responsibility to promote evidence-based recommendations based on sound scientific research, and assisting the media in reporting research findings is another way to provide nutrition education. As an added benefit, the media will credit their source, thereby providing an opportunity to promote the image of the nutrition division within your agency.

One way to establish positive relationships with the media is to offer to write copy for a particular topic area of interest to the media organization. For example, if new research findings are published on the benefits of

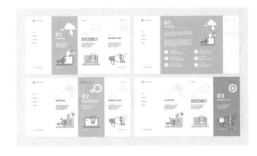

Sample of a press kit.
© PureSolution/Shutterstock.

cruciferous vegetables for reducing cancer risk, you could suggest writing a piece summarizing the evidence and providing tips for preparing cruciferous vegetables for the newspaper's health section. In your correspondence to the editor, outline a few nutrition-related topics you consider to be newsworthy and would be willing to research in order to write an educational piece for the paper. This provides a service to the media, who are often under pressure to meet deadlines, while promoting the image of the nutrition division within your agency as a credible source for health-related information.

Maintain records of newspaper and web articles, letters to the editor, public service announcements, and any other correspondence the nutrition division has with the media. Review social marketing activity, such as Twitter™ retweets or **HootSuite**™ analytic reports. Estimate the impact of your message by tracking the reach, such as checking the number of views on a webpage, or counting the number of "likes" on a Twitter™, Instagram™, or Facebook™ posting. If the message was part of a particular nutrition program or service, include these data when writing up the impact evaluation for the project. Repost abbreviated content on your social media and encourage others to repost in order to increase the audience.

HootSuite® A social media management system for brand management that supports multiple social media integrations.

Obtaining Financial Support for Nutrition Programs and Initiatives

As the nutrition division reaches out to the community, it is likely that gaps in the public health infrastructure will be identified that are not addressed in the planning documents of the agency. Possible reasons the problem was not addressed in the strategic plan include lack of awareness, no known solutions, or emergence after the development of the strategic plan. In discussing the problem with the administrator, you may both agree that the problem is important and that a workable solution has been proposed, but the administrator does not have the funds to allocate to the proposed program. Discuss the possibility of applying for grants to address the problem. The administrator will likely support proposal writing as a mechanism to increase revenue and appreciate the initiative displayed by the nutrition division. Obtaining funding from a range of sources also increases the stability and capacity of the nutrition division to provide programs and services.

The administrator may direct you to funding sources that will likely be interested in reviewing your proposal. Potential funding sources include the government, foundations, corporations, or charges for services rendered. Several web-based resources are available to identify funding agencies and provide guidance in preparing applications. Given the time-sensitive nature of requests for proposals, searching online funding databases is often more productive than searching through paper-based directories. **Table 18–2** provides a list of available Internet resources for identifying grant opportunities.

Summary

It is important to be professionally competent in what you know; however, who you know may be just as vital to accomplishing your objectives in promoting better health and nutrition. Networking includes relationships built at both personal and professional levels. These associations may range from informal interactions with individuals and groups of people for information, ideas, and resources, to semi-official alliances, and then on to structured coalitions that were purposefully organized to address a particular nutrition problem or need in the community. Numerous networking strategies were outlined in the chapter. Once you realize the benefits of networking, it is

TABLE 18–2
Internet Resources for Identifying Grant Opportunities

Organization	Website
U.S. Department of Health and Human Services	http://www.grants.gov/
Catalog of Federal Domestic Assistance	http://12.46.245.173/cfda/cfda.html
Food and Nutrition Service	http://www.fns.usda.gov/fns/
National Institutes of Health	http://grants.nih.gov/grants/oer.htm
Academy of Nutrition and Dietetics	http://www.eatright.org/
Foundation Center	http://fdncenter.org/
Robert Wood Johnson Foundation	http://www.rwjf.org/index.jsp

<u>More Resources</u>

Centers for Disease Control and Prevention, National Center for Chronic Disease Prevention and Health Promotion. *Physical Activity*. Accessed January 7, 2021. Available at http://www.cdc.gov /physicalactivity

Endsley DS. *Innovation in Action: A Practical Guide for Healthcare Teams*. St. Louis, MO: Wiley-Blackwell; 2010.

Liebler JG, McConnell CR. Planning. In: Liebler JG, McConnell CR, eds. *Management principles for health professionals*. 12th ed. Jones & Bartlett Learning; 2007:114-121.

U.S. Department of Health and Human Services. *Healthy People 2030*. Accessed January 7, 2021. http:// www.healthypeople.gov

(See chapter 15 for further strategies around grant writing.)

helpful to then develop a professional networking plan, either for yourself and/or your community organization.

This chapter also covers the benefits of gaining administrative support when planning programs. Earning administrative support is a necessary component in public health nutrition, since this can be the key to whether a program is successful. The support can be financial, as well as providing other kinds of resources. This chapter outlined several strategies to help ensure that your efforts are effective. Having a clear understanding of your agency's vision and strategic plan, partnering with your organization and its policy board, and obtaining support through media are all ways that you can set the stage for program development. You can further this momentum by using appropriate communication methods with key stakeholders. With careful attention and planning, these strategies can help you maximize success and get your program off the ground.

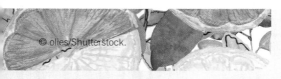
© olies/Shutterstock.

Learning Portfolio

Key Terms

	page
Federation	570
Network	570
Alliance	570
Coalition	570
Consortium	570
Social Networking	570
Social Media	570
Instagram™	570
TikTok™	570
Facebook™	570
Twitter™	570
LinkedIn™	570
Listserv	570
Cooperative Extension Service	571
HootSuite®	582

Issues for Discussion

1. How do the benefits of networking justify your investment of time and effort?
2. How can professional networking relationships benefit you personally?
3. Where do you want to go in your professional career? How can networking help you to achieve that goal?
4. Discuss why getting internal support for nutrition programs is as important as controlling external variables.
5. Describe how internal marketing is different from external marketing.
6. What is the competition that public health nutrition faces, and why should public health nutrition be maintained?

Practical Activities

1. Have students create a LinkedIn™ profile if they haven't already done so. In pairs, have them critique each other's profiles. Encourage them to start connecting with each other on LinkedIn™ to build their networking contact list.
2. Have students present a hypothetical proposal for a nutrition program that they would submit to the administration of a public health agency. The proposal should include goals and objectives, resources, estimated costs, and timelines. In addition, the proposal should identify the benefits to the consumer as well as to the public health agency.
3. Break students into small groups of 3–4. Have students find one user on social media—Instagram, Twitter, TikTok, or Facebook—whose content aligns with their own nutritional values. Have them write out why they chose this particular person on social media and how that person uses social media as a nutrition resource. Have each student share with their group.

Case Study 1: New RDN

A new dietitian has recently moved to a new city and would like to find a job in community nutrition. What are some ways they can get started with this endeavor? Make a list of specific strategies they can use to network and search for the perfect job.

Case Study 2: Experienced RDN

A dietitian who has practiced in public health for 5 years is interested in making a career change to work in weight management. Make a list of useful resources that this dietitian can use to learn more about the field. What are some ways this dietitian can learn more about weight management and gain useful networks?

References

1. Howard J. *Families*. New York, NY: Simon and Schuster; 1978.
2. Nutrition Jobs and Job Ventures, LLC. *Nutrition Jobs: dietetic career tools, coaching, and jobs*. Accessed January 7, 2021. http://www.nutritionjobs.com
3. U.S. Department of Agriculture. Approved Federal Funds for Supplemental Nutrition Assistance Education by Fiscal Year. Accessed January 7, 2021. https://snaped.fns.usda.gov/program-administration/funding-allocations

4. U.S. Department of Agriculture. *Supplemental Nutrition Assistance Program Education SNAP-Ed Plan Guidance.* Accessed January 7, 2021. https://snaped.fns.usda.gov/program -administration/snap-ed-plan-guidance-and-templates

5. *Merriam-Webster Online Dictionary.* Accessed January 7, 2021. http://www.m-w.com

6. Center for Science in the Public Interest. National Alliance for Nutrition and Activity (NANA). Accessed January 7, 2021. http://www.cspinet.org/nutritionpolicy/nana.html

7. The Stephen Korman Nutrition Center. *Metropolitan Area Neighborhood Nutrition Alliance (MANNA).* Accessed January 7, 2021. http://www.mannapa.org

8. U.S. Department of Health and Human Services. *Healthy People 2030.* Accessed January 7, 2021. http://www.healthypeople.gov

9. Wolff T. Community Tool Box. *QuickTips: Principles for Coalition Success.* University of Kansas. Accessed January 7, 2021. http://ctb.ku.edu/en

10. Cohen L, Baer N, Satterwhite P. *Developing Effective Coalitions: An Eight Step Guide.* Accessed January 7, 2021. https://www.preventioninstitute.org/publications/developing-effective-coalitions-eight-step-guide

11. Academy of Nutrition and Dietetics. Accessed January 7, 2021. http://www.eatright.org

12. American Public Health Association. *About APHA.* Accessed January 7, 2021. http://www.apha.org

13. Society for Nutrition Education and Behavior. *Identity Statement.* Society for Nutrition Education. Accessed January 7, 2021. http://www.sne.org

14. WetFeet. *Networking Works!* San Francisco: WetFeet Inc.; 2004.

15. Shortell SM, Kaluzny, AD, eds. *Healthcare Management: Organization Design and Behavior.* 6th ed. Delmar Cengage Learning; 2012.

CHAPTER 19

Marketing Nutrition Programs and Services

Federika Garcia Muchacho, MS, RDN, LDN
Gisela Alvarez, RDN, LDN

(We would like to acknowledge the work of Debra Silverman, MS, RDN; Nancie Herbold, EdD, RDN; and Paul N. Taylor, PhD, in past editions of Nutrition and Public Health.)

Learning Outcomes

AFTER STUDYING THIS CHAPTER AND REFLECTING ON THE CONTENTS, YOU WILL BE ABLE TO:

1. Compare and contrast business marketing and social marketing.

2. List and define the four Ps of marketing and some additional Ps of social marketing.

3. Discuss types of market research and how they can be used in planning a public health nutrition program or when promoting nutrition services.

4. The role of social media and technology in promoting nutrition services and programs.

5. Understand the ethics of marketing.

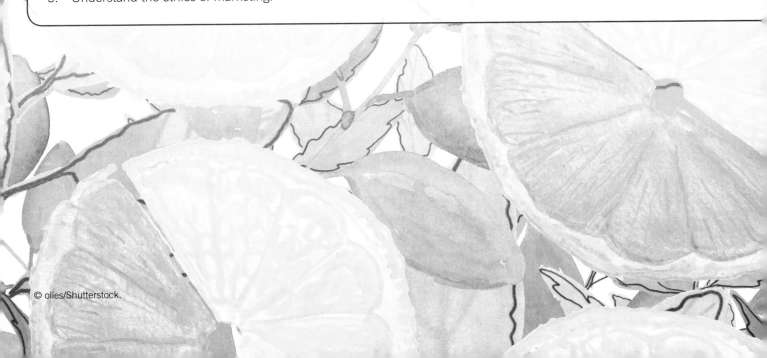

Introduction

Today's crowded food messaging environment requires that nutritionists understand mass personalized marketing communications. In the era of social media and technology, consumers turn to the Internet for guidance on common health conditions and answers to nutrition-related questions. Nonetheless, individuals are faced with an array of nutrition misinformation as spokespersons in the media seldom are nutrition professionals, with the knowledge and experience behind to safely, and effectively, educate the public. By having a thorough understanding of the power and value of marketing as a tool, nutritionists can use marketing concepts to chrome online leaders and effectively inform and educate the public as part of successful nutrition programs, while also promoting nutrition services.

The PHCN Guide for Practitioners provides a comprehensive definition of how Registered Dietitians (RDs) and nutritionists can gain knowledge and develop marketing skills to implement effective programs:

> "Identifies and utilizes principles of marketing for use in the food, nutrition, and physical activity components of health promotion/ disease prevention programs and services, including social marketing, messaging/countermessaging, behavioral economics, and electronic social networks."[1]

In this chapter, the focus is on distinguishing between business and social marketing, defining marketing tools, use of social media platforms, and how nutrition professionals can use the aforementioned to effectively create and promote nutrition programs and services at an individual level, community level, or mass scale.

Business Marketing Versus Social Marketing

Business marketing is "the process of creating, distributing, promoting, and pricing goods, services, and ideas to facilitate satisfying exchange relationships with customers in a dynamic environment."[2] In business marketing, an exchange of goods or services occurs between a buyer and a seller such that both buyer and seller are satisfied. The dynamic environment in which these exchanges occur consists of uncontrollable forces (consumers, competition, the economy, politics, government, the media, and technology) that affect the *marketing mix*. Because the marketing environment is dynamic, the most successful marketers continually evaluate their marketing plans and change them as necessary to ensure that their product is available at the right time, in the right place, and at an acceptable price for consumer satisfaction. In contrast, social marketing not only focuses on products but also on the promotion of services, and uses the marketing mix to promote behavior change.

The definition of **social marketing** has evolved from an individual to a systems-based focus since its introduction in 1971. The concept of social marketing has expanded to look at not only how to target individuals but also how to target those individuals in the context of the population as a whole, promoting collective action and ultimately leading to behavior change.[3]

> "Social marketing is a process that uses marketing principles and techniques to change target audience behaviors to benefit society as well as the individual. This strategically oriented discipline relies on creating, communicating, delivering, and exchanging offerings that have positive value for individuals, clients, partners, and society."[4]

Business marketing The process of creating, distributing, promoting, and pricing goods, services, and ideas to facilitate satisfying exchange relationships with customers in a dynamic environment.[2]

Social Marketing The process of combining commercial marketing methods with public health approaches in order to achieve significant, large-scale public benefits.[1]

These definitions describe the activities of nutritionists, public health agencies, and other government and private agencies (e.g., the Centers for Disease Control and Prevention [CDC], the Robert Wood Johnson Foundation) who desire to change behaviors and habits within a target population. Whereas business marketing focuses on maximizing the organization's profits, social marketing focuses on using commercial marketing tools and techniques to achieve various social objectives, such as to voluntarily change human behavior to benefit general society.[5]

The change of focus in social marketing from a "'downward stream'" to an "upstream,'" practice helped broaden the scope of social marketing and how it can influence behavior.[3] The original six benchmarks of social marketing proposed by Andreasen in 2002 are the following: Social marketing (1) is customer oriented, (2) has a clear behavior change focus, (3) incorporates an exchange analysis, (4) takes into account competition (both internal and external), (5) uses segmentation and targeting to select the intervention target group and (6) uses several elements of the **marketing mix** (product, price, place, and promotion), not just communications.[4] These benchmarks have been criticized in the past to be individual-focused; new proposed benchmarks as noted by Lee, et al.,[4] include: (1) a network perspective on behavior and structural change, (2) value creation in context, (3) facilitate participation through customer orientation and engagement, (4) competition and collaboration within value networks, (5) segmentation is driven by a relational, customized approach, (6) a service-driven framework. These proposed benchmarks look to move social marketing to a more systems-based approach, or an upstream marketing strategy, which seeks to influence the individual by also targeting "those who shape the structural and environmental conditions within society, including politicians, policy makers, civil servants, decision makers, regulators, managers, educators."[6] Many other theories have been proposed in recent years to look at the target individual in the context of the general population.[7]

Regardless of the line of thought that one follows or wishes to adopt, the use of social marketing to develop a nutrition program plan requires commitment from top-level management, adequate funding and personnel, marketing skills, and vision. As with the development of any nutrition program, the foundation to a successful program is thorough research, beginning with defining the problem one wishes to address in the public health arena. Once data has been collected and analyzed, recommendations can be made to form the outline of the program and to delineate the marketing plan.

Marketing mix A marketing strategy tool used to position a product or service to help meet the needs and demands of your target population (4 Ps: product, price, place, and promotion).

Pandemic Learning Opportunity

How did the Covid-19 pandemic change business and social marketing?

Marketing Research

Marketing research is necessary to plan, develop, and implement a successful social marketing program for an organization. Market research begins with defining the problem and gathering data to understand all aspects that need to be tackled to address said problem, a process that is similar to a nutrition assessment. As a Registered Dietitian/Nutritionist seeks to assess, diagnose, intervene, and monitor/evaluate in a clinical setting, similar concepts apply to marketing research; data collection, marketing segmentation, and the marketing mix are all steps to develop and promote nutrition programs and services.

Conducting marketing research allows for discovery of the psychosocial aspect of the targeted population, such as the knowledge, beliefs, and attitudes. Data collected will include both subjective and objective information, and the better the problem is understood given the data collected, the greater the likelihood of developing and implementing a successful plan that leads to behavior change.

Data Collection

Secondary Data

Secondary data are information collected by other groups and agencies for another primary purpose. In the context of nutrition research, health indicators collected by the federal government, such as the National Health and Nutrition Examination Survey (NHANES) data, are one example of secondary data. State Departments of Public Health collect state health statistics, such as infant mortality rate, teen pregnancy rate, and chronic disease incidence and prevalence, which are other examples of secondary data. Secondary data allows for a systematic research method to further evaluate a topic of interest. There are many helpful websites for data collection (**Table 19-1**) to further enhance nutrition program/service development.

Secondary data collection utilizes existing data for research purposes. Due to the vast amount of data compiled and archived, secondary data analysis has become a pertinent first step in developing social marketing campaigns. By developing research questions, identifying datasets, and thoroughly evaluating these, one can further define the focus of the campaign.[8] As more secondary data are gathered in the initial stages of research, time, money, and efforts are saved as it is highly likely either less primary data will need to be collected, or a more focused approach to primary data collection will be implemented.

TABLE 19-1
Helpful Websites for Data Collection

Website	Sponsoring Organization
www.eatright.org	Academy of Nutrition and Dietetics
www.apha.org	American Public Health Association
www.diabetes.org	American Diabetes Association
www.heart.org	American Heart Association
www.ama.org	American Marketing Association
www.restaurant.org	National Restaurant Association
www. adage.com	Advertising Age
www.adweek.com	Adweek
www.fao.org	Food and Agriculture Organization of the United Nations
www.ift.org	Institute of Food Technologists
www.who.int	World Health Organization
http://www.cdc.gov	Centers for Disease Control and Prevention
www.cdc.gov/mmwr/	Morbidity and Mortality Weekly Report
www.cdc.gov/nchs/	National Center for Health Statistics
www.cdc.gov/healthcommunication/	CDC's Health Communication Gateway
www.census.gov/	U.S. Census Bureau
www.cdc.gov/chronicdisease/	CDC's National Center for Chronic Disease Prevention and Health Promotion (NCCDPHP)

www.healthleadership.org	Center for Health Leadership and Practice
www.fda.gov	U.S. Food and Drug Administration
www.fedstats.sites.usa.gov	U.S. Federal Statistics
www.hhs.gov	U.S. Department of Health and Human Services
www.usda.gov	U.S. Department of Agriculture
www.ropercenter.cornell.edu	Roper Center for Public Opinion Research
www.cdc.gov/brfss/	Behavioral Risk Factor Surveillance System (BRFSS)
https://www.cdc.gov/kidneydisease/	Chronic Kidney Disease (CKD) Surveillance System
https://www.cdc.gov/hrqol/	Health Related Quality of Life (HRQOL)
https://www.cdc.gov/art/	National Assisted Reproductive Technology Surveillance System (NASS)
https://www.cdc.gov/tobacco/	National Tobacco Survey (NATS)
https://www.cdc.gov/nchs/nhis/	National Health Interview Survey (NHIS)
https://www.cdc.gov/nchs/nhanes/	National Health and nutrition Examination Survey (NHANES)
https://www.cdc.gov/cancer/uscs/	United States Cancer Statistics (USCS)
https://www.cdc.gov/reproductivehealth/	Pregnancy Mortality Surveillance System (PMSS)
https://www.cdc.gov/prams/	Pregnancy Risk Assessment Monitoring System (PRAMS)
https://www.cdc.gov/diabetes/data/index.html	US Diabetes Surveillance System
https://www.cdc.gov/fluoridation/	Water Fluoridation Reporting System (WFRS)
https://www.cdc.gov/healthyyouth/	Youth Risk Behavior Surveillance System (YBRSS)
https://www.aicr.org/	American Institute of Cancer Research

A professional literature review is a valuable example of secondary data collection that allows for a comprehensive pool of data from multiple credible sources (i.e., journals, articles, books) pertinent to the research question. For example, if one were to conduct a literary review on flaxseed's effect on cardiovascular health, one might find that in addition to fiber, flaxseed's high omega-3 content from ALA, as well as dietary lignans, help improve blood pressure, reduce total cholesterol levels, and improve HDL cholesterol.[9] Uncovering flaxseed's vast effects on different aspects of cardiovascular health can further help narrow the focus of the initial research question and bring a focus on one of the aforementioned aspects of flax and heart health. Reviews help synthesize what is known on a specific topic. Once secondary data is gathered and gaps in the collected data are identified, primary data collection begins.

Primary Data

Primary data are types of information collected from focus groups, observations, mail or telephone surveys, interviews, and the like. Primary data helps to further focus the problem and define targeted audiences. For example, after interviewing Hispanic mothers about the importance of family mealtime, Hammons AJ et al.,[10] found that technology is greatly accepted at the dinner table. While the parents did not lack knowledge about the effects of technology as a distraction during meals, the presence of technology during meals seemed ubiquitous. These findings can be addressed in existing culturally tailored obesity prevention programs to help families create healthier eating habits among the Hispanic population.[10] Collecting primary data can provide insight on the attitudes, beliefs, and consequent nutrition and health behaviors of a population.

Qualitative and Quantitative Data

Qualitative data Unmeasurable data collected to obtain descriptive information (i.e., beliefs, feelings, attitudes).

Primary information includes qualitative and quantitative data. **Qualitative data** are usually obtained from small samples of the targeted group; they help offer a perspective to explore and understand human behavior that arises from a different philosophy than a quantitative data design.[11] Open-ended questions and in-depth interviews with key informants may be conducted to obtain knowledge about the problem or topic of interest. *Key informants* are individuals who are knowledgeable about the targeted population and can provide insight and history on the specific problem such as agency representatives or community leaders. *Stakeholders* should also be interviewed. These are individuals who are interested in addressing the problem, such as the community health educator, the school nurse, or the area Director on Aging. Questions used during the qualitative data collection process seek to answer broad questions and understand human experiences and how they influence behavior in the context of the research questions. One of the downfalls of qualitative data is that it does not provide numerical, measurable data. Hence, limit the ability to generalize the results to the larger target population; this makes quantitative data as important in the research process.

Quantitative data Measurable data collected to obtain objective information (i.e., statistics, numbers, percentages).

Quantitative data are objective indices from a selected sample where results are expressed in numerical terms. Data collected from governmental agencies, for example, can help inform and create food and nutrition policy, such as the data analysis conducted to create the Dietary Guidelines for Americans 2020-2025. By using nationally representative data, the USDA provided national guidelines that are practical, relevant, and achievable.[12] Both qualitative and quantitative data add perspective and comprehensive information valuable to the creation of social marketing campaigns.

Discussion Prompt

Describe some quantitative and qualitative data examples.

Market Segmentation

Market segmentation is used to target a social marketing strategy to a particular audience or group.

Market segmentation is based upon[1]:

- *Demographics:* Age, race, sex, income, education
- *Geographics:* Country, state, urban/rural, climate
- *Psychographics:* Attitudes, values, beliefs, personality traits
- *Behavior:* Benefits wanted, usage

To best tailor your marketing strategy, it is important to identify the market segment. In the 2019 National Eating Disorders Association (NEDA) campaign during eating disorder awareness week, "Come As You Are," NEDA invited individuals at all stages of body acceptance and ED recovery. The campaign sought to "promote inclusivity in the greater eating disorder community," with a focus on diversity and inclusion.[13] The campaign used storytelling through various platforms such as social media, to highlight the intersectionality of eating disorders. "Call to Action," an activity component of the campaign, encouraged audiences to actively participate in spreading awareness. The first step included taking the "Body Acceptance Challenge," to pledge and reject diet culture, which was signed by more than 287 million people through 25 placements (NBC news, Yahoo, Teen Vogue, etc.).[14] The second part of the campaign asked audiences to take a photo of themselves holding a piece of paper/wearing a t-shirt/showing body art that stated something they liked about themselves. Audiences posted the picture on social media with the hashtag #ComeAsYouAre in the name of the NEDA campaign. At the end of 2020, more than 400,000 posts on Instagram use the hashtag #ComeAsYouAre. By the end of the campaign, donations to NEDA increased by 244%.[15]

The "California Children's Power Play! Campaign," aimed to improve fruit and vegetable intake and physical activity among 4th- and 5th-grade students. The campaign used a 10-week educational intervention during and after school, alongside social marketing interventions in the classroom, cafeteria, home, and community settings. These interventions reinforced the importance of a healthy balanced diet and physical activity for good health among low resource public schools. The intervention group significantly increased intake of fruits and vegetables and physical activity during recess and lunch at follow-up compared to the control group.[16]

By using market segmentation, a customized plan and strategy can be developed that increases the likelihood of yielding greater campaign success. Narrowing the target audience aids in the planning stages of the marketing mix, as well as defining strategies and media platforms to be used for message delivery. Given the advancement of technology during the past decade, social media has become an effective medium for the promotion of nutrition services, products and social campaigns. Nutrition professionals should be familiar with social media platforms and their potential role in developing health promotion and disease prevention campaigns. The applications of market segmentation and marketing mix within social media platforms will be discussed further in the chapter.

The Social Marketing Mix

In traditional business marketing, the specific combination of marketing elements used to achieve objectives and satisfy the target market is known as the *marketing mix*. Those variables over which an organization has control include the four Ps of marketing: product, place, price, and promotion, used at the initial planning stage once data collection has been completed.[17] Social marketing plans use the "4 Ps," to voluntarily change human behavior for social benefit. Throughout history, social marketing campaigns have played a significant role in the public health system. The COVID-19 pandemic outbreak has forced government agencies to leverage the use social marketing campaigns in an effort to raise awareness on the necessary measures to prevent spread such as proper hygiene, mask usage, and social distancing.[5] Product, place, price and promotion are key elements to carry through social marketing objectives and help solve social issues.

Product

In traditional business marketing, the *product* is either tangible (a good) or intangible (a service or an idea).[5] Community and public health nutrition products are usually intangible (e.g., distributing weight-control counseling, consulting on developing food service menus). Tangible community and public health nutrition products might include such things as humanitarian rations distributed to populations in disaster-stricken areas or surplus dry milk powder distributed to low-income populations. In stark contrast to business marketing, the social marketing product/service is intended to be used to ensure that the target population uses products or services in a way that promote behavior change. Social marketing seeks to provide target audiences with tools and skills that lead to behavior change for the greater good.[18]

Designing a nutrition program product that will have maximum potential for success requires careful planning. Some factors to consider include:[18]

- Naming the product (establishing a brand)
- Product packaging
- Differentiating the product from its competitors
- Considering product lifetime
- Continually revising to adapt to a changing market environment

As an example, consider the updated Nutrition Facts Label. The label intends to empower consumers to make informed food choices that positively impact their health and wellbeing.

In re-packaging the product (Nutrition Facts Label) for the first time in over 20 years, experts considered updating serving size and calories to a larger and clearer font, updating daily value percentages, distinguishing between total and added sugars, and adding nutrients of concern for public health purposes such as vitamin D and potassium.[19] Given the constant changing marketing environment, the Nutrition Facts Label changes now reflect realistic serving sizes based on realistic consumer consumption.

When developing a nutrition product, include long-range planning to ascertain the probable lifetime of the product. Remember that the marketing environment is dynamic, and that today's ideal product may be obsolete in the future due to changes in, for example, technology, public policy, or consumer awareness/interest.

Place

Place denotes the location where tangible goods are offered and also includes the product's distribution system, that is, the channels through which the product is offered to the target market (including storage, transport, sales, and delivery). For intangible products, place may denote the location where a service is offered, including the channels through which the target market will be reached (e.g., clinics, hospitals, daycare centers, congregate meal sites, shopping malls, agricultural fairs, in-home demonstrations).[18] When considering a place, remember to ensure that the product will be accessible to the target market and that product delivery is of high quality.

The FDA launched the "What's in It for You?' campaign to promote the new Nutrition Facts Label. The educational campaign included outreach through many channels including, but not limited to, social media, indoor/outdoor advertising, and downloadable educational material. Given that the campaign aimed to target not only consumers, but also healthcare professionals, educators, and food companies, the *place* was mainly technological avenues, which led to greater outreach.[20,21]

Price

Price is perhaps the most critical component of the marketing mix for both traditional business and social marketing, because price is the component most evident to the consumer in the target market. In business marketing, *price* is often a competitive tool. Commercial businesses must adopt the right pricing to ensure new customers, hold on to existing customers, and satisfy both groups' needs.[5] In most cases, business marketers establish a product's price so that the business will profit, and the consumer will be happy with the value received. Social marketing efforts, however, are not usually focused in generating a profit.

Social marketing projects must aim to reward the desired behavior change and discourage competing for undesirable behaviors, given that the ultimate objective *is* behavior change itself.[18] The target audience can exchange their monetary or non-monetary resources for benefits that can be either tangible or intangible. "Costs can include money, time, opportunity, energy, social, behavioral, geographical, physical, structural, psychological factors and convenience or pleasure."[18] Given that a price component is often not monetary in social marketing campaigns, the consumer has to perceive the benefits greater than the cost, otherwise the product's value will be perceived as low, and may lead to a decrease in participation.

In social marketing situations where money is involved as part of the exchange between both parties, program managers may want to recover all or a portion of their costs for goods or services. A pricing strategy that will not negatively affect participation in the program must be created prior to implementation of a campaign. Options range from full-cost recovery through sliding-scale fees to «suggested donations"

As part of their big-picture Nutrition Innovation Strategy (i.e., pricing strategy), launched in 2018, the FDA "What's In It For You" campaign aimed to reduce preventable death and disease related to poor nutrition.[18] This public health strategy is an on-going campaign to support consumer education using new innovative ways to reduce the burden of chronic disease. As part of the strategy, the FDA announced key activities that included an updated ingredient and Nutrition Label, modernized nutrition and health claims, modernized standards of identity of products, reduced sodium, and accessible nutrition education. Through said efforts, the FDA seeks to both facilitate industry innovation towards healthier foods and empower consumers at the same time. These efforts will help reduce nutrition-related chronic health conditions.

Promotion

Promotion is the means to introduce the product to the targeted audience. Promotion involves communicating a message through a variety of media to create awareness and promote action. The "What in It for You?" campaign, as mentioned, used multiple media to create awareness on the updated label. In their efforts to create greater outreach, the FDA created social media toolkits for professionals. The toolkits, available both in English and Spanish, consist of newsletters, texts, social media posts for Facebook and Twitter, images, videos, and educational resources. The pre-made posts included the hashtag #NewNutritionFactsLabel to facilitate a search for the content and further promote engagement in social media platforms.[19]

In this new age and era, nutrition professionals have had to become innovative in the design and delivery of nutrition programs, products and campaigns. A vast amount of learning opportunities has resulted following the COVID-19 pandemic. Technology and virtual programs have turned into the first (and at times, the only) option to reach large audiences given social distancing guidelines in effect. One such resource that is ready-to-use by nutrition professionals to deliver virtual interventions can be found on the webpage of the Supplemental Nutrition Assistance Program Education Toolkit (SNAP-Ed) (See **Table 19–2**). "SNAP is a federal program that helps millions of low-income Americans put food on the table. Across the United States there are 9.5 million families with children on SNAP. It is the largest program working to fight hunger in America."[22] These toolkits

Discussion Prompt

Identify online nutrition influencers. How important should it be that these influencers have nutrition credentials?

TABLE 19-2
SNAP-Ed Toolkit - Virtual Interventions to Engage and Reach SNAP-Ed Clients[23]

Intervention Name	Overview	Considerations for Online Delivery
Common Threads: Small Bites Program	The Common Threads: Small Bites Program is a direct nutrition intervention designed to increase nutrition knowledge, vegetable consumption, and variety of vegetables consumed.	Small Bites is a digital nutrition curriculum. To access the Small Bites digital resources, visit https://www.commonbytes.org/#!/resources/40.
EatFresh	EatFresh.org is a mobile-friendly website that was created for the SNAP-Ed population and the organizations that serve them. It provides practical resources and encouragement for individuals with varying levels of digital literacy, internet access, health awareness and culinary skills.	EARS data and pre-post surveys are built-in, along with a referral code system that allows SNAP-Ed Implementing Agencies to track their participants.
Eat, Move, Win	Eat, Move, Win is a direct education intervention, which consists of five online lessons that seek to improve high school students' awareness of their food environment and the link between food and health.	Eat Move Win is entirely online and available for virtual learning. There are a few features that work best in a classroom setting but can easily be adapted to online delivery or do not affect the fidelity of the program if not used.
FNV (Fruits n vegetables)	The FNV Campaign is a social marketing and PSE change intervention that aims to present fruits and vegetables in a way that is both fun and cool, ultimately shifting attitudes, behavior and social norms relative to healthy eating.	FNV can successfully be implemented as a digital campaign solely.

Reproduced from Online Interventions. SNAP. Accessed September 5, 2020. https://snapedtoolkit.org/online-interventions/

are created for professionals to use and further spread campaign awareness through the use of technology.

Evaluation

In social marketing campaigns, program effectiveness or success is assessed by a campaign's potential to improve an individual's health and/or behaviors.[24] Key components of any social marketing effort are tracking trends, performing frequent evaluations, and estimating success. Evaluation is an ongoing process and should stay at the forefront during planning stages of a social marketing campaign. In his book, "Social Marketing and Public Health: Theory and Practice," Jeff French[25] describes the means by which evaluations play a pivotal role in social marketing interventions:

1. Develop ideas that inform interventions (formative evaluation).
2. Assess progress of a project or program in order to improve it as it develops (process evaluation).
3. Learn whether the program has been effective (impact or summative evaluation).
4. Determine whether one program or intervention is worth investing in, by comparison with an alternative program or the status quo, depending on the resources and level of change achieved (cost-effectiveness or economic evaluation).[25]

The following questions are important to consider at the beginning of the evaluation process:

- How do we define the problem?
- What are our goals and objectives?
- Who is the market we want to reach?
- How will our target market find out about the product/campaign?

- What information do we have about the problem and the target market?
- What is our message?
- Who will benefit from the program or campaign?
- How will the target audience benefit?
- What media platform will we use?
- Who will be our partners and influencers to help deliver an effective program?
- Will they be cost effective?
- What is the timeframe?
- Which will be indicators of outcomes?
- How will we measure our goals and objectives?
- How will we evaluate the program?
- What is the end goal of the evaluation? Why is an evaluation being performed?

Three types of evaluations should be considered when assessing a social marketing campaign: formative evaluation, process evaluation, and outcome evaluation.

Formative Evaluation

Formative evaluation begins during the development of a social marketing program or campaign and during its implementation, it can also be considered as a "'front end' element of evaluation… with the aim of improving the project's design and performance."[25] Formative evaluation helps to define the problem and to refine possible interventions. It includes establishing the goals and aims of the campaign, including the marketing mix, pre-testing of ideas, procedures, and materials, and using focus groups, surveys, and interviews. For example, you may ask, "Did the target market understand the PSA message?" "Was the print material at a readability level appropriate to the audience?" "Was the social media channel used appropriate for our target audience and message?" "Was the action requested of the target market realistic?" This type of information allows revisions to be made before the full program is implemented.

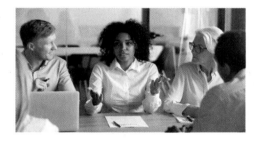

Focus groups allow professionals to get primary data and formative evaluation.

© Fizkes/Shutterstock.

Process Evaluation

Process evaluation assesses the implementation and function of the social marketing program, it helps distinguish and evaluate results of the planned vs. actual intervention. Main components of the process evaluation are the context, reach and delivery of the program or campaign.[26] In the setting of social marketing across social media platforms the analytics related to engagement can also be considered part of the process evaluation such as the reach of posts/stories/videos, etc. which help assess exposure, reach, and engagement.[27] Process evaluation uses continuous quality improvement (CQI) to monitor progress. CQI is a tool based on the premise that there is always room for improvement. Customers are asked how satisfied they are with the services, materials, venues, and costs associated with a program. CQI has been used in health care, including nutrition services, since the 1990s.[28]

Outcome Evaluation

Outcome evaluation (sometimes referred to as summative evaluation) determines the impact of the program or campaign, and whether the goals and objectives of the social marketing campaign are met. It is important that the goals and objectives are well defined at the inception of the social marketing process, otherwise it is difficult to measure the success of meeting them. Goals and objectives should be specific in order for them to be effectively evaluated. An example of an objective that can be measured is: "Twenty percent of the target audience/market will increase fruit and vegetable consumption by 1 serving within 3 months of initiating the campaign." Outcome evaluations make use of quantitative and qualitative methods to complete a comprehensive analysis of the impact and changes resulting from an intervention.[25]

Social Media and Technology; Opportunities for Business and Social Marketing for Nutrition Professionals

The power of **social media** has grown exponentially over the past decade; from Facebook to Twitter to TikTok, words, video, and images have now become the primary way to communicate, express and connect. Nutrition marketers and educators can make use of social media to broaden their reach to their target audience, as well as implement, manage, and evaluate their business, marketing campaigns, and programs.

There are six main platforms that claim to have over 1 billion daily active users of which four are owned by Facebook.[29] From 2012 to 2018, Facebook has remained the primary platform for the majority of Americans with roughly two-thirds of U.S. adults (68%) being active users. Younger audiences have leaned towards Instagram at around 71% of 18-to-24-year-old, and an even younger crowd of 16-to-24-year-old use the new video app TikTok.[29,30] It is vital for RD's and nutritionists to have a clear focus on their target audiences and become experienced in the use of social media platforms in order to create effective communication strategies and ensure audience's needs and interests are met.

Social media provides nutrition professionals with an avenue to apply marketing principles both in business marketing and social marketing. Customer's perceptions, attitudes and awareness towards a specific product, brand or campaign, can be positively influenced by making use of the diverse social media platforms. In this day and age, being social media savvy is a must for nutritionists and RDNs. Social media has become a platform to connect with others. The principles of business marketing when applied in the online realm for product placement purposes, can yield greater sales, and greater brand visibility thanks to advertising opportunities and word-of-mouth.[31]

The well-known yogurt brand Chobani® developed the #SwitchTheChobaniFlip challenge to celebrate Opposite day (January 25) and promote a limited-edition flavor in 2021. The brand created the hashtag challenge #SwitchTheChobaniFlip and introduced it on TikTok which consists of having influencers and users alike create a video dancing to Missy Elliot's 2002 song, "Work It," which said "I put my thing down, flip it and reverse it."[32] The brand reached out to influencers, nutrition professionals and experts for further promotion. The users who participated had a chance to win a case of their new limited-edition flavor dropped only on TikTok, consisting of cookie dough crunch in the larger compartment and Greek yogurt in the smaller section of their unique Chobani® Flip® line product. The campaign ran from January 25, 2021-February 28th, 2021, and for the first two days the hashtag had 958.4 million views on TikTok.[33]

Instagram's story features were used by the brand to promote an earlier line of products launched in July 2020, Chobani® Complete and Chobani® Probiotic.[34] The Instagram story feature posted on the company's profile, encouraged audiences to "tap to solve" a puzzle that highlighted Chobani®

Complete's ingredients.[35] By making social media a great part of their business marketing strategies, Chobani® is likely to leave a longer lasting impression on their audience and engage a variety of users through various platforms, that ultimately lead to more brand exposure and sales.

Nutrition professionals can take advantage of the growing online interest in nutrition and wellness topics in the community as a whole. Social media is a forum where information and misinformation are quickly spread, providing nutrition professionals with the unique opportunity to educate the masses using content created with evidence-based nutrition information. Nutrition professionals serve as a credible and trustworthy source on health and nutrition communications and marketing campaigns.[36] As such, they can offer creative content creation, recipe development, product consulting, experiential marketing strategies such as events or demos, speaking engagements, social media campaigns, among many other opportunities.

As the nutrition experts, RDN's can collaborate with brands to help develop healthier products, apply concepts from Medical Nutrition Therapy to adapt product composition to meet the needs of individuals with specific health conditions, as well as help educate clients and audiences on the health benefits of the product or brand. Examples of brands that have partnered with, or currently have RDN's on staff include Egg Nutrition Center, Sargento®, Kelloggs®, Banza, Kind®, Manitoba Harvest, Epicured® and the American Beverage Association, among many others. RDN's can work as employees, consultants, spokespersons, advisors, and ambassadors for food brands nationwide.[37] The meal delivery service Epicured® first introduced in 2016 was launched with the purpose to create meals for patients with Gastrointestinal Disorders.[38] The brand encouraged RDN's and other clinicians to join their nutrition collaborative program "Partners in Health,"[39] where they provide free CEU opportunities, samples, and workshops for greater brand visibility and community trust.

RDN's can also use the various forms of social media to promote their own counseling services. Social media provides a platform where RDN's can engage with a broader audience in a way that they can show their philosophy, personality and viewpoints on topics of interest. In this way, RDN's can find clients that connect with their content and continue engaging with existing clients "out of office."[36] The use of social media platforms in an interconnected way might lead to greater engagement and reach instead of only focusing solely on a single platform, given that a diverse audience exists in all platforms and all platforms serve a different purpose.[40,41]

> "Facebook is good for connecting with fellow dietitians, clients, and potential clients; Pinterest is best for recipes and workout ideas. RDNs setting up a counseling service can refer clients to the latter, once they've come in for a consultation. Twitter is more for professional-to-professional communication; and Instagram works well for food bloggers. One will have to zero in on how to make the best use of various social media outlets, including Foursquare Swarm, YouTube, LinkedIn, and Google+, based on your client base. Have social media accounts set up and ready to go," Jessica Crandall Synder RDN, CDE, AFAA told Today's Dietitian.[42]

RDNs can better understand their audiences' needs through social media engagement, and in this way tailor their services and their communication and outreach strategies. The Academy offers many resources in their Marketing Center including communication tips, radio scripts, downloadable content, and more.[43]

Social marketing principles can also be applied to social media. The Partnership for a Healthier America launched the Fruits and Veggies Campaign

Strategy Tip

Is it better to have a RDN on staff or consulting a fast-food giant or should it be boycotted by nutritional professionals?

(FNV) to promote greater intake of fruits and vegetables among moms and teens in two California and Virginia pilot markets.[43] The campaign used integrated marketing communication strategies with a social media component, alongside television, radio, and print publications. After the FNV Campaign launched, 650 million people engaged in the media with 350 million being solely on social media. After evaluations, researchers found that participants had a positive shift towards the attitudes and intention behind fruit and vegetable consumption.

Social media became indispensable for most during the COVID-19 pandemic in 2020. Platforms have been important for the spread of information about the novel Coronavirus, of which at times can include a lot of misinformation.[44] The World Health Organization has deemed social media a "misinfodemic – a vector for sharing low-quality content – misinformation, conspiracy theories, scams, geopolitical manipulation and other malicious activities – all of which could lead to unhealthy behaviors and loss of life."[45] Social media platforms have played an active role in helping stop the spread of both the virus and misinformation. Facebook used its news feed function to direct users to WHO website and websites of local health authorities, Twitter and other platforms similarly pointed users who frequently search for COVID-related content to reliable sources.[46] Through this strategy social media platforms ensure that users are reaching similar, credible information more often than not. Influencers, healthcare professionals, and celebrities have also posted content related to the novel virus and help spread reliable information to the general public.

Social Media Analytics

Social media marketing would not be possible without data to measure engagement and campaign outcomes. All social media platforms have analytics tools, some available to users, for example Instagram analytics are available to users who report their profile as a "business profile." These analytics take a look at engagement, impressions and reach, and audience demographics alongside other useful data for marketing professionals.[47] Many useful tools exist to track further analytics, help prepare posts that can be automatically shared, and create analytic reports.[48] These tools provide users with a cost-effective way to maximize social and business marketing, as shown in **Table 19–3**.

TABLE 19–3
Top 5 Free Social Media Analytics Tool[48]

NAME	FEATURES	COMPATIBILITY
Buffer Analyze	-Create professional reports -Track key engagement metrics and audience demographics -Posting strategy recommendations	-Facebook -Instagram -Twitter
Sprout Social	-Analyze paid campaigns -Analyze team's performance (task performance, response rates, etc.) -Create culture strategies	-Facebook -Twitter -Instagram -LinkedIn -Pinterest
Hootsuite	-Measure customer care team response -Track brand mentions -Customize and export reports to different formats	-Facebook -Instagram -YouTube -LinkedIn -Twitter -Pinterest

Zoho Social	-Differentiate between fans vs. other-user engagement -Detailed reports -Get detailed breakdown of content formats used by users	-Facebook -LinkedIn -Twitter -Instagram
Sendible	-Easily accessible report -Measure track team performance and response times -Notifications of reactions and engage with multiple social profiles across networks from a single dashboard	-Facebook -LinkedIn -Twitter -Instagram -You Tube

Compiled by the authors from: Lee K. 27 Free and Paid Social Media Analytics for Marketers. Buffer Library. Accessed December 30, 2020. https://buffer.com/library/social-media-analytics-tools/. Published June 30, 2020.

Social and business marketing through social media can lead to greater brand and campaign exposure. By embedding links to websites in social media posts/profiles, one can direct audiences to campaign or brand websites in real-time for further information. Through search engine marketing (SEM) and search engine optimization (SEO) social marketing efforts can better drive traffic to websites; the main difference between SEO and SEM being that SEO uses organic efforts while SEM consists of paid search engine advertising. Both strategies seek to gain greater website visibility and "clicks."[49]

RDN's can take advantage of other forms of media to support their business and social marketing campaigns. By using print, television, radio, and other forms of media can help reach a greater audience, reinforce messages and network with other professionals. Many dietitian nutritionists have chosen nontraditional career paths thanks to advancements in technology and the media. From freelance writing, consulting, recipe development to becoming a media spokesperson, can take advantage of the media to spread their message or find fulfillment outside of the clinical realm.[50,51]

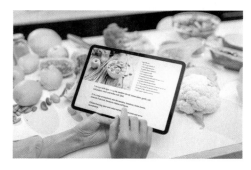

The internet allows RDNs to profile healthy recipes and other information on the internet. Millions of viewers can be reached.

© RossHelen/Shutterstock.

Marketing Ethics

Involvement of nutrition professionals in product development and brand partnership has undoubtedly raised concerns regarding marketing ethics. There is a fine line between recommending beneficial products to patients, clients, and the community as a whole and promoting products for the sole purpose of financial gains with disregard for the client's health and wellbeing. Transparency and disclosure will always prevail as a starting point when questions over whether or not an action is ethical arise.[52] Whether engaging in business or social marketing, the marketer must begin with a strong code of personal **ethics**. With a good sense of the moral principles and values that determine individual and group behavior within a society, one can reliably choose the right and just action when faced with a moral dilemma.

As the dimensions of marketing ethics in both traditional business and social marketing contexts are explored and debated, nutrition professionals, drawing on a strong personal code of ethics, would do well to follow the guidelines of the Academy of Nutrition and Dietetics Code of Ethic. The Code of Ethics is "based upon four key principles of ethical principles of ethical theory: autonomy, non-maleficence, beneficence, and justice."[52]

Ethics Moral principles and values that determine individual and group behaviors.

- Autonomy: represents the idea that patients should have as much input and control of their health as possible
- Non-maleficence: health care providers should hold as a priority the avoidance of harm to patients

- Beneficence: providers should keep the patient's best welfare as a ruling priority
- Justice: relates to the treatment of all patients equally regardless their individual characteristics or socio-economic circumstances

The principles of ethics can be applied to all aspects of the dietitian nutrition profession, not only clinical work. To further reinforce the importance of ethics in the profession, the Academy has mandated 1 Continuing Education Unit per cycle be completed on an ethics-related presentation.[53]

The Academy's Practice Paper: Social Media and the Dietetics Practitioner: Opportunities, Challenges, and Best Practices, is a guide for professionals to understand best practices when using social media.[54] Nutrition professionals should not only look for The Academy's Code of Ethics to develop their social media persona and content, but also be aware of the resources and advice provided by the Federal Trade Commission on social media transparency.[55] Even if the intention behind promotional posts is not monetary compensation, it is important to note that referral bonuses, discounts and samples can be seen as an incentive and conflict of interest if not disclosed properly. Professionals should be aware of the suggested social media disclosures:

- #ad
- #sponsored
- #paid
- #client
- "Company X gave me this product to review"
- "I was compensated X to write this blog post"[54]

Although exceptions exist, nowadays, most traditional business marketing ethics are guided by the principle that the customer's wants and needs are paramount, and profit-generating activities are aimed at customer satisfaction. Social marketers, too, are focused on the customer, but with the ultimate aim of improving their personal welfare and that of their society. The social marketer thus faces ethical challenges that are not seen in traditional business marketing; challenges that are only now being identified and studied.

In closing this overview of marketing ethics, we must point out that many of the ethical dilemmas that a public health nutritionist or RDN is likely to face will arise from cultural differences between the nutritionist and the client or the population being served.[56] The United States is a multicultural land with minority ethnic populations from most parts of the world. When serving those whose ethnic backgrounds differ from your own, make an effort to understand the societal culture and norms that govern them, as well as those that underlie the prevailing U.S. societal culture and norms. When entering into partnerships with multinational or global organizations, be sure to consider the often-great differences in marketing ethics of the cultures represented. Nutrition professionals should be comfortable with recognizing their own biases, learning about different cultures, connecting with other professionals for further learning opportunities, sharing their experiences and teachings, and asking questions.[56]

Discussion Prompt

Do you still feel that RDNs should represent fast-food giants after reading the ethics section? Why or why not?

Summary

Knowledge on social and business marketing can empower nutrition professionals to effectively reach and impact audiences such as consumers, clients, patients, and the community as a whole. While evidence-based research is key to developing and delivering campaigns supported by science, understanding of and presence in social media is pivotal to a campaign's success in this new era of technology and virtual connections. Nutrition professionals have been faced with multiple challenges to deliver campaigns due to social distancing regulations because of the COVID-19 pandemic. Nonetheless, these regulations have also led to learning opportunities and advancement in technology to better reach audiences and impact society for the greater good.

Social media has become a platform by which to connect with others. It is vital for nutrition professionals to have a clear focus on their target audiences and to become experienced in the use of social media platforms to create effective communication strategies and to ensure that the audience's needs and interests are met. Customer's perceptions, attitudes, and awareness toward a specific product, brand, or campaign, can be positively influenced by making use of the diverse social media platforms. At the same time, the dissemination of information through online platforms to the masses undoubtedly raises concerns over ethics, which nutrition professionals need to be aware of, and abide by, such as The Academy of Nutrition and Dietetics' Code of Ethics.

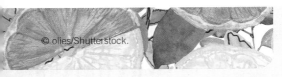
© olies/Shutterstock.

Learning Portfolio

Key Terms

Key Terms	page
Business marketing	588
Social Marketing	588
Marketing mix	589
Quantitative data	592
Qualitative data	592
Social media	598
Ethics	601

Issues for Discussion

1. How can a nutritionist promote healthful eating practices to people who are convinced that a currently popular diet plan is appropriate for everyone?

2. Find a problem you would like to improve in your University or within the community. How would you create a social marketing campaign to address the problem, what avenues would you use, and how would you incorporate social media and technology in your campaign?

3. You have been hired by WIC to provide an innovative social marketing campaign to support breastfeeding initiatives at a national level. Who would be your target population? What is the desired behavior change? How would you evaluate the success of your campaign?

4. How can and should a dietitian/nutritionist approach promoting healthful eating practices for children in partnerships with multinational fast-food and toy companies?

5. How can social media be used to create a viral campaign discouraging teenagers from drinking sugar-sweetened beverages? What platform would you use to best reach teens?

6. You have a successful social media account (i.e., on Instagram, Facebook, etc.), which you use to educate others about nutrition, health, and wellness. A yogurt company is interested in partnering up with you to help promote their new high-protein yogurt line through your social media account. What ethical considerations do you need to keep in mind? Is there a difference in ethical concerns based on whether you receive monetary payment for the promotion? Are there any disclosures you need to provide online?

7. How would you educate young adults on the topic of supplementation and the prevention of diseases through an online platform using evidence-based research? Which platform is most appropriate to deliver your campaign for your target market? How would you analyze your reach and engagement?

8. Which traditional and social media interventions would be beneficial in marketing a new community farmers' market and local, organic food hall?

Case Study: RDN Represents a Healthy Gut Bar

A startup company that makes granola bars and cereals has contacted you, a RDN, to help them in the final stages of product formulation, marketing, and promotion on the company's social media platforms to young adults working from home with an interest in gut health. They want to develop a grab-and-go product that is both nutritious and delicious, while also including at least five ingredients that support gut health such as traditional grains, nuts, and seeds with minimal added sugars. Some of the product ingredients are oats, almonds and chia seeds.

1. What type of evidence-based research on gut health would you use to support the company's recommendations for use of these ingredients?

   Now that the product is formulated and ready to launch, the company shows you their social media account on Instagram. They want you to come up with innovative ideas to reach their target market, young adults working from home with an interest in gut health. They provide you with freedom to open accounts in other social media platforms to best reach the audience if you feel like Instagram alone is not sufficient. They also encourage ideas to best use the platforms and methods to analyze the outcomes of the posts/videos/stories.

2. Would you recommend the company to use more than one social media outlet to promote their program? Why, why not? Which other(s) social media platforms would you recommend for them to use? What innovative ideas can you think of to best reach their target market on each of the platforms? What recommendations can you give them on how to best use each platform and how to analyze campaign outcomes?

Case Study: "Supplemental" Income

Joe Jones, RDN, has been employed for the past year as a clinical dietitian in an acute care hospital. Needing to make some extra income for his young family, Joe recently took a second job as a health coach and personal trainer at a wellness center. The wellness center earns a significant percentage of its profit by selling dietary supplements. Joe has been assigned an aggressive monthly sales quota that he must meet to maintain employment. He is eager to start promoting these supplements to his clients since he stands to make substantial additional commission income. However, Joe has minimal knowledge of dietary supplements and has never recommended them to his inpatients per hospital policy.

1. Does the Academy of Nutrition and Dietetics Code of Ethics permit Joe to sell dietary supplements?

Resources

1. Kaimal MM, Sajoy PB. Use of social marketing in the public health sector. *Perspectives on Business Management & Economics*. 2020;2:46-53. doi: http://www.pbme.in/papers/28 .pdf

2. Brychkov D, Domegan C. Social marketing and systems science: past, present and future. *Journal of Social Marketing*. 2017;7(1):74-93. doi: https://doi.org/10.1108/JSOCM-10 -2016-0065

3. Serrat O. The Future of Social Marketing. In: Knowledge solutions: tools, methods, and approaches to drive organizational performance. S.l.: Springer Verlag, Singapore; 2017.

4. Shams M. Social Marketing for Health: Theoretical and Conceptual Considerations. In: *Selected Issues in Global Health Communications*. London: IntechOpen; 2018.

5. Haber S. Dietitians on social media: making connections for better health. *Food&Nutrition*. 2017. https://foodand nutrition.org/blogs/the-feed/dietitians-social-media-making -connections-better-health/

6. Farr LT. Self-promotion, branding, and attracting buyers: I am convinced that you have the power to persuade and influence those who choose your services, how you will provide those services and how much you will be compensated for thos services. *J Acad Nutr Diet*. 2020;120(11):1789-1790. doi: https://doi.org/10.1016/j.jand.2020.09.018

7. Hart K. A practical guide to Instagram analytics for business accounts. Jumper Media. https://jumpermedia.co/instagram -analytics-for-business/. Published December 16, 2019.

8. Lee K. Know what's working on social media: 27 paid and free social media analytics tools. Buffer Library. https:// buffer.com/library/social-media-analytics-tools/. Published June 30, 2020.

9. Varagouli E. SEO vs. SEM: what is the difference and how it affects you. Semrush Blog. https://www.semrush.com /blog/seo-vs-sem/?kw=&cmp=US_SRCH_DSA _Blog_Core_BU_EN&label=dsa_pagefeed&Network=g &Device=c&utm_content=484020092625&kwid=aud -296306606820%3Adsa-1057183189355&cmpid=1176 9537497&agpid=117334838871&BU=Core&extid=15 0515357194&adpos=&gclid=CjwKCAiAu8SABhAxEiw AsodSZGcZCfvvXZAoxXmSnCXzUcJxdX9ELFmgFRkg ZN58S1jFKOMJFu1gsRoCka8QAvD_BwE. Published December 15, 2020.

10. Boyce B. The balance of professional ethics. *J Acad Nutr Diet*. 2017;117(7). doi: https://jandonline.org/article/S2212 -2672(17)30101-6/fulltext

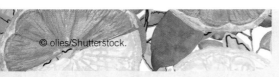
© olies/Shutterstock.

Learning Portfolio

11. Commission on Dietetic Registration the Credentialing Agency for the Academy of Nutrition and Dietetics. Ethics requirement for recertification. https://www.cdrnet.org/news/ethics-requirements-for-recertification

12. Helm J, Miller Jones R. Practice paper of the academy of nutrition and dietetics: social media and the dietetics practitioner: opportunities, challenges, and best practices.

References

1. Sisk K, Conneally A, Cullinen K. *Guide for developing and enhancing skills in public health and community nutrition.* 3rd Ed. Public Health/Community Nutrition Practice Group of the Academy of Nutrition and Dietetics, and the Association of State Public Health Nutritionists; 2018. Accessed February 18, 2021. Available at: www.phcnpg.org

2. Pride WM, Ferrell OC. *Marketing,* 18th ed. Boston: Cengage Learning; 2016:4.

3. Luca NR, Hibbert S, McDonald R. Towards a service-dominant approach to social marketing. *Marketing Theory.* 2016;16(2):194-218. doi: 10.1177/1470593115607941

4. Lee NR, Kotler P. Social Marketing: Changing Behaviors for Good, 5th ed. Los Angeles: Sage; 2016:9.

5. Kaimal MM, Sajoy PB. Use of social marketing in the public health sector. *Perspectives on Business Management & Economics.* 2020;2:46-53. doi: http://www.pbme.in/papers/28.pdf

6. Key TM, Czaplewski AJ. Upstream social marketing strategy: an integrated marketing communications approach. *Business Horizons.* 2017;60(3):325-333. doi: https://www.sciencedirect.com/science/article/abs/pii/S000768131730006X?via%3Dihu

7. Brychkov D, Domegan C. Social marketing and systems science: past, present and future. *J Soc Market.* 2017;7(1):74-93. doi: https://doi.org/10.1108/JSOCM-10-2016-0065

8. Johntson MP. Secondary data analysis: a method of which the time has come. *Qualitative and Quantitative Methods in Libraries (QQML).* 2017;3(3):619-626. doi: http://www.qqml-journal.net/index.php/qqml/article/view/169

9. Hadi A, Askarpour M, Salamat S, Ghaedi E, Symonds ME, Miraghajani M. Effect of flaxseed supplementation on lipid profile: an updated systematic review and dose-response meta-analysis of sixty-two randomized controlled trials. *Pharmacol Res.* 2020;152. doi: https://doi.org/10.1016/j.phrs.2019.104622

10. Hammons AJ, Villegas E, Olvera N, et al. The evolving family mealtime: findings from focus group interviews with Hispanic mothers. *JMIR Pediatr Parent.* 2020;3(2):e18292. doi: 10.2196/18292

11. Portney LG, Watkins MP. Foundations of clinical research: applications to practice. 3rd ed. Harlow: Pearson Education; 2015.

12. U.S. Department of Health and Human Services and U.S. Department of Agriculture. *2015 – 2020 Dietary Guidelines for Americans.* 9th Edition. December 2020. https://health.gov/our-work/food-nutrition/previous-dietary-guidelines/2015

13. Come As You Are this National Eating Disorders Awareness Week National Eating Disorders Awareness Week is Feb. 25 - March 3. National Eating Disorders Association. Accessed September 20, 2021. https://www.nationaleatingdisorders.org/come-you-are-national-eating-disorders-awareness-week-national-eating-disorders-awareness-week-feb. Published February 21, 2019.

J Acad Nutr Diet. 2016;116(11):1825-1835. doi: https://doi.org/10.1016/j.jand.2016.09.003

13. Fair L. Planning a social media marketing campaign? Read this first. *Federal Trade Commission.* November 2018. https://www.ftc.gov/news-events/blogs/business-blog/2018/11/planning-social-media-marketing-campaign-read-first

14. National Eating Disorders Association (NEDA). Momentum CG. Accessed September 20, 2020. http://www.momentum-cg.com/what-we-do/work/case-studies/national-eating-disorders-association-neda/

15. Winner: Momentum Communications Group with National Eating Disorders Association. Advocacy or Awareness Campaign. PR Daily. Accessed September 20, 2021. https://www.prdaily.com/awards/nonprofit-pr-awards/2019/winners/advocacy-or-awareness-campaign/. Published November 4, 2019.

16. Keihner A, Rosen N, Wakimoto P, et al. Impact of California children's power play! Campaign on fruit and vegetable intake and physical activity among fourth- and fifth-grade students. *Am J Health Promot.* 2017;31(3):189-191. doi: 10.4278/ajhp.141125-ARB-592

17. Serrat O. The future of social marketing. In: Knowledge Solutions: Tools, Methods, and Approaches to Drive Organizational Performance. S.l.: Springer Verlag, Singapore; 2017.

18. Shams M. Social marketing for health: theoretical and conceptual considerations. In: *Selected Issues in Global Health Communications.* London: IntechOpen; 2018:43-63.

19. U.S. Food & Drug Administration.. Social media toolkit on the new nutrition facts label. Accessed August 5, 2020. https://www.fda.gov/food/new-nutrition-facts-label/social-media-toolkit-new-nutrition-facts-label

20. U.S. Food & Drug Administration. Accessed August 10, 2020. https://www.fda.gov/food/nutrition-education-resources-materials/new-nutrition-facts-label

21. U.S. Food & Drug Administration. FDA nutrition innovation strategy. Accessed September 5, 2020. https://www.fda.gov/food/food-labeling-nutrition/fda-nutrition-innovation-strategy

22. Feeding America. Understanding SNAP, the Supplemental Nutrition Assistance Program. Accessed September 5, 2020. https://www.feedingamerica.org/take-action/advocate/federal-hunger-relief-programs/snap

23. Snap-Ed Toolkit. Online Interventions. Accessed September 5, 2020. https://snapedtoolkit.org/online-interventions/

24. Centers for Disease Control and Prevention. Research & Evaluation. Accessed September 30, 2020. https://www.cdc.gov/healthcommunication/research/index.html. Published October 6, 2016.

25. French J. *Social Marketing and Public Health: Theory and Practice.* Oxford, United Kingdom: Oxford University Press; 2017.

26. Cheng KK, Metcalfe A. Qualitative methods and process evaluation in clinical trials context: where to head to? *Int J*

Qual Methods. 2018;17(1). doi: journals.sagepub.com/home/ijq

27. Hasenbank T. Kansas State University. Office of Educational Innovation and Evaluation. Utilizing social media analytics to demonstrate program impact. Accessed September 20, 2020. https://blogs.k-state.edu/oeie/2019/06/20/utilizing-social-media-analytics-to-demonstrate-program-impact/. Published December 10, 2019.

28. Harvey G, Lynch E. Enabling continuous quality improvement in practice: the role and contribution of facilitation. *Front Pub Health.* 2017;5. doi: https://doi.org/10.3389/fpubh.2017.00027

29. Smith A, Anderson M. Social Media Use in 2018: Pew Research Center. Accessed December 10, 2021. https://www.pewresearch.org/internet/2018/03/01/social-media-use-in-2018/. Published July 31, 2020.

30. Mohsin M. 10 TikTok Statistics That You Need to Know in 2021. Oberlo. Accessed December 30, 2021. https://www.oberlo.com/blog/tiktok-statistics. Published January 21, 2021.

31. Liu Y, Lopez R. The impact of social media conversations on consumer brand choices. *Marketing Letters.* 2014;27:1-13. doi: https://doi.org/10.1007/s11002-014-9321-2

32. Koltun N. Chobani dips into TikTok with first hashtag challenge for Opposite Day. Marketing Dive. Accessed January 30, 2021. https://www.marketingdive.com/news/chobani-dips-into-tiktok-with-first-hashtag-challenge-for-opposite-day/593750/. Published January 25, 2021.

33. #SwitchTheChobaniFlip Hashtag Videos on TikTok. TikTok. Accessed January 30, 2021. https://www.tiktok.com/tag/SwitchTheChobaniFlip?is_commerce=1&name=SwitchTheChobaniFlip&sec_user_id=MS4wLjABAAAA7yR0Ik02YCLHqQxHFJOjcImsTm3WqJ8_HYhraDZge_k7EEBKOmiqL96SE7kNAxqD&share_link_id=5BDAA3B3-7A2F-49D8-BCA8-AF97EE491305&tt_from=whatsapp&u_code=dbd0b6e3fmdb10&user_id=6805940431538897925&utm_campaign=client_share&utm_medium=ios&utm_source=whatsapp&source=h5_m

34. Watson E. Chobani moves into functional beverage category with Chobani Probiotic; unveils new high protein Complete yogurt range. FoodNavigator-USA. Accessed January 20, 2021. https://www.foodnavigator-usa.com/Article/2020/07/21/Chobani-moves-into-functional-beverage-category-with-Chobani-Probiotic-unveils-new-high-protein-Complete-yogurt-range. Published July 21, 2020.

35. Williams R. Chobani gamifies Instagram story in multichannel push for new yogurt. Marketing Dive. Accessed January 20, 2021. https://www.marketingdive.com/news/chobani-gamifies-instagram-story-in-multichannel-push-for-new-yogurt/584490/. Published September 1, 2020.

36. Haber S. Dietitians on social media: making connections for better health. *Food&Nutrition.* May 2017. Accessed December 20, 2020. https://foodandnutrition.org/blogs/the-feed/dietitians-social-media-making-connections-better-health/

37. Palmer S. Dietitians' food industry relationships: what is ethical and what is not? *Today's Dietitian.* 2015;17:44.

38. Wilson D. Get "Epicured!" – An Interview with Richard Bennett, CEO of The First Low FODMAP Meal Delivery Service in the U.S. FODMAP Everyday. Accessed January 31, 2021. https://www.fodmapeveryday.com/interview-richard-bennett-epicured/. Published August 26, 2020.

39. Epicured. Partners in Health. Epicured's clinician community: partners in health. Accessed January 5, 2021. https://mmm.epicured.com/partners-in-health

40. Feeding America. Understanding SNAP, the Supplemental Nutrition Assistance Program. Feeding America. Accessed September 5, 2020. https://www.feedingamerica.org/take-action/advocate/federal-hunger-relief-programs/snap

41. Webb D. Creating your personal brand — tips from RDs in the trenches. *Today's Dietitian.* 2019;21(7):20.

42. Farr LT. Self-promotion, branding, and attracting buyers: I am convinced that you have the power to persuade and influence those who choose your services, how you will provide those services and how much you will be compensated for those services. *J Acad Nutr Diet.* 2020;120(11):1789-1790. doi: https://doi.org/10.1016/j.jand.2020.09.018

43. Englund TR, Hedrick VE, Duffey KJ, Kraak VI. Evaluation of integrated marketing communication strategies used for the Fruits & Veggies Campaign in California and Virginia. *Prev Med Rep.* 2020;18:101062. Published 2020 Feb 11. doi: 10.1016/j.pmedr.2020.101062

44. Tangcharoensathien V, Calleja N, Nguyen T, et al. Framework for managing the COVID-19 Infodemic: methods and results of an online, crowdsourced WHO technical consultation. *J Med Internet Res.* 2020;22(6):e19659. doi: 10.2196/19659

45. Broniatowski DA, Kerchner D, Farooq F, et al. Debunking the misinfodemic: Coronavirus social media contains more, not less, credible content. *arXiv*; 2021. PPR270042.

46. Merchant RM, Lurie N. Social media and emergency preparedness in response to novel Coronavirus. *JAMA.* 2020;323(20):2011-2012. doi: 10.1001/jama.2020.4469

47. Hart K. A practical guide to Instagram analytics for business accounts. Jumper Media. Accessed December 31, 2020. https://jumpermedia.co/instagram-analytics-for-business/. Published December 16, 2019.

48. Lee K. Know what's working on social media: 27 paid and free social media analytics tools. Buffer library. Accessed December 31, 2020. https://buffer.com/library/social-media-analytics-tools/. Published June 30, 2020.

49. Varagouli E. SEO vs. SEM: What is the difference and how it affects you. Semrush Blog. Accessed January 31, 2021. https://www.semrush.com/blog/seo-vs-sem/?kw=&cmp=US_SRCH_DSA_Blog_Core_BU_EN&label=dsa_pagefeed&Network=g&Device=c&utm_content=484020092625&kwid=aud-296306606820%3Adsa-1057183189355&cmpid=11769537497&agpid=117334838871&BU=Core&extid=150515357194&adpos=&gclid=CjwKCAiAu8SABhAxEiwAsodSZGcZCfvvXZAoxXmSnCXzUcJxdX9ELFmgFRkgZN58S1jFKOMJFu1gsRoCka8QAvD_BwE. Published December 15, 2020.

50. Gorrin A. The best part of becoming a registered dietitian… for me, it's being a media dietitian. *Amy Gorin Nutrition.* Accessed December 20, 2020. https://www.amydgorin.com/becoming-a-registered-dietitian-media-rd/

51. Caplan H. "I don't want to be a dietitian anymore." *Heather Caplan, Registered Dietitian, Fan of Real Talk.* October 2017.

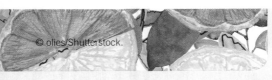
© olies/Shutterstock.

Learning Portfolio

Accessed December 20, 2020. http://heathercaplan.com/nutrition/i-dont-want-to-be-a-dietitian-anymore/

52. Boyce B. The balance of professional ethics. *J Acad Nutr Diet.* 2017;117(7):1120-1123. doi: https://jandonline.org/article/S2212-2672(17)30101-6/fulltext

53. Ethics Requirement for Recertification. Commission on Dietetic Registration the credentialing agency for the Academy of Nutrition and Dietetics. Accessed December 20, 2020. https://www.cdrnet.org/news/ethics-requirements-for-recertification

54. Helm J, Miller Jones R. Practice paper of the Academy of Nutrition and Dietetics: social media and the dietetics practitioner: opportunities, challenges, and best practices. *J Acad Nutr Diet.* 2016;116(11):1825-1835. doi: https://doi.org/10.1016/j.jand.2016.09.003

55. Fair L. Planning a social media marketing campaign? Read this first. *Federal Trade Commission.* November 2018. Accessed December 10, 2020. https://www.ftc.gov/news-events/blogs/business-blog/2018/11/planning-social-media-marketing-campaign-read-first

56. Robinson S. Doubling down on diversity: the journey to a more diverse field. *Food&Nutrition.* 2018.

CHAPTER 20

Striving for Excellence and Envisioning the Future

Christina Ypsilantis, RDN, LDN

(We would like to acknowledge the work of Jennifer Hughes, MS, RD, LDN; Marcia Thomas, MS, MPH, RDN; Pamella Darby, MS, MPH, RDN; and Elizabeth Barden, PhD, in the past editions of Nutrition in Public Health.)

Learning Outcomes

AFTER STUDYING THIS CHAPTER AND REFLECTING ON THE CONTENTS, YOU SHOULD BE ABLE TO:

1. Identify the multidisciplinary roles of the public health dietitian/nutritionist.
2. Describe the ways in which such roles help to advance community and public health nutrition efforts.
3. Suggest strategies for successful professional development.
4. Describe future challenges and ethical considerations facing public health dietitians/nutritionists.

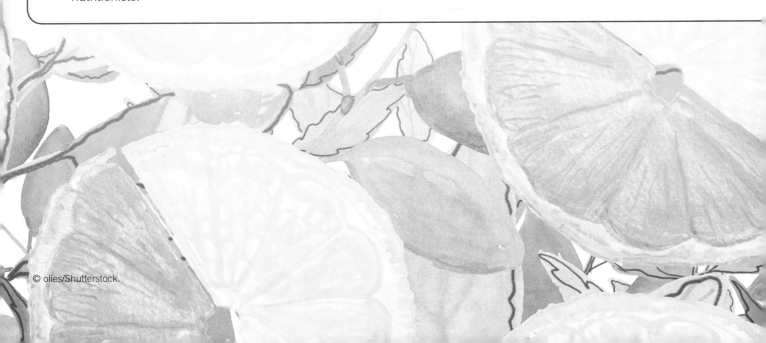

Introduction

The public health dietitian/nutritionist has stepped into the second decade of the 21st century which is full of both opportunities and challenges. On the one hand, there are an assortment of innovative technologies at our fingertips, technological advances in medicine, and improved methodologies for implementing and evaluating public health interventions. On the other hand, we still live and work in communities struggling with obesity, food insecurity, chronic disease, lack of medical insurance, and health disparities. The current health environment leaves us with no other choice but to challenge ourselves professionally, constantly striving for excellence in the field of public health so that we may meet such challenges and advance our efforts.

The motivation to achieve excellence in our field should stem from an understanding that existing opportunities must be embraced in such a way as to foster collective action toward improving the nutritional status of populations. Such opportunities include utilization of innovative technologies, enhanced modes of communication and education, collaboration, advocacy, professional development, and academic training. Globally, health is on the forefront of political and social agendas, with an ever-increasing awareness and interest in food and nutrition. This chapter seeks to encourage today's dietitians/nutritionists to confront with confidence the professional demands that arise, prepared to take on the many challenges of our field.

Multidisciplinary Roles of the Community and Public Health Dietitian/Nutritionist

Community and public health dietitians/nutritionists work in many different environments from community health centers to congregate meal sites and group care facilities. Despite the multitude of settings that we work in, our objectives are the same. Most of us enter the field of community and public health nutrition with the goal of educating the public about healthy eating to prevent and manage illness and disease. What we find when we begin our work is that there is so much more than just food involved in teaching people how to eat well.

The Institute of Medicine's initial report in 2003, *The Future of the Public's Health in the 21st Century*, encourages a broad training and practice of public health "because integrated interdisciplinary teaching is important to the preparation of a well-trained workforce that is capable of addressing today's broad array of public health issues...."[1] To be effective leaders in today's dynamic health environment, public health dietitians/nutritionists must take on multidisciplinary roles, often wearing different hats at the same time. Success in the field, which translates to community and public health action, requires that dietitians/nutritionists be ready to serve as educators, researchers, and advocates throughout the course of their careers.

Nutrition Educator

A hat we all wear is that of nutrition educator, even though efforts occur on many levels and the characteristics of communities and population groups may vary. Needs-assessments, therefore, prove invaluable to community nutrition activities and help to provide a framework for program planning and evaluation. From considering the location of supermarkets to cultural beliefs about food and health, ongoing assessment is necessary to understand how to begin and maintain work within populations and communities.

In a time when such huge health disparities exist, community and public health dietitians/nutritionists must take on the role of educating the public about those inequalities and helping to move communities toward healthier behaviors. When reviewing the Healthy People 2030 objectives, there are over 20 objectives regarding nutrition. This further cements the need for public health dietitians/nutritionists to help the communities at large feel empowered and have adequate tools to make dietary changes to optimize their health.[2] Dietitians are equipped with the tools they need, thanks to the latest and evolving **Standards of Practice (SOP)** in Nutrition Care.[3] The SOP is updated every 7 years to reflect current data and best practices, so dietitians within the Academy can catapult public health and nutrition-related issues to the forefront.[3] Furthermore, nutritionists in public health are in the uniquely qualified position not only to educate the lay public but also to educate other health professionals, policymakers, the media, and private organizations about evidence-based practice.

Nutrition Researcher

Dietitians/nutritionists in public health settings should also wear the hat of researcher. Investigation is critical to our understanding of the many nutritional concerns and risk factors facing our communities and vital to the development of effective public health practice and interventions. By disseminating research, we can reach a larger audience (via publications, presentations, and media) by sharing findings and recommendations for practice with colleagues, policymakers, and the general public.

Not all dietitians/nutritionists focus full-time on research or become part of large, multidisciplinary studies, such as working as epidemiologists, in academia, or in research centers. Although many more are now working in research areas than ever before, historically, many are involved in research activities that are intertwined in ongoing work such as program evaluation, assessment of intervention effectiveness, or focus groups to qualitatively assess a population of interest. The information collected from dietitians/nutritionists working within small, local community programs can be extremely valuable to others working within similar environments and may direct work done within a larger population. Frequently, public health dietitians/nutritionists collect data, but their results are not shared with others. Program evaluations, small quality-assurance projects, and lessons learned from building partnerships should all be shared with the rest of the field and may be just what is needed to help drive future research. In almost all settings, dietitians/nutritionists can engage in various levels of research, either independently or collaboratively. Dietitians/nutritionists are encouraged to collect data because data directs policy and policy drives action. It is our responsibility as public health professionals to ensure that policy favors optimal nutrition for all populations. **Evidence-based practice** is the cornerstone of all health-related initiatives and; therefore, the successful community and public health dietitian/nutritionist should look at research as a means to turn obstacles into opportunities.

The hallmark of public health inquiry is **community-based participatory research (CBPR)**. CBPR emerged in the past few decades to become a focus of public health research. CBPR differs from community research in that partnerships are built among multidisciplinary teams, where members of the community are active partners in all aspects of the research and have equal weight in the research process. Partners bring their own expertise and interest to the group and view the health problem from their own perspective. By looking at health problems from the community level, we can focus on the social, cultural, and physical environment and, hopefully, come closer to creating healthy and sustainable communities.[4]

Standards of practice A resource for credentialed registered dietitian/nutritionists (RDN) and nutrition and dietetic registered technicians (NDTRs) for self-evaluation and maintaining competent practice.

Discussion Prompt

From what you have learned in previous chapters, discuss the differences between registered dietitians and nutritionists?

Evidence-based practice Utilizing nutritional information that is based on scientific studies from reputable sources.

Strategy Tip

Search for dietitians or nutritionists in www.pubmed.gov and discover a plethora of research published in community and public health by these professionals.

Community-based participatory research An applied collaborative approach that allows residents of the community to be active participants and collaborators in research aimed at improving the health of their own community.

Nutrition Advocate

A third hat worn by dietitians/nutritionists is that of advocate. Dietitians/nutritionists have the responsibility to push their ideas forward. For example, these professionals advocate for the following:

- Elimination of health disparities
- Equal access to nutrition services for all who need them
- Inclusion of nutrition professionals in multidisciplinary teams
- Improved nutrition reimbursement for services
- Increased funding for nutrition programs and community resources

For dietitians/nutritionists to be heard, we need to stand up for our services and ensure that nutrition professionals are in the position of providing necessary information to the public.

Education in Public Health and Nutrition

Given the advances in public health and the complexity of our nutrition environment, a formal education in both nutrition and public health prepares professionals to meet the dynamic challenges presented locally and internationally. Increasingly, community nutrition jobs seek candidates who are registered dietitian/nutritionists (RDNs) and who possess advanced training in community and public health. This combination ensures that the professional has a rooted knowledge of nutrition science, expertise in clinical assessment and nutrition education, and can combine such principles with socioeconomic determinants to improve nutrition in community settings. Although degrees in both nutrition and public health are not required to work in the field of public health, such credentials will increase one's credibility in the job market and allow for advancement in the field.

Both schools of public health and programs in public health provide the primary professional degree for dietitian/nutritionists seeking public health training, the Master of Public Health degree (MPH). The MPH degree trains professionals to approach health problems with an ecological framework, wedding biological risk factors with behavioral, social, and environmental determinants. Although they vary by program, areas of specialization are available, and several programs offer a concentration specifically in public health nutrition. In addition to one's area of specialization and fieldwork, there are five core components of a public health degree: biostatistics, epidemiology, health services administration, environmental health, and social and behavioral sciences. Many programs have already incorporated these new areas of public health into their existing coursework, and it is likely that in the future, all public health programs will be required to include these components in their curriculum. (In addition, several other college degrees and university programs have been developed that also share the goals of health promotion and public health.) For those wishing to pursue further advanced training in public health research and leadership, doctoral degrees are available (either PhD or DrPH).

Several systems are in place to monitor and assess the quality of public health educational programs. The Council on Education for Public Health (CEPH) was created in 1974 by the American Public Health Association (APHA) and the Association of Schools of Public Health (ASPH) to accredit schools and programs of public health.[5] CEPH is recognized by the U.S. Department of Education and was established to serve the community by ensuring that graduates of public health programs are adequately prepared to serve as leaders in public health.

In response to an increasing need for adequate education of our future public health workforce, the Council on Linkages between Academia and

Public Health Practice (composed of public health leaders in the community and academia) developed Core Competencies for Public Health Professionals in 2001. These competencies have been revised twice since in keeping up with current needs in public health.[6] The skill set provides specific competencies in the following eight areas:

1. Analytical assessment
2. Policy development/program planning
3. Communication
4. Cultural competency
5. Community dimensions of practice
6. Public health sciences
7. Financial planning and management
8. Leadership and systems thinking

The skill sets are further divided by professional-level—frontline (tier 1), program management/supervisory (tier 2), and senior management/executive level (tier 3),—and have been acknowledged by the Centers for Disease Control and Prevention (CDC) and the APHA.[6]

Maintaining Currency in the Profession

As with all health professionals, it is imperative that dietitians/nutritionists working in public health stay abreast of current events, advancements in nutrition knowledge, and ongoing public health activities in order to serve the community effectively. It is especially important to be aware of where the public is getting their nutrition information from in order to be able to speak to current news events in the areas of public health and nutrition. Although nutrition and public health education provides the necessary foundation upon which to build a successful career, the dietitian/nutritionist is held accountable for maintaining and enhancing professional practice. This involves ongoing continuing education and participation in professional development. For example, the Commission on Dietetic Registration (CDR) requires that all dietitians report continuing professional development activities to maintain registration status. Through individualized self-assessment, dietitians identify ongoing strategies to ensure professional competence.

Examples of new and emerging areas of nutrition research that the public health dietitian/nutritionist should become versed in include:

- Epigenetics
- Nutrigenomics
- The human microbiome
- Functional and integrative nutrition
- Pandemic and other effects on food supplies

Strategies for ongoing professional development include the following.

Membership in Professional Organizations

Membership in professional organizations such as The Academy of Nutrition and Dietetics (AND) and the APHA provides public health professionals with numerous opportunities for professional development through:

- Continuing education activities
- Professional committees
- Discussion groups
- Professional meetings
- Scholarly publications
- Professional resources and networks

Pandemic Learning Opportunity

What can community and public health dietitian/nutritionists learn about supplying adequate and safe food to the public?

The AND supports numerous professional interest groups (dietetic practice groups or DPGs), which allow nutrition professionals to be active in specific areas of nutrition. Several DPGs of the AND may be of particular interest to community and public health professionals, including Hunger and Environmental Nutrition, Nutrition Education for the Public, Public Health/Community Nutrition, and School Nutrition Services.[7] Aside from the aforementioned DPGs, the AND is actively involved in public policy, most notably the Academy of Nutrition and Dietetics Political Advocacy Committee (ANDPAC). ANDPAC and APHA members can choose from 31 primary sections that represent major public health programs or disciplines. These sections include the APHA's Food and Nutrition Section and the Public Health Education and Health Promotion Section.[8] In addition to national organizations, there are numerous state and local professional societies, including affiliates of both the AND and the APHA. Through professional memberships, dietitian/nutritionists not only stay informed of current events in the field but also build lasting professional and social networks.

Conferences, Lectures, and Workshops

Conferences, lectures, and workshops are another way to stay abreast of the latest news and research in the field; gain insight into new, innovative public health interventions and activities; network and build valuable resources; and share best practices among colleagues. In addition to annual meetings of larger organizations, nutritionists should take advantage of the many workshops, meetings, and lectures that take place on a variety of public health topics throughout the year.

Journals and Public Health Publications

Peer-reviewed articles and other public health publications provide a rich source of knowledge on the latest research, insights, and lessons learned in practice. To engage in interdisciplinary dialogue, dietitians/nutritionists should embrace a wide variety of topics and be aware of the various perspectives shaping public health systems in the current social, medical, and political environment. Furthermore, by keeping up with recent publications and media news stories, the dietitian/nutritionist can help to separate fact from fiction when nutrition information reaches the general public.

Academic Courses and/or Programs

Community and public health nutrition is an evolving discipline with ever-emerging methodologies and practices. Whenever possible, the public health dietitian/nutritionist should consider strengthening their current state of knowledge with additional coursework in community and public health or nutrition programs. For example, you might enhance your current job performance through additional training in language and culture, computer and Internet technologies, communications and media, or research and statistical methodologies. If you do not have formal training in community and public health as mentioned previously, you should strongly consider advanced training through graduate or certificate public health programs. Formal education in public health prepares the nutrition workforce to meet the challenges of complex health issues facing communities, adds credibility and marketability to professional pursuits, and provides the skills necessary to advance to leadership roles in agencies or organizations.

Maintaining Political Awareness

Much of community and public health action is influenced by politics, so it is critical that dietitians/nutritionists stay abreast of current events and the political environment. Although some dietitians/nutritionists may be directly

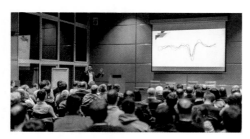

© Matej Kastelic/Shutterstock.

involved in the political scene through advocacy and grassroots efforts, all are affected in some way by political agendas, perhaps through funding, changes in school policies, insurance reimbursement, or community resources. Many professional organizations provide resources through websites and listservs that keep members informed of political action and policy development. The AND website offers an action center where nutrition professionals can take action and send letters to their state and federal representatives regarding issues that are important to the profession of public health nutrition.[9] The AND also offers public policy workshops and runs a donation-funded political action committee called ANDPAC that is broadly focused on food, nutrition, and health.[10] Within the academy, state affiliates take on the role of nutrition advocate on a local governance level. Dietetics professionals have the opportunity to join state public policy committees to take on an active role in nutrition & public policy. The state affiliates often promote "Action Alerts" through the academy, which serves as a way for AND members to send letters to their members of state government officials, regarding pressing nutrition issues. On the national level, ANDPAC provides individual members along with state affiliates copious resources for nutrition advocacy.

Utilizing Technology

Technological improvements have made the 21st century an exciting time to practice public health. In addition to new advancements in science and medicine, the public health workforce is witnessing innovations in surveillance, communication, and geographic information systems (GIS). As they become mainstream, utilization of such technologies will be important for all public health professionals to fully participate in professional activities. Based on the IOM report on preparing the public health workforce, it is likely that more and more educational programs in public health will require such instruction as part of their curriculum. The current era of booming social media is an opportunity for dietetics professionals to access a larger audience, to promote evidence-based nutrition.

Collaborations

One of the most significant strategies for professional advancement is through partnerships and collaboration. Collaboration allows for a synergistic approach to public health issues, pulling together the skills and resources of multiple parties to improve the health of populations, which is the ultimate goal of public health professionals. Through professional and community partnerships, dietitians/nutritionists can augment individual resources, ideas, and political momentum to accomplish a greater good than by acting alone. Such collaborations lead to creative, comprehensive, practical, and transformative thinking.[11] In addition, partnering with the community helps to foster trust and empowerment, thereby allowing for the implementation of community-based interventions that improve health outcomes. As the health of communities improves, especially when the community members themselves actively participate in the process, trust between the health professional and the community is likely to be further strengthened. The cycle thus continues, leading to the potential formation of additional collaborations.

To encourage sustainable action, partnerships should exist beyond the professional circle to welcome community participation. Depending on the desired outcome and goal, dietitians/nutritionists should seek collaborations with community leaders and community-based organizations, school administrators, universities, government officials and policymakers, parent groups, primary-care providers, and private organizations and businesses. The more

Strategy Tip

Go to the AND website at www.eatright.org and discover the pressing nutrition political issues by using the site's search engine. What did you find?

Strategy Tip

Search the Internet for blogs by dietitians/nutritionists. What did you find?

Discussion Prompt

Is it better for dietitians/nutritionists to partner with business and industry, for example fast food franchises, or steer clear of them? Why or why not?

people on the same team, the easier it will be to build trust, and the more consistent the messages to the public.

Future Challenges in Public Health Nutrition

As we move into the future and find an older, more inactive population, higher rates of chronic disease, and enormous health disparities, dietitians/nutritionists must serve as authorities on nutrition issues and be ready to work toward the solutions of the health problems facing our world today. As we forge ahead with scientific and technological advances in health improvement, ethical issues emerge in many aspects of public health practice. As we decide on a research objective or a treatment/prevention protocol, we must think about the moral values and implications involved in the decisions. We should know the issues, the differing opinions, and where we and the community stand on these ethical questions.

According to the University of Pittsburgh's Center for Bioethics and Health Law,[12]

> technology has changed the very boundaries and possibilities of life. Scientific discoveries have blurred the traditional distinctions among birth, life, and death as well as giving us a vast array of new treatments to combat pain and suffering.

For example, as we move forward with genomics, what will that mean for nutritional science? Will we no longer need to change our behaviors to prevent disease? Will parents want to test their unborn babies for unwanted chronic diseases?

Many current-day issues, not quite as obvious as the aforementioned questions, provide examples of ethical dilemmas that we face on a regular basis:

1. Who should provide nutrition education to the public: nutrition professionals, the media, government, physician groups, or private industry? What is the responsibility of government to ensure appropriate nutrition care for the public?
2. Given the increasing rates of childhood obesity, what are the implications for children of food advertising on television? Should the food industry have a role in the prevention of childhood obesity?
3. Despite the rise in obesity, there are still a large number of food-insecure households. Who is responsible for ensuring that all Americans have access to enough food?
4. Given technological advances, should genetically modified foods be sold in the marketplace? If so, does the public have the right to know if their food is genetically altered?
5. As we face a new era where the public health workforce is increasingly involved in bioterrorism preparedness, how are public health dietitians/nutritionists being trained to ensure the safety of our food and water supply?
6. What role does the government play in regulating our food choices? Does the government have an obligation to step in and, if so, how far?
7. In an aging society with rising healthcare costs, are the elderly being forced to choose between adequate nutrition and health care? How are community and public health dietitians/nutritionists working as advocates for our seniors?

Community and public health nutrition is a dynamic and exciting field. Its issues challenge us daily and allow us to grow and develop in ways we may not have imagined when we selected this career path as students. Public health allows us to deal with complex issues, technology, an ever-changing environment, and ethical issues, all of which present new opportunities. In order to meet the demands of the field, we need to be prepared for the associated challenges. Our work places us in a unique position where we are able to inform on food and nutrition policy, advocate for nutrition services, serve as media spokespeople, and help create healthier communities. Rigorous training and life experiences should enable us to survive and thrive in this dynamic field.

Summary

This chapter focuses on the roles of a public health nutritionist and the involvement required to remain current in the profession. As a professional in this field, you will wear many "hats" in whatever role you take on. To excel as a public health nutritionist, you must be multifaceted and willing to seek out opportunities for continuing education and interdisciplinary collaboration. In order to serve the public interest, it is vital that you stay engaged in the newest nutritional science as well as share best practices with your colleagues and community. There are many ways to stay involved both digitally and in person. The job of the public health nutritionist requires a dynamic personality and is not for the unmotivated or those who prefer a more obstinate career. The opportunities for service, learning, and advancement are boundless if you are willing to challenge yourself.

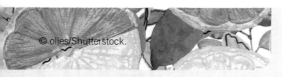

© olies/Shutterstock.

Learning Portfolio

Key Terms   page

Standards of practice   611

Evidence-based practice   611

Community-based participatory
research   611

Issues for Discussion

1. What community resources or professional affiliations are you aware of in your community that you can collaborate with in order to advance public health nutrition?

2. What steps can you take to become more aware of the social, cultural, physical, and environmental climate of the community/population that you intend to work with?

3. Log on to the AND advocacy website. Find one political issue relating to public health nutrition that is important to you. Go through the process of writing to your elected representative in support of this issue. What did you learn about the advocacy process?

4. Choose one emerging issue impacting community and public health nutrition. Research graduate programs, certificates, or continuing education available in this area. What did you find?

Practical Activities

1. Visit a job search website and search for "community and public health nutrition" jobs. Look at the positions posted and the job duties. Can you identify any of the "hats" mentioned earlier in this chapter that you would be expected to wear in this position?

2. Reflect on some of the skills mentioned in the continuing education section of this chapter. Are there any areas that you would like to gain additional proficiency in? Review several programs in higher education to identify which programs (degree or certificate) may meet your identified need.

3. Identify one listserv that you would benefit by being a member. Go through the process of enrolling in the listserv.

Case Study: Global Pandemic

In the year 2020, the world was hit with a pandemic that reached each continent, making significant global impacts. As referenced earlier in this chapter, public health dietitians/nutritionists wear many different hats, and this is certainly relevant in a pandemic. Let's set an example as to how a dietitian can step in to help in a pandemic and also see how you would transform your practices in a situation like this. Brainstorm the different hats of a community and public health dietitian/nutritionist, as evidenced earlier in this chapter. What were the roles of the public health dietitian/nutritionist during an unprecedented pandemic?

Case Study: Program Evaluation

You are the community nutritionist at a local community health center and you have just been awarded a grant to implement a nutrition and physical activity program for overweight youths in your neighborhood. This is an 8-week program for children and their families to learn about healthy eating and physical activity. The program is part of a pilot study for the rest of the city to determine whether it is worth investing in at all of the community health centers throughout the city.

Part A: List all the "hats" you will wear as the coordinator in the implementation, execution, and evaluation of this program.

Part B: Your program has come to an end and you have determined that it was successful. How can you use some of the tools that were discussed in the *Importance of Professional Development* section to promote this program and share your results?

Online Resources

1. View the variety of available DPGs at http://www.eatright.org.
2. Selection of Online Newsletters and Listservs
   a. Agency for Healthcare Research and Quality: http://www.ahrq.gov/
   b. The Academy of Nutrition and Dietetics: For members only, http://www.eatright.org/
   c. The Centers for Disease Control and Prevention: Includes the Morbidity and Mortality Weekly Report and National Health and Nutrition Examination Survey, https://www.cdc.gov
   d. International Food Policy Research Institute: http://www.ifpri.org
   e. National Institutes of Health: http://list.nih.gov
   f. U.S. Department of Health and Human Services: http://www.usda.gov
   g. U.S. Food & Drug Administration: http://www.fda.gov
   h. World Health Organization Weekly Epidemiological Record: http://www.who.int/wer/en/
3. Calendars of Events
   a. AND: http://www.eatrightpro.org/resources/news-center/member-updates/events-and-deadlines
   b. APHA: http://www.apha.org/events-and-meetings/apha-calendar
4. Listing of accredited Public Health Schools and Programs: http://ceph.org/
5. Listing of graduate programs in nutrition: http://www.nutrition.org/education-and-professional-development/graduate-program-directory/

References

1. Committee on Assuring the Health of the Public in the 21st Century. The future of the public's health in the 21st Century. In: *Board on Health Promotion an Disease Prevention*. 2002:366. doi: 10.17226/10548
2. Healthy People 2030. Accessed January 09, 2021. https://health.gov/healthypeople/objectives-and-data/browse-objectives/nutrition-and-healthy-eating
3. The Academy Quality Management Committee. Academy of Nutrition and Dietetics: Revised 2017 Standards of Practice in Nutrition Care and Standards of Professional Performance for Registered Dietitian Nutritionists. *J Acad Nutr Diet*. 2018;118(1):132-140.e15. https://doi.org/10.1016/j.jand.2017.10.003
4. Bruening M, Udarbe AZ, Yakes Jimenez E, Stell Crowley P, Fredericks DC, Edwards Hall, LA. Academy of Nutrition and Dietetics: standards of practice and standards of professional performance for registered dietitian nutritionists (competent, proficient, and expert) in public health and community nutrition. *J Acad Nutr Diet*. 2015;115(10):1699-1709.e39. https://doi.org/10.1016/j.jand.2015.06.374
5. Council on Education for Public Health (CEPH) History. Accessed December 12, 2020. https://ceph.org/about/org-info/
6. Public Health Foundation. Core competencies for public health professionals. Accessed October 7, 2021. phf.org/corecompetencies
7. Academy of Nutrition and Dietetics. Eat Right Pro. Dietetic Practice Groups. http://www.eatrightpro.org/resources/membership/academy-groups/dietetic-practice-groups
8. American Public Health Association. Member Sections. Accessed May 12, 2021. https://www.apha.org/apha-communities/member-sections/
9. Academy of Nutrition and Dietetics. Eat Right Pro. Advocacy. Accessed August 12, 2021. http://www.eatrightpro.org/resources/advocacy/action-center
10. Academy of Nutrition and Dietetics. Advocacy. *EatrightPro*. 2015. Accessed August 12, 2020. http://www.eatrightpro.org/resources/advocacy
11. Institute of Medicine. *Primary Care and Public Health: Exploring Integration to Improve Population Health*. Washington, DC: The National Academic Press; 2012. doi: 10.17226/13381
12. University of Pittsburgh. The Center for Bioethics and Health Law (CBHL): About. Accessed December 12, 2015. http://www.bioethics.pitt.edu/about/

Glossary

Activities of daily living (ADLs) Activities such as bathing, dressing, grooming, transferring from bed or chair, going to the bathroom (toileting), and feeding oneself.

Advocacy The act of supporting or promoting a particular cause or policy.

Affordable Care Act (ACA) The Affordable Care Act refers to two separate pieces of legislation—the Patient Protection and Affordable Care Act (P.L. 111–148) and the Health Care and Education Reconciliation Act of 2010 (P.L. 111–152). Its goal is to provide Americans with better health security by putting in place comprehensive health insurance reforms to expand coverage, hold insurance companies' accountable, lower healthcare costs, guarantee more choice, and enhance the quality of care for all Americans.

Aging-in-place A concept that describes how a growing number of aging adults prefer to grow old at home.

Agroterrorism The deliberate introduction of a disease agent, either against livestock or into the food chain, for purposes of undermining the socioeconomic stability and/or generating fear.

Alliance A merging of efforts or interests from representatives of different organizations with similar goals.

Annotated budget A budget with critical or explanatory notes.

Autocratic A leadership style that does not encourage employee input. The manager makes all decisions. Employees are expected to obey management decisions without asking any questions.

Baby boomers One-third of the U.S. population is composed of baby boomers, defined as older adults born between 1946 and 1964.

Biologic toxin The toxic material of plants, animals, microorganisms, viruses, fungi, or infectious substances of a recombinant molecule, whatever its origin or method of production, including (1) any poisonous substance or biological product engineered as a result of biotechnology produced by a living organism; or (2) any poisonous isomer of biologic products, homolog, or derivative of such a substance.

Blood lipid profile A group of blood tests often ordered to determine risk of coronary heart disease. The lipid profile includes total cholesterol, high-density lipoproteins (HDLs), low-density lipoproteins (LDLs), and triglycerides.

Body mass index (BMI) = mass (kg) mass (lb) (height (m))^2 or (height (in))^2 × 703.

Carriers Infected humans who can transmit contagious diseases to other humans.

Causality The ability of a variable in a study to be so strongly linked to the result that it can be determined that the variable caused the result. This can only be determined in a randomized, controlled type of study with all other types falling into a hierarchy.

Caveat emptor The principle in commerce that the buyer alone is responsible for assessing the quality of a purchase before buying.

CDC bioterrorism agents/diseases *Category A:* Can be easily disseminated or transmitted from person to person, result in high mortality rates, and have the potential for major public health impact, might cause public panic and social disruption, require special action for public health preparedness; *Category B:* Are moderately easy to disseminate, result in moderate and low mortality rates, require specific enhancements of the CDC's diagnostic capacity and enhanced disease surveillance; *Category C:* Emerging pathogens that could be engineered for mass dissemination in the future because of availability, ease of production and dissemination, and potential for high morbidity and mortality rates and major health impact.

Center for Nutrition Policy and Promotion United States Department of Agriculture (USDA) center where scientific research is linked with the nutritional needs of the American public. Projects include, but are not limited to, the Dietary Guidelines of Americans, MyPlate, MyWins, SuperTracker, the Healthy Eating Index, the USDA Food Patterns, and the USDA Food Plans: Cost of Food.

Chronic care model (CCM) An organizing framework for improving chronic illness care at both the individual and population levels, typically has six parts: self-management support; a well-designed healthcare delivery system; assistance with healthcare decision making; good clinical information (documentation) systems; organized healthcare; and supportive community stakeholders.

Chronic disease management Refers to the oversight of treatments, therapies, and education activities conducted by healthcare professionals to help patients with chronic disease and health conditions live with their illness and maintain motivation to manage their illness.

Chronic diseases Also known as noncommunicable diseases; they are not passed from person to person. They are of long duration and generally slow progression. The four main types of chronic diseases are cardiovascular, cancers, chronic respiratory diseases, and diabetes.

Coalition A formal, structured group that forms for a specific purpose or cause; an alliance, sometimes temporary, of people, factions, or parties.

Cohort study Study design in which populations (called cohorts) are followed prospectively or retrospectively with status evaluations with related to a disease or other outcome to determine which risk factors are associated with that outcome.

Community food security The state in which all persons obtain a nutritionally adequate, culturally acceptable diet at all times through local nonemergency sources.

Community-based participatory research An applied collaborative approach that allows residents of the community to be active participants and collaborators in research aimed at improving the health of their own community.

Community-oriented primary care (COPC) A system of identifying and addressing the health problems of a defined population using the resources of the community and the input of health professionals and community members; the health professionals and community members "treat" the community similarly to how patients are treated individually by physicians.

Community Any grouping of individuals who have a shared sense of identity or a common thread that draws all members together.

Comprehensive Primary Care Initiative (CPCI) A 4-year (2012–2016), multi-payer initiative through the Centers for Medicare and Medicaid Services (CMS) with a defined payment model to help redesign practice, support improved care, provide better health for populations, and lower health costs through improvement.

Confounder A variable associated with both the exposure and the outcome that skews the results of the study.

Congregate meals Meals provided in group settings.

Consequence management Includes measures to protect public health and safety; restore essential government services; and provide emergency relief to governments, businesses, and individuals affected by the consequences of terrorism. A consequence management response will be managed by FEMA using structures and resources of the Federal Response Plan (FRP).

Consortium Large groups of organizations, formed to undertake enterprises beyond the resources of any one member.

Consumer sovereignty Alludes to the power consumers have in directing market economies because goods and services are produced and exchanged mostly to satisfy consumer desires.

Consumer-based model Projects based on consumer inputs and designed with consumers in mind.

Contingency theory The belief that performance is a result of interaction between two factors: leadership style and situational favorableness.

Cooperative Extension Service A research-based program that provides outreach services and education to consumers.

Cost-effectiveness evaluation Determines if outcomes could be achieved at a lower cost and deals specifically with cost benefit.

Crisis management Crisis management is predominantly a law enforcement function and includes measures to identify, acquire, and plan the use of resources needed to anticipate, prevent, and/or resolve a threat or act of terrorism.

Cross-sectional study Observational study that involves collection and analysis of data from a population at one point in time. The National Health and Nutrition Examination Survey is an example of a cross-sectional study. These studies are used to generate hypotheses, not to test them.

Debarment Authorizes the FDA to debar (prohibit from importing food) persons who have been convicted of a felony relating to the importation of any food or who have engaged in a pattern of importing adulterated food that presents a threat of serious adverse health consequences or death to humans or animals.

Democratic This style is also called participative, because it encourages employee participation in decision making. The manager checks with the employees before making a decision and can act as a coach or problem-solver for the group.

Developmental origins of health and disease A field of inquiry that aims to identify, quantify, and evaluate strategies to modify prenatal and perinatal determinants of adverse adult health outcomes.

Dietary Guidelines for Americans (DGA) Evidence-based recommendations for food (and some nutrient intake) designed to promote health and reduce the risk of chronic disease for healthy Americans 2 years of age and older. They are the foundation of federal nutrition policy, nutrition education programs, and information activities.

Dietary Guidelines for Americans Guidelines provided by the Department of Health and Human Services and the United States Department of Agriculture every 5 years on the various nutrients found in foods and their recommended daily allowances, which will ensure a nutritionally balanced dietary intake to promote health and prevent occurrence of disease.

Dietary Reference Intakes (DRI) A system of nutrition recommendations from the Institute of Medicine's Food and Nutrition Board (now the Health and Medicine Division of the National Academies of Sciences, Engineering, and Medicine). Introduced in 1997, the DRIs were developed to broaden the Recommended Dietary Allowances.

Disaster field office (DFO) An office established in or near the designated area to support federal and state response and recovery operations. The disaster field office houses the federal coordinating officer (FCO), the emergency response team, and, where possible, the state coordinating officer and support staff.

Ecological model Projects based on explaining health-related behaviors and environments.

Emergency Operations Center (EOC) Site from which civil government officials (municipal, county, state, and federal) exercise direction and control in an emergency.

Emergency public information Information that is primarily disseminated in anticipation of an emergency or at the actual time of an emergency; in addition to providing information, it frequently directs actions, instructs, and transmits direct orders.

Emergency response team A team composed of federal program and support personnel, which FEMA activates and deploys into an area affected by a major disaster or emergency.

Emergency support function A functional area of response activity established to facilitate coordinated federal delivery of assistance required during the response phase to save lives, protect property and health, and maintain public safety.

Environmental justice Ensuring that all population groups are considered equally when decisions are made that affect the environment. For example, dump sites are often located in low-income or minority communities.

Epidemiology Assesses the occurrence of a disease within a set population. This field also looks at the factors that prevent and hasten the disease's development.

Evacuation Organized, phased, and supervised dispersal of civilians from dangerous or potentially dangerous areas, and their reception and care in safe areas.

Evidence-based practice Utilizing nutritional information that is based on scientific studies from reputable sources.

Evidence-based Analysis based on scientific proof.

Facebook An online social networking service.

Federal coordinating officer (FCO) Person appointed by the FEMA director, following a declaration of a major disaster or of an emergency by the president, to coordinate federal assistance.

Federal policy Policies made by the government of, relating to, or denoting the central government of the United States.

Federal Response Plan (FRP) Plan designed to address the consequences of any disaster or emergency situation in which there is a need for federal assistance.

Federally qualified health centers (FQHCs) Reimbursement designation significant for several health programs funded (by Bureau of Primary Healthcare and CMS) under the Health Center Consolidation Act (Section 330 of the Public Health Service Act), including community health centers, Migrant Health Program, Public Housing Primary Care Program, and Healthcare for the Homeless Program. FQHCs provide comprehensive primary care services.

Fetal alcohol syndrome (FAS) Mental and physical deficits caused by alcohol intake of the mother, primarily during the first trimester.

Fidelity Assurance that a project or program is implemented or delivered as planned or as designed.

First responder Local police, fire, and emergency medical personnel who first arrive on the scene of an incident and take action to save lives, protect property, and meet basic human needs.

Food away from home Meals and snacks eaten outside of the home, which comprise 40 to 50% of weekly meals and snacks for the average American. These foods tend to be higher in calories and fat, lower in fiber, and larger in portion sizes; consumption of food away from home has been associated with obesity.

Food insecurity A term used to convey the idea that the availability of nutritionally adequate and safe foods or the ability to acquire acceptable foods in socially acceptable ways is limited or uncertain.

Food insufficiency An inadequate amount of food intake due to a lack of resources.

Food security Access by all people, at all times to sufficient food for an active and healthy life . . . [and] includes at a minimum: the ready availability of nutritionally adequate and safe foods, and an assured ability to acquire acceptable foods in socially acceptable ways.

Formative evaluation Assesses whether a problem is occurring in a program, the extent of the problem, and if corrective action is necessary.

Fresh Fruit and Vegetable Program Originally created in 2002 through the Farm Bill, this program provides a fresh fruit or vegetable snack to all students in participating schools. The program goals include increasing the variety of fruits and vegetables children consume, creating healthier school food environments, and positively influencing the nutrition of students and their families.

Galactosemia Digestive problem resulting from absence of the enzyme that breaks down galactose.

Goal Desired result that an entity hopes to achieve.

Good Manufacturing Practices The U.S. Food & Drug Administration (FDA) adopted stringent regulations that require manufacturers of dietary supplements to use quality and purity testing.

Group visits or shared medical appointments (SMA) An innovative and often cost-effective method in which patients with common needs are brought together in a group setting with one or more healthcare providers to offer education and peer-to-peer support.

Guidelines Information intended to advise people on how something should be done or what something should be.

Guillain-Barré syndrome An inflammatory disorder of the peripheral nerves that is characterized by the rapid onset of weakness and, often, paralysis of the legs, arms, breathing muscles, and face.

Health Care for the Homeless (HCH) program HRSA grantee program that recognizes the unique needs of homeless persons, focusing on provision of coordinated and comprehensive healthcare; often includes substance abuse and mental health services.

Health disparities Refers to the inequalities that occur in the provision of health care and access to healthcare across different racial, ethnic, and socioeconomic groups.

Health maintenance organization (HMO) An organization that provides or arranges managed care for health insurance and acts as a liaison to healthcare providers (hospitals, doctors, etc.) on a prepaid basis; these providers have been paid by the HMO and are ensured consistent patients.

Health promotion Refers to activities that help individuals to improve their health via behavior modification as well as appropriate environmental interventions to reduce risky unhealthy behaviors associated with disease.

Health and nutrition educator An education specialist who designs, implements, and assesses health and nutrition educational activities for individuals and communities.

Health-related quality of life A scientific concept that describes a person's perception of their health, well-being, and ability to function.

Healthcare quality The measured value of providing healthcare services. In health care, quality could be related to improved quality of life, effectiveness of treatments, or decreased mortality.

Healthy Eating Index (HEI) Developed to provide a single measure to assess diet quality through adherence to the Dietary Guidelines for Americans for the U.S. population and the low-income subpopulation.

Healthy People 2030 A comprehensive health promotion and disease prevention agenda for the nation established by the Department of Health and Human Services.

Healthy People (HP) 2030 An initiative involving collaboration between the U.S. Department of Health and Human Services, other federal agencies, and public stakeholders with a vision to facilitate long and healthy lives for all people.

Healthy, Hunger-Free Kids Act of 2010 Now part of the Child Nutrition and WIC Reauthorization Act, the 2015 reauthorization requires all school districts to adopt wellness policies and increases funding available for fresh, healthy school food.

Hertzberg's two-factor theory A theory regarding motivation, also called the two-factor theory. Work characteristics causing dissatisfaction (i.e., work conditions, pay, and interpersonal relationships) are quite different from those causing satisfaction (i.e., achievement, recognition, and opportunity for growth).

Hierarchy of evidence Reflects the relative weight of different types of studies when making decisions about evidence-based practice or clinical interventions. There is no single accepted version of the hierarchy of evidence, but there is general agreement that systematic reviews and meta-analyses rank the highest, followed by randomized controlled trials, cohort studies, and expert opinions; anecdotal experience ranks at the bottom.

Hierarchy The ability of a type of study to determine causality based on the strengths and weaknesses of its inert design.

High-risk factor A greater-than-usual likelihood that a negative outcome may be caused or will happen.

Homelessness Condition of people without a regular dwelling; often unable to acquire and maintain regular, safe, secure, and adequate housing or a lack of "fixed, regular, and adequate night-time residence"; may reside during the night in a public or private facility or in transitional housing.

Hunger The uneasy or painful sensation caused by a lack of food. The recurrent and involuntary lack of access to food . . . [which] may produce malnutrition over time.

Impact evaluation Assesses whether interventions are producing desired outcomes.

Incidence The development of new cases of a disease over a period of time.

Incrementalism Policy-making in small steps rather than with large comprehensive reforms.

Incubation period Time between exposure and appearance of symptoms of a disease, syndrome, or illness.

Indemnity insurance Also known as "fee-for-service" insurance; indemnity plans allow freedom in choosing healthcare providers, and the insurance company establishes a set dollar amount for the services they will cover.

Indian Health Service (IHS) An agency within the Department of Health and Human Services responsible for providing federal health services to American Indians and Alaskan Natives; IHS is the primary federal healthcare provider and health advocate for Indian people, and they seek for these individuals to have optimal health status.

Institutional Review Board (IRB) Also known as an independent ethics committee, ethical review board, or research ethics board, an IRB is a committee that has been formally designated to approve, monitor, and review biomedical and behavioral research involving humans.

Instrumental activities of daily living Activities such as food preparation, use of telephone, housekeeping, laundry, use of transportation, responsibility for medication, managing money, and shopping.

Integrated marketing communications Integrates all the elements of the promotional mix-sales, marketing, public relations, advertising, and publicity to coalesce in a unified customer-focused message as a way to achieve an organization's objectives.

Key informants People who provide information about events.

Laissez-faire A leadership style also known as the "hands-off" style. The manager provides little or no direction and gives employees as much freedom as possible. All authority or power is given to the employees, and they must determine goals, make decisions, and resolve problems on their own.

Lead agency The federal department- or agency-assigned lead responsibility under U.S. law to manage and coordinate the federal response in a specific functional area.

Let's Move! Campaign Program developed by First Lady Michelle Obama to address the childhood obesity epidemic; components include educating parents on healthy eating; increasing physical activity among youth; increasing available healthy food options in schools; and ensuring that families have access to healthy and affordable food.

Life course approach Study of long-term effects on chronic disease risk of physical and social exposures during gestation, childhood, adolescence, young adulthood, and later adult life.

LinkedIn An online professional networking service.

Listserv An application that distributes messages to subscribers on an electronic mailing list.

Literacy Ability to read and write; have competence or knowledge in a specific area.

Local government Any county, city, village, town, district, or political subdivision of any state, Indian tribe or authorized tribal organization, or Alaska Native village or organization, including any rural community or unincorporated town or village or any other public entity.

Logic model Framework for building a common language for accountability and evaluation across the organization.

Longitudinal studies Follow a cohort of individuals over time, performing repeated measurements at prescribed intervals.

Low-density lipoproteins (LDLs) Protein molecules that carry cholesterol in the blood and around the body for use by various cells.

Majority-minority community Town or city in which the majority of citizens come from a racial or ethnic minority.

Maslow's hierarchy of needs theory The needs of an individual exist in a logical order (physiological, safety, belonging, esteem, and self-actualization); the basic root needs must be satisfied first.

McClelland's motivation theory An individual's motivation and effectiveness in certain job functions are influenced by three needs: achievement, affiliation, and power.

McGregor's X theory Managers believe that workers are motivated by only one thing: money. They are selfish, lazy, and hate work. The manager believes that workers need to be closely controlled and directed.

McGregor's Y theory Managers believe that workers are motivated by many different factors apart from money. They enjoy their work. The manager believes that employees will happily take on responsibility and make decisions for the business.

Medicaid U.S. government program that pays for medical assistance for certain individuals and families with low incomes. Learn more at http://www.cms.gov/medicaid.

Medical nutrition therapy (MNT) A therapeutic approach to treating medical conditions and their associated symptoms that may involve changes to diet or nutrition support and is typically administered by a Registered dietitian/nutritionist (RDN) or a physician.

Medically underserved areas/populations Areas or populations designated by the U.S. Health Resources Service Administration (HRSA) as having too few primary care providers, high infant mortality, high poverty, or a high elderly population. Often associated with Health Professional Shortage Areas (HPSAs) or areas/facilities where there are shortages of primary medical care and dental or mental health providers.

Medicare U.S. government medical benefit program for certain individuals when they reach age 65. Learn more at http://www.medicare.gov.

Migrant Health Program (MHP) Provides support to health centers so that they can provide appropriate and comprehensive preventative and primary healthcare to migratory and seasonal agriculture workers and their families; focuses on the occupational health and safety needs of this population.

Mini Nutritional Assessment (MNA) A validated nutrition screening and assessment tool that can identify geriatric patients age 65 and above who are malnourished or at risk of malnutrition.

Motivational interviewing (MI) A directive, client-centered counseling style for eliciting behavior change by helping clients to explore and resolve ambivalence. Compared with nondirective counseling, it is more focused and goal directed. Motivation to change is elicited from the client and not imposed by the counselor.

MyPlate, MyWins The "visual translation" of the Dietary Guidelines for Americans for the public.

National Health and Nutrition Examination Survey (NHANES) A program of studies designed to assess the health and nutritional status of adults and children in the United States. The survey is unique in that it combines interviews and physical examinations.

National Nutrition Monitoring and Related Research Program (NNMRRP) Established in 1990 (PL 101–445), this is a comprehensive, coordinated program for nutrition monitoring and related research to improve health and nutrition assessment in U.S. populations.

Neophobia Reluctance to try new foods.

Network A group of people who form relationships to share ideas, information, and resources.

Nutrition education Provision of knowledge of foods as it relates to their nutritive content and their relationship to maintaining good health and preventing the occurrence of chronic diseases. The acceptance and voluntary inclusion of this knowledge into dietary behavior is an integral component of effective nutrition education.

Nutrition/health assessment In-depth evaluation of objective and subjective data related to an individual's nutrition and health status, including all biological, environmental, social and nutrition factors to identify the specific needs of a person and determining how those needs will be addressed.

Nutrition monitoring Collecting nutrition and health-related information from a population is critical for designing and evaluating policies and programs that improve health status and decrease risk factors.

Nutrition policy A set of concerted actions, based on a governmental mandate, intended to ensure good health in the population through informed access to safe, healthy, and adequate food.

Nutrition programs Initiatives with the role of fostering behavior change toward food and nutrition and supporting caring practices.

Nutrition-focused Physical Exam A physical exam used to accurately identify and grade malnutrition by identifying fat loss, muscle loss, and/or edematous conditions associated with or affecting nutrition status.

Nutritional epidemiology Utilizes the processes of epidemiology to look at the influence of dietary factors on a disease or health condition in the population.

Nutrition security The provision of an environment that encourages and motivates society to make food choices consistent with short- and long-term good health.

Obesity In adults aged 20 years and older, a body mass index (BMI) greater than or equal to 30 kg/m².

Obesigenic An environment that encourages obesity through features such as unlimited quantities of a variety of foods high in caloric density together with minimal energy expenditure.

Opinion leaders Those who are experts in a given field and communicate their findings.

Overweight In adults aged 20 years and older, a body mass index (BMI) ≥25 kg/m² but <30 kg/m².

Patient-centered care The provision of health care that is respectful of and responsive to individual patient preferences, needs, and values; the patient has a significant role in determining their course of care.

Patient-centered medical home (PCMH) A model or philosophy of organizing primary care into a multidisciplinary, team-based approach to allow for better communication and coordination of care; focused on meeting the needs of the patient "right where they are"; significant emphasis on quality and safety.

Peer-reviewed literature Articles that have been subjected to scholarly review by experts in the field and revision by the author to address any comments or concerns of these scholars prior to publication in a scientific journal or textbook.

Perishable food Food that is not heat-treated, frozen, or otherwise preserved in a manner so as to prevent the quality of the food from being adversely affected if held longer than 7 days under normal shipping and storage conditions.

Point-of-service (POS) A managed healthcare insurance plan that offers lower healthcare costs but limited options.

Population-based medicine Assessing the healthcare needs of a specific population (groups of individuals who have one or more personal or environmental traits in common) and making healthcare decisions for the population as a whole rather than for individuals.

Population All of the inhabitants of a given region (e.g., the U.S. population, or the population of California).

Prebiotics Substances that induce the growth or activity of microorganisms (e.g., bacteria and fungi) that contribute to the well-being of their host.

Preeclampsia A hypertensive disorder of pregnancy characterized by the presence of protein in the urine and swelling, putting both mother and infant in danger.

Preferred provider organizations (PPO) A type of health plan that contracts with medical providers, such as hospitals and doctors, to create a network of participating providers. The insured pays less to use providers that belong to the plan's network.

Prevalence (prevalence proportion) The proportion of people in a population who have a disease.

Prevalence Indicates how many individuals within a population have a disease or health condition at one moment in time.

Prevention Those interventions that occur before the initial onset of disorder.

Probiotics A preparation (such as a dietary supplement) containing live bacteria that is taken orally to restore beneficial bacteria to the body.

Process evaluation Assesses the effectiveness of administrative activities and program implementation.

Project planning team The project team includes the manager and the group of individuals who work together on a project to achieve its objectives.

Public health nutritionist An expert in food and nutrition who applies this expertise to nutrition research, practice, and policy to improve the health of populations.

Public Housing Primary Care (PHPC) program Provides residents of public housing with increased access to comprehensive primary healthcare services; services are provided at public housing developments or at other locations immediately accessible to residents.

Public policy Rule, guideline, or practice established by an elected or appointed authority, administration, or management. Policy interventions targeting communities and organizations have a much greater potential impact or reach than individual or interpersonal/groups interventions.

PubMed The premiere database for peer-reviewed articles on nutrition and medicine. Many citations in PubMed include links to full-text articles from PubMed Central or publisher websites.

Qualitative data/research Any method of data collecting that generates narrative data or words rather than numerical data or numbers. The words must reflect the study participant's perspective. The Internet has provided a platform for community development when you search for shared characteristics of the community.

Quantitative data/research Hypothesis-testing research that gathers numerical data or data that can be quantified.

Randomized controlled trials A type of scientific study design in which the individuals being studied are randomly assigned to different treatments under study. The most rigorous of these trials is a double-blind, placebo-controlled trial in which neither the investigator nor the study participant knows the treatment type. Results from these studies provide strong evidence in the hierarchy of evidence. This study design allows for testing of hypotheses.

Recall bias Inaccurate reporting by a study participant that leads to less accurate study results.

Recovery As defined here, includes all types of emergency actions dedicated to the continued protection of the public or to promoting the resumption of normal activities in the affected area.

Registered dietitian/nutritionist A food and nutrition expert who has met academic and professional requirements set forth by the Commission on Dietetic Registration to earn the credential of Registered Dietitian/ Registered Dietitian Nutritionist.

Reiter syndrome A peripheral arthritis lasting longer than 1 month.

Reliability The extent to which, when tested, the same result will occur consistently.

Requests for Proposals (RFPs) Invitations to suppliers to bid on supplying products or services that are difficult to describe for a company, or in this example, a public agency.

Response Those activities and programs designed to address the immediate and short-term effects of the onset of an emergency or disaster.

Retrospective studies These studies examine events that have occurred in the past or they represent attribute variables that cannot be manipulated; therefore, the researcher does not have direct control of the variables under study.

Risk factors Specific characteristics associated with an increased chance of developing a chronic disease.

Socialecological model An approach in which interventions not only address individual intentions and skills but also the social and physical environmental context of a desired behavior, considering as well all social networks and organizations that share that environment, which will have the most potential for population-wide impact.

Social media Websites and applications that enable users to create and share content or to participate in social networking.

Social networking The use of dedicated websites and applications to interact with other users, or to find people with similar interests to oneself.

Stakeholder An entity that has an interest in something.

Strategies An evidence-based method or plan of action designed to achieve a particular goal.

Summative evaluation Focuses on program impact and program effectiveness.

Supercentenarians The classification of the older adult population over the age of 110.

Surveillance The continuous, systematic collection of data, as well as its timely interpretation regarding the current and changing condition of a population.

Syndromic surveillance Surveillance activities that enable early detection of epidemics with data analysis for patterns of prodromal illnesses including the use of medications, illness syndromes, or events.

Target population The group that is the focus of an assessment, a study, an intervention, or a program.

Telehealth or Telemedicine The use of telecommunication and information technologies to provide clinical care when distance is a barrier; may also be more convenient as the healthcare provider and patient can set up a time to communicate that is flexible for both parties.

Teratogenic Causing birth defects.

Terrorism The unlawful use of force or violence against persons or property to intimidate or coerce a government, the civilian population, or any segment thereof, in furtherance of political or social objectives.

Theory X Managers believe that workers are motivated by only one thing: money. They are selfish, lazy, and hate work. The manager believes that workers need to be closely controlled and directed.

Theory Y Managers believe that workers are motivated by many different factors apart from money. They enjoy their work. The manager believes that employees will happily take on responsibility and make decisions for the business.

Transformational A leadership style that emphasizes creating relationships among staff. The manager instills confidence and promotes staff respect that results in higher productivity, job satisfaction, and improved communication.

Transmissibility Ease with which disease is transmitted by victims. Methods may be direct (personal contact), indirect (through material contaminated by the infected person), or secondary (through particles spread by coughing or sneezing).

Trends Annual rates reported over a period of time, usually in terms of years.

Triangulation The process of using a range of methods and integrating multiple sources of data to gain a more complete picture of relevant health issues, potential solutions, and effective program evaluation.

Triglycerides These store energy, which is housed in fatty tissue and is gradually released between meals to meet the body's needs. High levels of triglycerides in the blood may be associated with coronary artery disease.

Twitter An online social networking service that enables users to send and read short 280-character messages called "tweets."

U.S. Pharmacopeia Dietary Supplement Verification Program A voluntary testing and auditing program that ensures the safe manufacture of dietary supplements providing approval seals on products to signify passage of laboratory tests for potency, purity, and freedom from harmful contaminants.

Underemployment Employment that is insufficient in some important way for the individual, including individuals who are highly skilled but working in low-paying jobs and part-time workers who would prefer to work full-time.

Validity A test designed to measure what it set out to measure.

Vectors Infected animals or insects that serve as hosts to the organism.

Virulence The relative severity of the disease produced by a pathogen.

Vroom's expectancy theory Assumes that behavior results from conscious choices among alternatives whose purpose is to maximize pleasure and minimize pain. The key elements to this theory are referred to as *expectancy*, *instrumentality*, and *valence*.

Worksite interventions Healthy lifestyle programs delivered at the workplace, including health education, cafeteria modifications, dietary consultations performed by registered dietitians, and physical education.

Index

24-hour diet recall, 13, 15, 23, 57, 140
5 As (assess, advise, agree, assist, and arrange), 376
6 Ms of management (manpower, market, machine, method, material, and money), 529

A

Academy of Nutrition and Dietetics (AND), 12, 92, 112, 559
ACE inhibitor, 370
Acquired Immune Deficiency Syndrome (AIDS), 333
additives, 430
adequate intake (AI), 28, 29
Administration on Aging (AoA), 355
Administration on Community Living (ACL), 355
adolescence, 266
adolescent pregnancy, 259
Adult Treatment Panel (ATP), 322
advertising, 234
advertising, food, 278
advertising, truth in, 236
advocacy, 88, 93
Affordable Care Act (ACA), 198, 372, 373, 378
aflatoxin, 447
after-school care, 295
Agency for Healthcare Quality and Research (AHQR), 11, 371
aging-in-place, 349
agricultural chemicals, 453
Agricultural Research Service (ARS) (USDA), 17, 105
agrosystems, 105
Agroterrorism, 456
air quality, 198
alcohol, 257
Alcohol and Tobacco Tax and Trade Bureau (TTB), U.S. Department of, 428
alkaloids, 448
alliance, 570
alternative sweeteners, 450
Alzheimer's disease, 347
American Academy of Pediatrics (AAP), 260
American Association of Retired People (AARP), 92
American Diabetes Association (ADA), 12, 92
American Heart Association (AHA), 273, 374
American Public Health Association (APHA), 92, 559, 575
American Society for Nutrition (ASN), 559
amnesic shelling poisoning (ASP), 448
analogy, 55
analytical-study design, 53
animal studies, 24
annotated budget, 507
anthrax, 461

anthropometric assessment, 137, 138, 317
antidiabetic agents, 370
antioxidants, 450
arthritis, 348
Assessment Protocol for Excellence in Public Health (APEX-PH), 162
Association of State and Territorial Public Health Nutrition Directors (ASTPHND), 131
Association of State Public Health Nutritionists (ASPHN), 558
asymptomatic, 442
at-risk factors, 200
atherosclerosis, 319
ATP III Classification, 322
Atwater, Wilbur O., 114
autocratic, 536
autonomy, 73
Avian Influenza, 437

B

baby boomers, 345
bacteria, 435, 439
Behavioral Anchored Rating Scale (BARS), 531
behavioral health practitioners, 369
Behavioral Risk Factor Surveillance System (BRFSS), 19, 131
Best Bones Forever!, 238
bill, 82, 83
biochemical assessment, 137, 138
biochemical data, 317
bioengineered foods, 455
biological gradient, 55
biological hazards, 434, 435
Bioterrorism, 456
bioterrorism agents, 461
bioterrorism diseases, 461
Bioterrorism Preparedness and Response Act (2002), 464
blockchain, 454
blood pressure, 23
Body Mass Index (BMI), 6, 256, 268, 350
Bogalusa Heart Study (BHS), 21, 51
botulism, 461
bovine spongiform encephalopathy (BSE), 439, 440, 447
brainstorm, 135
breastfeeding, 260, 261, 372
Bright Futures, 293
brucellosis, 462
budget, 504
Bureau of Primary Health Care (BPHC), 379
business marketing, 588

C

calcium, 267, 331, 351
calories, 257
Campylobacter, 434
Campylobacter coli, 439
Campylobacter jejuni, 439, 439
cancer, 5, 6, 307, 325, 347
cardiovascular disease (CVD), 21, 23, 50, 56, 319
case-control, 53
causality, 52
CDC Evaluation Wheel, 176
CDC Organizational Chart, 119
CDCynergy model, 166
Center for Disease Control and Prevention (CDC), 6, 77, 100, 116, 176, 348
Center for Nutrition Policy and Promotion (CNPP), 14, 29, 100, 103
Center for Science in the Public Interest (CSPI), 92
certified dietary manager (CDM), 549
certified dietitian nutritionist (CDN), 548, 549
certified food protection professional (CFFP), 549
certified health education specialist (CHES), 549
certified nutrition specialist (CNS), 549
CHANGE Model, 171
Chemical Composition of American Food Materials, USDA, 114
chemical hazards, 447
Child and Adolescent Trial for Cardiovascular Health (CATCH), 223
Child and Adult Care Food Program (CACFP), 193, 195, 359, 360, 415,
Child Nutrition Programs, 111
childcare programs, 271
childhood, 266
cholera, 463
cholesterol, 7, 321
Chronic Care Model (CCM), 379
chronic disease, 306
chronic kidney disease (CKD), 331
chronic wasting disease (CWD), 439
clean eating, 218
Clean Water and Safe Drinking Water Act, 119
clinical assessment, 139
clinical controlled trial, 54
clinical trials, 24
Clostridium parvum, 463
Clostridium perfringes, 434
Clostridium perfringes, epsilon toxin of, 462
coalition, 91, 570
Coastal Zone Act Reauthorization Amendments (1990), 119
Code of Federal Regulations (CFR), 74
coherence, 55
cohort studies, 12
cohort study, 54
cohort study, prospective, 55

cohort study, retrospective, 54, 55
collaborations, 615
Color Additives Amendment, 429
Color Additives Amendment (1960), 431
colors, 452
Commission on Dietetic Registration (CDR), 613
Commodity Supplemental Food Program (CSFP), 359
community food security, 406
Community Health Assessment and Group Evaluation (CHANGE), 170
community health worker (CHW), 549
community interventions, 230
community-based participatory research, 611
community-oriented primary care, 384
complementary foods, 263
complementary medicine, 349
computer-based model, 166
Concept Paper, 502
Concepts of Operations Plan (CONPLAN), 459, 469
confounding variable, 59
consistency, 55
consortium, 570
consultant, 552
consumer advocacy group, 92
Consumer Expenditure Survey, 17
Consumer Price Index (CPI), 185
consumer-based models, 161
contact tracing, 444
contingency theory, 536
continuing education credit, 557
Continuing Survey of Food Intakes by Individuals (CSFII), 16, 17
Cooperative State Research, Education, and Extension Services (CSREES), 105
coronary artery disease (CAD), 319
Coronavirus Disease 19 (COVID-19), 6, 48, 56, 74, 82, 90, 101, 103, 112, 186, 187, 189, 191, 193, 216, 217, 233, 254, 315, 334, 351, 361, 370, 392, 408, 428, 442, 443, 539,
Coronavirus Pandemic, 33
Cost-Effectiveness Analysis (CEA), 177
cost-effectiveness evaluation, 175
Coxiella burnetiid, 463
Creutzfeldt-Jakob disease (CJD), 446
critical control points (CCPs), 434
cross-sectional studies, 12, 51
cross-sectional study, 53, 55
Cryptosporidium, 436
Cryptosporidium parvum, 446
cultural barriers, 189
cultural competency, 613
Current Population Survey, 409
Customs and Border Protection (CBP), 427
Cyclospora cayetanensis, 436, 446

D

data collection, 147, 590
daycare, 294
Delaney Clause, 431
democratic, 536
dental hygienist, 554
dentist, 554
Department of Health and Human Services (HHS), 16, 114, 220
Department of Homeland Security, U.S. (DHS), 426, 427
Department of Treasury, U.S., 426
descriptive studies, 51
descriptive-study design, 53
Determine Your Nutritional Health, 358
Developmental Origins of Health and Disease (DOHaD), 310
diabetes mellitus, 5, 6, 307, 322, 327, 332, 347, 372
dialysis, 383
Diet and Health Knowledge Survey (DHKS), 18
Dietary Approaches to Stop Hypertension (DASH), 23, 24, 218, 321
dietary assessment, 57, 59, 139
dietary goals, 75
Dietary Guidelines, 118
Dietary Guidelines Advisory Committee (DGAC), 104
Dietary Guidelines for Americans (DGA), 11, 30, 31, 61, 76, 104, 112, 212, 220, 308, 559,
Dietary Guidelines for Disease Prevention, 312
Dietary Reference Intakes (DRI), 11, 25, 28, 29, 331, 375,
Dietary Supplement Health and Education Act, 429
Dietary Supplement Health and Education Act (1994), 431
Diffusion of Innovation Theory, 211
director of nutrition services, 528
disciplinary action, 531
disease management, 377, 378
Division of Diabetes Treatment and Prevention, HIS, 386
doctors of osteopathy (DOs), 368
dysentery, 463

E

E. coli 0157, 436, 439
Early Childhood Longitudinal Studies (ECLS) Program, 409
Eat Less, Move More toolkit, 377
eating disorders, 282
ecological (correlational) study, 53, 55
ecological models, 161
Economic Research Service, USDA (ERS), 105, 110, 129
economics, 288
Economy Food Plan, 185
Elderly Nutrition Program, 352, 355
Elderly Nutrition Program (ENP), 357
Electronic Benefit Transfer (EBT), 101

Emergency Use Authorization (EUA), 446
energy, 266
energy balance, 289
environmental influences, 289
environmental justice, 272
Environmental Protection Agency, U.S. (EPA), 100, 118, 427, 431
EPA Organizational Chart, 120
Epi-pen, 432
Epidemiologic Studies, 21
epidemiology, 48
epinephrine, 432
Escherichia Coli (E. coli), 434, 439
Escherichia Coli (E. coli) 0157:H7, 462
essential businesses, 443
estimated average requirement (EAR), 28, 29
ethics, 199, 601
evaluation, 175, 514
Evidence Analysis Library (EAL), 12
evidence-based, 287
evidence-based practice, 8, 37, 387, 611
Expanded Food and Nutrition Education Program (EFNEP), 113, 415, 559
experiment, 55

F

Facebook, 570
Fair Packaging and Labeling Act, 429
Families First Coronavirus Response Act (FFCRA), 445
Families First Coronavirus Response Bill, 103
family mealtime, 284
Farm Bill (1933), 75
fast foods, 273
fast-food, 348
FDA CFSAN Organizational Chart, 117
FDA Modernization Act, 38
Federal Emergency Management Agency (FEMA), 443, 469
Federal Food, Drug, and Cosmetic Act, 429
Federal Food, Drug, and Cosmetic Act (1938), 430
federal grants, 497, 498
Federal Meat Inspection Act (1906), 428, 429
Federal Poultry Products Inspection Act, 429
Federal Trade Commission Act, 429
Federal Trade Commission (FTC), 426, 427
Federally Qualified Health Center (FQHC), 388
federation, 570
fee for services, 500
fee-for-service, 380
Feeding America, 416
fetal alcohol syndrome, 252, 258
Five Food Groups, 75
flavors, 452
fluoride, 265
focus groups, 144, 212
folic acid, 372

Food Access Research Atlas, 131
food additives, 114, 449
Food Additives Amendment (1958), 429, 430
Food Allergen Labeling and Consumer Protection
        Act (2004), 429, 432
food allergens, 432, 272
food allergies, 272
Food and Agricultural Act (1977), 112
Food and Drug Administration, U.S. (FDA), 37, 100,
        105, 114, 347, 425
Food and Nutrient Database for Dietary Studies
        (FNDDS), 108
Food and Nutrition Assistance Research Reports
        Database, 112
Food and Nutrition Services (FNS), 100
food biosecurity triad, 465, 468
Food Composition Database, USDA, 107
food defense, 433
Food Distribution Program on Indian Reservations, 195
food distribution programs, 416
Food Economics Division (FED), 111
Food Emergency Response Network (FERN), 467
food fads, 217
food fraud, 433
Food Frequency Questionnaires (FFQ), 13, 15, 58, 59, 140
Food Guide Pyramid, 32
food insufficiency, 407
food label, 18, 31, 35
food labeling, 432
food modifications, 273
Food Nutrition and Consumer Services (FNCS), 100
Food Pyramid, 113
Food Quality Protection Act (1996), 429, 431
food records, 57
food safety, 424, 463, 559
Food Safety and Inspection Service, USDA (FSIS), 105, 425
Food Safety Institute, 110
Food Safety Modernization Act, 429
Food Safety Modernization Act (FSMA) (2011), 429, 433
food sanitation codes, 428
food security, 192, 406, 410
food security measurement, 409
food security, high, 410
food security, low, 410
food security, marginal, 410
food security, United States, 411
food security, very low, 410
Food Stamp Act (1969), 112
Food Stamp Program (FSP), 100
Food Surveys Research Group (FSRG), 107
Food, Conservation, and Energy Act (2008), 429, 432
foodborne pathogens, 427
formative evaluation, 175, 597
formula feeding, 262
fortification, 75
foundation grants, 497, 499
Framingham Heart Study (FHS), 22, 50, 51

Fresh Fruit and Vegetable Program, 224
Fuel Up/Lift Off!, 238
fungi, 435

G

galactosemia, 261
Gantt Chart, 173
gastroenteritis, 443
Generally Recognized as Safe (GRAS) food, 430
genetically engineered foods, 455
Genetically Modified Organisms (GMOs), 455
genetics, 328
genotypes, 108
gestational diabetes, 259, 328
Giardia lamblia, 439, 446
Global Branded Food Products Database
        (Branded Foods), 108
glucose metabolism, 328
glycoalkaloids, 448
good food manufacturing practices
        (GMP), 347, 425, 434
government programs, 382
grant proposal, 518
grants, 497
green spaces, 199
grievance, 531
Guide for Effective Nutrition Interventions
        and Education (GENIE), 170
Guide to Strategies to Support Breastfeeding Mothers
        and Babies, CDC, 118
Guillain-Barre syndrome, 439

H

H1N1 virus, 437
H5N1 virus, 437
Hatch Act (1887), 113
Have a Plant campaign, 290
Hazard Analysis and Critical Control Points
        (HACCP) programs, 114, 425, 433, 466
Hazard Analysis Critical Control Point (HACCP), 114
Head Start, 196, 294, 385
Health and Human Services, U.S. Department
        of (HHS), 425, 426
Health and Urban Development, U.S. Department
        of (HUD), 390
Health Belief Model, 212
Health Care for the Homeless, 389
Health Communication Planning Guide, 177
Health Communication Process, 167
health determinants, 315
health disparities, 184, 288, 308, 384
health literacy, 374, 385
health maintenance organization (HMO), 349, 381, 382

Health People (HP) 2030, 11, 25–27, 76, 78, 219, 252–253, 307, 309, 369, 406
Health Professionals Follow-Up Study (HPFS), 51
health promotion, 308
Health Promotion and Prevention Action (HPA) model, 307
Health Resources and Services Administration (HRSA), 387
health risks, 318
healthcare quality, 371
Healthy Eating Index (HEI), 34, 104
Healthy Eating Plate, 334
Healthy, Hunger-Free Kids Act of 2010 (HHFKA), 224, 275
heart disease, 6, 347
hepatitis A, 443
Herzberg's two-factor theory, 536, 537
hierarchy, 51
hierarchy of evidence, 12
high blood pressure, 372
Hispanic Health and Nutrition Examination Survey (HHANES), 17
HIV/AIDS, 348, 387
holistic approach, 308
Homeland Security Act, 429
homelessness, 190, 191, 391
homeopathic, 349, 352
HootSuite, 582
Household Food Security Survey Model, 408
Human Nutrition Information Service (HNIS) (USDA), 17
human subjects, 516
hunger, 192
hypertension, 5, 319, 321, 332

I

impact evaluation, 175
incidence, 52, 56
indemnity insurance, 377, 380
Indian Health Care Improvement Act (1976), 385
Indian Health Service (IHS), 384
Industrial Internet of Things (IIoT), 455
infancy, 260
infancy, nutritional assessment, 265
Infant Feeding Practices Survey, 18
Infant Formula Act, 429
infant growth and development, 263
influenza, 347
Instagram, 570
Institute of Food Technologists (IFT), 558
Institute of Medicine (IOM), 7, 28, 78
Institutional Review Board (IRB), 516
integrative medicine, 349
International Convention for the Prevention of Pollution from Ships, 119

International Micronutrient Malnutrition Prevention and Control (IMMPaCt), 118
Internet, 240, 361
Intervention Mapping, 170
iron, childhood and adolescence, 267
iron, infancy, 265

J

job description, 535

K

key informant, 146
kidney disease, 6
kidney failure, 347
Knowledge-Attitude-Behavior Model (KAB), 212

L

laboratory assessment, 137, 138
laissez-faire, 536
Land-Grant College Systems, 113
law, 83
lead exposure, 271
leadership, 613
leading health indicators (LHIs), 369
legislation, 81, 86, 89
legislative authorization, 113
licensed dietician nutritionist (LDN), 548, 549
Limey, 50
LinkedIn, 570
lipid-lowering drugs, 370
Listeria, 436, 439
listserv, 570
literacy, 188
lobbying, 90, 91
Logic Model, Simplified, 162
Logic Models, 161
London Dumping Convention, 119
longitudinal studies, 259
low-density lipoprotein (LDL), 321
low-FODMAP diet, 218
Low-Rent Housing Act (1937), 390

M

mad-cow disease, 447
managed care, 381
MAP-IT Model (Mobilize, Access, Plan, Implement, Track), 169
MAPP Model, 169
Marine Plastics Pollution Research and Control Act, 119
Marine Protection, Research and Sanctuaries Act, 119

market segmentation, 592
marketing, 235
marketing ethics, 601
marketing mix, 589
marketing research, 589
Maslow's theory, 536
master certified health education specialist (MCHES), 549
Maternal Infant and Child Health (MICH), 252
McClelland's theory, 537
McGregor's X and Y theories, 536
Meals on Wheels, 356, 416
media, 221, 581
Medicaid, 103, 198, 360, 391
medical (licensed) social workers (MSWs/LMSWs), 368
medical doctors (MDs), 368
medical nutrition therapy (MNT), 310, 359, 382
Medically Underserved Area (MUA), 389
Medically Underserved Population (MUP), 389
Medicare, 198, 361, 370, 382
Medicare+Choice plan (M+C), 383
MEDLINE, 9
metabolic diet studies, 23
micronutrients, 267
mid-arm circumference, 350
Migrant Health Center, 389
Migrant Health Program (MHP), 390
milk-processing plant, 428
minerals, 267
Mini Nutritional Assessment (MNA), 349
Minority-Serving Institutions (MSIs), 109
Mobilizing for Action Through Planning & Partnerships (MAPP), 168
molds, 447
mortality rates, 307
motivational interviewing, 231
Multilevel Approach to Community Health (MATCH), 165
multivitamin supplements, 351
mycotoxins, 447
MyPlate, 15, 25, 30–33, 85, 104, 113, 308, 334

N

National Academy of Medicine, 7, 368
National Academy of Science (NAS), 92
National Agricultural Library (NAL), 106
National Agricultural Statistics Service (NASS), 105
National Ambulatory Medical Care Survey (NAMCS), 369
National Cancer Institute (NCI), 14
National Cancer Institute (NCI) Dietary Assessment Primer, 15
National Center for Health Statistics (NCHS), 16, 27, 129, 131, 306
National Cholesterol Education Program, 322
National Emergencies Act (NEA), 442

national emergency, 442
National Health and Nutrition Examination Survey (NHANES), 6, 14, 16–17, 19–20, 131, 210, 217, 287, 409
National Health and Nutrition Examination Survey (NHANES) I, 17
National Health and Nutrition Examination Survey (NHANES) II, 17
National Health and Nutrition Examination Survey (NHANES) III, 17
National Health Care for the Homeless Council (NHCHC), 393
National Heart, Lung, and Blood Institute (NHLBI), 12, 13, 223
National Initiative for Children's Healthcare Quality (NICHQ), 375
National Institute of Food and Agriculture (NIFA), 105, 109
National Institutes of Health (NIH), 371
National Kidney Disease Education Program (NKDEP), 332
National Nutrient Data Bank, 18
National Nutrition Monitoring and Related Research Program (NNMRRP), 16
National Oceanic and Atmospheric Administration (NOAA), 427
National Resource Center on Nutrition and Aging (NRCNA), 356
National School Lunch Program, 75, 101, 111, 193–194, 416
National Shellfish Sanitation Program (NSSP), 448
National Vital Statistics System, CDC, 159
Nationwide Food Consumption Survey (NFCS), 17
needs assessment, 128–129, 133, 148, 150, 160, 508
network, 570
networking, 574
niacin, 5
NIH Consensus Statement on Osteoporosis, 331
Norovirus, 434
nurse practitioners (NPs), 368
Nurses Health Study (NHS), 50–51
Nurses Health Study (NHS) II, 61
nutrient intake, 257
nutrigenomics, 8
nutrition, 290, 315, 350
nutrition advocate, 612
nutrition assessment, 13
Nutrition Assistance Program: Puerto Rico, American Samoa, and the Commonwealth of the Northern Marianas Islands, 196
nutrition counseling, 370
Nutrition Education and Training Program (NET), 113
Nutrition Education for Practicing Physicians (NEPP), 374
Nutrition Education Programs, USDA, 113
Nutrition Evidence Systematic Review (NESR), 12, 104

Nutrition Facts Label, 36–37, 85, 118
Nutrition in Medicine (NIM), 374
Nutrition Labeling and Education Act (1990), 35, 431
nutrition monitoring, 12, 515
nutrition policy, 74, 76, 80
nutrition program, 306
Nutrition Program for the Elderly, 196
nutrition screening, 13
nutrition surveillance, 515
Nutrition-Focused Physical Exam, 350
nutritional additives, 452
nutritional assessment, 270
nutritional assessment, adolescence, 281
nutritional assessment, school-aged children, 274
Nutritional Education and Labeling Act, 429
nutritional epidemiology, 48–49, 60–61
nutritionist, 547

O

obesity, 6, 130, 210, 315, 348, 372
Obesity Intervention Plan, USDA, 114
occupational therapist, 554
Ocean Dumping Ban Act, 119
Office of Water, EPA, 118
Offspring Study, 23
older adults, 345
Older Americans Act (OAA), 352
Older Americans Act Nutrition Services Program, 30
Older Americans Nutrition Program, 359
Organic Foods Production Act, 429
osteopathic physicians, 368
osteoporosis, 330, 372
out-of-pocket, 377
outcome evaluation, 597
overweight, 210, 289, 293
overweight children, 283, 286

P

P Process Model, 167
pandemic, 442
Panel Study of Income Dynamics, 409
paralytic shellfish poisoning (PSP), 448
Partnership for a Healthier America (PHA), 386
patient-centered primary care, 368
Patient Education Protocols and Codes (PEPC), 385
patient-centered care, 368
patient-centered medical home (PCMH), 390
pellagra, 5
perishable foods, 464
pharmacist, 554
Pharmacopeia Dietary Supplement Verification Program, U.S., 347

physical activity, 7, 282, 323, 348, 351
physical education, 284
physical hazards, 453
physical inactivity, 283
physical therapist, 554
physician assistants (PAs), 368
plague, 461
Planned Approach to Community Health (PATCH), 162
plant-based diet, 326
plant-derived substances, 327
plausibility, 55
pneumonia, 347
point-of-service plan (POS), 381
policy, 79–80, 87, 89
population-based medicine, 377
poverty guidelines, 185
prebiotics, 350
preconceptual period, 255
Predisposing, Reinforcing, and Enabling Constructs in Education/Environmental Diagnosis-Policy, Regulatory, and Organizational Constructs in Educational and Environmental Development (PRECEDE-PROCEED) Model, 164
preeclampsia, 259
preferred provider organization (PPO), 381
pregnancy, 329
Pregnancy Nutrition Surveillance System (PNSS), 19
pregnancy, nutritional assessment, 258
pregnancy, weight gain, 256
prenatal care, 256
preschool, 294
preservatives, 453
press kits, 581
prevalence, 51, 56, 133
prevention, 306
primary, 368
primary care physician (PCP), 381
primary care provider (PCP), 553
primary data, 129, 141, 591
probiotics, 350
program evaluation, 357
Program Evaluation and Review Technique (PERT), 172
program implementation, 172
project models, 161
Protocol for Assessing Community Excellence in Environmental Health (PACE-EH), 171
protozoan, 446
psychologist, 555
puberty, 279
public health manager, 528
Public Health Security and Bioterrorism Preparedness and Response Act (2002), 429, 432
Public Housing Primary Care (PHPC) Programs, 391
Public Housing Primary Care Programs, 389
public policy, 72
Pure Food and Drugs Act (1906), 114, 429

Q

Q fever, 463
qualified health claims (QHC), 38
qualitative data, 592
quantitative data, 592

R

Rapid Eating and Activity Assessment for Patients (REAP), 375
recall bias, 57
registered dietician (RD), 549
registered dietician/nutritionist (RDN), 549
registered dietician/nutritionists (RDNs), roles and responsibilities, 532
registered nurses (RNs), 368
reimbursement, 377
Reiter syndrome, 439
reliability, 139
request for proposal (RFP), 498
Research, Education, and Economics, USDA (REE), 105
Resource Conservation and Recovery Act, 119
respiratory diseases, 347
Revitalizing Quality Nutrition Services (RQNS), 103
ricin toxin, 463
rickets, 5
Robert Wood Johnson Foundation (RWJF), 379
rural health clinic services, 383

S

Safe Drinking Water Act, 429
safe food handling, 437
Salmonella enterica, 440
Salmonella, 434, 440, 462
Salmonella Bongori, 440
Scantrack, 18
School Breakfast Program, 111, 193–4, 416
School Health Index (SHI), 276
school meals, 274
School Nutrition Association (SNA), 558
School Nutrition Association Certificate Program, 549
School Nutrition Dietary Assessment Study (SDNA), 18
school nutrition specialist (SNS), 549
school wellness, 276
schools, 223
schools, nutrition education, 277
scrapie, 439
screen time, 277, 285, 290
screening, 310
Seafood Inspection Program, 427
secondary data, 590
secondary datasets, 129

secondary prevention, 309
secondhand smoke, 348
sedentary lifestyle, 348
segregation, 191
self-quarantine, 444
self-regulation, 228
Senior Farmer's Market Nutrition Program (SFMNP), 195, 359, 360, 417
sequestrants, 453
sexually transmitted diseases (STDs), 347
shared medical appointments (SMAs), 379
Shiga toxin-producing E. coli (STEC) 0157:H7, 439
Shigella, 436, 441, 463
Shore Protection Act, 119
skin-fold thickness, 350
smallpox, 461
SMART (Self-Monitoring and Recording Using Technology) trial, 239
smoking, 7, 257, 324
snacking, 280
Social Cognitive Theory, 213
social determinants of health, 199
social distancing, 443
social isolation, 197
Social Learning Theory, 213
social marketing, 237, 588, 593
social media, 240, 361, 570, 598
social media analytics, 600
social networking, 570
Social Security program, 352
social workers, 555
Society for Public Health Education (SOPHE), 92
socioeconomic indicators, 149
socioeconomic status (SES), 286
Special Diabetes Program for Indians (SDPI), 385
special interest group, 72
Special Milk Program, 194
Special Supplemental Nutrition Assistance Program for Women, Infants, and Children (SNAP), 30, 75, 77, 85, 100, 102, 113, 129, 186, 193, 194, 286, 311, 359, 393, 416
specificity, 55
stabilizers, 453
staffing, 530
stakeholder, 144
Standard Reference Legacy Release (SR Legacy), 108
Staphylococcal enterotoxin B, 463
Staphylococcus aureas, 434
state grants, 499
States of Change Model, 215
stay-at-home order, 444
strength, 52
stroke, 6, 307, 347
Strong Heart Study, 51
substandard housing, 190
sugar intake, 222

sugar intake, children, 273
summative evaluation, 175
Summer Food Service Program (SFSP), 193, 194, 417
Supplemental Nutrition Assistance Program Education
    (SNAP-Ed), 31, 101, 559
Supplementary Supplemental Income, 352
supplements, 37
surface-active agents, 453
sugary beverages, 285
Survey of Program Dynamics, 409
Swine flu, 437
SWOT (strength, weaknesses, opportunities, threats)
    technique, 529
syndromic surveillance, 467

T

target population, 128, 132, 134, 137, 141, 147
Team Fruits and Vegetable (FNV) campaign, 290
Team Nutrition Initiative, 559
technology, 615
telehealth, 382
temporality, 55
tertiary prevention, 310
Theory of Planned Behavior, 215
Theory of Reasoned Action, 215
Theory X, 536
Theory Y, 536
therapeutic lifestyle changes (TLC), 323
thickeners, 453
third-party payer, 377
third-party reimbursement, 500
Thrifty Food Plan, 104
Thrifty Meal Plans, 186
Tiktok, 570
toolkits, 375
Total Diet Study (TDS), 17
toxicants, 447
transformational, 537
Transtheoretical Model, 215
traumatic brain injury (TBI), 393
trends, 511
triad of food security, 464
triangulation, 513
Trichinella spiralis, 446
tularemia, 461
Twitter, 570

U

U.S. Census Bureau, 131
U.S. Department of Agriculture (USDA), 12, 14, 16, 75,
    80, 100, 131, 359, 425, 426
U.S. Department of Health and Human Services (DHHS), 76

U.S. Preventive Services Task Force (USPSTF), 371
unchlorinated water, 439
underemployment, 187
unemployment, 187
unpasteurized milk, 439
upper intake Level (UL), 28
USDA Organizational Chart, 115

V

vegetarian eating practices, 281
VERB Campaign ("it's what you do"), 237
very low-density lipoprotein (VLDL), 324
veterans, 392
Veterans Affairs, U.S. Department of (VA), 393
veterinarians, 555
Vibrio cholerae, 463
viral hemorrhagic fevers, 461
virulence, 460
vitamin D, 5, 264, 331, 351
vitamins, 267
Vroom's theory, 537

W

Wagner-Steagall Housing Act (1937), 390
walking, 290
waterborne pathogens, 427
weigh screening, 269
weight, 268
weight loss, 372
weight management, 317
Weight, Activity, Variety, and Excess (WAVE), 375
Well-Integrated Screening and Evaluation for Women
    Across the Nation (WISEWOMAN), 380
wellness interventions, 349
wellness screening, 349
Wholesome Meat Act, 429
Wholesome Poultry Products Act, 429
WIC, 294
WIC Food Package, 292
WIC Nutrition Education, 293
WIC Program (Special Supplemental Nutrition
    Program for Women, Infants, and Children),
    18, 291, 417
worksite, 228
worksite interventions, 226

Y

Yersinia enterocolitica, 437
Youth Risk Behavior Surveillance System (YRBSS), 19,
    129, 131